DUMBARTON OAKS PAPERS
NUMBER THIRTY-EIGHT

DUMBARTON OAKS SYMPOSIUM

1983

BYZANTINE MEDICINE

Dumbarton Oaks Papers

NUMBER THIRTY-EIGHT

1984

SYMPOSIUM ON BYZANTINE MEDICINE

John Scarborough
Editor

Dumbarton Oaks Research Library and Collection

Washington, District of Columbia

All correspondence and orders should be addressed to
Dumbarton Oaks Publications Office
1703 32nd Street, N.W.
Washington, D.C. 20007

Library of Congress Cataloging in Publication Data

Symposium on Byzantine Medicine (1983: Dumbarton Oaks)
Symposium on Byzantine Medicine.

(Dumbarton Oaks papers; no. 38)
Papers from a symposium held in 1983 at Dumbarton Oaks,
Washington, D.C.
Includes index.
1. Medicine, Medieval—Byzantine Empire—History—
Congresses. 2. Physicians—Byzantine Empire—Congresses.
3. Veterinary medicine—Byzantine Empire—Congresses.
I. Scarborough, John. II. Dumbarton Oaks. III. Title.
IV. Series. [DNLM: 1. History of Medicine, Medieval--
congresses. WZ 54 S989s 1983]
R141.S95 1983   610′.9495   84–25967   ISBN 0-88402-139-4

Composition by Graphic Composition, Inc.
Printed by Meriden-Stinehour Press

to Owsei Temkin

CONTENTS

SYMPOSIUM ON BYZANTINE MEDICINE

INTRODUCTION*

Among medical historians, the commonly held opinion of Byzantine medicine is one of stagnation, plagiarism of the great medical figures of classical antiquity, and a somber boredom that seemingly awaited the Italian Renaissance. Even in his carefully researched and generally incisive essay on Byzantine medicine,[1] Temkin states as a fundamental premise that "Byzantine medicine . . . represents the formation as well as the continuation of a tradition, broken and unbroken."[2] But Temkin's views are cautious and salutary compared with accounts found in most contemporary histories of medicine, which say that Galen's compilation was the last contribution to medical knowledge in the West until the Renaissance. Typical is Majno's ". . . after Galen, the history [of medicine] grinds to a halt for at least one thousand years. Europe sank into the Dark Ages."[3] Garrison writes that "[Byzantine] medicine had become an affair of salves and poultices, talismans and pentagrams, with a mumbling of incantations and spells very like the backwoods pranks of Tom Sawyer and Huckleberry Finn, or some of the vagaries of Christian Science."[4] Singer and Ashworth note that "[Byzantine] medical writers became mere compilers from

the works of former authors."[5] German medical histories are not free of this anti-Byzantine prejudice,[6] but the classic lines are in Allbutt's prolix and diffuse *Greek Medicine in Rome*:

> Medicine of any pretence to a scientific quality thus passed . . . into slumber. The germ, in suspended animation, was enclosed in . . . a huge and cumbrous and somatic envelope . . . Byzantine medicine . . . had become a tradition, a burial of talents. The culture of the mistress of the world in this period was imitative, hoarding, and stereotyped.[7]

Fortunately, a slowly growing number of scholars have challenged this Gibbonesque attitude toward the medicine of a millennium, in one of the great civilizations of world history. The collection of papers in this volume follows the paths cut through the negatives by a few modern historians of medicine, especially Owsei Temkin. One may, moreover, borrow the insight of Alexander Kazhdan, who has recently written that the ". . . Byzantine literati, or at any rate the greatest among them, [were] involved in the real life of their time."[8] So also, one may presume that the physicians and medical writers of the Byzantine Empire were likewise embroiled in the issues and debates of their day, and that any consideration of Byzantine medicine must assume a firm historical and social context. For example, although the modern physician will immediately reject any notion that magic and

[The reader is referred to the list of abbreviations at the end of the volume.]

*A revised version of the "Introductory Remarks" given on 29 April 1983 at the Dumbarton Oaks Symposium on Byzantine Medicine

[1] O. Temkin, "Byzantine Medicine: Tradition and Empiricism," *DOP*, 16 (1962), 97–115 = Temkin, *Double Face of Janus*, 202–22.

[2] *Ibid.*, 97 = *Double Face of Janus*, 202.

[3] G. Majno, *The Healing Hand: Man and Wound in the Ancient World* (Cambridge, Mass., 1975), 417. The book, however, is generally an excellent example of superb medical history. See reviews by John Scarborough in *AHR*, 82 (1977), 66–67, and *CJ*, 72 (1976), 80–82.

[4] F. H. Garrison, *An Introduction to the History of Medicine*, 3rd ed. (Philadelphia, 1921), 111.

[5] C. Singer and E. A. Underwood, *A Short History of Medicine*, 2nd ed. (New York, 1962), 67.

[6] E.g., T. Meyer-Steineg and K. Sudhoff, *Illustrierte Geschichte der Medizin*, 5th ed., rev. R. Herrlinger and F. Kudlien (Stuttgart, 1965), 101: "Mit Galenos hatte der forschende und erkennende Griechengeist in der Heilkunde seinen letzten grossen Zeugen verloren."

[7] T. C. Allbutt, *Greek Medicine in Rome* (London, 1921; rptd. New York, 1970), 394.

[8] A. Kazhdan, in collaboration with S. Franklin, *Studies on Byzantine Literature of the Eleventh and Twelfth Centuries* (Cambridge and Paris, 1984), vii.

astrology might be useful in medical practice, many of our sources for Byzantine medicine show a strong influence of both, ranging from the religious-medical cures of pilgrims' tokens examined by Vikan below[9] to a continued employment of the medical astrology of the quasi-mythical Hermes Trismegistus and the firm belief in demonology.[10] One should not, therefore, be surprised that one of the greatest Byzantine medical practitioners, Alexander of Tralles, sanctioned magic, particularly when the patient's belief aided a cure.[11] Moreover, the student of Byzantine medicine must not attempt to impose a "modern view" that would excise the so-called non-rational elements of medical practice, since this would wrest medicine from its matrix, thereby warping the conclusions to suit modern pre-conceptions.

MEDICINE AND BYZANTINE SOCIETY

Medicine figures quite commonly in Byzantine history and culture, and when one examines the full range of sources, they reveal a vibrant civilization that incorporated the entire compass of human activity, including medicine. Importantly, non-medical sources show a general awareness of medicine and medical practice. The hagiographical literature has repeated allusions to doctors,[12] some well known, some almost ignored until consideration in this volume.[13] The modern observer soon

detects a lively mixture of Greek medical theory, venerated notions of magic, and hoary traditions of folkmedicine, a medley characteristic of Byzantine medicine as a whole. Yet even the modern concept of "medical advance" must admit the vital importance of Byzantine hospitals, which were taken for granted long before the medieval West adopted and adapted similar institutions.[14] Nothing quite comparable had existed before the fourth century,[15] after which the Christian *xenodochia* slowly began to evolve into carefully staffed, well organized hospitals, in full development by the twelfth century.

Literary sources further verify the typical presupposition of a sophisticated medical knowledge, widely diffused among the upper strata of the Byzantine Empire; such medicine was practiced by skilled professionals, well schooled in the theory of medicine. Illustrative are the following: Procopius' *Wars* and *Anecdota* contain numerous instances of medical knowledge, often on a rather high plane;[16] Photius' review of important books includes Dioscorides, among other medical authors;[17] Psellus' *Chronographia* gives details of the illness and death of Romanus III that rest upon close acquaintance with technical medical theory as well as with everyday knowledge of physicians and their approaches to treatment;[18] Anna Comnena's *Alexiad* not only has many examples of medicine and medical learning,[19] but also the "death scene" of Alexius Comnenus, which suggests a long-standing awareness of therapeutics and medical theory;[20] and John

[9] Gary Vikan, "Art, Medicine, and Magic in Early Byzantium," in this volume.

[10] E.g., "Hermes Trismegistus" in *Catalogus Codicum Astrologorum Graecorum*, Vol. IV: *Codices Italicos*, ed. D. Bassi, F. Cumont, A. Martini, and A. Olivieri (Brussels, 1903), 134–36. Cf. A.-J. Festugière, *La Révélation d'Hermès Trismégiste*, Vol. I: *L'Astrologie et les sciences occultes* (Paris, 1950; rptd. 1983), 146–60. For Byzantine demonology, see L. Delatte, *Un office Byzantin d'exorcisme (Ms. de la Lavra du Mont Athos, Θ 20)* (Brussels, 1957).

[11] E.g., Alexander of Tralles VIII, 2 [*On Colic*] (ed. Puschmann, II, 376).

[12] In the fairly abundant literature on this topic, one can consult: H. J. Magoulias, "The Lives of the Saints as Sources for the History of Byzantine Medicine in the Sixth and Seventh Centuries," *BZ*, 57 (1964), 127–50 (not always reliable); P. Charanis, "The Monk as an Element of Byzantine Society," *DOP*, 25 (1971), 61–84, esp. 74; D. J. Constantelos, "Physician-Priests in the Medieval Greek Church," *Greek Orthodox Theological Review*, 12 (1966–67), 141–53; Mary E. Keenan, "St. Gregory of Nazianzus and Early Byzantine Medicine," *BHM*, 9 (1941), 8–30, and "St. Gregory of Nyssa and the Medical Profession," *BHM*, 15 (1944), 150–61; and Evelyne Patlagean, "Birth Control in the Early Byzantine Empire," in R. Forster and O. Ranum, eds., *Biology of Man in History*, trans. [from the French] by E. Forster and P. M. Ranum (Baltimore, 1975), 1–22.

[13] See Vivian Nutton, "From Galen to Alexander," John Duffy, "Byzantine Medicine in the Sixth and Seventh Centuries," and Susan Harvey, "Physicians and Ascetics in John of Ephesus," in this volume.

[14] Many references conveniently collected in D. Constantelos, *Byzantine Philanthropy and Social Welfare* (New Brunswick, New Jersey, 1968), ch. 11: "Hospitals." But see Timothy Miller, "Byzantine Hospitals," in this volume.

[15] Scarborough, *Medicine*, 76–93, and "Roman Medicine and Public Health," in T. Ogawa, ed., *Public Health: Proceedings of the 5th International Symposium on the Comparative History of Medicine . . . 1980 . . . Susono-shi, Shizuoka, Japan* (Tokyo, 1981), 33–74, esp. 56–57 with nn. 217–28.

[16] E.g., Procopius, *History of the Wars: The Persian War* I, 6.17–18 [Persian method of blinding].

[17] Photius, *Library* 178: Dioscorides (ed. R. Henry, *Photius: Bibliothèque*, Vol. II [Paris, 1960], pp. 182–84); *Library* 164: Galen (ed. Henry, Vol. II, pp. 135–36); *Library* 72: Ctesias (ed. Henry, Vol. I [Paris, 1959], pp. 105–47); *Library* 216–19: Oribasius (ed. Henry, Vol. III [Paris, 1962], pp. 131–39); *Library* 221: Aetius of Amida (ed. Henry, Vol. III, pp. 140–52).

[18] Michael Psellus, *Chronographia* III, 24–26 (ed. E. Renauld, *Michel Psellos: Chronographie ou Histoire d'un siècle de Byzance (976–1077)* [Paris, 1926–28; 2 vols.; rptd. 1967], Vol. I, pp. 49–52).

[19] Georgina Buckler, *Anna Comnena* (Oxford, 1929; rpt. 1968), 215–21.

[20] Anna Comnena, *Alexiad* XV, 11 (ed. B. Leib, *Anne Comnène Alexiade* [Paris, 1937–45; 3 vols.; rptd. 1967], Vol. III, pp. 230–43). Comparable are the accounts of the death of Theodora.

Tzetzes' *Letters* show a deeply embedded expertise in "ancient" medical writings, particularly Galen.[21] These five authors are merely indicative of the continual context of a sophisticated state of medicine through the millennium of Byzantine culture. And one can cite Chrétien de Troyes (*Cligès*, 5699–6050) to show that Byzantine physicians were widely respected in the twelfth century, as contrasted to "progressive" physicians from Salerno.

BYZANTINE MEDICINE: THE PRIMARY SOURCES

The medical sources also disclose a lively and constant activity. Old traditions and fresh observations are reworked, recombined, and reorganized according to the shifting needs of Byzantine society. Veterinary medicine provides a clear example of this continual adaptation, and one needs to recall that "horse medicine" was an integral part of the newly fashioned army based on cavalry, created in the late third and early fourth century, becoming standard with Constantine I (A.D. 324–37). The new demands of the military produced tracts on veterinary medicine by Apsyrtus (? *fl.* under Constantine),[22] and Hierocles (? *fl.* c. A.D. 360),[23] which formed major sources for the extant collection of veterinary materials known as the *Corpus hippiatricorum Graecorum*, probably compiled in the reign of Constantine VII Porphyrogenitus (A.D. 913–59).[24] Both Apsyrtus and Hierocles appear to have been "physicians in the field," and their descriptions of equine disorders (glanders, for example) occasionally match and surpass anything before the nineteenth century.[25] Recent studies by Fischer have detailed how innovative were these

veterinary authors, as they struggled with the old nomenclature and how to "fit" it within new conclusions based on personal observations.[26]

The old Roman civilization was securely based on an agricultural ideal, and the Romans had established their mastery of farming—both in practice and theory—with the farming manuals by Cato the Elder (234–149 B.C.), Varro (116–27 B.C.), and Columella (his *De re rustica* was written c. A.D. 60–65). Unlike the normal practice of taking Greek medical writings and putting them into Latin (as in the case of the beautifully written *De medicina* by Cornelius Celsus [*fl.* A.D. 14–37]),[27] the Latin veterinary works were soon rendered into Greek. Byzantine physicians and students of natural history fused the old Roman tradition of agricultural treatises with botany, and as early as A.D. 360, Didymus of Alexandria wrote a *Georgica* as well as an *Octatomus*;[28] the *Georgica* became a source for the extant *Geoponica*, and the details of various remedies in the *Octatomus* were combined in the writings of Anatolius of Beirut (*fl.* c. A.D. 365), who composed a medico-agricultural work that was also incorporated into the *Geoponica*. An important aspect of "medical" literature in the Byzantine Empire consisted of farmers' applications and observations in terms of their crops and animals, and a consideration of Byzantine medicine should include how botanicals and therapeutics functioned on the farm, where the vast majority of the citizens resided.

Byzantine medical sources provide evidence of a perpetual activity. Philagrius (*fl.* c. A.D. 375) made

---

Victor Tonnennensis, *Chronica*, sa. 549 (ed. T. Mommsen, *Chronica Minora*, II, 202): "*Theodora Augusta Chalcedonsis synodi inimica canceris plaga corpore toto perfuse vitam prodigiose finivit.*" Malalas 484, and Procopius, *Wars* VII, 30.4, add nothing further. Simple "cancer:" Tony Honoré, *Tribonian* (Ithaca, New York, 1978), 12. Syphilis: J. Körbler, "Die Krebserkrankung der byzantinischen Kaiserin Theodora," *Janus*, 61 (1974), 15–22.

[21] E.g., John Tzetzes, *Letters* 81 (ed. P. A. M. Leone, *Ioannis Tzetzes Epistulae* [Leipzig, 1972], p. 121). Cf. C. Harder, *De Ioannis Tzetzae historiarum fontibus quaestiones selectae* (Kiel, 1886), esp. 71.

[22] R. E. Walker, "Roman Veterinary Medicine," appendix in J. M. C. Toynbee, *Animals in Roman Life and Art* (London, 1973), 303 with n. 3, p. 404.

[23] H. Gossen, "Hierokles," *RE*, Vol. XVI (Stuttgart, 1913), cols. 1713–15. See also K. Hoppe, "Theomnestos," *RE*, Supplementband VII (Stuttgart, 1940), cols. 1353–54.

[24] Walker, "Veterinary Medicine" (n. 22 above), 404 n. 6.

[25] *CHG*, II, 1–9 [Apsyrtus]; II, 10–17 [Hierocles]; II, 18 [Theomnestus] (ed. Oder and Hoppe, Vol. I, pp. 13–23). Glanders was one of the first diseases of horses and donkeys to be

observed in Greek antiquity. Aristotle, *Historia Animalium* 605a16–19, is one of the earliest records. The μᾶλις of Apsyrtus, Hierocles, and Theomnestus becomes *maleus* in Vegetius, *Mulomedicina* I, 10 (ed. Lommatzsch, pp. 21–23), from which name is derived the modern nomenclature of the causative bacilli (*Malleomyces*), particularly *Actinobacillus mallei*.

[26] K.-D. Fischer, "Wege zum Verständnis antiker Tierkrankheitsnamen," *Historia Medicinae Veterinariae*, 2 (1977), 106–11; "*Philimelia* und *phlemina*," *Hermes*, 107 (1979), 495; "Three Lexicographical Notes," *Glotta*, 57 (1979), 224–26; and "Palladius, de vet. med. 14. 15. 5," *Liverpool Classical Monthly*, 4 (1979), 73–74. See also Anne-Marie Doyen-Higuet, "The Hippiatrica and Byzantine Veterinary Medicine," in this volume.

[27] Scarborough, *Medicine*, 59–63.

[28] M. Wellmann, "Didymos," *RE*, Vol. II (Stuttgart, 1894), col. 2073. Meyer, *Botanik*, II, 256–57. Anatolius of Beirut: *Geoponica* II, 10; V, 10 and 18; VI, 3.4 and 13; VII, 28; X, 8, 18.72 and 85; XI, 20; XII, 7 and 36; XIII, 17; XIV, 21; and XVIII, 17. Meyer, *Botanik* II, 258–59. E. Oder, "Beiträge zur Geschichte der Landwirthschaft bei den Griechen," *RhM*, 45 (1890), 212–22. For the *Geoponica*, see: W. Gemoll, *Untersuchungen über die Quellen, den Verfasser und die Abfassungszeit der Geoponica* (Berlin, 1883; rptd. Wiesbaden, 1972); and N. G. Wilson, *Scholars of Byzantium* (London, 1983), 143. The *Geoponica* was compiled under the orders of Constantine VII Porphyrogenitus, to whom the collection is dedicated: *Geoponica*, Prooemium, 2 and 11.

original observations on diseases of the spleen,[29] and a certain Posidonius (? *fl.* c. A.D. 390) investigated the brain, in what appears to be an attempt to "localize" brain function.[30] Natural philosophy, physiology, and medicine were amalgamated in *On the Nature of Man* by Nemesius of Emesa (*fl.* c. A.D. 400),[31] and Galen is a basic foundation in this very influential treatise. Famous are the medical encyclopedias of Oribasius (c. 325–400),[32] Aetius of Amida (*fl.* under Justinian [A.D. 527–65]),[33] Alexander of Tralles (c. 525–605),[34] and Paul of Aegina (*fl.* c. A.D. 640 in Alexandria).[35] And these are but the major names in a continuing catalogue that would include Nicetas (c. A.D. 800),[36] Theophanes "Nonnus" (*fl.* A.D. 912–59),[37] Damnastes (*fl.* A.D. 1050),[38] Stephen Magnetes (c. 1050),[39] Michael Psellus (1018–78),[40] Symeon Seth (*fl.* under Michael VII Ducas [1071–78]),[41] John Tzetzes (? *fl.* c. 1130),[42] Hierophilus the Sophist (c. 1350),[43] and John Actuarius (c. 1320).[44]

The would-be student of Byzantine medicine is thus faced with an overabundance of source materials, with some of the texts basically in the form of unedited manuscripts, or in printed texts edited in the eighteenth and nineteenth centuries that do not reflect high standards of textual criticism, collation of manuscripts, and the essential firsthand command of anatomy, medicine, and pharmacology. Many of our printed editions emerge from the pioneering collections of Dietz, Ermerins, and Ideler, as well as more recent texts on Byzantine botany and pharmacology by Delatte and Thomson.[45] Sometimes there are glaring interpolations in the nineteenth-century editions which can be rectified only through a fresh series of readings in the various manuscripts. Two examples will serve to illustrate the state of our printed sources. Theophilus Protospatharius (*fl.* in the reign of Heraclius [A.D. 610–41]) composed tracts entitled *On Pulses, On Urines,* and *On Defecation,* and the "best" texts of these treatises are in Ermerins and Ideler,[46] while Theophilus' *On the Constitution of the Human Body* was last edited and translated (into Latin) by the admirable physician-classicist W. A. Greenhill in 1842.[47] John Actuarius, a crucial source for the understanding of Byzantine medical knowledge as it was transmitted into the Renaissance, remains generally unedited in the Greek, but as Hohlweg's essay below suggests,[48] there is now a concerted effort to determine the best witnesses in the tradition for John Actuarius and to place him securely into the history of late Byzantine medicine and pharmacy on the basis of well-edited Greek texts.

Reliable, modern texts do exist, but only in a small minority of cases. Well-edited Greek texts are available for Oribasius,[49] Paul of Aegina,[50] Alexander of Tralles,[51] Aetius of Amida (through Book VIII),[52] Stephen of Alexandria's *Commentary on the Prognosticon of Hippocrates,*[53] Philaretus' *On Pulses,*[54]

[29] T. Puschmann, ed. [Latin text], *Nachträge zu Alexander Trallianus* (Berlin, 1887; rptd. Amsterdam, 1963), 74–129 ("Fragmente aus Philagrius").

[30] A. Lewy and R. Landesberg, "Über die Bedeutung des Antyllus, Philagrius, und Posidonius," *Janus,* 2 (1847), 758–71, and 3 (1848), 166–84. O. Temkin, "Das 'Brüderpaar' Philagrios und Poseidonios," *SA,* 24 (1931), 268–70.

[31] ed. Matthaei.

[32] H. O. Schröder, "Oreibasios," *RE,* Supplementband VII (Stuttgart, 1940), cols. 797–812. B. Baldwin, "The Career of Oribasius," *Acta Classica,* 18 (1975), 85–97.

[33] ed. Olivieri.

[34] ed. Puschmann; French trans. by Brunet.

[35] ed. Heiberg.

[36] Sarton, *Introduction,* I, 608. J. Kollesch and F. Kudlien, eds., *Apollonii Citensis in Hippocratis De articulis commentarius* (Berlin, 1965 [*CMG* XI 1, 1]): illustrations probably by Nicetas and his assistants.

[37] J. S. Bernard, ed., *Nonni Epitome De curatione morborum* (Gotha, 1794–95; 2 vols.). But see Joseph Sonderkamp, "Theophanes Nonnus: Medicine in the Circle of Constantine Porphyrogenitus," in this volume.

[38] Sarton, *Introduction,* I, 727. Hunger, "Medizin," 310.

[39] Meyer, *Botanik,* III, 365–79. Sarton, *Introduction,* I, 727.

[40] Psellus, *Medical Poem:* Ideler, I, 203–43. Psellus, *On the Bath:* Ideler, II, 193. Meyer, *Botanik,* III, 350–56.

[41] B. Langkavel, ed., *Simeonis Sethi Syntagma De alimentorum facultatibus* (Leipzig, 1868). *Philosophy and Medicine:* Ideler, II, 283–85. Meyer, *Botanik,* III, 356–65. Hunger, "Medizin," 308–9.

[42] See n. 21 above.

[43] Hierophilus, *On Diet:* Ideler, I, 409–17, and probably unnamed works by Hierophilus in Ideler, I, 423–29, and II, 257–81. L. Oeconomos, "Le calendrier de régime d'Hiérophile d'après des manuscrits plus complets que le Parisinus 396," *Actes du VI° Congrès International d'Études byzantines* (Paris, 1948 [1950]), I, 169–79. Another version of the Greek text of *On Diet* by Hierophilus is in Delatte, *Anecdota,* II, 456–66. Hunger, "Medizin," 309.

[44] Hunger, "Medizin," 312–13. See also Armin Hohlweg, "John Actuarius' "De methodo medendi"—On the New Edition," in this volume.

[45] Delatte, *Anecdota,* II, 273–499. Margaret H. Thomson, ed. and trans., *Textes Grecs inédits relatifs aux plantes* (Paris, 1955).

[46] *On Pulses:* Ermerins, 1–77. *On Urines:* Ideler, I, 261–83. *On Defecation:* Ideler, I, 397–408. *Commentaries on Hippocrates' Aphorisms:* Dietz, II, 236–544 (probably conflated with Damascius, Stephen of Athens, and Meletius).

[47] Oxford: 'E Typographeo Academico.'

[48] Hohlweg, "John Actuarius" (n. 44 above).

[49] ed. Raeder.

[50] ed. Heiberg.

[51] ed. Puschmann.

[52] ed. Olivieri.

[53] J. M. Duffy, ed. and trans., *Stephanus the Philosopher: A Commentary on the Prognosticon of Hippocrates* (Berlin, 1983 [*CMG* XI 1, 2]).

[54] J. A. Pithis, ed., trans., and comm., *Die Schriften ΠΕΡΙ ΣΦΥΓΜΩΝ des Philaretos* (Husum, 1983).

Leo the Physician,[55] Pelagonius,[56] and Palladius[57] (the last two in Latin). One can generally trust the texts of the *Geoponica*,[58] Eutecnius' *Paraphrases of Nicander and Oppian*,[59] the veterinary material in the *Corpus hippiatricorum Graecorum*,[60] but we are still most puzzled by John of Alexandria (c. A.D. 627–40), even though well-edited texts of Latin translations of John's *Commentary on Hippocrates' Epidemics* and *Commentary on Galen's On Medical Sects* are now available.[61] Iskandar's summary of the Arabic transmission of the "Sixteen Galenic Categories" in late Alexandrian medicine shows some of the problems in untangling Byzantine from Arabic traditions,[62] also noted from another aspect by Lieber.[63]

An enormous lacuna exists in our comprehension of cross-cultural medical transmissions. Baader's essay below[64] addresses some of the problems in how Byzantine medical works eventually made their way into the early medieval West, and Dols' study of concepts of insanity[65] poses some fresh questions to what might appear to be mutually exclusive Greek and Arabic sources. We are reasonably well informed about Ḥunain ibn-Isḥāq's many excellent translations of Greek medical texts into Syriac and into Arabic,[66] but earlier and later translations and adaptations remain foggy. We would, for example, like to know far more about Sergius of Resaina (d. in Constantinople, A.D. 536;

fl. at Raʿs al-ʿain somewhat earlier) and his translations of Greek works into Syriac.[67] Myerhoff examined Sergius' link with Ḥunain ibn-Isḥāq,[68] and Budge's text of the *Syrian Anatomy* has other connections,[69] but the essential character of these Syriac renditions remains quite uncertain. Harvey's examination of Syriac texts of John of Ephesus' medical opinions[70] illustrates the rich lore of material extant in this generally unexplored aspect of Byzantine medical influences, and this is coupled with the extensive number of manuscripts of Syriac translations of Galen.[71] One presumes such translation was fundamental for the medical teaching at Jundishapur under the Sassanians (especially in the reign of Nūshīrwān the Just [A.D. 531–79]),[72] where multi-cultural medical traditions mixed into an amalgam; with the expulsion of the Nestorians from Edessa in 489, and the banishment of the neo-Platonists from Athens in 529, one also assumes these refugee-scholars enriched the "school" at Jundishapur with further Greek heritages, which, in turn, became melded with Hindu, Jewish, Christian, Syriac, and Persian sources. In their turn, all these traditions would have heavy impact on Arabic medicine. On the "other side" are the works by Symeon Seth, whose *Philosophy and Medicine* appears in Ideler,[73] and whose *Properties of Foods* was last edited by Langkavel.[74] In the works of Symeon Seth one meets—presumably for the first time—Arabic and Hindu spices and drugs in a Greek medical text. One may wonder why such influ-

[55] ed. Renehan.

[56] ed. Fischer.

[57] ed. Rodgers.

[58] ed. Beckh.

[59] Isabella Gualandri, ed., *Eutecnii Paraphrasis in Nicandri Theriaca* (Milan, 1969). M. Geymonat, ed., *Eutecnii Paraphrasis in Nicandri Alexipharmaca* (Milan, 1976). M. Papathomopoulos, ed., *Eutekniou paraphrasis eis ta Nikandrou Thēriaka kai Alexipharmaka* (Ioannina [Greece], 1976) and ed., *Anōnymou paraphrasis eis ta Oppianou halieutika* (Ioannina, 1976). See reviews of Papathomopoulos and Geymonat by G. Giangrande in *JHS*, 98 (1978), 181–82.

[60] ed. E. Oder and C. Hoppe.

[61] C. D. Pritchet, ed., *Iohannis Alexandrini Commentaria in sextum librum Hippocratis Epidemiarum* (Leiden, 1975), and ed., *Iohannis Alexandrini Commentaria in librum De sectis Galeni* (Leiden, 1982).

[62] A. Z. Iskandar, "An Attempted Reconstruction of the Late Alexandrian Medical Curriculum," *Medical History*, 20 (1976), 235–58.

[63] Elinor Lieber, "Galen in Hebrew: The Transmission of Galen's Works in the Medieval Islamic World," in Nutton, ed., *Galen: Problems*, 167–86 (esp. 172–79).

[64] Gerhard Baader, "Early Medieval Latin Adaptations of Byzantine Medicine in Western Europe," in this volume.

[65] Michael Dols, "Insanity in Byzantine and Islamic Medicine," in this volume.

[66] M. Meyerhoff, "New Light on Ḥunain Ibn Ishāq and his Period," *Isis*, 8 (1926), 685–724. Ullmann, *Medizin*, 115–19. Sezgin, *Geschichte*, III, 247–56.

[67] Sarton, *Introduction*, I, 310 and 423–24. Sezgin, *Geschichte*, III, 177. Ullmann, *Medizin*, 22 and 100. A. O. Whipple, "The Role of the Nestorians as the Connecting Link between Greek and Arabic Medicine," *Annals of Medical History*, n.s. 8 (1936), 313–23.

[68] Meyerhoff, "New Light" (n. 66 above), 703. Meyerhoff's listing of the 129 works, translated by Ḥunain, include the following which had been previously translated into Syriac by Sergius: Nos. 4, 6–8, 11–20, 49, 53–54, 66, 71, and 80. Lieber, "Galen in Hebrew" (n. 63 above), 174–75.

[69] E. A. Wallis Budge, ed. [Syriac] and trans., *Syrian Anatomy Pathology and Therapeutics or "The Book of Medicines"* (London, 1913; 2 vols.), I, clvix–clxxii. The compiler says he "studied in Alexandria," etc. Sergius was a friend of the Byzantine historian Agathias, and much of the information in Agathias' accounts of the Sassanian court, customs, and the like, was drawn from data ". . . procured for him by his friend and interpreter Sergius from the Persian Royal Annals . . ." (Averil Cameron, *Agathias* [Oxford, 1970], 39).

[70] See n. 13 above.

[71] R. Degen, "Galen im Syrischen," in Nutton, ed., *Galen: Problems*, 131–66. See also A. Merx, "Proben der syrischen Uebersetzung von Galenus' Schrift über die einfachen Heilmittel," *ZDMG*, 39 (1885), 237–305.

[72] Ullmann, *Medizin*, 22 and 100. Whipple, "Nestorians" (n. 67 above), 314–19. Sarton, *Introduction*, I, 435–36.

[73] Ideler, II, 283–85.

[74] *Ibid.*

ences and counter-borrowings did not appear sooner in Byzantine medicine. Study of Seth's *Philosophy* and *Properties of Foods*, as well as the unedited *Lexicon of Botany*,[75] and his *Compendium of Urines*[76] might show how deeply Arabic and Indian ideas had penetrated into Byzantine medicine by the eleventh century.

THE STUDY OF BYZANTINE MEDICINE: PROSPECTS AND QUESTIONS

Temkin has provided an exemplary method to follow, as we formulate the initial stages of the opening of the medical history of Byzantium to modern students of the History of Medicine. We must employ a carefully balanced approach to Byzantine medicine, that will necessarily include medicine and allied areas, philology, and history. All three must be present to prevent anachronism, and all three broad categories will provide context.

Medicine. Here one focuses on the practice of medicine and how it "works" in society, and the researcher must pose questions to the sources that will elucidate the texts in their own terms. What assumptions (regarding theory and technical matter, for example) are taken for granted by the physician? What assumptions are taken for granted by patients? What is the definition of a "professional" physician? What is the actual status of the practicing physician in Byzantine society? What role does tradition play in the practice of medicine in the Byzantine Empire? Is Temkin correct as he emphasizes the twin notions of "tradition and empiricism"? What are the basic sources of medical knowledge? Texts? How is a physician trained? Apprenticeships? Lectures? Institutional settings?

In Byzantine medicine, the historian needs to clarify various particular aspects of medicine as they were, asking a basic "what is it"? Generally lacking in secondary scholarship are specifics on Byzantine medical theory, herbs and drugs used in pharmacy, the ingredients of compound drugs, Byzantine surgical tools as distinguished from Greek and Roman types, and the regulations of medical institutions. With the publication of Gautier's text of the *Typikon*, and Miller's discussion of Byzantine hospitals below,[77] this omission has been partially filled.

Bliquez' analysis and catalogue of Byzantine surgical instruments below[78] is the first of its kind, and in the essays by Stannard and Scarborough below,[79] one can begin to perceive basic classes of drugs, as well as generally preferred drugs and changes in those choices in Byzantine pharmacy. Each paper, however, represents a beginning stage in modern scholarship.

Linked with the basics of "what is it?" are questions of "specialties" in medical practice. In Byzantine medicine, how were such specialties connected with the traditions of antiquity? How did they change over the ten centuries of Byzantine history? What would constitute a "specialty" in Byzantine medicine? Renehan and Savage-Smith analyze the theory and practice of ophthalmology respectively below,[80] and demonstrate that eye diseases demanded a specialized expertise, somewhat akin to ancient *kollyria* compounders but rather more sophisticated in Byzantine times. "Faith healing" is another "specialty"—elucidated by Vikan below[81]—and one would welcome a full study of how gynecology and/or midwifery functioned in Byzantine society.[82] Théodoridès' essay on rabies in this volume indicates a specialized expertise in the symptomatology of rabies, and the papyri show a common knowledge of pharmaceutical specifics,[83] perhaps not expected in light of modern preconceptions. It is one of the important tasks of future research in Byzantine medicine to see and read the texts as they are, with a continual effort to avoid

---

[75] Meyer, *Botanik*, III, 356–65. Sarton, *Introduction*, I, 771. Hunger, "Medizin," 308–9.

[76] G. Harig, "Von den arabischen Quellen des Symeon Seth," *Medizinhistorisches Journal*, 2 (1967), 248–68.

[77] P. Gautier, ed. and trans., *Le Typikon du Christ Sauveur Pantocrator* in *REB*, 32 (1974), 1–145. Timothy Miller, "Byzantine Hospitals," in this volume.

[78] Lawrence Bliquez, "Two Lists of Greek Surgical Instruments and the State of Surgery in Byzantine Times," in this volume.

[79] Jerry Stannard, "Aspects of Byzantine Materia Medica," and John Scarborough, "Early Byzantine Pharmacology," in this volume.

[80] Robert Renehan, "Meletius' Chapter on the Eyes," and Emilie Savage-Smith, "Hellenistic and Byzantine Ophthalmology," in this volume.

[81] Gary Vikan, "Art, Medicine and Magic in Early Byzantium," in this volume.

[82] For short, suggestive and synoptic accounts, see P. Diepgen, *Zur Frauenheilkunde im byzantinischen Kulturkreis des Mittelalters* (Wiesbaden, 1950 [Akademie der Wissenschaften und der Literatur in Mainz, Abh. geistes- und sozialwissenschaftlichen Kl., Jhrg. 1950, Nr. 1: pamphlet of 14 pp.]), and *Über den Einfluss der autoritativen Theologie auf die Medizin des Mittelalters* (Wiesbaden, 1958 [Akad. Wiss. Lit. Mainz, Abh. g.-soz. Kl., Jhrg. 1958, Nr. 1: pamphlet of 20 pp.]). Diepgen's *Die Frauenheilkunde der alten Welt* (Munich, 1937) also has many "pointers." For the broader contexts, see Judith Herrin, "In Search of Byzantine Women: Three Avenues of Approach," and Susan Ashbrook Harvey, "Women in Early Syrian Christianity," in A. Cameron and A. Kuhrt, eds., *Images of Women in Antiquity* (Detroit, 1983), 167–89 and 288–98.

[83] Jean Théodoridès, "Rabies in Byzantine Medicine," and John Scarborough, "The Papyri and Byzantine Medicine on Multi-Ingredient Incense," appendix to "Early Byzantine Pharmacology," both in this volume.

modern assumptions which do not apply, for example, regarding the role of anatomy learned from dissection.

Philology. We must have well-edited Greek, Arabic, Latin, Syriac, and Hebrew texts which result from the best modern techniques of philological criticism. Lieber's study of Asaf below indicates how careful editing of a medieval Hebrew text may well alter our basic views of medieval medical theory generally,[84] and Riddle's analysis of the scholia attached to Dioscorides delineates how Byzantine herbal lore and pharmacy actually differed from, and occasionally improved upon, classical models and texts.[85] Hohlweg's essay on John Actuarius shows why reliance upon Renaissance printed texts is fraught with dangerous misrepresentation, especially if one relies on Latin translations of scattered Greek texts of unproven worth, and Todd's paper below indicates how a careful study of texts of philosophical commentary can yield much information on Byzantine medical theory.[86] At the present stage of the study of Byzantine medicine the manuscripts are fundamental. Those manuscripts also show a Greek that is a living, changing language, as Temkin and Fischer have demonstrated for Byzantine anatomy and veterinary medicine.[87] One also should recognize that Galen's Greek may provide the "formal," intentionally archaic language of many medical authors, paralleled by historical writers like Procopius and Anna Comnena, who intentionally aped Thucydides in several sections of the *Wars* and *Alexiad*. Byzantine pulse lore,[88] uroscopy, pharmacy, veterinary medicine, and many other particular aspects, indicate how Byzantine medical writers took their ancient language and invented new words and new approaches, much as had the Ptolemaic Alexandrian physicians when they invented technical terms from common words. One would also like to know what linguistic changes came into Byzantine medicine and science from the Arabic. The analysis of basic primary texts remains the essential problem of our

study of Byzantine medicine as a whole, and until we have more solidly edited editions and translations like those by Renehan and Duffy, our conclusions will be uncertain due to the gaps existing in reliable texts. Classical scholars looking for "new worlds to conquer" would be welcome to edit the numerous authors in Byzantine medicine and science awaiting competent philologists. Classicists uncomfortable with the purely scientific would still have many texts from which to choose that would be important to Byzantine medicine; for example, an explication of the genre of "medical poetry" would repay generous efforts by skilled classical philologists.[89]

History. In this broad category one should include all kinds of history in order to give context to medicine, a setting which is crucial to define how medicine functioned within Byzantine society. Subdivisions of Byzantine history suggest why each subtopic may be important, and why each has to be rejoined to the wider cultural and medical world of the Byzantine Empire. Political and military history, illustrated by Procopius and Anna Comnena, supply details of how military medicine operated and how doctors and medicine fit—or did not fit—into the public activities of politics and politicians. Not only does a Maurice show what medical care actually was available in the Byzantine army,[90] but analysis of how physicians took part in politics and struggles for power can give instances of doctors' abilities to shift from one calling to another, as indicated by Baldwin's essay below.[91] Cultural history can delineate changes in preferred notions of ideals, and one may be able to comprehend why there would be a revival of the "old" sources in the tenth century, seen both in the medical compilations of Theophanes "Nonnus" and the gathering of veterinary sources that constitute the *Corpus hippiatricorum Graecorum*, texts explicated by Sonderkamp and Doyen-Higuet in this volume.[92] Cultural history encompasses literature and what writers seek to

[84] Elinor Lieber, "Asaf's *Book of Medicines*," in this volume.

[85] John M. Riddle, "Byzantine Commentaries on Dioscorides," in this volume.

[86] Robert Todd, "Philosophy and Medicine in John Philoponus' Commentary on Aristotle's *De anima*," in this volume.

[87] O. Temkin, "The Byzantine Origin of the Names for the Basilic and Cephalic Veins," *XVIIe Congrès International d'Histoire de la Médecine*, Vol. I: *Communications* (Athens, 1961), 336–39 = Temkin, *Double Face of Janus*, 198–201. Fischer: n. 26 above.

[88] Pithis, ed., *Philaretos* (n. 54 above). See also M. Stoffregen, ed., trans., and comm., *Eine frühmittelalterliche lateinische Übersetzung des byzantinischen Puls- und Urintraktats des Alexandros* (Berlin, 1977 [Diss.]).

[89] See, e.g., F. O. Salinas, "Precetti di salute. Poemetto didascalico greco-bizantino del V secolo," *Pagine di Storia della Medicina*, 17, 3 (1973), 5–22.

[90] G. T. Dennis, trans., *Maurice's Strategikon* (Philadelphia, 1984), pp. 15, 29–30, 42, 59 and 77. Cf. B. Wassiliewsky and V. Jernstedt, eds., *Cecaumeni Strategicon* (St. Petersberg, 1896; rptd. Amsterdam, 1965), 125 [p. 53].

[91] Barry Baldwin, "Beyond the House Call: Doctors in Early Byzantine History and Politics," in this volume. Cf. V. Nutton, "L. Gellius Maximus, Physician and Procurator," *CQ*, 21 (1971), 262–72, and Scarborough, *Medicine*, 112–13.

[92] Joseph Sonderkamp, "Theophanes Nonnus: Medicine in the Circle of Constantine Porphyrogenitus," and Anne-Marie Doyen-Higuet, "The Hippiatrica and Byzantine Veterinary Medicine," both in this volume.

portray about themselves and their society, and Kazhdan's essay below[93] gives hints of the wealth of information to be gleaned by study of non-medical authors for their views of medicine and physicians. Religious history in Byzantine times is a well-known trove of data, but not until recently have the hagiographical sources been tapped accurately for their details on the presumed conflict between the secular and spiritual approaches to medicine. In this collection of papers, Nutton, Duffy, and Harvey delve into this broad genre,[94] and discern a constant debate, marked by fuzzy borders between the two supposedly opposed views.

Art history has much to teach us regarding manuscript illuminations of plants and medical practice,[95] and legal history incorporates what was thought "right" in medical practice, and the penalties for practitioners who violated the customs embedded in law.[96] Desirable would be an examination of how Byzantine law treated doctors and medicine, and what regulations were placed on those who practiced.[97] Social history shows how one lived in an ordinary way, somewhat removed from the Great Names and battles that festoon the historical accounts, and we can thereby perceive the "sense of medicine" accepted among those classes of people who did not record their ideas or impressions. Folkmedicine is present in all cultures and societies, and Vikan's examination of "amuletic drugs" in this volume gives clear glimpses of a folkmedicine, Christian in its forms but displaying a venerated heritage from a pagan past. Finally, even economic history can lend specifics to our attempts to understand Byzantine medicine, much as the listing of drugs and spices in Diocletian's *Price Edict* suggests not only why certain imported medicines were so expensive, but that they were also highly esteemed by pharmacologists in late Roman and early Byzantine medicine.[98]

The twenty-one papers assembled here in *Byzantine Medicine* all attempt to address basic issues in the study of the medical history of Byzantium, and they represent a collective effort to establish the consideration of Byzantine medicine and allied sciences on sure foundations. It is hoped that this volume will engender interest in a neglected area of the History of Medicine, and that Byzantine medicine can take its place as one more facet that illumines the fascinating, turbulent, and important millennium of the history of Byzantium.

We contributors extend our deep gratitude to the Dumbarton Oaks Research Library and Collection for hosting the 1983 Symposium on Byzantine Medicine, where earlier versions of these papers were presented. One could not overpraise the gracious attention by the staff, nor could one say too much in thanks to Giles Constable, Peter Topping, and others of the Senior Fellows of the Center for Byzantine Studies at Dumbarton Oaks. We all benefited greatly from discussions and suggestions, both from our colleagues in the Symposium and from members of the audience. We furthermore extend our appreciation to Dumbarton Oaks for undertaking to publish our papers as a volume in the *Dumbarton Oaks Papers*, thereby giving the collection of essays a unity which would have been lost had the participants published their contributions separately in scattered journals.

John Scarborough

---

[93] Alexander Kazhdan, "The Image of the Medical Doctor in Byzantine Literature of the Tenth to the Twelfth Centuries," in this volume.

[94] See n. 13 above.

[95] Byzantine manuscript illuminations are distinctive and important. See, e.g., Soranus (ed. Ilberg), plates 1–60 (MS illuminations for Soranus' *Bandages* from Cod. Laur. 74, 7); Apollonius of Citium (ed. Kollesch and Kudlien [n. 36 above]), plates I–XXX (MS illuminations for Apollonius' *On Hippocrates' Joints* from Cod. Laur. 74, 7), color reprod. of Cod. Laur. 74, 7, fol. 200 (reduction of dislocated vertebrae by ladder-jolting) in L. MacKinney, *Medical Illustrations in Medieval Manuscripts* (Berkeley, 1965), plate 91A. A selection of color plates from the beautiful sixth-century Vienna Codex of Dioscorides is in O. Mazal, *Pflanzen, Wurzeln, Säfte, Samen: Antike Heilkunst in Miniaturen des Wiener Dioskurides* (Graz, 1981), and various miniatures of the insects, arachnids, and animals described by Nicander, Dionysius, Dioscorides, Oppian, and others, are given in color by Z. Kádár, *Survivals of Greek Zoological Illuminations in Byzantine Manuscripts*, trans. T. Wilkinson [from the Hungarian] (Budapest, 1978). How much the sensitive skills of art historians can aid us in understanding these "pictorial guides" to both ancient and Byzantine medicine can be gauged by the numerous studies by K. Weitzmann, which include medical and scientific illuminations, e.g., "The Greek Sources of Islamic Scientific Illustrations," *Archaeologica Orientalia in Memoriam Ernst Herzfeld* (Locust Valley, New York, 1952), 244–66 (rpt. in H. L. Kessler, ed., *Kurt Weitzmann: Studies in Classical and Byzantine Manuscript Illumination* [Chicago, 1971], 20–44) and *Illustrations in Roll and Codex*, 2nd ed. (Princeton, 1970), esp. 134–37 and 143–47. See also K. Weitzmann, *Late Antique and Early Christian Book Illumination* (New York, 1977), 61–71 with plates 15–20, and (ed.) *Age of Spirituality* (New York, 1979), 199–200. Cf. Gary Vikan, ed., *Illuminated Greek Manuscripts from American Collections: An Exhibition in Honor of Kurt Weitzmann* (Princeton, 1973), 66–69.

[96] For doctors and Roman law, see K.-H. Below, *Der Arzt im römischen Recht* (Munich, 1953).

[97] Byzantine law provides some of the foundations for the preliminary study by Aristotelis C. Eftychiadis, Ἡ ἄσκησις τῆς βυζαντινῆς ἰατρικῆς ἐπιστήμης καὶ κοινωνικαὶ ἐφαρμογαὶ αὐτῆς κατὰ σχετικὰς διατάξεις (Athens, 1983).

[98] Siegfried Lauffer, ed., *Diokletians Preisedikt* (Berlin, 1971), 36, 26–119 [pp. 195–99].

FROM GALEN TO ALEXANDER, ASPECTS OF MEDICINE AND MEDICAL PRACTICE IN LATE ANTIQUITY*

Vivian Nutton

When, in the sixteenth century, the monks of the Great Lavra on Mt. Athos commissioned a new scheme of paintings for their refectory, one wall was covered with a magnificent tree of Jesse, with, at its foot, various pagan sages who, in some way, had foretold the truth of Christian doctrine. Prominent among them, between Aristotle and the Sibyl, stands Galen the righteous healer.[1] How this physician, born in A.D. 129, came to figure in such a parade of witnesses is a long and complicated story which, at its lowest level of explanation, graphically illustrates the place of medicine in Byzantine society as subordinate to theology, yet necessary. Byzantine medicine, which is traditionally taken to mean the medical theories and practices which are found in the Roman Empire from the fourth century onwards, is by no means easy to categorize. Few handbooks give it more than a passing mention, usually in despair at the paucity of accessible material, and even modern scholarly articles are depressingly few. The old survey by Iwan Bloch still retains its value as a description of a slowly changing system of medicine allegedly embedded in an almost equally static society.[2] Yet this state of affairs is a measure of our failure to exploit an abundance of material from a variety of sources, pagan and secular, Greek, Syriac, and Arabic, medical, theological and historical. Above all, with but rare exceptions, historians of medicine have been content to go over the same ground and to reach the same conclusions, without looking beyond a few limited sources or employing their critical faculties as historians.

My survey of the medicine in late antiquity has two aims: first, to suggest some guidelines for the study of Byzantine medicine; and secondly, to locate the medicine of late antiquity firmly within its social and intellectual context. Such a programme would be indeed vast, yet because several of the papers in this volume will take up and develop many of the particular points I wish to make in this introduction, I shall confine myself to setting out some of my general conclusions and leave the detailed discussion to others. This has the advantage that the links and interactions between the various aspects of medicine and medical practice may stand out clearer in this broad survey, and that general considerations that affect the whole of the medicine of the Byzantine world can be spelled out before some of their particular emphases are described. A chronological division in the mid-sixth century also allows the historian to observe both short- and long-term trends, which can become obscured or disappear if viewed in the context either of a single generation or of the many centuries that separate the foundation of Constantinople from the Muslim Conquest. The neglect of Byzantine medicine owes not a little to this chronological com-

[The reader is referred to the list of abbreviations at the end of the volume.]

*I am grateful to John Scarborough and Ihor Ševčenko for help and advice. My greatest debt is to the late A. H. M. Jones, who first introduced me to the problems and delights of late antiquity.

[1] Photographs in G. Millet, *Monuments de l'Athos*, I, *Les peintures* (Paris, 1927), pl. 151; P. Huber, *Athos* (Zürich, 1969), pl. 193; P. Yiannias "The Wall Paintings of the Lavra" (Diss., Univ. of Pittsburgh, 1971), pl. H.1 (curiously calling Galen Palenos, p. 289). A much earlier painting, "in Byzantine style," from the cathedral at Anagni in Southern Italy shows both Hippocrates and Galen; A. Cherubini, *I medici scrittori dal XV al XX secolo* (Rome, 1977), 27. On the function of pagan sages in such paintings, see, e.g., C. Mango, "A Forged Inscription of the Year 781," *Zbornik Radova*, 8 (1963), 201–207; G. Nandris, *Christian Humanism in the Neo-Byzantine Mural Painting of Eastern Europe* (Wiesbaden, 1970), 24–44, but this account is somewhat confused.

[2] Iwan Bloch, in M. Neuburger, J. Pagel, *Handbuch der Geschichte der Medizin* I (Jena, 1902), pp. 481–588. The survey of medical literature by Hunger, "Medizin," 263–320, updates Bloch for the purely literary medical evidence.

pression of a millennium or more into a few pages, in which, almost inevitably, slow developments of doctrine or therapies are transformed into a solid, unyielding and unchanging monolith. By being viewed within a particular historical context, Byzantine medicine takes on a more dynamic form, and some of the anachronisms that have bedeviled its study can be eliminated.

The most obvious difference between the medicine of the second and that of the sixth century A.D. can be summed up in one word, Galenism, in both its positive and its pejorative meanings. Instead of the variety of great names that can be cited for the second century—Galen, Rufus, Soranus, Antyllus, maybe even Aretaeus—and the evidence from both literary and epigraphic texts for new interests and ideas on surgery, the fourth and later centuries present us with a dull and narrow range of authors—the summarizers, the encyclopaedists—who have been studied not for themselves but for the earlier sources they happen to encapsulate. Oribasius, Aetius, Alexander, Paul are the medical refrigerators of antiquity: we are concerned with their contents, not their mechanics or their design. Yet this is our fault, not theirs. Ancient historians have long enjoyed the advantages of Whiggishness, without its reproaches. We can happily talk about Hippocratic medicine and its medical achievements in the same breath, because almost everything in the Corpus counts as an achievement through being the earliest recorded example in Europe of, for example, the connection of tuberculosis and a hunched back. We can accept Galen almost without question at his own estimation, because his own ideas on medicine, on research, on progress, coincide to a great extent with our own; and we can warm to a man whose stated commitment to the truth above all else would not be out of place today. Yet, faced with the great compendia, we find it difficult to understand them, apart from noting the range of their sources. There is no obvious commitment to research, to private investigation, even to argument and criticism. In them medicine appears to stand still, somehow to be frozen, to return to my earlier metaphor of the refrigerator. We are in a quandary also because our conception of how medicine works has changed drastically; and it is not surprising that the last major work of medico-historical value to be done on them was over a century ago by Francis Adams, whose third and final volume of his great translation of Paul appeared in 1847. The reason for this is simple: to Adams, Paul was transmitting a living medicine, one that could still be used in his daily practice in Scotland, and it was precisely for this reason that Adams, on the basis of his own experience as a doctor, could reach such a sound judgment on the merits of this compiler.[3]

We should approach the problem of the medical learning of these encyclopaedists of late antiquity with a variety of questions. Obviously, we must be interested in the sources they had at their disposal, and it is entirely legitimate to draw conclusions from them as to the spread of Galenism in late antiquity. It is indeed a lengthy process, largely illuminated for us by Owsei Temkin, and its outlines are clear.[4] Galen already enjoyed a high reputation in his own lifetime, certainly in the Greek-speaking half of the Empire. Theodotus the shoemaker, Athenaeus of Naucratis, and Alexander of Aphrodisias, in their own ways, attest his influence among his contemporaries as doctor and philosopher.[5] Some of his philosophical writings enjoyed lasting fame. As late as the fifth century, Marinus of Sichem, the biographer and pupil of Proclus, is said to have dissented from his master's views on Plato's Parmenides in favor of the erroneous ones of Galen and Firmus.[6] Later still, Galen's scientific writings were known, in part, to Philoponus, and some of his little tracts on logic and morals have come down to us in Greek or in Arabic.[7] If Galenic philosophy retained some influence, Galenic medicine was far more important. It is clear that Oribasius, for example, took Galen as his main source, supplementing him, where necessary, as with his comments on the plague, from other authors such as Rufus of Ephesus.[8] This was not a purely personal decision by Oribasius, a mere whim. It reflected

[3] Paul (trans. Adams), *passim*. The German version of Paul, by J. Berendes, *Des besten Arztes sieben Bücher* (Leiden, 1914), though useful, lacks a substantial commentary. Recent scholarship has added little to the older assessment of Adams by C. Singer, "A Great Country Doctor: Francis Adams of Banchory," *BHM*, 12 (1942), 1–17.

[4] O. Temkin, *Galenism* (Ithaca and London, 1973). See also his articles: "Geschichte des Hippokratismus im ausgehenden Altertum," *Kyklos*, 4 (1932), 1–80; "Byzantine Medicine: Tradition and Empiricism," *DOP*, 16 (1962), 97–115 (= *The Double Face of Janus* [Baltimore and London, 1977], 202–22).

[5] O. Temkin, *Galenism*, 55–61: *contra*, J. Scarborough, "The Galenic question," *SA*, 65 (1981), 1–31. I shall confirm Temkin's assessment, with new material, in a forthcoming article in *BHM*, 1984.

[6] Damascius, *Vita Isidori*, in Photius, *Bibl.* 351B. For Galen and Hippocrates as philosophers, cf. Gregory Nazianzen, *Or.* VIII.20.

[7] For Philoponus, see R. B. Todd, "Philosophy and Medicine in John Philoponus' Commentary," in this volume; for the Arabs, cf. G. Strohmaier, "Galen in Arabic: Prospects and Projects," in Nutton, ed., *Galen: Problems*, 187–96.

[8] Cf. H. Mercurialis, *De peste . . . praelectiones* (Basle, 1577), 11.

the growing importance of Galen, and the belief, easily induced by Galenic rhetoric, that he had somehow defined and completed medicine. Hippocrates sowed, Galen reaped, says one commentator;[9] all that was left to others was thus gleanings from the stubble.

Yet the encyclopaedists were not just compilers; they had to select. They were constantly adding fresh material or compressing the old; they were not dumb copyists. My reading of Oribasius fills me with admiration for his broad knowledge of Galen, for his ability to summarize and yet keep in as much of the original as possible, and, most importantly in an age that valued rhetoric highly, for his skill in expressing its essentials clearly. It is this sort of categorization that we should employ when looking at the compendia, to try and see them on their own terms, and to judge them on their ability to put across an effective message. They must be seen as the equivalent of Osler's *Principles and Practice of Medicine*, not of a research monograph.

It is in this light, too, that we should approach such authors as Cassius Felix, Magnus of Nisibis and Caelius Aurelianus, enough of whose writings survive to enable us to form a reasonably critical judgment on them. They have in the past been dismissed crudely as translators, or mere abbreviators, of earlier writings by Galen or Soranus.[10] But this is far too simple. Jackie Pigeaud's recent work on Caelius has shown how that author adapts his material, occasionally criticizes it, and produces a large work of considerable elegance and effectiveness.[11] Magnus of Nisibis was celebrated for his rhetoric and his logic, though his practical abilities and experience, to say nothing of his character, were less impressive.[12] His book on urines, which survives in Arabic and in part in the second volume of Ideler's *Physici et Medici Graeci*, and which is a restatement of Hippocratic and Galenic doctrine, was highly regarded by succeeding generations. It was mentioned by Theophilus, for whom it was a major source, and by Johannes Actuarius; it was translated into Arabic, and, finally, excerpted by

Byzantine doctors.[13] Theophilus' mild criticism does not justify the almost total neglect of Magnus by modern scholars, and in fact it tells us what Magnus' audience was looking for. He is praised for his attempts to systematize and arrange in order the various urines, by their types and by their differences, but condemned for failing to include all their diagnostic and prognostic indications. His teaching was therefore left incomplete (partly from his lack of first hand experience), but his was the argument and organization followed by subsequent writers on the subject.[14] As Gerhard Baader his pointed out, in earlier diagnostic theory uroscopy plays a very minor part—although Galen's practice in no way neglected it—whereas late antiquity and the Middle Ages elevated it to being the major guide to diagnosis. In this development the role of Magnus may have been crucial.[15]

It would be wrong to conclude, too, that summaries, handbooks, and collections of drugs, such as we find with pseudo-Apuleius and Marcellus Empiricus, are new phenomena in late antiquity. One of the most important of the lost works of Rufus was his big compendium *For the Layman*, to which may be plausibly attributed many short excerpts preserved under his name by later encyclopaedists.[16] Galen summarized not only his own books on pulses but also the *Anatomy* of Marinus and various Platonic dialogues, and his *Therapeutics, for Glaucon*, was deliberately designed as a brief introduction to medicine for a layman.[17] Scribonius Largus and Marcellus Empiricus are separated as authors of recipe collections only by the centuries, not by any development in their aims and methods.[18] Yet one significant development which *can*

[9] Palladius, *In Epid. VI scholia*, p. 157 Dietz.

[10] E.g., I. E. Drabkin, "Soranus and His System of Medicine," *BHM*, 25 (1951), 503–18.

[11] J. Pigeaud, "Pro Caelio Aureliano," *Mémoires du Centre Jean Palerne*, 3 (1982), 105–17. A similar conclusion has been reached by G. Harig and D. Nickel in their preparatory studies for a new edition of Caelius in the *CML* series.

[12] Eunapius, *Vit. phil.* 497 ff.; Philostorgius, *Hist. eccl.* VIII.10; Libanius, *Ep.* 497; for his character, see Libanius, *Epp.* 1208, 1358.

[13] Theophilus, *De urinis*, pref. (p. 261 Ideler); Johannes Actuarius, *De urinis* I.2 (p. 5 Ideler). For manuscripts and the later revisions and editions, see Galen (ed. Kühn), XIX. 574–601, 602–608; Anonymous, *De urinis*, pp. 307–16 Ideler; H. Diels, *Die Handschriften der antiken Ärzte*, II (Berlin, 1906), 59 f.; F. Sezgin, *Geschichte des arabischen Schrifttums*, III (Leiden, 1970), 165 f.; M. Ullmann, *Die Medizin im Islam* (Leiden, 1970), 81 f.

[14] Theophilus, *De urinis*, pref. (p. 261 f. Ideler).

[15] G. Baader, "Early Medieval Latin Adaptations of Byzantine Medicine in Western Europe," in this vol. Hence the translation into Greek of Avicenna's chapters on urine, pp. 286–302 Ideler; and of similar books in Syriac and Persian, pp. 303–16 Ideler. For Galen's practice, cf. Nutton, ed., *Galen: On Prognosis*, 2 (*CMG* V 8,1, p. 80), but undoubtedly it is by the pulse that Galen mainly made his diagnoses, and his interest is more in the quantity and frequency of urination than in the quality of urine.

[16] So, rightly, J. Ilberg, "Rufus von Ephesos. Ein griechischer Arzt in trajanischer Zeit," AbhSächsAkadWiss (1931), 45 ff.

[17] Galen, XIX.25–30 K.; XIX.46 K.; XIX.31 K.

[18] The arguments of P. Brown, *The Cult of the Saints* (London and Chicago, 1981), 113 ff., on the place of Marcellus Empiri-

be discerned in late antiquity is the accentuation of the divorce between practical and theoretical texts. Magnus of Nisibis was clearly a theoretical professor, and recent studies on John of Alexandria and Agnellus have shown how their lectures became more and more devoted to extensions of theory, rather than to practical purposes.[19] But this tendency was not itself new; Galen complained about it in his own day, and the format of lectures and commentaries on particular texts only encouraged this sort of logical or philological specialization.[20] I wonder, too, whether the magnitude of Galen's own achievement, with its stress on the indissoluble unity of theory and practice, did not frighten succeeding generations of scholars with the thought of the learning needed to combat Galen *in toto* and, at the same time, console them by suggesting that a concentration on one aspect of medicine would necessarily bring about improvements in others.

Yet it would be foolish to deny the effect of Galenism, an effect so powerful that a poet could, in a wonderful trope, refer to Christ as a second (and neglected) Galen.[21] Hippocrates comes to be studied through Galen's eyes, even through Galen's text,[22] and the theories of his opponents are pushed to the fringes of the scientific community, to Latin-speaking Africa and the collectors of popular scientific curiosities, the *Problemata*, like pseudo-Alexander and Cassius the Iatrosophist.[23] Other medical sects passed peacefully away. The last recorded Greek doctor who claimed to be a follower of Asclepiades lived around 350 A.D., and I prefer to believe that those doctors on Byzantine epitaphs who call themselves "men of the spirit," πνευματι-κοί, are confessing their faith rather than their medical learning.[24] Not that we should regard the

medicine of the late antiquity simply as a degenerate form of Galenism. There were bold spirits prepared to put forward their own ideas—Alexander of Tralles, for example, and Jacobus Psychrestus. This great philosopher, beloved by emperor and people alike, honored with statues at Athens and Constantinople, who ordered the rich to aid the poor, who treated those in poverty without fee, relying only on the *annonae* given him as a civic doctor, this paragon of learning and experience gained his fame, his influence and indeed his nickname, Psychrestus, from a radical new technique. He treated his patients with cooling waters, as a means of reducing their tensions and worries about money.[25] Yet even here we may find an earlier precedent in the Augustan physician, Antonius Musa, whose cold water treatments succeeded in curing the emperor Augustus, but may have hastened the death of his favorite heir, Marcellus.[26]

Nor does experimentation cease immediately on the death of Galen or in the darkness of the third century. True, we no longer have records of the medical contests at Ephesus, but Nemesius of Emesa apparently preserves details of the anatomy of the tongue that derive from fourth-century Alexandria.[27] A similar conclusion might be drawn from the discussion of the tongue in the pseudo-Galenic *De motibus liquidis*, which, in the form in which it survives, is a Latin translation going back via Arabic to a Syriac original.[28] But both Nemesius and the Syriac author may be deriving their information direct from some lost tract of Galen, and the anatomical progress they show over Galen may therefore be illusory. A detailed programme of anatomical research such as we can see in Galen, and

---

cus in the Western world of healing are suggestive, but not conclusive. Cf. also B. Merlette et al., "Le manuscrit 420 de Laon et la médecine carolingienne," *Histoire des sciences médicales*, 14 (1980), 51–69.

[19] Agnellus of Ravenna, *Lectures on Galen's De sectis* (Buffalo, 1981); C. D. Pritchet, *Iohannis Alexandrini in librum de sectis Galeni* (Leiden, 1982); cf. O. Temkin, "Studies on Late Alexandrian Medicine," *BHM*, 3 (1935), 405–30 (= *The Double Face of Janus*, pp. 178–97).

[20] See, for example, Galen, *CMG* V 10,1, 420 f.; XVIIA.496–524 (*CMG* V 10,2,1, 10–26).

[21] George of Pisidia, *Hexaemeron*, 1.1588 f.

[22] B. Alexanderson, *Die hippokratische Schrift Prognostikon* (Göteborg, 1963), 169; J. N. Mattock, M. C. Lyons, eds. and trans. (Arabic) *Hippocrates: On the Nature of Man* (Cambridge, 1968), viii.

[23] See the evidence collected in my article "The Seeds of Disease: An Explanation of Contagion and Infection from the Greeks to the Renaissance," *Medical History*, 27 (1983), 9–13.

[24] From Cibyra Minor in Cilicia, DenkWien, 102 (1970), 65, n. 38 and pl. 52; on πνευματικοί, *CIG* 9578, 9792; cf. *Vita S. Marthae*, ed. P. Van den Ven (Brussels, 1970) ch. 51.17.

[25] *Chron. Paschale*, PG 92.824A; *Suda, s. Ἰάκωβος; Malalas, Chron.*, p. 370 Dindorf; Marcellus, *Chron.*, p. 88; Photius, *Bibl.*, 344A; *Suda, s. Σωρανός* (confusing Soranus of Ephesus and Soranus of Mallus ?); Alexander, II.163 Puschmann.

[26] Suetonius, *Aug.* 59; Cassius Dio, 53.30; cf. F. Atterbury, *Antonius Musa's Character Represented in the Person of Iapis* (London, 1742). A similar therapy was advocated by Charmis of Massilia, Pliny, *NH* 29.5.10, under the emperor Claudius, cf. *ib.* 29.8.22 and Galen, XIV.80.K.

[27] For Ephesus, J. Keil, "Ärzteinschriften aus Ephesos," *ÖJh*, 8 (1905), 128–38; *Die Inschriften von Ephesos*, VI, 1160–69. For Nemesius, *De nat. homin.* 8, 14 (pp. 195 ff., 208 f. Matthiae, cf. p. 404 f.), with the arguments of W. Telfer, *Nemesius of Emesa, On the Nature of Man* (London, 1955), 331.

[28] Ps.-Galen, *De motibus liquidis*, in Galen, *Opera omnia*, ed. R. Chartier (Paris, 1679), V, pp. 400, 403–405. On the question of authenticity, cf. Galen, II.443 K.; XVIIIB.931 K., and the summary of J. C. G. Ackermann, in Galen, I.clxii K. Cf. also the discussion of H. Baumgarten, "Galen, Uber die Stimme" (Diss., Göttingen, 1962), 88–93. The problem will be discussed in a forthcoming article by Dr. J. Wollock.

earlier in Rufus and Satyrus, cannot be shown to have survived the fourth century. But before we condemn late antiquity too harshly, we must note that Galen himself believed that anatomy had almost disappeared between the age of Herophilus and Erasistratus and that of Marinus, four hundred years later: the tradition of anatomical research is a very fragile thing.[29]

One should not, however, confuse the absence of experimental anatomy on the Galenic model with a declining interest in practical techniques, including surgery. John of Ephesus describes a surgeon relieving a painful condition by the permanent insertion of a drainage tube.[30] The medical reputation of Alexandria also rested on more than the theoretical content of its lectures. The fourth-century professor Ionicus, according to his biographer Eunapius, was skilled in knowledge of all parts of the body, and possessed great practical skills in surgery and bandaging.[31] A few years later, a lawyer friend of St. Augustine, Innocentius, who had rejected the advice of two distinguished local doctors at Carthage, was quite prepared to accept it when it came from an Alexandrian doctor, even though it entailed a complicated and painful operation.[32] Happily for him, God intervened, and his anal fistula was found to be miraculously healed.

The intervention of God brings me on to my second broad section, the position of medicine and medical men within a Christian society. In a recent article, Darrel Amundsen has strongly argued that, on the whole, Christianity was favorable to medicine, or at any rate, not hostile[33]—a conclusion with which I would agree—yet this argument is rather too bland, and misleading on one important point. As Harnack long ago showed, Christianity is a healing religion *par excellence*.[34] The New Testa-

ment emphasizes the power of Christ and his apostles to cure diseases, and this was one of the features that secured for Christianity the primacy among competing religions. Similarly, Ramsay MacMullen has recently pointed to the crucial significance of healing miracles in securing the allegiance of intellectual doubters and of the ordinary people to Christianity.[35] Yet this Christian healing was not that of the doctors. It succeeded where they had failed, often over many years and at great expense; it was accessible to all; it was simple. It was a medicine of prayer and fasting, or of anointing and the laying on of hands.[36] The power to heal was given to Christian elders, and they were to be consulted first in all cases of illnesses.[37]

There is, thus, a tension, to put it at its lowest, between the model of the New Testament and the real world outside. It is not that Christianity is necessarily opposed to secular healing; but it presupposes an alternative medicine on which true Christians may be expected to rely. How many Christians actually followed this expectation is unknown, and unknowable. But it is a doctrine that surfaces from time to time among the ascetics and among the more fundamentalist Christians like Tertullian, Tatian, Marcion, even Cyprian. But even those who, like St. Basil, knew and approved of secular medicine, were always careful to leave room for this peculiarly Christian type of healing. The tension was almost palpable, and we can find various theologians endeavoring to hold it in balance. One example, chosen at random, is St. Diadochus of Photike, a monk of northern Greece, who wrote his "On Spiritual Knowledge," about 480 A.D.[38] In Diadochus' view, there is nothing to stop a Christian calling in a doctor when he falls ill. Divine providence has implanted remedies in nature, and hence human experience has developed the art of medicine. But, all the same, our hope of healing should not be placed in doctors but in the true savior Jesus Christ. Ascetics in monasteries or in towns, because of their environment, cannot always maintain that perfect charity necessary for the efficacy of faith for healing. To them Diadochus recom-

---

[29] Galen, XV. 136K; cf. A. Vesalius, *De humani corporis fabrica* (Basle, 1543), fol. 3r.-v.

[30] John of Ephesus, PO 18, p. 643 f.; see below, pp. 88 f.

[31] Eunapius, *Vit. phil.* 499.; W. C. Wright, the Loeb translator, p. 537, confuses the issue further by translating ἡ καθ' ἕκαστον πεῖρα, not as "in every type of experience," but as "in every kind of experiment," with its implications of medical research. But πεῖρα is regularly used as the counterweight to λόγος, mere theory.

[32] Augustine, *Civ. Dei* XXII.8. Note also the hostile comment of Fulgentius, *Mitologiae*, p. 9 Helm (cf. c. 523), on an Alexandria whose streets were crammed with the stalls of surgical butchers, all killing their patients.

[33] D. W. Amundsen, "Medicine and Faith in Early Christianity," *BHM*, 56 (1982), 326–50. Both this article and the excellent collection of essays edited by W. J. Sheils, "The Church and Healing," *Studies in Church History*, 19 (1982), would have benefited from a closer attention to and exposition of the New Testament evidence.

[34] A. Harnack, "Medicinisches aus der ältesten Kirchengeschichte," Texte u. Untersuch. 8.4, 1892, pp. 37–152; H. J. Frings,

"Medizin und Arzt bei den griechischen Kirchenvätern bis Chrysostomos" (Diss., Bonn, 1959) is a very useful collection of primary material.

[35] R. MacMullen, *Paganism in the Roman Empire* (New Haven and London, 1982), 95 f., 135.

[36] E.g., Mark, 7.31, Luke, 5.18, 6.18, 8.41, 9.37, 11.14. Cf. Arnobius, *Adv. gent.* I.45–50.

[37] James, *Ep.* 5.13–18. A study of patristic exegesis of this passage would repay the effort.

[38] St. Diadochus of Photike, *On Spiritual Knowledge*, chs. 53–55.

mends that they should not succumb to the deceits and temptations of the devil, who has induced some of them to boast publicly that they have not needed a doctor for many years. But hermits in the desert can draw near the Lord, who heals all kinds of sickness. And moreover, the solitary hermit has the desert itself to provide consolation in his illness. Concern for the body, and worries about illness, indicate that the Christian has not yet emancipated himself from the desires of the flesh, has not yet cultivated the true dispassion that waits joyfully for death as the gateway to a truer life.

This rejection of doctors in favor of spiritual medicine is particularly marked in the Lives of the Saints. Not all of them are as hostile as the biographer of St. Artemius, but throughout there runs a current of dislike of doctors, overtly for their high fees and their failures, which is hardly to be found in similar healing stories from the pagan side.[39] Aelius Aristeides remained a personal friend of doctors like Satyrus, and doctors contributed generously to healing shrines.[40]

Besides, despite Arnobius' boast that doctors of genius were turning to Christianity, the medical profession was always suspect as a stronghold of paganism and heresy.[41] Oribasius, Agapius of Alexandria, Asclepiodotus of Aphrodisias, Jacobus Psychrestus and his father, these are but a few of the famous doctors of the fourth and fifth centuries whose paganism was overt.[42] As for Gesius, professor of medicine at fifth-century Alexandria, "whose rhetorical expertise removed all difficulties of medical exposition," and whose diagnosis was "a bright light that would bring a sure relief," he might be officially a Christian, but his sympathies were clearly with his pagan friends.[43] He protected the

pagan philosopher Heraiscus after he had tried to defend the oracle of Menuthis from Christian attack, and, says Sophronius, he treated his Christianity lightheartedly. His punishment for announcing that the cures of SS. Cyrus and John were purely natural and not miraculous was to be attacked by a disease that defied all treatment by the doctors. It was only removed after Gesius had made a contrite confession of his impiety.[44] Fifty years later, John of Ephesus denounced in the persecutions of Justinian an indiscriminate collection of grammarians, sophists, lawyers and, finally, doctors.[45]

Heresy was also linked with medicine. The Adoptionists, led by Theodotus the shoemaker, had even by 210 been led astray by Galen in applying logic (and textual criticism) to their sacred texts.[46] Later still, the career of Aetius, with its sudden switches from tinker to schoolmaster to doctor and to heretical theologian, offers an interesting example of the ease with which a man of ability and flair could set himself up as a doctor.[47] Yet even Aetius' bitterest opponent, Gregory of Nyssa, allows that he cured some of his patients and that he made a reputation by intervening in medical debates.[48] At times too, a priest might be protected by his medical skills, even if his morals were dubious and his theology unsound. Gerontius of Milan, doctor and deacon, defied St. Ambrose's instructions to remain in Milan and await investigation for his claim to have seen a demon, and fled to Constantinople. Powerful friends secured his prefer-

---

[39] *Miracula S. Artemii*, ed. A. Papadopoulos-Kerameus, *Varia graeca sacra* (St. Petersburg, 1909), *passim*, esp. pp. 3, 4, 24, 26. P. Hordern, "Saints and Doctors in the Early Byzantine Empire: the Case of Theodore of Sykeon," *Studies in Church History*, 19 (1982), 1–13, is an excellent and sober survey. H. J. Magoulias, 'The Lives of the Saints as Sources of Data for the History of Byzantine Medicine in the Sixth and Seventh Centuries,' *BZ*, 57, (1954), 127–50, adds some further details, but is very unreliable. As Hordern rightly emphasizes, not all Christian healers opposed secular healing: the biographer of SS. Cosmas and Damian is glad to acknowledge their expertise (ἐϰμελετήσαντες) in Hippocratic and Galenic medicine, although, of course, they regarded the healing sent from god as "safer" (ἀσφαλέστερον), Vita SS. Cosmae et Damiani, *AnalBoll*, 1 (1882), *sect.* 4.

[40] Aelius Aristeides, *Or.* 49.8–10.

[41] Arnobius, *Adv. gentes* II.5.

[42] See on this, A. Moffatt, "Science Teachers in the Early Byzantine Empire: Some Statistics," *Byzantinoslavica*, 24 (1973), 15–18.

[43] Photius, *Bibl.* 352B; *Suda, s.* Γέσιος; the quotations come from Aeneas of Gaza, *Ep.* 20, and Procopius of Gaza, *Ep.* 102.

Cf. also Aeneas, *Ep.* 19; Procopius, *Epp.* 16, 102, 122, 125; Zacharias Schol., *De opificio mundi*, PG 75.1016, including him as an interlocutor in his debate on creation, *ib.*, 1060–1106. Of his medical works nothing can be shown to have survived (but note Vatican, Pal. lat. 1090, ff. 1r.-42v., commentary on Galen's *De sectis*, elsewhere attributed to Agnellus). Traces of his activity as a commentator can be found in Dietz, II, 343, n. 4; and in G. Bergsträsser, "Ḥunain ibn Isḥāq, "uber die syrischen und arabischen Galen-Ubersetzungen", AbhKM, 17.2 (1925), p. 36, n. 101. His name also appears in connection with the vexed question of the *Summaria Alexandrina*, see E. Lieber, "Galen in Hebrew: The Transmission of Galen's Works in the Mediaeval Islamic World," in Nutton, ed., *Galen: Problems*, 167–86, esp. p. 177 with nn. on p. 185.

[44] Zacharias Schol., *Vita Severi*, PO, 1, 27–32, gives a graphic description of the attack on Menuthis, but without mentioning his friend Gesius. For his part, see Sophronius, *Mirac. SS. Cyri et Iohannis* 30: PG 73.3513–17.

[45] John of Ephesus, *Eccl. Hist.*, ROChr, 2 (1897), 481 f.

[46] Eusebius, *Eccl. hist*, V.28: H. Schöne, "Ein Einbruch der antiken Logik und Textkritik in die altchristliche Theologie," *Festschrift F. Dölger.* (Münster, 1939), 252–66; R. Walzer, *Galen on Jews and Christians* (Oxford, 1949), 75–86.

[47] Philostorgius, *Eccl. hist.* III.15; Sozomen, *Eccl. hist.* III.15.

[48] Gregory Nyss., *Contra Eunomium* I.42, 45, cf. Philostorgius, *loc. cit.*

ment to the bishopric of Nicomedia, and when the angry Ambrose gained the assistance of John Chrysostom, the patriarch of Constantinople, in deposing him, the inhabitants of Nicomedia made vigorous complaints, praising Gerontius' unstinting use of his abilities among them as a doctor.[49] They were clearly more concerned for their bodies than their souls, like the Christians who secured the deposition of the orthodox bishop Basil of Ancyra for failing to excommunicate a quack who had killed several patients.[50]

It should not be forgotten that, for long after Constantine's conversion, large parts of the empire remained steadfastly pagan, and that the traditional healing shrines continued for many years to attract large numbers of patients. In England, the shrine of Nodens at Lydney enjoyed its best days in the late fourth and early fifth century,[51] while the Lives of SS. Cosmas and Damian and, in particular, SS. Cyrus and John reveal the vigorous activities of such shrines in Asia Minor and Egypt.[52] The letters of Libanius make several references to the cult of Asclepius, while the Life of Damascius, from the late fifth century, often mentions pagan healing shrines and, in particular, theurgy, the pagan equivalent of Christian miracle.[53]

As is well known, Christianity took over from pagan healing cult not only its function as a source of medical treatment but also its language, its imagery, even its sites. *Christus medicus* is a metaphor that has been often studied, and Erich Dinkler has recently discussed the artistic borrowings of Christianity from Asclepius cult.[54] At Caesarea Philippi a statue traditionally supposed to represent Jesus and the woman with the issue of blood has been plausibly argued to have been either a statue of an emperor with the epithet *Soter*, Savior, or one of

Asclepius.[55] Pagan shrines became Christian temples. A Christian basilica was constructed at the Asclepieion at Epidaurus; the Asclepieion at Rome is now the church of S. Bartolommeo and the healing spring its font, and churches dedicated to St. Michael often replaced healing shrines to Heracles.[56] The Christian hatred of these pagan shrines is best attested at Pergamum, where there was a deliberate destruction of all the cult images, big or small, of Asclepius. The result is that our information on them depends on literary descriptions in Galen and on chance survivals of representations of the cult statue from the Black Sea region.[57]

There are borrowings too among pagans from Christianity. The increase in pagan miracles, in theurgy, that is associated with the philosophers and doctors of late antiquity, like the two Asclepiodoti, is in one sense a deliberate reaction against Christian doctrines, and Julian's attempts to impose the cult of Asclepius as the center of paganism can only be understood against a background of Christianity as a healing, missionary religion.[58] It was Julian also, who, in a famous letter to the high priest of Galatia, encouraged pagans to follow the examples of Jews and Christians in their practical efforts to remedy social problems. Pagans, like their opponents, were to look outwards, and to care for their friends and fellow believers; charity was a means of proselytism.[59]

The early centuries of the Christian empire show a reformation of problems about health and healing. Professor Amundsen has rightly emphasized the new attitudes towards sickness and suffering, which combine the Stoic doctrines of indifference

[49] Sozomen, *Eccl. hist.* VIII.6.

[50] *Ibid.*, IV.24. It is perhaps worth noting that, apart from the story told by Galen and preserved only in Arabic (M. Meyerhof, "Autobiographische Bruchstücke Galens aus arabischen Quellen," *SA*, 22 [1929], 83), there is no evidence for prosecution of quack doctors in antiquity, and it may be doubted whether that man was prosecuted or punished for selling dangerous poisons or for impersonating a pupil of the great Galen.

[51] R. E. M. and T. V. Wheeler, *Lydney* (London, 1932).

[52] J. Geffcken, *Der Ausgang der griechischen-römischen Heidentums* (Heidelberg, 1920) remains fundamental.

[53] R. Asmus, *Das Leben des Philosophen Isidoros von Damaskios aus Damaskos* (Leipzig, 1911); E. R. Dodds, *The Greeks and the Irrational* (Oxford, 1950), 283–311.

[54] E. Dinkler, "Christus und Asklepios," SBHeid, 1980.2; K. Hauck, "Gott als Arzt," in C. Meier, U. Ruberg, *Text und Bild: Zwei Aspekte des Zusammenwirkens zweier Künste in Mittelalter und früher Neuzeit* (Wiesbaden, 1980), 19–62. For literary references, see D. W. Amundsen, *BHM*, 56 (1982), 331.

[55] Eusebius, *Hist. eccl.* VIII.18; cf. the *Passio IV SS. Coronatorum, Acta Sanctorum*, Nov. 3, for the significance to Christians of statues of Asclepius.

[56] F. Robert, *Épidaure*, (Paris, 1935), 41; M. Besnier, *L'île Tibérine dans l'antiquité* (Paris, 1902), 184–246; J. P. Rohland, *Der Erzengel Michael* (Leiden, 1977), 75–104.

[57] G. Strohmaier, "Asklepios und das Ei," in *Festschrift F. Altheim*, 2 (Berlin, 1970), 143–53. A further study by Dr. Strohmaier on the artistic representations of the cult at Pergamum is scheduled to appear in the *Proceedings of the Twenty-sixth International Congress of the History of Medicine* (Plovdiv, 1978), but so far only Vol. I has appeared.

[58] R. Asmus, "Der Neuplatoniker Asklepiodotos der Grosse," *SA*, 7 (1913), 26–42, needs to be supplemented by the epigraphic evidence provided by L. Robert, *Hellenica IV* (Paris, 1948), 119–26. The article by G. Senn, "Asklepiodotos von Alexandreia, ein positivistischer Naturforscher des V Jahrhundert," *Archeion*, 21 (1938), 13–27, is full of errors and misconceptions. For Julian, see the material collected by the passionate P. Athanassiadi-Fowden, *Julian and Hellenism* (Oxford, 1981), 166–70.

[59] Julian, *Ep.* 22.

to the pains of the body with the idea of the nobility of suffering and of, in some way, it being a test of one's faith.[60] Suffering is to be more than endured, it is almost to be welcomed. I cannot find in pagan literature anything to compare with Tertullian's view of famine and pestilence as the acceptable will of God and as the rightful cure for the prosperity and population growth he saw around him.[61] Nor would a pagan have advised a frightened congregation, as Cyprian did in 252, to accept a plague joyfully as proof of God's love: for by it the wicked were sent swifter to Hell, and the just would more quickly obtain their everlasting refreshment.[62] It is true that plague in the pagan world was often seen as the result of divine displeasure, and that the measures taken against it were regularly religious—supplications, vows, public festivals, temple building, and so on—but I cannot imagine a pagan asking the question posed in the *Moral Questions* attributed to Athanasius and summarized in the later collection by Anastasius of Sinai, "Should a man rightly flee from the plague, if, as was possible, it was sent by the wrath of God?"[63] The theologians' answer neatly sidesteps the issue: yes, if the plague has a purely natural cause, in the filth and overcrowding of the towns or in the polluted air; but the wrath of God will seek out the sinner everywhere, even in the desert, and in such circumstances, flight is in vain.

The theologians' opening response to this question also indicates some of the dangers of Christianity to the scientific mind. They apologize for talking largely about natural plagues, for they might seem to some to doubt the providence and power of God, who oversees all things, and to deny that the plague is a sign of divine displeasure. Their message is largely secular and its advice medical, not theological, but it is given with a slightly worried glance at fellow and more fundamentalist theologians. I am reminded of Alexander of Tralles' comment that he could have included in his books many more sympathetic remedies, chants and charms, but was prevented from so doing—presumably by theological difficulties, rather than by the opposition of his medical colleagues.[64]

Alexander of Tralles, a member of a distinguished intellectual family, widely traveled, well read, and by no means uncritical in the selection of his material, reveals another side of medicine in the Christian empire—the emergence into acceptability of remedies that had earlier been excluded as "falling outside the profession of medicine." That phrase had been coined c. 60 A.D. by Scribonius Largus, rejecting a remedy for epilepsy that involved the blood of a gladiator. That was rejected also by Pliny, and by Galen, but it appears in Alexander[65] as a proven remedy, frequently given. Alexander also includes many other folk remedies, many spells, amulets and charms. These were not new—some can be found in the pages of Pliny—and the names of Pamphilus and Xenocrates remind us that not every doctor was as scrupulous as a Scribonius, a Dioscorides or a Galen. The papyri of Egypt, not to speak of the pages of Ammianus, show a growing acceptance, among all classes, of the power of such amulets and charms.[66] Sophronius, bishop of Constantia, was accused in 449 of astrology, phialomancy and other kinds of divination, and of corrupting thereby Peter the *archiatros*, who had read his books on astrology.[67] There is an obvious shift between Galen's time and that of Alexander in the definition of what is or is not medically and socially acceptable as a type of remedy. We should not regard the injunctions of Alexander to pick a mandrake with one's left hand, or the instructions he gives for the correct formula to be spoken over a sufferer from gout as being new or confined to him.[68] They can be found centuries earlier, but in what we would term magical texts, or in early Roman domestic medicine.[69]

[60] D. W. Amundsen, *BHM*, 56 (1982), 334–42; cf. the (indiscriminate) collection of material in F. Bottomley, *Attitudes to the Body in Western Christendom* (London, 1979), 59–96.

[61] Tertullian, *De anima* 30; contrast, *Anth. Pal.* VII.626.

[62] Cyprian, *De mortalitate* 9.

[63] Ps.-Athanasius, *Quaest. ad Antiochum* 103, 104 (PG 28.662); Anastasius of Sinai, *Quaest. moral.* 114 (PG 89.765 f.). On the relationship between the two collections, see M. Richard, *Opera minora*, 3 (Louvain, 1977), n. 64, pp. 43–56. Cf. also the fragment of (ps.?) Athanasius on illness, *OCA*, 117 (1938), pp. 5–9.

[64] Alexander, I.573 Puschmann. See also, on Alexander, J. Duffy, below, p. 25 ff.

[65] Alexander, I.565 Puschmann; cf. Celsus, *De med.* III.23; Scribonius Largus, *Comp.* 17.

[66] Ammianus, *Hist.* XVI.8.1; XIX.12.14; XXVI.3.1–4; XXVIII.1.26–29; cf. A. A. Barb, "The Survival of Magic Arts," in A. D. Momigliano, *Paganism and Christianity in the Fourth Century* (Oxford, 1963), 100–125; P. Brown, *Religion and Society in the Age of St. Augustine* (London, 1972), 119–46.

[67] E. Honigmann, "A Trial for Sorcery," *Isis*, 35 (1944), 281–84.

[68] Alexander, II.585 Puschmann.

[69] W. H. S. Jones, "Ancient Roman Folk Medicine," *JHM*, 12 (1957), 459–72. Cf. L. Edelstein, "Greek Medicine in Its Relation to Religion and Magic," *BHM*, 5 (1937), 201–46 (= *Ancient Medicine* [Baltimore, 1967], 205–46).

Christianity, by its emphasis on prayers and spiritual songs, gave a sort of sanction to this white magic, within limits.

It also introduced, or re-introduced, into medicine the idea of demons and demoniac possession. The wolf-man wandering half naked among the tombs at night, derives his characterization in part from the gospels, in part from earlier medical texts.[70] A somatic explanation for madness is regarded as unusual even among doctors, who instead invoke demonic possession.[71] We enter upon a world filled with angels and demons, in which sickness is viewed as a symptom of a battle between competing divine agents, and in which apparitions, sent by God or Satan, are common. It was the vision sent to the dying Theodoric that compelled him to express to his personal physician, Elpidius, his deep repentance for the murders of Boethius and Symmachus.[72] Elpidius, doctor and deacon, ambassador, traveler, and restorer of a public bathhouse at Spoleto, knew demons when he saw them.[73] He is said to have been attacked by them, not only outside as they lay in ambush for him, but within his house, into which they pursued him throwing stones. In answer to his prayers, S. Caesarius came and exorcised the spirits who were afflicting him.[74]

Whether or not one believes in this tale, it expresses one truth, that in late antiquity, medical men were willing to consider the intervention of demons and spirits as a cause of disease, and disease as some form of divine punishment for sins, far more openly than they had done in the time of Galen.[75] This change of perspective has never been satisfactorily investigated from the medical side, and

we should be wary of taking it as the result of such vague and unverifiable processes as Christianity's democratization of high culture.[76]

One institution, however, does seem to owe its origin to Christian charity: the establishment of hospitals open to all members of the community and providing medical treatment, alongside a variety of other services. As is well known, Roman hospitals were restricted either to estate or domestic servants, or to the members of the army.[77] And, despite the claims of S. W. Baron, Jewish hospitals until the middle ages were hostels or hospices for pilgrims,[78] and similar hostels could be equally found at most pagan shrines, where, at great festivals, a city would also secure the attendance of doctors to look after its visitors.[79] But the Christian hospital, that combination of medical center, poorhouse, old folks home, hostel and meeting place, does seem, both from its size and the variety of its functions, to be a new creation. The earliest is traditionally that of St. Basil at Caesarea in the 370s, almost a new city outside the walls, and his example was quickly followed: by Eustathius in Pontus, Pammachius at Ostia, Fabiola in Rome, Chrysostom in Constantinople.[80] There was a hospital in Hippo, and another at Ephesus, in the early fifth century, which had over seventy beds in the poorhouse alone. Indeed, the impact of the hospitals was such that by the end of the fourth century a learned cleric, St. Nilus of Ancyra, could devote a

---

[70] Paul of Aegina, III.16, with Adams' commentary *ad loc.*: cf. also Luke, 8.27.

[71] Philostorgius, *Hist. eccl.* VIII.10; I am not entirely persuaded by Edelstein's arguments, *Ancient Medicine*, 219.

[72] Procopius, *Hist.* V.1.38.

[73] *Vita Aviti*, p. 181, calls him a deacon at Lyons; Avitus, *Ep.* 38; Ennodius, *Ep.* 384, calls him a doctor, cf. also *Epp.* 312, 437. The reference to his "Pontic rudeness," Ennodius, *Ep.* 445, may imply a visit to Constantinople, for he certainly knew Greek well, *ibid.* 384. Nevertheless, I think it unlikely that he is the Elpidius mentioned by Aeneas of Gaza, *Ep.* 19, as a well-known doctor at Gaza, *pace* L. M. Positano in her edition of Aeneas (Naples, 1950), *comm. ad loc.* On the bathhouse at Spoleto, Cassiodorus, *Var.* IV.24.

[74] *Vita S. Caesarii*, I.41.

[75] O. Böcher, *Christus Exorcista: Dämonismus und Taufe im Neuen Testament* (Stuttgart, 1972); A. J. Festugière, "Épidémies hippocratiques et épidémies démoniaques," *WSt*, 79 (1966), 157–64; together with the articles cited in nn. 66 and 69 above.

[76] H. Gertler, "Ärztliche Betrügereien im Rom der späten Kaiserzeit," in V. Beševliev and W. Seyfarth, *Die Rolle der Plebs im spätrömischen Reich* (Berlin, 1969), 77–80; contrast the wise words of A. D. Momigliano, "Popular Religious Beliefs and the Late Roman Historians," *Studies in Church History*, 8 (1972), 1–18.

[77] G. Harig, "Zum Problem 'Krankenhaus' in der Antike," *Klio*, 53 (1971), 179–95.

[78] S. W. Baron, *The Jewish Community* (Philadelphia, 1948), 91 f.; *id.*, *A Social and Religious History of the Jews*, 8 (New York, 1958), 239.

[79] A. Hug, in *RE*, 18.3, 1949, cols. 520–29, *s.v.* Pandokeion; *Inschr. Olympia* I.62; *Inschr. Priene* 111; *Inschr. Ilion* 3. Healing shrines, both pagan and Christian, can be considered a primitive form of hospital, in that they provided a form of medical assistance particularly for the poor, but long stays there are uncommon, and the amount of medical attention and treatment open to question.

[80] For Basil, see T. Miller, below, p. 54; for Eustathius, Epiphanius, *Haer.* III.1 (PG. 42.504), almost simultaneously with Basil, and possibly even earlier; Pammachius, Jerome, *Ep.* 66; Fabiola, Jerome, *Ep.* 77; Chrysostom, Palladius, *Dial.* (PG 47.20), cf. Chrysostom, *Ad Stag.* III.13 (PG 47, 490), cf. *id.*, *Hom. in Matt.* 56 (PG 58.630). Note also the emergency and temporary actions of St. Ephraim at Edessa during a plague c. 370, Sozomen, *Hist. eccl.* III.16.

long simile to detailing the various medical activities found within the hospital.[81]

That the hospitals in some way answered a need is obvious from the comments of their founders, and I wish only to raise two caveats. While Temkin is surely right to stress the importance of Christian hospitals as centers for medical advice and even for instruction, evidence for a recognizable teaching function in the hospital, which we know of in eighth- and ninth-century Islamic hospitals, is hard to find before eleventh-century Constantinople.[82] The Lives of Isaac the Protector and of Marathonius, which portray their heroes as leaving high society for menial tasks in a hospital, do not suggest a high degree of medical expertise or knowledge, even for the head of a hospital. But one should remember that in the Roman army, a man could equally move from being in charge of the camp hospital to being in charge of the military jail, and that administrative experience mattered perhaps more than acquaintance with Galen.[83] The introduction of formal teaching into the Byzantine hospital may thus owe much, if not all, to influence coming from the Arabs. Similarly, despite Dr. Miller's arguments,[84] material is still lacking that will enable us to judge whether the complexities of the Pantocrator hospital were the result of a natural development within the Byzantine hospital which in turn was adopted by the Arabs, or whether, as I think more likely, they were taken over from an Arabic tradition, perhaps itself deriving from Gondeshapur.[85]

My second point is a plea for help. The chronicle of Joshua the Stylite is our best ancient evidence for the effect of famine and plague on a local community, and it graphically describes how in the years around 500 Edessa was hit by a series of natural calamities. The reaction of the authorities

was to set up more and more temporary hospitals, in the army camp, in the stoas, in the baths, to cope with the influx of patients from the town and its countryside.[86] An explanation purely in terms of filling a need is not enough to explain this change of attitude, which, within the space of a century, set the hospital in the front line of defence against illness. Medical historians need to look far more closely than they so far have at the sermons and literary texts about hospitals, and also at the various structural changes in society that may determine this new attitude.

One explanation may be that, after the chaos of the later third century, many of the former social and political ties, at both local and provincial level, had disappeared, and were replaced by a variety of different and overlapping systems of authority. In the West, we have the growth of big landed estates, with peasants being brought into almost fortified townlets. In the East, bishops like Gregory Thaumaturgus, Cyprian, or, later, St. Basil, take over some of the roles of the local aristocracy, for good or ill.[87] In the great Justinianic plague, St. Nicholas of Sion was suspected by the inhabitants of Myra in Lycia of engineering a food shortage in the town by banning the farmers from coming thither to market their produce. The local and provincial officials could not believe that this prudential decision was that of the farmers alone, and an unsuccessful attempt was made to arrest the saint.[88] We may be also getting a progressive fragmentation within the medical profession, between high and low class practitioners. The law codes indicate a growing power and influence for the court physician and his peers while the humbler local physician tries desperately to keep even the small privileges he has.[89] True, there is a constant tension between the financial needs of a community and a doctor's enjoyment of some degree of tax immunity at the community's expense, but the split between the court physicians, with their immense wealth and titles, and the lower men only adds to

---

[81] Augustine, *Serm.* 356.10; Ephesus, *Acta Conc. Oec.* II.1.405 (A.D. 451); Nilus, *Ep.* III.33 (PG 79.397).

[82] D. J. Constantelos, *Byzantine Philanthropy and Social Welfare* (New Brunswick, 1968), 152–84, gives a useful survey; Temkin, "Byzantine Medicine," 114 (= *The Double Face of Janus*, p. 220), but although there are doctors attached to hospitals, e.g., *CIG* 9256, I can find no secure evidence for formal teaching before the middle Byzantine period. A man like St. Sampson, *ActaSS*, June 27 (cf. PG, 115, 277–308), could have picked up his medical skills outside the hospital.

[83] John of Ephesus, *Lives* (PO 18.669); Sozomen, *Hist. eccl.* IV.27. For the careers of the (earlier) *optiones valetudinarii*, *ILS* 2117, 2437.

[84] In his article, "Byzantine Hospitals," in this volume.

[85] On the Pantokrator, see now P. Gautier, "Le typikon du Christ Sauveur Pantokrator," *REB*, 32 (1974), 1–145. On Islamic hospitals, a short introduction is S. Hamarneh, "Development of Hospitals in Islam," *JHM*, 17 (1962), 366–84.

[86] Joshua Stylite, *Chron.* XXVI, XXVIII, XLI–XLIII ed. Wright; cf. Sozomen, *Hist. eccl.* III.16; Hydatius, *Chron.* II.17–18.

[87] P. Brown, "The Rise and Function of the Holy Man in Late Antiquity," *JRS*, 61 (1971), 80–101; F. Millar, "Paul of Samosata, Zenobia and Aurelian: The Church, Local Culture and Political Allegiance in Third-Century Syria," *ibid.*, 1–17.

[88] *Vita Nicolai Sionitae*, ed. G. Anrich, *Hagios Nikolaos* (Leipzig, Berlin, 1913, 1917), I, p. 40; II, p. 243 f.

[89] *CTh* XIII.3; *CIC, CI* X.53; K. H. Below, *Der Arzt im römischen Recht* (Munich, 1953), 41–55; and the references in the next note.

this tension. The proud claim of Libanius, arguing on behalf of a civic doctor at Rhosus in Syria, that, though Philo himself is weak, the law is strong, rings somehow false against the implication of the law codes, that this law at least was eminently flexible.[90]

There are other indications of a growing, formal series of hierarchies among what was still an open profession which anyone might join. I merely note: the foundation of the Roman College of doctors in 368, the first example of self-selection for a medical elite, but which I would interpret less as a gesture of imperial philanthropy than as another attempt by Valentinian to reduce senatorial patronage;[91] the creation, both for Rome and for Constantinople, of a "count of the doctors" to take charge of all the doctors of the city;[92] and, the legal division of even *archiatri* into various grades of social eminence.[93] The result will be, as we learn from a letter of Theodore of Studion, a whole variety of different grades and statuses for the medical profession,[94] which may indeed correspond more closely to the realities of a practice of healing whose providers ranged from the local barmaid up to the doctor to the emperor.[95]

It would be wrong to conclude from this that late antiquity was in any way unusual. Recent studies of fourteenth-century France, sixteenth-century Norwich, and seventeenth-century Tuscany have alerted us to the possibility of the coexistence of a wide variety of healers, with different levels of expertise, wealth and status.[96] True, there is in late antiquity a general expectation that doctors will make money, even if they come from humble backgrounds, and patients were at times wary of offers of assistance from doctors whom they suspected of planning to fleece them.[97] True, we have several examples of really wealthy doctors: Pegasus of Laribus, who could ransom a governor's nephew for fifty *solidi*, about ten years' pay for a soldier,[98] or two chief doctors of Africa whose annual retainers were of seventy or ninety-nine *solidi*, which, in exceptional circumstances, might be topped up with fees and gifts to equal the income of a major bishop;[99] Phoebammon of Antinoopolis had an annual retainer from the hospital of sixty *solidi*, boats, vineyards and other pieces of property.[100] Doctors donated mosaics at Cartenna, Tralles, Furni and Mactar, and paid towards a church at Aphrodisias.[101] There were other local worthies: Alexander of Ephesus, whose statue stands proudly in the street of the Kouretes;[102] Dionysius, doctor, priest and philanthropist, captured and then released by the Goths;[103] not to mention Scantia Redempta, whose merits surpassed the capacity of men to record them, and who numbered among her activities the practice of medicine.[104] Below them, we have

---

[90] Libanius, *Ep.* 723, referring to Julian, *Ep.* 75b. On the relationship between this letter and *CTh* XIII.3.4., see J. Gothofredus, *Codex Theodosianus* (Lyon, 1665), V, p. 30; W. Ensslin, "Kaisar Julians Gesetzgebungswerk und Reichsverwaltung," *Klio*, 18 (1922), 147 f.; V. Nutton, "Archiatri and the Medical Profession in Antiquity," *PBSR*, 45 (1977), 147 f.

[91] *CTh* XIII.3.8, with my comments at "Archiatri," pp. 207–208, 217 f. It is worth stressing that the legal position of doctors in Rome before Valentinian was unique, and that there is no evidence for the creation of an exactly similar college, chosen from doctors by doctors, elsewhere in the Byzantine or Roman worlds. It may be significant that in the reconstituted *CIC, CI* XII.40.8, there is specific mention of the doctors at Rome, but not at Constantinople. It is unwise to posit on the evidence of a law directly relating to Rome that there must have been a replica of the college, founded and organized on exactly similar lines, at Constantinople, and, still more so, in cities elsewhere. Cf. also my article, "Continuity or Rediscovery? The City Physician in Classical Antiquity and Mediaeval Italy," in A. W. Russell, *The Town and State Physician in Europe* (Wolfenbüttel, 1981), 16–21.

[92] Cassiodorus, *Var.* VI, 19; but the title of Vindicianus as *comes archiatrorum* (in Marcellus, *De medicamentis*, ed. Liechtenham [*CML* V, 2nd ed.], I, p. 46), may imply a creation for Rome under Valentinian. L. Deubner, *Kosmas und Damian* (Leipzig, 1907), 160. Himerius, *Or.* 34.

[93] *CTh* VI.16 (= *CIC, CI* XII.13.1); XIII.3.17–19.

[94] Theodore Stud., *Ep.* II.162 (PG 99, 1907–09).

[95] For the barmaid-midwife, Eunapius, *Vit. phil.* 463; on the variety of types of practitioner, Hordern, "Saints and Doctors," 10 f., has sound things to say, against H. Evert-Kappesowa, "The Social Rank of a Physician in the Early Byzantine Empire," *Mélanges I. Dujčev* (Paris, 1980), 139–64, whose article is based on a limited number of sources and contains many errors of interpretation.

[96] D. Jacquart, *Le milieu médical en France du XIIᵉ au XVᵉ siècle* (Geneva, 1981); M. Pelling, C. Webster, "Medical Practitioners," in C. Webster, *Health, Medicine and Mortality in the Sixteenth Century* (Cambridge, 1979), 165–235, extended in M. Pelling, "Tradition and Diversity: Medical Practice in Norwich, 1550–1640," in *Scienze, credenze occulte, livelli di cultura* (Florence, 1982), 159–71; C. M. Cipolla, *Public Health and the Medical Profession in the Renaissance* (Cambridge, 1976), 67–124.

[97] Libanius, *Epp.* 1018, 1523 (where the οὔπω is significant); Sozomen, *Hist. eccl.* III.16.

[98] Procopius, *Hist.*, IV.17.14.

[99] *CIC, CI* I.27.1.41. Three other doctors received retainers of fifty *solidi* a year. Professors and teachers at Carthage were to receive seventy *solidi*, lawyers from fifty to seventy-two. On the possibility of extra from fees, see the comments of S. L. Greenslade, *JThS*, n.s. 16 (1965), 222. A contemporary bishop of Anastasiopolis, a middle-ranking see, had an income of 365 *solidi* a year, *Vita Theodori Syk.* 78.

[100] P. Cairo Maspéro 67151, A.D. 570; Phoebammon was the son (and brother ?) of a civic physician.

[101] *CIL* VIII. 9633 (*ILChV* 614), of A.D. 357; H. Grégoire, *Recueil des inscriptions grecques chrétiennes d'Asie Mineure* (Brussels, 1922), n. 123; *CIL* VIII.25811 (*ILChV* 606b); *AEpigr*, 1952.49; Grégoire, *Recueil*, n. 272.

[102] Good photograph in *ÖJhBeibl*, 352 (1959), 363.

[103] *ILChV* 1233.

[104] *CIL* X.3980 (*ILS* 7805).

the wandering doctors: an Egyptian astrologer and doctor died at Ragusa in Sicily; another Egyptian after many journeys found his rest in Milan; a doctor from Claudiopolis in Asia Minor is buried at Verona; a Syrian, a Spaniard and two Gauls are recorded as *medici* in the Roman catacombs; and a Greek physician turns up in Spain at the end of the fourth century.[105] Nor can one say much about those doctors, both men and women, of whom nothing is known save their name, profession and place of burial, except that they existed, even in humble communities.[106] Poverty might even force a doctor to flee his responsibilities and disappear from the gaze of the taxman.[107] At the very bottom, there are the slaves, and here we have a serious problem. Excepting the παῖδες ἰατρῶν, who are far more likely to be apprentices, assistants, or even the doctors themselves than slaves,[108] I know of no text later than the third century which refers undisputedly to a slave or an ex-slave doctor, with the exception of two laws, of 530 and 531. These fix the maximum price for a slave doctor at sixty *solidi*, ten more than a secretary, and double the maximum for an unskilled slave.[109] Was Justinian legislating then for a nonexistent problem? Is this a piece of antiquarianism, like some of the laws reiterated later in the *Basilica*?[110] The numbers of such slaves may well have been very small, certainly by comparison with the first century A.D., yet the context of these laws suggests that such slaves did exist. The first law is eminently practical, setting the maxi-

mum price to be paid by an owner who wishes to manumit a slave held in common, and here Justinian expressly imposes a solution upon an old and much discussed question. The second again deals with the price to be paid to co-owners, in this case for a slave left as a joint legacy, whom one owner wishes to purchase entirely for himself. Although the numbers of such disputed slaves cannot be known, and it may be doubted whether they were high even in the days of slave doctors in the first century, the law and Justinian's decision do suggest that they existed and had not disappeared entirely from the social scene.

The evidence I have put forward hardly permits firm conclusions about the status, or even about the practice, of medicine in late antiquity.[111] At best one can point to long-term trends, or to areas which seem worthy of further investigation, and this essay has aimed to sketch possible developments rather than establish unshakable conclusions. Yet there is one final impression that can be set forward, if only briefly. Compared with the first three centuries of the Roman Empire, the doctor in late antiquity has a much greater public profile beyond the confines of his city and civic life. He becomes a bishop, a church leader, even a saint; an ambassador, a provincial governor, even the Master of Offices.[112] Although I do not believe in the ancient tradition that associated the founding of the great medical school of Gondeshapur (Iran) with Greek physicians sent by the Emperor Aurelian in 271 or 272 to accompany his daughter to the Sassanian

[105]*Epigraphica*, 12 (1950), 99 (= S. L. Agnello, *Silloge di iscrizioni paleocristiane della Sicilia* [Rome, 1953], n. 68); *Epigraphica*, 10 (1948), 62 f., with the corrections of W. Peek, *ibid.*, 12 (1950), 27 f.; *IG* XIV. 2310a; *CIG* 9777; *CIL* VI.9597; *CIG* 9578; *AE* 1939, 162; *Vitae SS. Patr. Emeritensium*, ed. Garvin, IV.11.

[106]E.g., *MAMA*, III.167, 409, 528b, 617; VII.233: VIII.118; *RBibl.* (1905), 248; *Sammelbuch* 7316, 7488, 7491, 7493; *BCH*, (1880), 199; *Inscr. Syria* 1528; J. Jalabert, *Mél. fac. or. Beyrouth* (1906), 146; V. Beševliev, *Spätgriechische Inschriften* 98, cf. 184a; *CIG* 9209, 9669, 9792, 9977; *Epigraphica*, 6 (1944), 6; *ICVR* 1041, 5695; *ILChV* 255, 607, 608, 609, 613; *IG* XIV.604, 1529, 2406; *PBSR*, 37 (1969), 97 f.; G. Lefebvre, *Receuil des inscriptions grecques chrétiennes d'Egypte*, nos. 4, 496, 799. This list is not complete, and I have not listed clerics who are also physicians, e.g., *Inschr. Erythrae* 142.

[107]C. Wessely, *Stud. Pal.* 20.129 (A.D. 497), cf. Libanius, *Ep.* 756.

[108]Although, as Professor Renehan has shown, *Greek Lexicographical Notes* (Göttingen, 1975), 156 f., the phrase is regularly used as a circumlocution for "doctors," e.g., PG 59.137; 62.437; Aeneas Gaz., *Ep.* 20; *Suda, s. ἀποπληξία*, it can have a more specific use, e.g., Aristides, *Or.* 39.14; Julius Africanus, 20 Vieillefond; Origen, *Entretiens avec Héraclide* (P. Fouad), p. 162; Epiphanius, *Haer.* 51.1.

[109]*CIC, CI* VI.43.3.1; VII.7.1.5a; Below, *Der Arzt*, 9–11.

[110]H. J. Scheltema, *CMH*, IV.2 (Cambridge, 1967), 66 f.

[111]I remain sceptical about almost all attempts to define the status of doctors in antiquity, since, for the most part, they are based on a few scattered pieces of literary evidence. In the absence of quantitative records, such as the sixteenth-century taxation lists, reliance on qualitative sources—i.e. comments by doctors, poets, historians—is essential. But great caution is necessary, and few of the essays at delineation have covered more than a fraction of the existing sources, or made satisfactory comparisons between medical and other similar groups like those of the *professores* and *grammatici*. The evidence of epigraphy has been largely neglected, and the criterion of judgment adopted has all too often been dependent on an anachronistic definition of who a doctor was. On the problems of interpretation, see my forthcoming article, "Verso una storia soziale della medicina antica," and "Murders and Miracle Cures: Lay Views of Medicine in Classical Antiquity," in R. S. Porter (ed.), *The Patient's View* (Cambridge, 1985).

[112]Respectively, Basil of Ancyra, Jerome, *Vir. ill.*, 89; Hieracas the heretic, Epiphanius, *Haer.* 67; St. Caesarius, Gregory Naz., *Or.* VII.; Maruthas of Martyrpolis, Socrates, *Hist. eccl.*, VII.8, with J. S. Assemani, *BO*, 1725, III.1.73; Vindicianus, Augustine, *Conf.*, IV.3, cf. *id.*, *Ep.* 138; Theoctistus, Zacharias Schol., *Chron.*, V.1; V.4, cf. Photius, *Bibl.*, cod. 220. W. A. Fitzgerald, "Medical Men, Canonized Saints," *BHM*, 22 (1948), 635–46, is a useful, if somewhat uncritical, listing.

court,[113] there can be no doubt of the significance of medical men in late antiquity as envoys and mediators between Byzantium and Persia.[114] They appear in political negotiations between emperors, or between city and emperor, and the machinations of Joseph, doctor, politician and Catholicos of Seleucia, were notorious on both sides of the political frontier.[115]

Even a translator, Sergius of Resaena, turns out to have had a more than minor role to play in ecclesiastical diplomacy. Born at Antioch, he studied medicine at Alexandria before becoming civic physician at Resaena, on the Syrian frontier.[116] It cannot be excluded that he spent some time also at the Persian court, for Agathias mentions a Sergius who translated into Greek a history of the kings of Persia.[117] He was probably also a deacon, a friend of the great Patriarch of Antioch, Severus, and sufficiently acquainted with theological writers like Origen and Dionysius the Areopagite to compose his own tract on "Faith."[118] He was also a distinguished translator, mainly of medical and philosophical writings, and it was largely through his versions that the Syriac and, indirectly, the Arab physicians derived their acquaintance with Galenic medicine.[119]

Denunciations of him as "lustful after women, incontinent and greedy for money" or "a eunuch, corrupt and immoral" are perhaps to be treated less as fact than as the judgment of his opponents on his theological maneuvers.[120] In 535, having fallen out with Asylus, bishop of Resaena, he visited Ephraem, Patriarch of Antioch, to complain of his ill-treatment. Ephraem, concerned at the rising tide of Monophysitism, sent Sergius to Rome with a letter for Pope Agapetus, accompanied by a young architect from Amida, Eustathius. He was cordially received in Rome. But, on a second mission in 536 to the Patriarch of Constantinople, he was struck down with an unmentionable disease and died there in what his opponents regarded as deserved agony.[121]

Doctors are undeniably prominent in political and ecclesiastical negotiations in the fifth and sixth centuries, and it would be tempting to ascribe this feature to either a growth in the importance of physicians, or, with perhaps greater plausibility, to their abilities as bilingual (or even multilingual) men of culture, able to cross political frontiers and yet communicate in a shared language, usually Syriac. But court doctors have always been prominent or suspected of having a hand in political and dynastic dealings, and travels of physicians between the Greek world and the courts of the Near East had been known since the time of Democedes and Ctesias.[122] The increased profile of the physician may perhaps be due as much to the bias of the sources—which reveal far more information about diplomacy than a Livy, a Tacitus or an Appian—as to any sudden rise of physicians as a class to historical eminence.

This survey ends tentatively, and with good reason, for much work still remains to be done before a proper history of medicine and medical ideas in late antiquity can be written. Yet, despite its essentially preliminary nature, it points to a series of truths that not all medical historians have been willing to believe. There is, for the period of late antiquity, a great variety of evidence, in both quantity and quality, which deserves study in its own right

[113] The tradition, which is found in Arabic and Syriac authors, e.g., Barhebraeus, *Chron.*, p. 56 Budge, is accepted by C. Elgood, *A Medical History of Persia*, (rev. ed. Amsterdam, 1979), 46, and, with varying degrees of scepticism about the influence of the school before the sixth century, by A. Siassi, "L'Université de Gond-i Shāpūr," *Mélanges H. Massé* (Teheran, 1963), 366–74; F. R. Hau, "Gondeschapur—eine Medizinschule aus dem 6. Jahrhundert n. Chr.," *Gesnerus*, 36 (1979), 99; H. H. Schöffler, *Die Akademie von Gondischapur* (Stuttgart, 1979), 29 f. The serious weakness of this late tradition is easily demonstrated: according to the Roman sources, the emperor Aurelian had no daughter, cf. *Vita Aureliani* 42. In its place I would set a gradual accretion of medical learning across a political, though, significantly, not a cultural or linguistic, frontier over several centuries.

[114] I have not yet seen the article by R. C. Blockley, in *Florilegium*, 2 (referred to by Professor Baldwin, below, p. 17). The importance of doctors as ambassadors is acknowledged both by Greek historians, like Procopius and Menander, and by writers of Syriac chronicles. See, e.g., J. B. Chabot, "Synodicon Orientale," *Notices et extraits*, 37 (1902), 352, n. 1; *Chron. of Sirt*, PO, 7, pp. 136, 148, 161, 524. For the importance to a city of its doctor, Procopius, *Hist.*, XXVI.31 f. Cf. also N. M. Garsoian, "Le role de l'hiérarchie chrétienne dans les relations diplomatiques entre Byzance et les Sassanides," *REArm*, n. s. 10 (1974), 119–38. A J. Butler, *The Arab Conquest of Egypt*, 2nd ed. (Oxford, 1978), 135.

[115] Zach. Schol., *Chron.* XII.7; *Chron. of Sirt*, PO, 7, pp. 176–81 (cf. p. 192, for another court doctor meddling in high ecclesiastical politics); Assemani, *BO*, III.1.433.

[116] Zach. Schol., *Chron.* VII.10.

[117] Agathias, *Hist.* IV.30, but this may be another Sergius.

[118] Severus, *Epp.*, PO, XII.2, nos. 31, 85, 86; C. Brockelmann, *Geschichte der christlichen Literatur des Orients* (Leipzig, 1907), 42.

[119] R. Degen, "Galen im syrischen," in Nutton, ed., *Galen, Problems*, 131–66.

[120] Zach. Schol., *Chron.* VII.10; Barhebraeus, *Hist. Patr.*, ed. Assemani, *BO*, II, p. 323. The Jacobite chronicle of 724 is a little milder, tr. J. B. Chabot, CSCO, *Script. Syr.*, ser. 3, IV.170.

[121] *Ibid.*

[122] Democedes, Herodotus, *Hist.* III.129–37; Ctesias, *FGrHist* (repr. Leyden, 1954), no. 688. For even earlier movement of "palace doctors," cf. E. Edel, *Ägyptische Ärzte und ägyptische Medizin am hethitischen Königshof* (Opladen, 1976).

and not just for its part in the transmission of Galenic ideas from the second century to the Arabs and the Renaissance. It reveals a medical world somewhat different from the static and forbidding picture painted by Bloch and even A. H. M. Jones—with new problems, and with new solutions. It represents a challenge to the historian, yet its rewards are substantial. Later essays in this volume will exemplify how much can be learned from even small sectors of a vast field, which still awaits its harvesters. The brevity of this exposition can thus be justified in the words of a late Alexandrian commentator on *Epidemics VI*, for, like Hippocrates, I am sowing the seed, and my selection of topics has been deliberately restricted in order to encourage others to use their judgment and their own powers of discovery.[123]

The Wellcome Institute for the
History of Medicine, London

[123] Palladius, *In Epid. VI scholia* (p. 157 Dietz).

BEYOND THE HOUSE CALL: DOCTORS IN EARLY BYZANTINE HISTORY AND POLITICS

BARRY BALDWIN

First, a brief survey of the doctor's role in Graeco-Roman history and literature, to put the attitudes and careers of late antiquity in perspective. We may begin Byzantinely with Homer. In *Iliad* 11.514, rescue of the wounded physician Machaon is an Achaean priority on the grounds that a man who can pull out arrows and heal with his ointments is worth many men. This pragmatic view is reinforced in *Odyssey* 17.382–85, where doctors are registered as craftsmen along with seers, carpenters, and minstrels, a classification echoed in Plato's *Gorgias*, where they are compared to shipwrights (455b). In his recent and monumental—in size, at any rate—volume on ancient class warfare,[1] the marxist Geoffrey de Ste. Croix rather snidely juxtaposes them with whores and "other providers of essential services."

The elder Pliny would have liked that! In his captious history of medicine (*NH* 29.1.1–28), he clearly has Homer in mind when he says that, despite Asclepius and other alleged resurrections, medicine was famous in Trojan times *only* for the treatment of wounds.[2] He goes on to remark the curious (*mirum dictu*) lack of evidence for the history of medicine down to the Peloponnesian War.[3] We may gloss his account by remarking the significant failure of doctors to bulk large in Old Comedy. Yet the extended medical simile whereby Euripides describes his treatment of tragedy in the *Frogs* (939 f.) implies some public awareness of the art, and is comparable to the analogy between medicine and kingship drawn in the sixth-century Byzantine treatise *On Political Science*.[4] And Aristophanes' occasional allusions[5] to doctors' greed set the pace for centuries to come.

From this time, Pliny continues, the profitability of medicine knew no bounds, and the tale of Hellenistic and Roman doctors is told in terms of their moneygrubbing, making fame as well as fortune out of fads and gimmicks, and of quarreling amongst themselves like philosophers. We need not follow him in detail, though notice his singling out of Erasistratus in the light of that worthy's disparagement by Galen and consequent mockery in the twelfth-century Byzantine satire *Timarion*;[6] also Vettius Valens, said to be as famous for his eloquence as his science, and so looking to the future connection between medicine and rhetoric; and the pugnaciously heterodox Thessalus of Nero's time who proclaimed himself Conqueror of the Physicians (*Iatronikes*), a title that vaguely prefigures such Byzantine pomposities as *Didaskalos ton iatron* and *Hypatos ton philosophon*. At the other end of the labeling scale is Archagathus, the first doctor to come to Rome (219 B.C.), whose relentless use of knife and cautery earned him the nickname Executioner (*carnifex*), a sobriquet used many centuries later by Theodore Prodromos as the title of his satire against doctors.[7]

We take our leave of Pliny with the reflection that his espousal of old Cato's John Birch-like view of Greek doctors as a conspiracy to kill off the Romans may have been prompted in part by contem-

---

[The reader is referred to the list of abbreviations at the end of the volume.]

[1] G. de Ste. Croix, *The Class Struggle in the Ancient Greek World* (London, 1981), 271.
[2] *. . . fama clarior, vulnerum tamen dumtaxat remediis* (29.1.3).
[3] Though notice Theognis, fr. 432, for an early connection between Asclepiadae and large fees.

[4] See E. Barker, *Social and Political Thought in Byzantium* (Oxford, 1957), 70; cf. A. R. Littlewood, "The Midwifery of Michael Psellus: an Example of Byzantine Literary Originality," *Byzantium and the Classical Tradition*, ed. M. Mullett and R. Scott (Birmingham, 1981), 136–42.
[5] *Av.* 584; *Plut.* 407; cf. V. Ehrenberg, *The People of Aristophanes* (Oxford, 1951), 134.
[6] *Timarion* 28, ed. R. Romano (Naples, 1974).
[7] Ed. G. Podestà, *Aevum*, 21 (1947), 12–25.

porary gossip over the part played by the physician Xenophon in the death of Claudius.[8] Pliny does not say as much, but could be dropping a hint when he quotes[9] the gloomy epitaph, "It was the crowd of physicians that killed men," a sentiment that is ubiquitous, from a line of Menander (fr. 1112), to a situation in Petronius (*Sat.* 42.5: *medici illum perdiderunt*), to the lips of the dying Hadrian.[10] Hence the image of the deadly doctor in epigrams of the Greek Anthology (11.112–26), their unfavorable role in the jests of the *Philogelos*,[11] that delightful jokebook compiled in (probably) the fifth or sixth century, and what is perhaps the most crushing comment of all, that of Athenaeus: "Were it not for the doctors, there wouldn't be anything stupider than the professors" (*Deip.* 666a).

That conjunction is a good cue for the vexed issue of iatrosophists. Medicine, of course, often went together with philosophy and rhetoric. Galen is the outstanding example,[12] but the combination is implicit in some of the characters chronicled by Philostratus. The Pergamene, who is in Athenaeus if not Philostratus, enjoyed the accolade *protos kai monos* (the first and only), concerning which we should note and savor the droll remark of a late Byzantine savant, Michael Italicus: εἰ πρῶτος, πῶς μόνος; καὶ εἰ μόνος, πῶς πρῶτος;[13] Eunapius (*VS* 497, 499) may treat doctors and philosophers as separate categories, but he still thought them part of the same story. Indeed, one of his stars, Ionicus, is perhaps the most breathtakingly versatile on record: as well as his skills in anatomy, pharmacy, amputation, dissection, and post-operative bandaging, he was philosopher, orator, poet, and diviner! Such combinations help us see how medicine came to be a standard ingredient in Byzantine higher education, as the statements of didactic intent in Psellus' *Carmen de re medica* and similar works[14] make clear. In the fifteenth-century satire *Mazaris*,[15] Holobolos is asked whether he is rated as a top doctor or top orator down in Hades, or whether he follows both callings as on earth, where greed drew him to medicine.[16]

Yet "iatrosophist" is a word tossed around textbooks without due regard for its history and usage. Bowersock[17] is a prime offender, adducing as he does *Anth. Pal.* 11.281 (Palladas on Magnus) where the word is only in the lemma, and Dio Chrysostom 33.6 where it appears by courtesy of a von Arnim emendation. LSJ cite only a fragment of Damascius on Gesius (to whom we shall recur); their Supplement adds ps.-Callisthenes 1.3, of magicians. Lampe (*PGL*) gives two examples from Epiphanius, two from Sophronius; notice the cognate adjective, not in LSJ, used by the former of a quack physician. The *Philogelos* in two jokes (175, 183) has a doctor addressed as σοφιστά. Some allowance has naturally to be made for different ways of saying the same thing. When Stephanus of Byzantium calls Gesius ὁ περιφυὴς τῶν ἰατρῶν σοφιστής, that is pretty much the same as using the compound. But when all is said and done, the rarity of *iatrosophistes* remains a striking and unappreciated fact.[18]

One more matter will complete the setting. In pagan times there had been a conflict of vested interests between Asclepius and the medical profession. But this can be exaggerated. Aelius Aristides is witness to the fact that some doctors preferred co-existence, even co-operation.[19] As with so many

[8] Tacitus, *Ann.* 12.67; for Xenophon and doctors like him at Rome, cf. S. Treggiari, *Roman Freedmen during the Late Republic* (Oxford, 1969), 129–32. Cato's views are cited *in extenso* by Pliny, *NH* 29.1.14.

[9] *NH* 29.1.11: *hinc illa infelix monumentis inscriptio, turba se medicorum perisse.*

[10] Dio Cassius 69.22.4, albeit not in *HA, Hadr.* 25.9, where instead there are the famous verses on Hadrian's soul, on which see now A. Cameron, "Poetae Novelli," *HSCPh*, 84 (1980), 167–72.

[11] Ed. A. Thierfelder (Munich, 1968). Doctors feature in various jokes (139, 142, 174–77, 183–85, 221), mainly for greed and incompetence, but sometimes for bad temper or gluttony. On the social tensions reflected in the *Philogelos*, cf. R. Browning, "The Low Level Saint's Life in the Early Byzantine World," *The Byzantine Saint*, ed. S. Hackel (Birmingham, 1981), 121.

[12] See G. W. Bowersock, *Greek Sophists in the Roman Empire* (Oxford, 1969), 66 f.

[13] *Ep.* 13, ed. J. A. Cramer, *Anecdota Graeca* 3 (Oxford, 1836), 188: on the title, cf. J. Duffy, "Philologica Byzantina," *GRBS*, 21 (1980), 267.

[14] Such as the iambic poems On the Sacred Art by, respectively, Archelaus, Hierotheus, and Theophrastus, edited along with Psellus' poem and sundry other works by Ideler (*Physici et Medici Graeci Minores* [Berlin, 1842]).

[15] Written, it may be noted, in the reign of Manuel II, who left one quarter of his fortune to his doctors; Sphrantzes, *Chron. Min.* 15.

[16] In the *Mazaris*, doctors are constantly upbraided as killers and vampires, stronger stuff than the *Timarion*, whose mockery of medical theory is in a more literary and chaffing style. Incidentally, I cannot agree with O. Temkin, "Byzantine Medicine," *DOP*, 16 (1962), 115, that the *Timarion's* audience would need "a remarkable medical knowledge" to enjoy it, or with its editor Romano who thinks it must have been written by a doctor (he suggests Nicolas Callicles, against which notion I am writing elsewhere). Any educated Byzantine could appreciate a comic routine about doctors, just as we can today, without a deep professional knowledge.

[17] *Greek Sophists*, 67, n.3.

[18] It may be added that the word occurs in garbled Latin form (*eotrosuliste*) in *Corpus Glossariorum Latinorum* (ed. Goetz, Leipzig, 1892) 3.600.32 as a gloss on *medicus sapientissimus*, a different shade of meaning.

[19] Cf. C. A. Behr, *Aelius Aristides and the Sacred Tales* (Chicago, 1968), 162–70.

Byzantine things, this debate carried on under changed names. The rivalry was now between greedy, incompetent doctors and the efficient medicare of the Christian healing saints, as admirably documented for the East by H. J. Magoulias[20] and for the West by Peter Brown.[21] It is notable that some saints developed very professional-sounding expertises, such as St. Artemius[22] who specialized in genital tumors, in obvious rivalry with the earthly *kelotomos* prescribed (for example) in John II Comnenus' *typikon*[23] for his monastery hospital.

In what follows, I more or less cover the ground of the first two volumes of *PLRE*, A.D. 260–527. In seeking to include all doctors, that compilation may be thought to overvalue the profession in historical and social terms, especially as other classes who sometimes had more obvious impact on their times—charioteers being a case in point—are just as routinely excluded. But that is a topic for another occasion.[24]

Oribasius is the obvious starting point. But to find room for others, I will stick to wondering about the exact nature of his role in raising Julian to the throne.[25] For in an enigmatic sentence (*VS* 476), Eunapius says he worked in concert (συνήδεσαν) with a certain Euhemerus[26] the Libyan to allow Julian to overthrow the tyranny of Constantius. Eunapius refers the reader to his fuller account in the History, which we do not have. But since we know that his chief source was Oribasius' own memoir, the version there offered will have been what the doctor chose to reveal. Significantly, Eunapius drops his remark about Oribasius in the long section on Maximus, not in the doctor's own notice where (*VS* 498) it is said with deliberate vagueness that he so shone in every virtue as well as medicine as to disclose[27] Julian as emperor.

Two more things about Oribasius. First, he may have held no formal office of state; various late sources claim a quaestorship, but this is not believed in by *PLRE*.[28] Second, his exile after Julian sent him to unspecified barbarian courts. If this is taken to include Persia, Oribasius may have helped to form the taste for Byzantine doctor-diplomats that characterizes eastern potentates in the sixth century.[29]

As far as we can see, Oribasius stood uniquely close to an emperor in the fourth century. This may well have to do with the religious history of the times. Of the doctors whom we glimpse, a goodly number are clearly pagan. Eustochius, for notable instance, a disciple of Plotinus and the only one present at the master's death; Heraclides, also an epic poet, and Olympius who combined with his medicine the arts of grammar, rhetoric, and philosophy, both men frequent in the letters of Libanius; Zeno of Cyprus, along with his pupils Ionicus, Magnus, Oribasius, and Theon, who together constitute the block of medical men in Eunapius' Lives; and Dysarius at Rome, lauded by Symmachus and a character in the *Saturnalia* of Macrobius. In general terms, the label of Asclepiad[30] that attached to doctors at least until the twelfth century[31] will have kept them identified with paganism in the public mind. Before Constantine and in Julian's reign, this will naturally have been an advantage. Otherwise, although pagans were far from being shut out of office in the early centuries of Christian rule, the connection started to become harmful, being no doubt one reason for the castigation of doctors in the Lives of the Saints.[32] Not that there is any straight line in all of this. After all, Oribasius was allowed back from exile, and was still deemed a good marital prospect by the lady of wealth and pedigree who became his wife and the mother of

---

[20] "The Lives of the Saints as Sources of Data for the History of Byzantine Medicine in the Sixth and Seventh Centuries," *BZ*, 57 (1964), 127–50.

[21] *The Cult of the Saints* (Chicago, 1981), 4.

[22] *Miracula S. Artemii*, ed. A. Papadopoulos-Kerameus, *Varia Graeca Sacra* (St. Petersburg, 1909), 26.

[23] Ed. A. Dimitriovsky (Kiev, 1901), 682 f.

[24] See my two articles, with general discussion and lists of addenda and corrigenda in *Historia*, 25 (1976), 118–21; 31 (1982), 97–111. To avoid superfetation of footnotes, readers should assume that *PLRE* furnishes basic references and material for the individual doctors dealt with in the balance of this paper. However, *PLRE* has (inevitably) many errors of omission and commission, and I have always indicated these in my text and/or notes.

[25] For his career, see my "The Career of Oribasius," *Acta Classica*, 18 (1975), 85–97.

[26] About whom we know nothing more; *PLRE* omits him.

[27] The verb used is ἀποδείκνυμι, a favorite of Eunapius in such contexts, e.g. frs. 4, 39, 42; a full conspectus of references

is provided by J. C. Vollebregt, *Symbola in novam Eunapii Vitarum editionem* (Amsterdam, 1929), 39.

[28] It cites only *Suda* 0 543 (Adler) for the claim; the quaestorship is also given by Philostorgius, *HE* 7.77 (= *Passio Artemii* 35) and Cedrenus 1.532 (Bonn).

[29] See R. C. Blockley, "Doctors as Diplomats in the Sixth Century A.D.," *Florilegium*, 2 (1980), 89–100.

[30] Bowersock, *Greek Sophists*, 65, n. 2; cf. L. Cohn-Haft, *The Public Physicians of Ancient Greece* (London, 1956), 30.

[31] E.g. Constantine Manasses, *Hodoiporikon* 3.73, ed. K. Horna, *BZ*, 13 (1904), 313–55; the *Timarion* also links doctors with Asclepius.

[32] In addition to the eastern material assembled by Magoulias (note 20 above), notice the incident in Gregory of Tours, *Vita Martini* 2.50.194, where the local *Jewish* doctor says of the dead saint, "Martin will do you no good whom the earth now rests, turning him to earth . . . ."

his four children. Yet it remains striking that the two doctors most conspicuous in high places come late in the fourth century: Vindicianus, proconsul of Africa (379/82), who placed the crown of rhetoric on the young Augustine's head and who also dissuaded him from astrology;[33] and Marcellus of Bordeaux, named *magister officiorum* in the East (394/5) whilst Theodosius I was on the throne. Neither can have been the sort of doctor eulogized by Eunapius.

Earlier ages again provide the perspective. Of the 563 new men registered by T. P. Wiseman[34] as entering the senate 139 B.C.–A.D. 14, only one may have had medical connections, being possibly the son of Augustus' physician M. Artorius Asclepiades. This latter in turn is only one out of two in Crook's[35] list of 360 members of the *consilium principis* from Augustus to Diocletian. The other is L. Gellius Maximus, *archiatros* and friend of Caracalla.[36] His son, an officer of the Fourth Legion in Syria, was one of a crop of pretenders liquidated around 218/9. Dio Cassius (80.7.1) remarked that his attempt showed how topsy-turvy (πάντα ἄνω κάτω) the world had become. The same combination of medicine and military recurs in the West in a certain Dorus, former surgeon of the *scutarii*, whom Magnentius had promoted to night-watch commander in charge of public buildings. Having tried c. 350 to convict the city prefect Adelphius of treason, he made a similar attempt[37] in 356 against the powerful Arbetio. However, the hearing was mysteriously suppressed at the last minute and, in the splendid phrase of Ammianus (16.6.3) *Dorus evanuit*—no doubt in the Orwellian sense! Finally, on a still more odious note that helps us appreciate the hagiographic attacks on doctors, let us quickly shuffle on and off the stage a certain Aristo who cut out the tongue of the martyr Romanus in the Galerian persecution,[38] hoping that he deserves the asterisks and obeli of disbelief with which *PLRE* adorns him.

The fifth and sixth centuries also fail to come up with a kingmaker of the Oribasian style.[39] What *is*

notable in the light of previous discussion is the much higher tally of Christian doctors. Even more to the point, a good number of these were converts. The most colorful case is Gesius (or Gessius) of Petra, famous in Zeno's reign as both practitioner and teacher of medicine, by which he won not only great wealth but also what Damascius (fr. 35) vaguely calls "unusual honors from the Romans." His ultimate[40] conversion came after the miraculous healing of a disease his own skills had failed to combat. A common, and most understandable, reason for conversion, especially in the case of Probianus, a palace doctor of the fifth century, who was cured of gout, a remission for which most sufferers would think any price worth paying.[41] Some conversions will have been expedient, but we need not be cynical about them all, certainly not in such cases as the Alexandrian medicals Cyrus and Stephanus who became monks.[42]

The most spectacular success story is that of Jacobus, nicknamed Psychristus, a very rare Greek word[43] presumably alluding to his cold bath treatments, a tradition going back to Antonius Musa under Augustus. Son of a doctor, the rackapelt Hesychius, Jacobus joined his father in Constantinople where the latter had recurred after being missing for nineteen years.[44] It was no doubt his father's contempt for rivals that gave Jacobus his notorious brusqueness and scorn of court etiquette which he did not even set aside when tending the emperor Leo. This lack of a bedside manner did him no more harm than his paganism: he was *comes* and *archiatros*, and much honored by statues erected by senators.

Since *PLRE* overlooked him, let us at least notice a doctor-philosopher said to have been a legate

---

[33] *Conf.* 4.3.5; 7.6.8; *Ep.* 138.3.

[34] *New Men in the Roman Senate* (Oxford, 1971); cf. no. 106 in Wiseman's register for the possible medical relations of A. Cascellius.

[35] J. A. Crook, *Consilium Principis* (repr. New York, 1975), nos. 35, 161.

[36] For his career and titles, *PIR*[2] G 131.

[37] In cahoots with a *comes* inaptly called Verissimus.

[38] Prudentius, *Perist.* 10.896 f.

[39] *PLRE* is right to find the homonym addressed by Isidore of Pelusium, *Ep.* 1.437, too late to be the great man: a relation?

[40] In baldly stating that he remained a secret pagan after baptism, *PLRE* neglects the splendid detail in Sophronius whereby Gesius arose from the baptismal waters with a parody of *Odyssey* 4.509, 511, to the effect that "this is a bath which takes one's breath away," on his lips; cf. K. Holum, *Theodosian Empresses: Women and Imperial Dominion in Late Antiquity* (Berkeley and Los Angeles, 1982), 175. One might have thought this homeric rather than biblical utterance a clue to his unregenerate paganism.

[41] It was their failure to cure his gout and migraine that moved Libanius, *Or.* 1.140–41, to harsh criticism of his doctors. For a variant on this cause of conversion, notice the *archiater* Dioscorus who came over as an old man in gratitude for his daughter's recovery from illness.

[42] Nor in the case of the Jewish convert Adamantius.

[43] In the Latin Glosses, it is equivalent to *refrigeratum*.

[44] A Damascene, Hesychius had got married at Drepanum, after which he abandoned wife and child and spent the missing years in Alexandria and Italy. Apart from the necessary mobility of an errant husband and father, his travels recall those of many a poet, or other *literati* of the times.

(ὑπάρχων) in high favor with Zeno. His name is suspicious, being Galen, and his source more so, namely the *Patria Cpoleos*.[45] But even if he is a fiction, it is an instructive one.

When sources dub Jacobus a philosopher, that need not mean much, stemming no doubt from his successful treatment of the neo-platonist Proclus. But the linkage of medical with other skills is still evident.[46] Petrus of Constantia in Osrhoene may seem unusual as a doctor-astrologer, but that is certainly no odder than the philosopher-dancer Memphis[47] of the Antonine Age. Also apparent is what we might loosely call Christian *iatrosophia*: Dionysius, Helpidius, and Julianus were doctors and deacons, whilst a certain Joannes was both physician and treasurer (*syncellus*) to Cyril of Alexandria.

Careers and sympathies of a very different sort provide balance. One Anthimus was arrested in Constantinople in 478, flogged, and exiled for supporting Theodoric Strabo. The unfortunate deacon-doctor Dionysius was taken prisoner by the Goths, amongst whom he continued to practice: was that why they took him? In 448 a certain Eudoxius was involved with the Bacaudae, and only escaped by fleeing to the Huns.[48] Thus, doctors were as caught up as any other profession in the vicissitudes of late Roman and early Byzantine life, at many levels of society and achievement.

In brief finale, the situation was largely then as now. Despite the hostile jokes, which we need not always take more seriously than modern routines about doctors on golf courses or flubbing diagnoses, the medical man was needed, and was known to be needed. In the hagiographies the healing saint is often the last resort, not the first. And the tradition of do-it-yourself medicine was for people far away from urban centers, who clearly went primarily to man's medicine.[49] Doctors were generally learned men, if not always in medicine first. To quote a modern iatrosophist, Jonathan Miller,[50] "I wasn't driven into medicine by a social conscience, but by rampant curiosity." Hence they were in line for the usual preferments given in late antiquity to the erudite. As Symmachus put it with unwonted brevity: *vetus est sententia artes honore nutriri*.[51] Jones,[52] then, was quite wrong when he concluded: "The little that we know of a doctor's life is derived mainly from the papyri and from hagiography. The former suggest that their principal activity was signing medical certificates for the use of the courts and the administration, the latter that their fees were exorbitant and their cures few." And when doctors were attacked, we should recall how Petronius at once qualified his standard joke about them having killed the patient with the reflection that it was really the fault of destiny: to blame the doctor was only *animi consolatio*.

The University of Calgary

[45] Ed. T. Preger (Leipzig, 1901–7) 45.10.175.1; Galen was powerful enough to resist a prosecution by a *kapelos* called Callistratus.

[46] Sometimes manifest not so much in the individual as in his genes: witness Stephanus, father of Alexander of Tralles, also of Dioscorus the doctor, Metrodorus the grammarian, Olympius the jurist, and the famous architect of St. Sophia, Anthemius; Agathias, *Hist.* 5.6.3.

[47] In full, L. Aelius Aurelius Apolaustus Memphis; *PIR*[2] A 148.

[48] He was not the only such case of a fugitive from the empire; the Greek merchant with whom Priscus of Panium (fr. 8) had his famous conversation in Attila's camp will be thought of.

[49] On this, cf. Brown, *Cult of the Saints*, 116, with special reference to Marcellus of Bordeaux, whose compliment (*De med.* 23.77) to the Jewish patriarch Gameliel's amateur knowledge of empiric medicine is worth noting. Also observe such phenomena as the Theodorus disclosed in an inscription from Aphrodisias as a κηρωματίτης. The word is in no Greek lexicon; L. Robert, *Hellenica*, 13 (1965), 167–70, explains it as a species of osteopath. One wonders also if the explosion of veterinary writers in the fourth century—Apsyrtus, Papyriensis, Pelagonius, Secundus—had anything to do with the greater use of cavalry in the late Roman world.

[50] Now as familiar in North America as in Britain for his skills in medicine, satire, writing, acting, and direction both of Shakespeare and the ballet. The quotation appeared in the London *Observer*, February 6, 1983.

[51] *Ep.* 1.43. Libanius, *Or.* 18.158, is (predictably) eloquent on the subject of Julian's preferment of poets and historians; cf. W. E. Kaegi, "The Emperor Julian's Assessment of the Significance and Function of History," *PAPS*, 108 (1964), 33. Anastasius, on the evidence of John Lydus, *De Mag.* 3.50.3, deemed only literary men suitable for the praetorian prefecture. John himself is a perfect example of the system: vain about his own learning, he regularly evaluates other officials on the basis of their education. For many other texts, and criticism of the principle, cf. A. Alföldi, *A Conflict of Ideas in the Late Roman Empire* (Oxford, 1952), 106 f. In his novel *The Masters* (Penguin ed., 28), C. P. Snow (himself a product of the system) quips nicely on the survival of the principle in Britain: "He's thought to stand a chance of the colonial service if he can scrape a third. Of course, I'm totally ignorant of these matters, but I can't see why our colonies should need third class men with some capacity for organised sports."

[52] A. H. M. Jones, *The Later Roman Empire* (Oxford, 1964), 1012–13. He went on to surmise that "these impressions" were no doubt unjust," but did not go beyond the limited view of his adminstrative evidence.

BYZANTINE MEDICINE IN THE SIXTH AND SEVENTH CENTURIES: ASPECTS OF TEACHING AND PRACTICE

JOHN DUFFY

In the period we are considering—the sixth and seventh centuries—there were two ways of acquiring a medical training in the Greek East: by apprenticeship to a practicing physician and by attendance at the lectures of a professor of medicine. The first was the time-honored one, enshrined for us in the Hippocratic *Oath*, and no doubt the more accessible of the two. But it would not necessarily have been the more desirable way, because higher education through the book, at least until the middle of the seventh century, was an important avenue in the Byzantine world to the professions and to positions in both the civil and the ecclesiastical services.[1] Certainly the more formal study of medicine, particularly in a city like Alexandria, must have given a badge of distinction to a young man which would stand him in good stead for setting up practice and attracting a clientele. We may also remark that those medical men who were sometimes called upon by the state for diplomatic missions probably owed their selection not least to education; they would have belonged to the well-trained elite and the pool of talent available to the authorities for special service.[2]

We may be sure that it was possible to sit at the feet of a medical sophist in a number of places in the Byzantine Empire, though, if we were to rely on the literature, we would get the impression that it could be done only at Alexandria. This city, which enjoyed a remarkable association with medicine from the time of the first Ptolemies in the third

century B.C. until the Arab conquest nearly a thousand years later, completely drowned out the claims of other centers for a share of the limelight. Much more than, say, Beirut with law, Alexandria became synonymous with doctors and medical studies. If one had qualified in that city, it was something to be mentioned; otherwise, it seems, there was no point in identifying the place of study. Since practically all of our information derives from there, Alexandria of necessity becomes for us the representative of Byzantine medical education as a whole; other centers are not likely to have done much different or to have offered anything more.

To Alexandria students came from all corners of the East and, no doubt, from parts of the West too. In most cases they would have to have been from families who could afford to send a young man abroad, to maintain him away from home for about four years[3] and, possibly, to pay the teacher's fees.[4]

On looking into the classroom, we are not greatly surprised to find that the course of study consisted for the most part of reading from the works of Hippocrates and Galen and hearing them expounded by the teacher. Obviously not all of those two authors was read, but a traditional selection which focused on more or less eleven treatises from the Hippocratic Collection and fifteen or sixteen from the large corpus of Galen's writings. This syllabus, tackled in a definite order, was designed to acquaint the learner with the main areas of an extensive subject. In the case of Hippocrates, the reading ranged from the general principles of the

[The reader is referred to the list of abbreviations at the end of the volume.]

[1] On the role of higher education see the recent judicious remarks of C. Mango in his *Byzantium: The Empire of New Rome* (London, 1980), 35–36 and 128 ff.

[2] There is a short article on this topic by R. C. Blockley, "Doctors as Diplomats in the Sixth Century A.D.," in *Florilegium*, 2 (1980), 89–100.

[3] This estimate of the period of study is taken from L. G. Westerink's "Academic Practice About 500: Alexandria," a paper delivered at the Colloquium on the Transmission of Knowledge, Dumbarton Oaks (1977), and scheduled for publication by Dumbarton Oaks.

[4] The connection, if any, between salaried public doctors and teachers of medicine needs to be explored.

Aphorisms to the specialized discussion in *Women's Diseases*. The chosen works of Galen covered the broad areas of anatomy, physiology, etiology, diagnostics, and therapeutics.[5] From the point of view of quantity Galen certainly predominated, and even Hippocratic doctrine was presented through a Galenic filter. But in the eyes of the Alexandrians, the "father of medicine" was still very much the sacred figure, and it could be said with some fairness that for them the Hippocratic writings were the "Bible," while Galen by comparison was merely the best commentator.

The most important source for our knowledge of the details of the Alexandrian syllabus is the group of school lecture notes which survive from the sixth and seventh centuries. This corpus of commentaries, while relatively small in size, still gives us a good idea of classroom procedures and pedagogical method. It soon becomes clear to anyone reading this literature that the teacher relies heavily on deliberate repetition as a means to inculcate the central tenets of medical theory and lore. If the student, to give a few simple examples, is frequently reminded over the course of several years that "the natural faculties are four in number,"[6] or that "our bodies are composed of solids, fluids, and 'airs',"[7] or that "Hippocrates calls every kind of tumor a swelling,"[8] he is not likely to forget the in-

formation in a hurry. The same applies to more elaborate topics, such as the different types of fever or the process by which food is assimilated in the body.

Another salient feature of the lectures is the influence of methods borrowed from the philosophers.[9] We can see it in the widespread use of *diairesis*, i.e., in the division of a subject, let us say urines, into a widening series of subdivisions, based on differences such as color and sediment, until the topic is exhausted and felt to be under control. This too must have been a useful aid for memory. The syllogistic method is employed to unravel the tightly knitted thoughts of Hippocrates, who, as the commentators like to say, was "a man of few words." The Aristotelian four causes figure prominently in the lectures, and are put to good use in explaining the etiology of normal and abnormal conditions. In fact, the influence of Aristotle on one commentator was so great that he took the retrograde step of arguing for the heart, and against the brain, as the seat of sensation and the leading principle of the body.[10]

Some of the commentaries also reveal elements of what might be called an Alexandrian mode of exegesis. We have, for instance, the lecture notes of both Palladius and John of Alexandria on book six of the *Epidemics*, and from these it is clear that there was a definite procedure for handling the Hippocratic work. It consists of three steps, in which the following points are treated by the lecturer: (1) the wording of the text itself, i.e., variant readings and clarification of individual words; (2) the general meaning of the lemma as a whole; and (3) various explanations of the text by earlier commentators and how to decide between them. The terminology used to describe these distinct operations is very similar in both John[11] and Palladius.[12] And to prove that the approach is not peculiar to

---

[5] A handy and up-to-date version of the complete syllabus will be found in Appendix II of the Westerink article cited in n. 3. There is some question about whether *De sanitate tuenda* was included by the Alexandrians. It would appear that it did not formally belong to the reading list, but was a later addition, perhaps to a Syriac version of the canon, as argued by Elinor Lieber in her valuable paper "Galen in Hebrew: the Transmission of Galen's Works in the Mediaeval Islamic World," in Nutton, ed., *Galen: Problems*, 167–86, esp. 178–79. That the Alexandrians had already attached special importance to the treatise is suggested by the fact that John of Alexandria gives a kind of synopsis of its six books in his commentary on the Hippocratic *Epidemics VI*, 140b1–41 (ed. Pritchet, pp. 286–88). It is also mentioned by Palladius in his lectures on *Epidemics VI* (Dietz, II, 157.10–17). For an older discussion of the Alexandrian canon, see O. Temkin, "Geschichte des Hippokratismus im ausgehenden Altertum," *Kyklos*, 4 (1932), 1–80, esp. 76 ff.

[6] J. M. Duffy, ed. and trans., *Stephanus the Philosopher: A Commentary on the Prognosticon of Hippocrates* (Berlin, 1983) [*CMG* XI 1, 2]), 132.17 ff.; cf. Stephanus on the *Aphorisms*, Escorialensis Σ.II.10, fol.121ᵛ and Ambrosianus S 19 sup., fol. 45ᵛ. (Manuscript references are given, since this is for the most part an unpublished commentary; the first full edition, by L. G. Westerink, will appear in the *CMG*; I thank Professor Westerink for providing me with a typewritten copy of his edition).

[7] John of Alexandria on *Epidemics VI* 148c (ed. Pritchet, p. 402); Stephanus on Galen's *Therapeutics* (Dietz, I, p. 321); Stephanus on the *Aphorisms* (see n. 6), Ambrosianus S 19 sup., fol. 11ʳ.

[8] John of Alexandria on *Epidemics VI*, 120c 11–13 (ed. Pritchet, p. 9.); Stephanus on the *Prognosticon*, 126.19; Stephanus on the *Aphorisms*, Escorialensis Σ.II.10, fol. 69ᵛ. Westerink (note 3 above)

gives a good illustration of repetition from Stephanus on the *Aphorisms*.

[9] For the special ties between medicine and philosophy in the late Alexandrian period see L. G. Westerink, "Philosophy and Medicine in Late Antiquity," *Janus*, 51 (1964), 169–77 (reprinted in his *Texts and Studies in Neoplatonism and Byzantine Literature* [Amsterdam, 1980], 83–91).

[10] His view is cited in Stephanus' lectures on the *Prognosticon* (note 6 above), 126.1–14, where he is referred to as "the new commentator" (ὁ νέος ἐξηγητής).

[11] John of Alexandria's work in its complete form survives only in a medieval Latin version, edited by Pritchet. However, there are some fragments of the original in a number of Greek manuscripts; in Vaticanus gr. 300 (fol. 192ʳ) the three steps are given as: (1) σαφηνίζειν τὰς λέξεις, (2) ἡ διάνοια τοῦ παντὸς λόγου, and (3) ἡ διάκρισις τοῦ λόγου.

[12] Palladius' commentary is in Dietz, II, 1–204; for the point we are dealing with see pp. 5–6, 13, and 19.

a discussion of the *Epidemics*, we have the lectures on the *Aphorisms* by Stephanus of Athens, which show an almost identical scheme and several agreements in the technical terms used to describe the individual steps.[13]

As for the teachers themselves, anyone interested in their lives or personalities would be disappointed, because beyond the names of five or six whose works have partly survived we know very little.[14] Only the earliest of them for our period, Gesius, made any sort of name for himself outside the school environment. His fame was due in good part to his outstanding abilities as both teacher and practitioner, and it may be gauged by the fact that Sophronius of Jerusalem devotes a whole chapter of the *Miracles of Cyrus and John* to attacking the man and his reputation.[15] Gesius in his better light even made it into the Byzantine *Who's Who*, the *Suda* lexicon.[16] But this man is clearly an exception and, generally speaking, Alexandrian medical professors, the iatrosophists, were not likely to do anything which would catapult their names beyond the immediate time and place. Judged from their lecture notes they emerge as scholastics who handed on a traditional body of knowledge, based on the classics of ancient medicine. In the *auditorium* they gave their students a solid core of theory and helped them to master the basic tenets of Hippocrates and of the Galenic system. In this respect they were doing no more and no less than their colleagues in the other subjects of higher education.

And here there is a question to be asked about the iatrosophists which deserves some attention. To what extent were these teachers involved in the practice of medicine and, related to this, did their students get any firsthand experience during the period of training? Their contemporaries were inclined to take a negative view of the iatrosophists, and they did not often get a good press. They were targets for the traditional attack on sophists in general, which branded them as being good with words but useless in action. An iatrosophist who could display both qualities was regarded as something of a rare bird; Gesius, whom we have just met, is a case in point. The same attitude is apparent also

early in the seventh century in a poem on Emperor Heraclius by George of Pisidia: the emperor, in one of his decisive actions, is compared to a medical teacher who joins practice to his theory; in other words, an admirable combination and, we may suppose, one that could not be taken for granted.[17]

Now it is entirely possible that some teachers spent most of their time with the books and deserved the image of ivory-tower academics; it is conceivable too that some students read medicine as part of a liberal education and had no intention of becoming practicing physicians. However, there is enough evidence to assure us that not all Alexandrian teachers were isolated on an academic island, cut off from the realities of illness and disease, and we will see that it was possible for students also to get to the bedside of the sick. For a start, the teachers themselves were well aware of the difference between preaching and practicing, or, as they would put it, between οἱ λόγοι and τὰ ἔργα τῆς τέχνης. They sometimes protest their primary interest in the works of medicine, and even cite examples from their personal experiences. There is not, to be sure, a great deal of attention paid to the details of actual medical care, but more than enough to convince us that they were fully conversant with the common types of treatment, including drugs.

More impressive, however, is the testimony of Sophronius of Jerusalem, who had occasion himself, around the first decade of the seventh century, to seek help from Alexandrian medical professors for an eye ailment; they failed to cure him and were repaid by being constantly berated in his *Miracles of Cyrus and John*. From the picture of the situation presented by Sophronius there can be no doubt that the iatrosophists were regarded in Alexandria as the leaders of the medical profession,[18] and as such they were automatically consulted, especially in complicated cases. And Sophronius takes us a step further in two of the miracle accounts. In no. 60, concerning a certain Theodore laid low with a fever, we are informed that the patient had been visited by the iatrosophists, who were accompanied by young men. This indicates, firstly, that teachers went on sick calls and, secondly, that students did the rounds and got firsthand experience with the master. These points

---

[13] Dietz, II, p. 248; Stephanus inserts a fourth point on the usefulness of each aphorism, which he labels τὸ χρήσιμον τῆς ἐννοίας.

[14] They are discussed in: W. Bräutigam, *De Hippocratis Epidemiarum Libri Sexti Commentatoribus* (Diss., Königsberg, 1908); O. Temkin (note 5 above), 1–80, esp. 64–74; see also Appendix I of Westerink (note 3 above).

[15] Ed. N. Fernández Marcos, *Los Thaumata de Sofronio* (Madrid, 1975), no. 30; the older edition is in P G, vol. 87, part 3.

[16] *Suda* (ed. Adler), s. Γέσιος.

[17] *Expeditio Persica* II 191–92, ed. A. Pertusi, *Giorgio di Pisidia. Poemi I. Panegirici epici* (Ettal, 1959): ὡς οὖν σοφιστὴς τοῖς ἰατρικοῖς λόγοις / πεῖραν συνάψας. For a different view of what might normally be expected from iatrosophists, see Th. Nissen, "Medizin und Magie bei Sophronios" (= Sophronios-Studien III), *BZ*, 39 (1939), 351–52.

[18] This is well brought out by Nissen (note 17 above), 352–53.

are confirmed by miracle no. 33, which tells of a woman visited in a dream by the Saints Cyrus and John, disguised as medical personnel—one of them is said to be the teacher and the other his student. In a sense the only surprising thing about these details is that they are never mentioned in the school commentaries, probably because they were taken for granted. So, the image of the Alexandrian iatrosophist as an aloof, armchair doctor is not quite accurate, and the student got some practice, which enabled him to begin his career armed with more than a set of lecture notes.

Since we have introduced the work of Sophronius, it will be appropriate at this point to consider briefly the genre of miracle accounts, a branch of Byzantine literature which, apart from providing useful concrete details about the profession, commonly expresses views on conventional medicine. Here we will confine ourselves to confronting the attitudes projected by these texts, and to spelling out some of the assumptions made by the authors. Two groups of incubation miracles from the seventh century will be considered. One of them, the *Miracles of Cyrus and John*,[19] was written around the year 610 by Sophronius, before he became patriarch of Jerusalem. It describes seventy cases of cures produced at the shrine of the two martyr saints at Menuthis in Egypt, not far from Alexandria, and as we have seen, it throws valuable light on the iatrosophists of that city. The second set, the *Miracles of St. Artemius*,[20] is the work of an unknown author who was writing close to the year 660. This text presents forty-five miracles of the martyr Artemius, who had his shrine at the Church of St. John Prodromos in Constantinople and specialized, for an unknown reason, in cases of genital tumors, especially scrotal hernia. It has very interesting information on hospitals in the capital and some tidbits on the practice of surgery.

A composite picture of the medical profession based on these two writers is anything but flattering. At their most charitable they tell us that doctors, relying on the empty doctrines of Hippocrates and Galen, cannot even make a proper diagnosis and would be better off referring their patients to the care of the saints. On the blacker side we find that many physicians are little better than criminals: they are negligent and often make the patient's condition worse; they are only inter-

ested in the victim's money and are prepared, even when a fatal outcome is already certain, to continue treatment in order to collect their fees. The general message, then, is "Do not expect doctors to do anything for you except to take your money and abandon you as soon as your purse is empty." In the same vein the miracle accounts often ridicule the expensive and elaborate preparations of doctors which turn out to be useless, while the healing saints, who ask for no compensation, are able to work wonders with the most paltry substances— very often the candle wax taken from their own shrines.

Let it be said straightaway that this hostile attitude is a traditional pose and typical of the genre. It is a kind of artificial venom, discharged in greater or lesser quantity depending on the mood of the individual author, and, in a way, it is just a more aggressive form of the common pious sentiment that Christ is the real healer, while man's powers are useless compared to His. But the polemic is so relentless and the attacks so pointed that the modern reader may come away with a mistaken impression. He might suppose that the authors, even if not the Church itself, are at heart opposed to conventional medicine and reject the role of the physician. But this is not the case, as we will see by probing into the assumptions being made.

Sophronius and his fellows are not advocating a boycott of medicine; they are not encouraging their contemporaries in case of illness to pass by the doctor and to rely solely on the mercy of God. For a start, practically all the diseases in the miracle stories are presented as incurable conditions; in other words, the patients have first attended the doctor and only after failure there have they approached the saints as hopeless cases. Therefore, it is taken for granted, even by a Sophronius, that the sick normally seek medical help.

There were no doubt holy men and women who, even in serious illness, preferred to entrust themselves to God rather than to doctors, and on the surface the miracle writers may want to be seen as supporters of this ideal faith. But they are well aware of the facts of life, and assume that, ascetics excepted, in the event of injury or sickness the first impulse of the ordinary man is to look for medical help. The proof of this comes from three telling incidents which take place at the shrines themselves. In Sophronius' miracle no. 8 we are told that the steward (*oeconomos*) of the shrine falls ill and seeks medical attention before he realizes that he has the Saints close at hand; in no. 67 when a young

---

[19] See note 15 above.
[20] Ed. A. Papadopoulos-Kerameus in his *Varia Sacra Graeca* (St. Petersburg, 1909), 1–79.

pilgrim injures himself seriously in a suicide attempt, some of the attendants go out to the neighboring villages for a doctor and bring one back to the scene. In the miracles of St. Artemius we read of a priest attached to the church of St. John Prodromos who develops testicle problems, and visits a series of doctors before approaching St. Artemius, whose shrine is in that very church.

Naturally, enough, the authors present these as exceptional cases and as reprehensible lapses of faith. But it would not take much reading behind the lines to realize that the writers' shock at those happenings is little more than a formality and that, for all the hue and cry, there is nothing extraordinary in such behavior. In sum, we can say that though it is certainly not the intention of their authors, the miracle accounts show as well as anything else that for the average Byzantine there was no contradiction between piety and practicality. When the polemic is skimmed off the top, we are left with the stories of desperate cases who have tried all the conventional ways and now travel to the shrines for special help. As for the rest, the sick who are at home and hope to recover, we must imagine that they are still seeing the doctor.

And what do we know about this doctor? We could draw a sketch of him using the two kinds of literature which we have discussed so far—commentaries and miracle accounts—but it would not be easy to do a fuller portrait from them. Luckily there is someone who can help us to fill out the picture, a good guide to the everyday realities of Byzantine medical practice. He is Alexander of Tralles, born in the first half of the sixth century and member of a distinguished family from Asia Minor; his father was a doctor and his four brothers were also professional men, including the famous Anthemius who helped to rebuild St. Sophia in Constantinople. Alexander himself became a physician and spent much of his time abroad, and part of it in Rome. Towards the end of his life he wrote, for the use of doctors, a therapeutic handbook of a traditional kind, going from head to toe or, pathologically speaking, from baldness to gout.[21] Looked upon as a medical author of the Justinianic period and not, for example, as a minute figure in the grand pageant of Greek Science, Alexander deserves attention—and not a little admiration—on several accounts. For if we could entertain questions about the practical experience of the iatro-

sophists, we can have no doubts about this man's firsthand knowledge. The keynote of his work, already struck in the preface, and heard consistently throughout, is *peira*, experience, and he tells us that now, in his old age and unable to practice any more, he is setting down the cures and treatments which over the years he has found to be most effective. He is one of the very few Byzantine medical writers who bring us close to the physician in action, and he shares with us details of cases from his own practice. This alone is reason enough to look more closely at a few of his attitudes and approaches to the art.

Completely orthodox in theory, Alexander's main mentors among the older writers are Hippocrates and Galen. But when it comes to prescribing remedies, he is no blind follower of the ancients; he knows where to draw the line of respect and is not afraid to assert his independence, even if it means disagreeing with Galen.[22] He chooses truth over authority, and the deciding factor is always experience. His thinking on remedies may be summed up as follows: "If they don't work, it doesn't matter what the ancients say about them." He can be fairly critical of doctors in his own day and faults them for not being careful enough in the use of drugs: many physicians, he tells us, are only interested in combating the symptoms[23] and often cause more harm than good.[24] He himself, whenever possible, prefers to prescribe dieting or baths or exercise;[25] when he has to use drugs, he tries to avoid those that are harsh or known to be dangerous.[26] Again, with a glance perhaps at his less competent or less scrupulous colleagues, he reminds the reader that a drug does not have to be complex or expensive in order to be effective.[27] He finds it necessary, too, to warn about getting the genuine article, because some doctors are being sold counterfeit pills.[28] Finally, he is not at all bashful about recommending his own pills and preparations for the best results.[29]

Good doctor that he is, Alexander always has the patient uppermost in mind and is very sympathetic to individual feelings and fears. For the patient who does not like barley-gruel—and many people, he

---

[21] Ed. Puschmann, 2 vols.

[22] E.g., II, 83.15 ff.; 155.16 ff. Puschmann.
[23] I, 577.2–3 Puschmann.
[24] II, 5.2 ff. Puschmann.
[25] E.g., I, 601.10–11; II, 439.3 ff.; II, 457.14 ff. Puschmann.
[26] I, 609.22 ff.; II, 123.19–21 Puschmann.
[27] II, 205.12 ff. Puschmann.
[28] II, 207.13 ff. Puschmann.
[29] I, 547.19 ff.; II, 295.2 ff.; II, 345.6 ff.; II, 427.5 ff. Puschmann.

adds, can't stand the mention of the word—he is willing to substitute oatmeal juice, if it is available.[30] For gout sufferers who might not be able to take medicine orally, being suspicious of drugs, or squeamish, or suffering from a stomach ailment, he provides an alternate list of remedies to be applied externally.[31] In Alexander's book, cases of brain fever deserve special consideration and every effort is made to create a calm and soothing environment for them: the temperature and amount of light in the sickroom are controlled; visitors are screened and nobody, not even a relative, is allowed to enter who has upset the patient in the past; even the number of friends admitted is kept within limits, since a crowd tends to be disturbing and has a bad effect on the quality of the air in the room.[32]

In fact Alexander's concern for the treatment and welfare of his patients is so great that he is willing to accept and even to support the use of charms, amulets, and folk remedies. The subject first comes up, not surprisingly, in the part of the work dealing with epilepsy,[33] and is afterwards discussed on several occasions.[34] It must be admitted that Alexander is not entirely consistent in presenting his reasons for supporting these unorthodox methods, and it may well be that he felt uncomfortable in divulging his views. At any rate, in his first statements there is a note of defensiveness, and the use of charms and amulets seems to be condoned only in desperate cases when the scientific method has failed. It later transpires, however, that he can advocate their use in other circumstances, even when it seems to be only a matter of accommodating the needs and wishes of his patients. We get the flavor of his thinking from this passage which comes towards the end of recommendations for colic: "I know that anyone using the methods just mentioned would need no other help from outside. However, since many patients, and especially the wealthy ones, object to drinking medicine and to treating their bowels with enemas, they force us to cure the pain with the help of magical amulets. That is why I have thought it worthwhile to give you an account of those also, both the ones which I know from my own experience and those whose effectiveness is vouched for by trusted friends."[35]

It is usual to react with disappointment to this aspect of Alexander's work; it is seen as the flaw in what otherwise is a praiseworthy document, an embarrassing blot on a good record. But there is another way of looking at it. Even without arguing for what might be the psychological soundness of Alexander's approach, we may admire the man's candor. For it must have taken a certain amount of courage to openly associate oneself with such practices, at the risk of ridicule and loss of intellectual respectability. Apart from this, the student of the realities of Byzantine life in the sixth century has reason to be grateful to him, because he reveals quite a lot about the place of superstition and magic in a part of Byzantine society where we might not have expected it. We are apt to connect such phenomena more with the lower classes, but this work warns us against underestimating the role of so-called popular beliefs in the upper strata, where Alexander and his patients belong.[36]

More than many Byzantine authors, including those of technical works, Alexander of Tralles deserves to be taken at face value. Since such a statement cannot be made lightly for any Byzantine writer, I will support it with a few arguments. In the first place, Alexander's aim is severely practical and down-to-earth—to provide a handbook on therapy for the working physician; it is based on earlier material to be sure, but made much more alive than other compilations by incorporating the results of extensive personal experience. Secondly, the author makes a conscious effort to communicate, which is in keeping with his objective; he deliberately chooses, as he explains in the preface, to use clear language and common words, insofar as possible. Finally, if he were mainly in the business of impressing, he would have avoided a risky topic like magic, or at least he would have dissociated himself from its use. For these reasons, then, we would argue that Alexander should be trusted, and that his manual may be believed to contain genuine reflections of medical practice in the author's day.

In his discussion of doctors and other professionals in the later Roman Empire, A. H. M. Jones makes the following observation: "The little that we know of a doctor's life is derived mainly from the papyri and from hagiography. The former suggests that their principal activity was signing

---

[30] I, 523.13 ff. Puschmann.
[31] II, 573.25 ff. Puschmann.
[32] I, 519.6 ff. Puschmann.
[33] I, 557.13 ff. Puschmann.
[34] E.g., I, 571.21 ff.; II, 319.4 ff.; II, 473.30 ff.; II, 579.14 ff. Puschmann.
[35] II, 375.10–16 Puschmann.

[36] His patients carry sneezing ointment in ivory boxes (I, 493.19–20 Puschmann); they have large numbers of servants in their houses (I, 515.19–21 Puschmann); for certain types of gastric ailments they are advised to go to warm springs, take sea voyages, or travel on long trips (II, 249.22–25 Puschmann).

medical certificates for the use of the courts and the administration, the latter that their fees were exorbitant and their cures few. Both impressions are no doubt unjust."[37] This is a wise reservation.

On the question of fees we have nothing new to add, since we lack hard and reliable evidence for charges in individual cases; there are some figures mentioned in our two miracle sets, but these are likely to be fanciful exaggerations.[38] On the other hand, the texts that we have considered leave no doubt that the papyri—at least those read by Jones—create a very lopsided impression. We hope to have shown that other documents of the sixth and seventh centuries have much to tell us about the Byzantine medical man as teacher, student, and practitioner; they present the doctor of the period, as we could have expected, busily involved in diagnosing, prognosing, and treating all kinds of diseases and accidental injuries. Obviously it is not possible to measure in any way his rate of success. However, if we allow ourselves to be influenced more by the example of Alexander of Tralles than by the strictures of the miracle accounts, we can come away with the optimistic thought that he was likely to care and to try his best.

University of Maryland

---

[37] *The Later Roman Empire (284–602)* (Norman, 1964), vol. II, 1012–13.

[38] In Sophronius' miracle 40 a doctor asks three *solidi* from a kidney patient; in the *Miracula Artemii* (no. 36) two doctors offer to cure the sick boy of a poor woman, one for twelve, the other for eight *solidi*. An idea of value may be gained from the following: in the early seventh century a bath attendant earned a salary of three *solidi* per annum, and in the time of Justinian the cost of feeding the average working man for a year was five *solidi*. These figures are taken from Jones (note 37 above), vol. I, 447–48.

THEOPHANES NONNUS: MEDICINE IN THE CIRCLE OF CONSTANTINE PORPHYROGENITUS*

JOSEPH A. M. SONDERKAMP

The common opinion has it that in the realm of applied sciences Constantine VII not only initiated the famous handbook on agriculture but also commissioned a work on medicine which occasionally is even called a "medical encyclopedia."[1] The work in question is a little treatise on therapy, which its title says is dedicated to a Constantine Porphyrogenitus. For more than 300 years this addressee has been believed to be Constantine VII, although the evidence for this identification has never been thoroughly examined.[2]

The text, which was printed twice,[3] is designed for use in everyday medical practice. Some 300 short chapters, arranged in the traditional fashion from head to heels, deal with a great variety of diseases, their symptoms, causes, and treatment. At the end there are two special sections, one about diseases that may occur in any part of the body and the other about various kinds of poisoning.[4] Each chapter usually begins with a definition of the disease it deals with, combined in most cases with a brief description of its principal symptoms. It may continue with a short remark about the causes that are held responsible for the condition. The closing section, which usually is the largest, is concerned with therapy, giving a number of prescriptions in most cases, often complemented by bloodletting or dietetical suggestions. The prescriptions are very terse, concentrating on the ingredients and their proportions. Instructions for the application of the medicines are rare and hints for their preparation rarely go beyond a ἐνώσας, a μίξας ὁμοῦ or a similar phrase.

Thus the work is a practical vademecum, providing essential information in a condensed, readily accessible form, primarily—almost exclusively one might say—in the field of therapy.

This type of manual has a long tradition. Galen's vast "On the composition of medicines according to the seat of the diseases"[5] is but the most voluminous example (fig. 1). Other specimens, more similar to this text, are the pseudo-Galenic books "On medicines that are easily procured,"[6] parts of Oribasius' works for his son Eustathius and his friend Eunapius,[7] or the third, fourth and fifth books of Paul of Aegina,[8] to name but a few.

[The reader is referred to the list of abbreviations at the end of the volume.]

*I would like to acknowledge with gratitude my appointment to a Junior Fellowship at Dumbarton Oaks for the year 1981/82, during which much of the research on which this paper is based was carried out.

[1] See e.g., H. Haeser. *Lehrbuch der Geschichte der Medizin und der epidemischen Krankheiten*, 3rd ed., I (Jena, 1875), 477; G. Costomiris, "Etudes sur les écrits inédits des anciens médecins grecs, 3," *REG*, 4 (1891), 100–101; Krumbacher, 2nd ed., 263, 614; I. Bloch, "Byzantinische Medizin" in M. Neuburger-J. Pagel, *Handbuch der Geschichte der Medizin*, I (Jena, 1902), 560–61; P. Lemerle, *Le premier humanisme byzantin*, Bibliothèque byzantine, Etudes, 6 (Paris, 1971), 296; J. Théodoridès, *Les sciences biologiques et médicales à Byzance*, Les cahiers d'histoire et de philosophie des sciences, 3 (Paris, 1977), 31; Hunger, "Medizin," 305. The most recent contribution to this matter is L. Felici, "L'opera medica di Teofane Nonno in manoscritti inediti," *Acta medicae historiae Patavina*, 28 (1981–82; publ. 1983), 59–74.

[2] See p. 39 f., below.

[3] Noni, medici clarissimi, *De omnium particularium morborum curatione . . . liber*, nunc primum in lucem editus, et summa diligentia conversus per H. Martium (Strasbourg, 1568). Theophanis Nonni *Epitome de curatione morborum Graece ac Latine*, Ope codicum manuscriptorum recensuit notasque adiecit J. St. Bernard, I–II (Gotha-Amsterdam, 1794–95). Text and translation are a mere reprint of the 1568 edition. New is the large body of notes in which divergent manuscript readings are reported, problems of the text are discussed and many parallels in similar works are pointed out.

[4] Chapters 233–59 (II 216–84 Bernard) and 261–83 (II 290–356 Bernard), respectively.

[5] Galen (ed. Kühn), XII, 378 through XIII, 361.

[6] Galen (ed. Kühn), XIV, 311–581.

[7] Oribasius, (ed. Raeder) *Synopsis ad Eustathium, Libri ad Eunapium* (*CMG* VI 3). Parallel are mainly books 6 to 9 of the *Synopsis* and books 3 and 4 of the *Ad Eunapium*.

[8] Paul (ed. Heiberg [*CMG* IX]).

It is evident, then, that we are not dealing here with any kind of folk medicine but with a work that continues the practical tradition of ancient scientific medicine in the form it had taken in late antiquity.

As to the sources of this manual, the question seems to be rather complex. It is clear that the author does not follow one source only; he does not simply abbreviate or rewrite the work of one particular predecessor.[9] If the author was a compiler, he was certainly fully versed in the literature of his field. A number of chapters when analyzed turn out to be almost completely patchworks of brief quotations taken literally from various older—never acknowledged—works of the same kind, rearranged in order to suit the compiler's purpose. There are, however, paragraphs in these chapters, mainly prescriptions, that do not turn up in these older works, not, that is, in the parallel sections of those texts that are accessible in printed editions. Moreover, there are other chapters of which nothing resembles older available parallels more than very vaguely. As more hitherto unpublished parallels—like Paulus Nicaeus—become available and the time-consuming work of scanning the sections of older works that are not parallel to the chapter in question goes on, a number of these unparalleled passages will be linked to their sources. Still, the possibility cannot be ruled out that the author is more original than we might expect him to be. In this context it is important to note that there are no apparent traces of any influence of Islamic medicine on the work.

The little book met with considerable success. The first printed edition had been based on one manuscript only. The second took five more manuscripts into account.[10] So far I have discovered fifty

manuscripts, nearly all of which were copied in the fourteenth, fifteenth, or sixteenth century.[11] Most of these manuscripts contain the full text of the work. Within the families the text is surprisingly stable, but between them the differences are considerable. They may affect the micro-structure of the text—a specific ingredient of a prescription, for instance. More important for the textual physiognomy of the individual families, however, are the macro-structural divergences, consisting in the presence or absence of entire sections of the text—mostly prescriptions or groups of prescriptions. It is these features that determine the specific makeup of the families, which can, with respect to this, be called recensions in a way. Ten such recensions are now discernible. Six of these are attested by extant manuscripts for the fourteenth century, two more for the period around 1400. So the manuscript tradition seems to have been split up considerably even before the oldest extant witnesses were written, which shows that the text was widely used even before 1300.

The popularity of the text is also documented by the occurrence of a number of minor forms of transmission—typical for this kind of practical literature—in the manuscript tradition of this treatise. There is a carefully prepared version of the entire text in colloquial Greek of which we have a manuscript of the fourteenth century. In several instances parts of the work or a number of selected chapters are transmitted separately among other medical or non-medical texts; excerpts from the text are copied in the margins of parallel passages of other authors, just as this text itself attracts such marginalia, and it even occurs that parts of the work are transmitted in one and the same manuscript side by side with its full text.[12]

The next step also occurs: excerpts from this work are incorporated into similar texts. For instance the so called Ἀποθεραπευτική of Theophilus[13] con-

---

[9] Felici (note 1 above), 61, repeats the old but erroneous belief that Oribasius and more precisely his *Collectiones medicae* are the source (at least the main source) of this little book: "infatti l'ordine e il contenuto dei capitoli è lo stesso delle *Collectiones* di Oribasio" (she uses this as an argument later on, 62, 67, 70). Nothing, however, could be less true. As Freind (note 33 below) showed already in 1725, our text has absolutely nothing to do with the *Collectiones medicae*, except for the opening phrase of their preface (see also below). The *Eclogae medicamentorum*, on the other hand (not by Oribasius but based on his work: Oribasius [ed. Raeder (*CMG* VI 2.2)]), to which Felici by a slip attributes the preface to the *Collectiones*, though one of the sources on which it occasionally draws, provided neither in content nor in arrangement the guideline for our text.—I cannot enter here into a discussion of the priority of either our manual or Leo's Σύνοψις τῆς ἰατρικῆς (in Ermerins, 79–221), which often are very close. My impression is that Leo draws on our text; but a more detailed demonstration than I can give here would be required to prove this.

[10] Martius' text is a slightly corrected printing of the text as it is contained in his manuscript, Monac. gr. 362 (not 589 as Felici

[note 1 above], 60, says). Bernard, in addition to Martius' edition, made use—through transcripts—of Vindob. med. gr. 26, 27, 32 and 50, as well as Paris. Coislin 335 (see p. XVII–XIX of his *praefatio*).

[11] Paris. Suppl. gr. 764 may have been written in the late thirteenth century, Athen., Ἐθν. Βιβλ. 1502 was copied as late as the early seventeenth century. Felici [note 1 above], 61, listing ten manuscripts of the text, says that Paris. gr. 2091 contains "solo pochi capitoli"; it does, however, contain all the chapters from 134 (I 422 Bernard) on; likewise Vindob, med. gr. 26 contains the entire work, not "solo frammenti."

[12] For a detailed documentation of these points I must beg the reader's indulgence until my study of the manuscript tradition of Theophanes' works, which I have undertaken in preparation of a new edition, is published.

[13] A. P. Kousis has given a general idea of this compilation and published a number of excerpts in his "The Apotherapeu-

tains a chapter περὶ ἡμιτριταίου ("On semitertian fever") which is nothing more than the 142nd chapter of the treatise we are concerned with here.

In a number of manuscripts this therapeutic manual is accompanied by one or two[14] other texts, each of which is also transmitted independently from it. One is a treatise on foodstuffs of about thirty pages in print. It was published first by Ermerins[15] and a little later again by Ideler,[16] but from different versions: Ermerins' text ends in the middle of a chapter and omits all that follows in Ideler from p. 268, 24 τὰ στύφοντα on. Cohn showed that even Ideler's text is not complete, as there are manuscripts that divide the treatise into two books—p. 257, 7 to 268, 12 Ideler forming the first, p. 268, 13 to 281, 6 Ideler the second book respectively—and that each of these books has its own preface.[17] In addition to Cohn it should be noted, though, that although the majority of manuscripts of either version contain the preface to the first book, the number of manuscripts that have preserved the division into two books, and with it the preface to the second of them, is very small.

The first book deals with the nutritive values of foodstuffs under general headings, listing items which exhibit the respective qualities, and the first

seven chapters of the second book continue in the same fashion. The remainder of the second book forms a counterpart to what precedes in that here individual foodstuffs—first vegetables and after that animal products—are listed with remarks on their respective dietetic properties.

As Felici has pointed out,[18] the source of this text is Oribasius, *Collectiones medicae*, book three. This is true for all that is printed in Ermerins and even beyond that up to p. 270, 10 Ideler, for all the chapters, that is, dealing with specific qualities of foodstuffs. The long first chapter of our treatise is exceptional in that only very little of it is taken from the corresponding chapter in Oribasius (*Collectiones* 3, 15), whereas the bulk of the material must be derived from another source, which I have not been able to identify. From the second chapter on the text follows Oribasius exclusively and closely. The result is a considerably abbreviated version of his presentation consisting of literal borrowings for one half and of paraphrases of his text for the other. The arrangement of the chapters is, however, quite independent from the model.[19]

For the second part of the work, the chapters devoted to individual foodstuffs, the source is similarly Oribasius, *Collectiones*, books 1 and 2. The way in which the source is put to use is the same as before. Moreover, this time also the arrangement of the material follows the source with few exceptions. Many of Oribasius' chapters, however, have no equivalent in our treatise.[20]

---

tic of Theophilus according the (sic!) Laurentian Codex, plut. 75, 19" in Πρακτ.'Ακαδ.'Αθ., 19 (1944; publ. 1948), 35–45. The chapter referred to is contained on fol. 116ᵛ of the manuscript (42 Kousis).

[14] Felici (note 1 above), 61, maintains this to be the case only in Marc. gr. V 16 and Vatic. gr. 292. But there are at least six, perhaps even eight more manuscripts containing all three texts.

[15] Ermerins, 223–75 from Paris. gr. 2224; note, however, that his chapters 1–4 have nothing to do with our treatise (on which they follow in the manuscript) but were arbitrarily prefixed to it by the editor (see his note, p. 224).

[16] Ideler, II, 257–81, line 6 (281, lines 7–30 do not belong to this treatise, although they immediately follow it in this or a somewhat longer version in a number of manuscripts). Ideler's edition seems to have escaped Felici's notice. As the two other manuscripts she utilized (Marc. gr. V 16, Vatic. gr. 292) happen, like Ermerins' codex, to belong to the mutilated branch of the tradition, she is under the mistaken assumption that this treatise ends genuinely with σταφίδων 268, 24 Ideler.

[17] L. Cohn, "Bemerkungen zu den konstantinischen Sammelwerken," *BZ*, 9 (1900), 154–60 (only section 1, 154–58, deals with our texts), with edition of the prefaces to both books. Felici (note 1 above) is apparently unaware of this article, as she treats the preface of the first book (none of her manuscripts contains the second preface) as unpublished and gives a new edition of it, accompanied by an Italian translation, 67–69.—As early as 1498 Giorgio Valla published a Latin translation of this treatise in its full form, including both prefaces, from a manuscript (probably Mutinensis gr. 61 which belonged to Valla) in which Michael Psellus is credited with the authorship; see *Georgio Valla . . . Interprete. Hoc in volumine hec continentur, Nicephori logica, Georgij valle libellus de argumentis . . . Venetiis per Simonem Papiensem dictum Beuilaquam. 1498. Die ultimo Septembris, y IIᵛ-VIᵛ.* This translation was reprinted under Psellus' name in the fifteenth and sixteenth centuries. The false attribution to Psellus has lived

on to the present day. Not only Bloch (note 1 above), 561, listed it among his works but so does Hunger, "Medizin," 307 with note 24 (the texts are not "only similar" but identical, if one allows for contemporary editing).

[18] Felici, 69, following M. Formentin, "I codici greci di medicina nelle Tre Venezie," *Studi Bizantini e Neogreci*, 5 (1978), 93.

[19] Oribasius (ed. Raeder), I, 67–91. Our treatise uses the following chapters of book 3: 15, 17–20, 24, 25, 29, 30, 16, 8–10, 5, 6, 22, 23, 3, 13, 14, 11, 12, 2, 31–34, 27, 28, 26, 21. Book 3 of the *Collectiones* is repeated, except for the first chapter, in book 4 of Oribasius' *Synopsis ad Eustathium*, chapters 1–34 (123–45 Raeder), and with a number of minor abbreviations and transpositions in book 1, chapters 17–51, of his *Libri ad Eunapium* (332–47 Raeder). From a comparison, however, of the texts as printed in Raeder's and Ideler's editions, respectively, it is evident that our text is based on the *Collectiones*, not on the minor books, let alone on Aëtius of Amida, book 2, chapters 239–71, where Oribasius' text recurs again (Aetius [ed. Oliveri], I–IV [*CMG* VIII 1], 237–55).

[20] I, 4–65 Raeder. The following chapters are used: book 1: 15, 16, 5, 17, 18, 20–24, 28, 32, 35–42, 49–57, 60, 61, 64, 65; book 2: 1–4, 12, 13, 17, 22–28, 30, 31–36, 39–44, 46–50, 52–57. Felici goes at some length to explain the peculiarities of the *De alimentis* in Vatic. gr. 292, which follows Oribasius much more closely than the text does in her other two manuscripts, so that it looks almost like a simple excerpt from Oribasius, *Collectiones* 3. Her hypothesis is that the Vatican manuscript contains a first rough draft of the treatise, whereas the other codices present

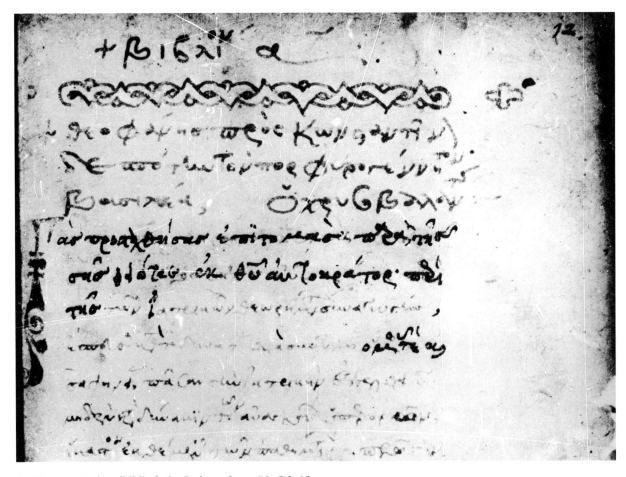

1. Munich, Staatsbibliothek. Cod. gr. 362, fol. III[v]

2. Vienna, Nationalbibliothek. Cod. med. gr. 50, fol. 12

The other text occurring occasionally together with the therapeutic manual is a pharmacopeia, in which the indication and preparation of a large number of composite medicines are described. It is as yet unedited. In the manuscript tradition the text has undergone much editing, sometimes to an extent that renders it hard to follow the thread of what appears to have been the original version. The complete text of this might fill some seventy to eighty pages in print. The material is divided into a number of sections, the first and longest dealing with the antidotes. The remaining sections treat troches, lozenges, various oils, desiccative powders, and potions. The last section, quite large again, is devoted to plasters. The individual chapters first discuss the indications of the particular medicine and then give a detailed account of its ingredients and the way in which it is prepared.[21]

So far, I cannot say much about the sources of this text and the way in which they were used.[22] But it is clear that Islamic medicine has not exerted a discernible influence on this treatise. In the manuscript tradition these three texts are combined in various ways. All three may—in different arrangements—be contained in the same manuscript, or a combination of any two of them. Of course each of them may appear in a codex without any of the two

others. The total number of manuscripts of the *De alimentis* which I know of is twenty-eight, of the *De remediis* twenty-four. If these figures are less impressive than that of extant copies of the *De curatione morborum*, they still show that these two texts as well must have circulated quite widely.

It has been noted long ago—but sunk back into oblivion again—that there are indications which link the dietetical treatise to the manual on therapy. Since the time of Peter Lambeck and Charles Du Cange it has been known that for either text there is one witness crediting a certain Theophanes with the authorship.[23] We will have to come back to this later. In 1891 George Costomiris[24] maintained that the pharmacopeia belonged to the same author's oeuvre, without, however, corroborating this assertion with any argument beyond the fact that the treatises are—in a number of manuscripts—transmitted side by side. Jeanselme's remarks, likewise, did not go into the matter deeply enough.[25] From an analysis of the four little prefaces, however—the two books of the dietetical treatise each have their own proem—it becomes quite probable that indeed these three treatises have been written by one and the same author.

"In the abridgment," the proem of the manual on therapy begins, "commissioned by your godliness, Emperor by the grace of God, concerning the collection of medical teachings, it was my endeavor to treat the entire art of healing as succinctly and clearly as it might be done, without—if possible—overlooking any important point, setting forth each disease, naming clearly, in the first place, their causes, in the next place the symptoms by which they will be recognized easily, subsequently the therapy, by which we will cure each of them *secundum artem*, beginning at the head because the holy rational soul is located there."

This is the entire proem. From this text it becomes evident: that the author had been working

---

the final version, both going back to the same author. Now Vatic. gr. 292 (fourteenth century) is a most peculiar copy not only of the *De alimentis* but of *De curatione morborum* and the other text accompanying it as well. It is also, as far as I can see, the only witness presenting these peculiarities in any of the treatises. As it is unlikely that the "first draft" of a text like the *De alimentis*, if ever it had been published, should have been preserved in a single manuscript four centuries younger than its compiler, I would rather suggest that Vatic. gr. 292 is, at least as far as our little corpus is concerned, the result of a medical man's attempt at creating a new work by rewriting these three texts. As he was aware of the source of the *De alimentis*, he placed a copy of that source at his side for reference and inspiration. The result is a sort of *Oribasius redivivus*. In his rewriting of the *De curatione morborum* his method had to be different, because there is no similar single source. His "new edition" of the third treatise is so different from the original that it renders it almost completely unrecognizable.

[21] In a number of manuscripts the first sections of the chapters are omitted. This was prompted by the example of chapters that never had a section specifying the indications of the *compositum* in question. This type of chapter was also traditional; compare e.g., Oribasius, *Synopsis* 3, 138 versus 3, 139 (both p. 103 Raeder).

[22] The method of compilation of this text is, it seems, eclectic, as in the manual on therapy. Paul (ed. Heiberg), book 7, chapters 11–20, and Oribasius, *Synopsis*, book 3 seem to be among its sources. They provide, however, only part of the material. Moreover it remains to be clarified whether the passages of our text that are more or less identical with either Paul or Oribasius were taken over directly from these authors or derived from an older common source.

[23] P. Lambeck, *Commentarii de Augustissima Bibliotheca Caesarea Vindobonensi*, VI (Vienna, 1674), 115–16, nr. 24, describing Vindob. med. gr. 50. C. Du Fresne, dominus Du Cange, *Glossarium ad scriptores mediae et infimae Graecitatis*, II (Lyon, 1688), in the preface to the Appendix (col. 1/2), quoting from Regius gr. 3496 (today Paris. gr. 2091) an anonymous text for its apology for the use of the vernacular. He adds that in Regius gr. 3502 (today Paris. gr. 1630) the author of the same text is called Theophanes.

[24] See note 1 above. Costomiris was the first to draw attention to this text in connection with Theophanes.

[25] E. Jeanselme, "Sur un aide-mémoire de thérapeutique byzantin contenu dans un manuscrit de la Bibliothèque Nationale de Paris" in *Mélanges Charles Diehl*, I (Paris, 1930), 147–70, particularly 164–67.

on commission of a Christian emperor, that he strove to be brief and clear, what the structure of the individual chapters is, and what the work begins with.[26] It also becomes clear that the author is not a man of many words.

Let us compare with this first the preface to the dispensatory,[27] which is equally short: "The science of antidotes, oils and plasters, which is difficult to understand for the general public, has been presented, though in this writing in a moderate fashion, which will be useful not only during travels but also during sojourns elsewhere. Although in comparison with the supernatural dimensions of our Emperor's learnedness/eloquence (λογιότης) it will appear unworthy, still, since it is of use for the public, I will—beginning with the most important and greatest antidote, I mean theriac—treat subsequently also the remaining medicines."

Again here an author is writing to an emperor, whose erudition is emphasized. If it was underlined in the first preface that the presentation would be brief and clear, it is stressed here that a subject which is hard to understand for most people has been set forth in a comprehensible manner. This will prove to be of use especially in situations in which reliable professional advice may not be easily obtained, as on travels. In conclusion it is said that theriac will be dealt with first, because it is the most important antidote.

This last remark is a striking parallel with the preface of the manual on therapy. In both cases the remark is superfluous as in either book the arrangement of the material has not been devised by the author but simply follows a traditional pattern. The fact that in the foreword to the pharmacopeia a structurally identical remark is made in exactly the same place as in the introduction to the therapeutical treatise strongly suggests that both prefaces—and consequently both treatises—are products of the same mind.

The prefaces of the two books on foods at first sight make a quite different impression. The proem to the first book[28] reads:

> This again is a work resulting from your forethought and a commission originating from your noble design and love to man. Constantine, greatest and most godly

Emperor, that laymen should know in the same manner as the wise and learned/people of high station (ἐλλόγιμοι) how to use the best and useful foodstuffs and again how to be on their guard and to avoid those that are opposite to them. No one who is able to think a little will criticize us if he sees that we use in the present work words and phrases that carry the odor of the market and the street. For it is in no way because we are ignorant of the best words which are most commonly used among the Greeks that we use barbarous and distorted words—that would be quite absurd even for people who are but moderately educated—but in order that nothing might escape or remain unknown to him who has no share whatsoever in Greek education, we decided to transmit to him what is to be known and understood from the present writing in the most commonly used spoken language. We will put at the beginning the diet producing healthy humors, then the diet that makes neither slender nor fat, next to this the diet that is easily digested. . . .

After this follows the enumeration of the remaining chapters of the first book.

The preface of the second book reads:[29]

> Those foodstuffs, most serene and excellent Emperor Constantine, that belong to a wholesome diet, and the consumption of which is neither unfamiliar nor disgusting nor unsuited, have been made known in brief fashion in the book before this as completely and clearly as was possible. Since some short points remain to be dealt with which belong to a treatment of therapy rather than of hygiene—for instance which foods have a warming and desiccative effect, and so, according to the oppositions, those whose effect is cooling and moisturizing, which are easy of digestion, which are hard to digest and pass slowly through the body, and which even may cause certain diseases, like the foodstuffs that do damage to the head—I will also treat these for you. They are very short and would by themselves not fill a book. But if to them is added [the description] of the natural qualities of the individual foods this book might perhaps become even more voluminous than the first. We will try then, with the help of God and adhering to the former aim—I mean the layman-like and rather coarse presentation, in order to let nothing remain unknown to the common man, who has not tasted of Greek education at all—to deal with them also in the briefest manner.

What at first appears quite different, upon close examination reveals great similarity. The preface to the first book touches on three points: the imperial commission (a new commission!), the comprehensibility of the presentation for the general public, and the arrangement of the material. Exactly the same points are made in the preface to the manual on therapy and also—though in a different sequence—in the remarks introducing the

---

[26] The preface to our manual on therapy is echoed, including the rationale for the beginning at the head, in the prefatory remarks to books 1 and 2 of Leo's *Synopsis* (89, 109 Ermerins).

[27] *Editio princeps* with Italian translation by Felici (note 1 above), 63.

[28] Edited by Cohn (note 17 above), 156, and again, with Italian translation, by Felici (note 1 above), 67–69.

[29] Edited by Cohn (note 17 above), 156–57.

dispensatory. But it looks like the author here has been trying to produce a longer text. The *topos* about the language of the work, for instance, which very appropriately serves to emphasize the point that the book can be understood by anyone, is developed rather broadly. And instead of summarizing the first chapter of the book he bores his readers with a tedious enumeration of all the chapters. Evidently the author had difficulties in varying this preface. He tried to write something different, he tried to write more, but he was unable to produce more than a somewhat extended version of his already known set of ideas. The introduction to the second book with its reference to the first is much more felicitous. The idea, too, that on the one hand what is actually left to be dealt with is hardly enough to form a separate book, whereas on the other hand, if still another section is added, the book may end up exceeding even the size of the first, is a pretty device.

But by emphasis again on the comprehensiveness, conciseness, and clarity of the first book, it reiterates a theme that has played a conspicuous role in the introductory remarks to the manual on therapy. Clarity and brevity are underscored still another time, as characteristics of the second book as well at the end of its preface. Finally, the arrangement of the material is not forgotten; it has found a placc in the middle section and consists in a listing of some of the chapters, which reminds us of the long list at the end of the preface to the first book.

So this proem again moves in the same narrow circle of ideas as the others. The close resemblance of all four texts seems to me to suggest that they were all written by the same man, and consequently that all three treatises are indeed fruits of the same pen.

The reference to an earlier imperial commission in the opening phrase of the preface to the first book on foodstuffs gives us a hint as to the sequence in which the treatises have been written. For now that we know that all have been written by one and the same man, we understand that this remark refers to the manual on therapy and the dispensatory. Apparently these were composed— at about the same time—before the dietetical treatise. This indication is confirmed, moreover, by the observation that the dispensatory is a necessary complement to the manual on therapy, since in that treatise composite medicines are frequently prescribed of which just the names are quoted. The ingredients, however, are never given, nor is the

preparation of these medicines described. It seems impossible to me that this characteristic—which, of course, is caused by the peculiarities of the sources of the work—should have escaped the notice of the author, who, if not a man of much rhetoric, was by all means a very competent and conscientious specialist. So the dispensatory is called for if full use is to be made of the manual on therapy.[30]

Whether a separate treatise on composite prescriptions was envisaged from the outset or the idea developed during the writing of the therapeutical treatise, we cannot say. At any rate, the dispensatory and the manual on therapy form a dyad which was followed by the work on foods at a later stage. The idea of dividing the material of the dietetical work into two books may perhaps even have been prompted by the treatment of curative medicine in two separate writings.

The remark in the proem to the dispensatory that it will prove its usefulness on travels and during stays abroad clearly indicates that the book is intended to be used by laymen. Equally, the people referred to in the prefaces of the books on foodstuffs as lacking education would not seem to be professionals who did not receive sufficient literary

---

[30] Mainly for this reason Felici, 64–66, considers the *De remediis* not a separate treatise but a mere section of the *De curatione morborum*. Its separation might be due to a deliberate replacement of this too complicated part of the work by an abridged version of itself (represented by "the last chapters of the Vienna manuscripts used by Bernard for his edition" of *De curatione morborum*). It is more likely, however, she continues, that the *De remediis* became separated from the work it belonged to simply because its little preface made it look like a separate writing. The awkward gap thus caused motivated some *anonymus* to put together a new section containing the missing information and attach that to the text. First, however, neither does Bernard's edition contain any addition to Martius' text at the end of the *De curatione morborum*, nor do the Vienna manuscripts. Secondly, there are at the end of *De curatione morborum* a number of chapters, 284–97 (II 356–66 Bernard), that deal very tersely with the preparation of a few *composita*, mainly cathartics. Only these could be compared with the *De remediis*. The differences, however, in the number of drugs treated and the treatment itself, as well as the very inconsistent transmission of these chapters in the manuscripts, show clearly that they are neither an abridged version of the *De remediis* nor a makeshift for it but simply an accretion of the text developed in its manuscript tradition. The fact, on the other hand, that Felici, 66, compares the treatment of animal bites in the two treatises, shows that apparently she considers all from *De curatione* chapter 261 (II 290 Bernard) on as an equivalent of *De remediis*. But this section quite definitely belongs to the original text of *De curatione*, continuing a tradition of such sections in similar treatises (cf. e.g. Dioscorides, *De simplicibus*, 2, 120–68 [in Dioscorides (ed. Wellmann), III, 299–317]; Oribasius, *Ad Eunapium* 3, 63–72 [430–32 Raeder]; Aetius XIII [ed. Zervos], 268–92; Paul V, 1–58 (ed. Heiberg, II, 5–3g). The difference in treatment is due to the different point of view that governs each of the treatises. The remaining arguments Felici offers for her assumption are also not convincing.

training but rather people who are no experts in medicine.

The introductory remark to the therapy manual gives no indication about the public for which the booklet is written, except perhaps for the phrase that the symptoms of the diseases will be described in a way that will facilitate diagnosis. The close link, however, which exists between the manual on therapy and the dispensatory would suggest, in my opinion, that this treatise is meant to be used by laymen as well.

To sum up what we have been able to establish so far, we can say that we are dealing with a group of three interrelated treatises, intended for the general public, all three written by the same author on commission of the emperor.

Who is the author of these popular little books? Our handbooks call him Theophanes Nonnus. In doing so they follow John Stephen Bernard, who prepared the second of the two editions of the manual on therapy. It was Bernard who established a link between the two names under which the author had been known before.

In the edition of 1568, the author had been called Nonus (sic!), without the Theophanes, in accordance with what Jeremy Martius had found in the manuscript he had been using. Martius thought that this was a name of the old Roman type of counting praenomina like Quintus, Sextus, etc. And he seriously asked himself whether this Nonus had been a Roman by birth or just someone who had been given a Roman name. The misjudgment about the setting of the text implied in this consideration becomes even more striking when we read in the same preface that he opts for the son of Constantine X Ducas (reigned 1059–67) as the *porphyrogenitus* who commissioned the work.[31]

A little over a hundred years after Martius' edition Peter Lambeck in his description of the Greek medical manuscripts in Vienna made known that in one of the manuscripts of the text belonging to the imperial library the name of the author was given as Theophanes. Lambeck, however, did not identify the text of this manuscript as the treatise edited by Martius. Since most scholars, of course, knew about the work from Martius' edition rather than Lambeck's catalog, the author continued to be known and referred to as Nonus. Occasionally "Nonnus" occurs, and rarely "Nonius"—a rather

oversophisticated interpretation of the "Noni" in the title of the first edition.[32]

John Freind in his *History of Physick* seems to have been the first to take notice of the other name mentioned in connection with the text, without, however, discussing the problem arising from the discrepancy.[33] This was done at length by Bernard in the preface to his edition.[34] He proposes an interesting solution: "Theophanes" he says is the actual name of the author, whereas "Nonus" is an honorary title he had been given. It should be written "Nonnus," no matter what the manuscript may read. This honorific title used to be given to men and women of exemplary piety in ancient times in Egypt. That the author of this treatise has by all means a claim to such a religious title is apparent, Bernard says, from the fact that, speaking in a chapter about the laurel and the fig tree, he does not call them the sacred trees of Apollo and Artemis but prefers to say they are the sacred trees of the sun, a way of putting it which is much more appropriate for a Christian writer.[35] Similarly in another chapter, where he quotes a phrase from Paul of Aegina, he changes the improper κοτταβισμός into the less offensive γυμνάσια.[36] Should the reader not be convinced by this explanation but prefer to take "Nonnus" as a polite designation like "dominus," a meaning which is attested as Du Canges has shown—but in his dictionary of medieval Latin as Bernard himself points out!—this would be equally possible since in Byzantine letters doctors are frequently addressed as κῦρ ὅδε and referred to in the titles of their works in the same manner. So it is perfectly possible that the author of this text should have been designated in a similar way. On the basis of this remarkable argumentation the author has been called Theophanes Nonnus by everyone since Bernard's time.

In view of these various explanations and interpretations it seems advisable to take a fresh look at the original source material. Although in most manuscripts the therapeutical treatise lacks any indication of authorship, there are altogether four

[31] Page)(ij of the *Epistola dedicatoria*.

[32] For Lambeck see note 23 above. The various forms of the surname are mentioned by Bernard, p. X of the *praefatio*.

[33] J. Freind, *The History of Physick from the Time of Galen to the Beginning of the Sixteenth Century*, I (London, 1725), 253–57.

[34] P. VII–XI of the *praefatio*.

[35] *De curatione morborum* 260 (259 Bernard says by mistake; II 286–88 Bernard).

[36] *De curatione morborum* 185 (II 92 Bernard).

different names connected with the text in the manuscript tradition. As we have seen, in one manuscript each the name of the author is given as Theophanes or Nonus. In several other manuscripts two more names occur: Psellus and Oribasius.

The last two attributions are easily discarded. Constantine/Michael Psellus was a well-known polymath. There is hardly a subject he did not write about, and it must be admitted that usually he is well informed. He contributed to medical literature as well. I have no way of knowing whether the recension of Symeon Seth's manual of foodstuffs that bears Psellus' name[37] really has anything to do with him. As long as the manuscript tradition of that work has not been thoroughly investigated it seems best to be sceptical. But there is no reason to doubt that the *Carmen de re medica*[38] is indeed a product of his pen. And on reading this poem it becomes evident that Psellus was a man of encyclopedic learning and a brilliant writer but that he was not a doctor. In this didactic poem a layman imparts to laymen some rudiments of medical science as an element of their general education. It is not a primer for future physicians. On this general level Psellus was able to contribute to medical literature. An actual manual of medicine on a professional level, as our treatise in spite of its limitations doubtless is, lay beyond his qualifications. That, on the other hand, an anonymous medical writing should have been attributed to Psellus is not surprising if we consider his reputation.

Finally, if Psellus' name does indeed appear in a number of manuscripts, it has to be taken into account that all these codices belong to the same family. So we are not dealing here with a widespread tradition of venerable antiquity but just with a comparatively late reader's or scribe's ambitious conjecture.

No one will seriously consider Oribasius, whose name appears in several codices in the title of our treatise, as the author of this text. Moreover all manuscripts naming Oribasius belong to the same family and even to one of the two sub-families into which it is divided, which makes it clear that again this name is a relatively recent addition, based on the observation, of course, that the opening phrase of the preface is a quotation from that author.

Let us come back to Nonnus. Bernard's ingenuous interpretation will not satisfy us any more. So we will have to start again with Nonus, the name by which the author was usually referred to during the first two centuries of his printed existence.

This indication of authorship is indeed contained in the Augsburg manuscript on which the first edition was based. So Martius was by all means justified in publishing the text under this name. It was less appropriate, though perfectly understandable from the point of view of sales promotion, to qualify the author as "medicus clarissimus." This man was not so well known, after all. Actually, no one had ever heard of him before. Of course this made him all the more interesting. Every new figure in Byzantine and Greek literature was readily welcomed in an age that was still very incompletely informed about what had actually come down of this literature.

However, there is something special about this indication of authorship in the manuscript. The name does not form part of or an addition to the title proper of the treatise (fol. 6). Nor is it contained in the relevant lemma of the short table of contents which the scribe who contributed the lesser part to the manuscript has given a place on the verso facing the beginning of the text (fol. III^v, see fig. 1). There the text is likewise nameless. The name appears only in a note which a hand that does not recur elsewhere in the manuscript has added still above that table of contents. It reads: νόνου φιλοσοφικὸν μετὰ ἰατρικοῦ. This note has been written by someone well known: Andreas Darmarios, who between 1558 and 1587 copied innumerable manuscripts and sold still more on extended travels from Italy to Flanders and Spain. In 1566 he is known to have spent some time in Augsburg.[39]

His merchandise was not always beyond suspicion. It is known that a number of times he was unable to resist the temptation to offer his customers—whom he knew to be always keen on new discoveries—some authors whose claim to literary fame was not founded any better than that of, say, Aristeas or Dionysius Areopagita.[40]

---

[37] See lastly Hunger, "Medizin," 307.
[38] Ideler, I, 203–43.

[39] For Darmarios see *Repertorium der griechischen Kopisten 800–1600*, I: *Handschriften aus Bibliotheken Großbritanniens*, Österr. Akad. Wiss., Veröffentlichungen der Kommission für Byzantinistik, 3.1, A: *Verzeichnis der Kopisten*, von E. Gamillscheg und D. Harlfinger (Vienna, 1981), 29, where the relevant literature is given. Monac. gr. 362 is not listed among Darmarios' manuscripts; Prof. O. Kresten very kindly confirms my identification of Darmarios' hand in this codex.
[40] See O. Kresten, "Phantomgestalten in der byzantinischen Literaturgeschichte: Zu vier Titelfälschungen des 16. Jahrhunderts," *JÖB*, 25 (1976), 207–22, especially 213 ff.

So what are we to think of Nonus? As indicated above, the Augsburg manuscript is the only one containing this name. Not even the manuscript from which it was copied[41] has it. Darmarios cannot, therefore, have found this name in the manuscript tradition of our text. He must have taken it from some other source or fabricated it himself. As a name Νόνος is not attested. What is doubtless meant here is Νόννος. Bernard was quite correct in regarding this orthographical peculiarity as irrelevant. We are familiar with this name mainly through Nonnus of Panopolis, the Egyptian epic poet. From literary sources, inscriptions, papyri and seals we know of quite a number of people of this name from the second century A.D.[42] down to the early mid-Byzantine period. Nonnus of Panopolis seems to have been the only writer among them. Of a medical author of that name we hear nothing.

The name Νόννος associated with this particular treatise, however, raises still another improbability. One of the sources used for the compilation of this text is the work of Paul of Aegina, written in the middle of the seventh century. At this period the name Νόννος was past the peak of its popularity. I know of only two Νόννοι—at least as far as seals are concerned—who lived in the seventh century or around 700, respectively,[43] whereas for the earlier periods the name is much more often attested. After the early eighth century the name disappears altogether. It is therefore most improbable that this text should indeed be the authentic work of a late seventh- or eighth-, let alone ninth-century writer who is otherwise completely unknown and who, in addition to that, is supposed to have borne a name that was practically extinct in his time.

Moreover, where could Darmarios have found this information? Is it conceivable that he might still have been able to use sources that are lost to us today? No, there can be no doubt that we are dealing here with another of Darmarios' falsifications.

It is done most dexterously and quite clumsily at the same time. On one hand, in an age that was much interested in everything connected with late antique philosophy and "theosophy," of which Egypt was considered the principal focus, Darmarios could be sure to arouse interest with a name and an indication of content that pointed in that direction. Less felicitous was the idea to label this of all texts as φιλοσοφικὸν μετὰ ἰατρικοῦ, since anyone who read but one page of it would realize that the philosophical substance of this text is nil. Perhaps the Augsburg city fathers lacked the time for a proper examination so that they quickly bought what might turn out to be a spectacular find. Darmarios, at any rate, achieved his aim.

We are left, then, with the testimony of the Vienna codex. From the transcript of that manuscript which he obtained from Vienna, Bernard learned that the title of the work read not only Θεοφάνης πρὸς Κωνσταντῖνον δεσπότην τὸν πορφυρογέννητον βασιλέα, as Lambeck had written, but Θεοφάνης πρὸς Κωνσταντῖνον δεσπότην τὸν πορφυρογέννητον βασιλέα, ὁ Χρυσοβαλάντης. Whether Lambeck simply forgot to report this or scholarly vanity induced him to suppress what he did not understand need not concern us. Bernard, at any rate, did not know what to make of this and asked John Bolla, who had transcribed the manuscript for him, for his opinion.[44]

Bolla wrote him that he thought this was a personal name, perhaps the name of a scribe. As to what the name might be derived from, one could think of the monastery τοῦ Χρυσοβαλάντου, mentioned by (Pseudo-)Codinus,[45] although this was not very likely. More appropriately it might be derived from χρυσόβαλα or χρυσοβάλανον—that is, "golden suppository"—which would make a perfect epithet for a doctor. Finally, Bolla asks, could it not be an epithet of Theophanes which was added by someone subsequently? The comma preceding the name might indicate this. Bernard could not bring himself to like any of these ideas. So he reported them but left the matter at that.

If one looks at the manuscript,[46] which is of the fourteenth century, one realizes at once that this second name is not a later addition. The entire title has been written—in red—by the first hand. It is

---

[41] Laurent. Antinori 101 in all probability. Felici (note 1 above), 66, maintains that in Vatic. gr. 292 the *De alimentis* is attributed to "Teofane Nonno." The manuscript, however, contains no indication of authorship with any of the three treatises we are dealing with here. In all three cases the names have been supplied by the catalogers (see G. Mercati-P. Franchi de'Cavalieri, *Codices Vaticani Graeci*, I: *Codices 1–329* [Rome, 1923], 406).

[42] *SIG*, II, 559, no. 847.

[43] See G. Zacos-A. Veglery, *Byzantine Lead Seals*, I.2 (Bâle, 1972), 745, no. 1183 (Νόννου, seventh century) and V. Laurent, *Le corpus des sceaux de l'empire byzantin*, V.1 (Paris, 1963), 744–45, no. 942 (Νόννου μητροπολίτου, seventh/eighth century; in his publication of the Orghidan seals collection Laurent had dated this seal to the seventh century).

[44] Bernard's *praefatio*, XIII–XIV.

[45] He is thinking of the story in the Πάτρια Κωνσταντινουπόλεως 3.76 (*Scriptores originum Constantinopolitanarum*, ed. Th. Preger, II [Leipzig, 1907], 243) which he knew of through Du Cange's dictionary.

[46] Vindob. med. gr. 50, fol. 12; see fig. 2.

divided into three lines. The little fenestra between βασιλέα and ὁ Χρυσοβαλάντης in the third line is an indication neither for a subsequent addition nor for the omission of an illegible word which the model of the manuscript had in that place. It is simply due to the care devoted to the design of the title. The scribe wanted the last line to begin and end flush with the two above it. In order to obtain this graphic effect he moved apart the words in the line, joining, of course, the article to its noun. Likewise, the final punctuation does not stand in the margin by accident, because, say, an addition to the title turned out to be longer than was anticipated. A comparison with the little cross standing in the margin before the title will make clear that it was quite deliberately put in the place where it stands.

Finally, if ὁ Χρυσοβαλάντης were to be a later addition, βασιλέα would have to be followed by final punctuation. But what we see there is a comma, and nothing else has ever stood there; there are no traces of alterations. So the entire title, as it stands, must be considered genuine. In itself it should not cause the difficulties Bernard and Bolla had in interpreting it. The beginning and end of this title give us, in a typical Byzantine hyperbaton, the Christian name and the surname of the author. So, according to this manuscript, the author of the three treatises we are concerned with here seems to have been called Θεοφάνης Χρυσοβαλάντης.

There seems to be no trace of a Byzantine family bearing this name. But there is a family with a name that is very similar: the Χρυσοβαλαντίται.[47] Several members of this family are mentioned in sources of the eleventh to thirteenth centuries.[48] It could, therefore, be that our author was a member of the Χρυσοβαλαντίτης family.

Another possibility is that our Theophanes was somehow affiliated with the monastery τοῦ Χρυσοβαλάντου, in Constantinople. No hospital is mentioned in connection with this convent, but among its churches and chapels was one dedicated to St. Michael, and another dedicated to St. Panteleemon. This could reflect the existence of a hospital which may have been too insignificant to attract general attention. If such a hospital did indeed exist, Theophanes may have been given his surname because he served as a physician there.[48a]

As it is somewhat awkward that only a single manuscript should have preserved the name of the author of these relatively popular treatises,[49] it cannot be but welcome that at least his first name is confirmed by a second witness, referred to already by Du Cange.[50] Paris. gr. 1630 (fourteenth century) contains, among other medical texts, a fragment of the preface to the first book of the De alimentis (fol. 27ᵛ). It comprises only five lines and a half, the first sentence. As the remainder of the page is left blank, the model from which this text was copied seems to have been equally incomplete. Next to the title of this fragment, however, stands, in the outer margin but copied by the same scribe, a name: Θεοφάν(ους). It is hardly conceivable that this neither too common nor particularly prominent name should appear in connection with two different treatises, originating with the same author, by mere coincidence.

There is, to my knowledge, no testimony to the person, time of life, or work of Theophanes Chrysobalantes/Chrysobalantites except the treatises themselves. It is only a scholarly tradition by which our author is linked to Constantine VII. Martius thought that the son of Constantine X Ducas might have been the *porphyrogenitus* who commissioned the work, only because the prince's father was a patron of learning.[51] A hundred years later, Lambeck[52]

[47] I would like to thank professors A. Kazhdan and N. Oikonomidès for supplying references to members of this family.

[48] John Chrysobalantites, eleventh century: V. Laurent, *Le corpus des sceaux de l'empire byzantin*, II (Paris, 1981), 92–93, no. 200 (in the form Χρ(υ)σ[ο]βαλαντ(ίτης)); Constantine Chrysobalantites, second half of the eleventh century: *ibid*, 482–83, no. 910 (in the form Χρυσ[ο]βαλαντ(ί)τ[ης]); NN Chrysobalantites, mid-eleventh century, perhaps identical with the foregoing: referred to by Psellus, *ep. 64* (Μιχαὴλ Ψελλοῦ Ἱστορικοὶ λόγοι, ἐπιστολαὶ καὶ ἄλλα ἀνέκδοτα, ed. K. N. Sathas, Μεσαιωνικὴ βιβλιοθήκη, V [Venice-Paris, 1876], 296); Theodore Chrysobalantites, probably late eleventh or early twelfth century: N. Wilson-J. Darrouzès, "Restes du cartulaire de Hiéra-Xerochoraphion," *REB*, 26 (1968) 5–47, no. 9, p. 34, line 34 of the document (in the form Χρυ(σο)βαλαντίτ(ης)); Anna Chrysobalantitu, thirteenth century: mentioned in a document prepared by Demetrius Chomatenus, *Analecta sacra et classica spicilegio Solesmensi parata*, ed. J. B. Pitra, VI (Paris-Rome, 1891), 420.

[48a] For the monastery see R. Janin, *Géographie ecclésiastique*, I, 3: *Les églises et les monastères*, 2nd. ed. (Paris, 1969), 66, 154, 350, 387, 540–41.

[49] The testimony of the Vienna codex does not, however, have to be mistrusted for the sole reason that so far it is the only witness bearing this name, especially since Chrysobalantes/Chrysobalantites is not a name that would have come easily to the mind of anyone wishing to christen an anonymous text.

[50] See note 23 above. Cohn (note 17 above), 155, also referred to this manuscript as it is the model for many of the texts contained in Berlin, Deutsche Staatsbibliothek, Phillipp, 1566, including this fragment (together with the name) from *De alimentis* (fol. 32ᵛ).

[51] Unlikely as Martius' suggestion is in itself, it is ruled out by the fact that we now know that this prince's name was probably not Constantine but Constantius, see D. J. Polemis, *The Doukai* (London, 1968), 48.

[52] Not in the text but only in the indexes of his catalog of the Vienna medical manuscripts (note 23 above), 213, 215.

suggested that the *porphyrogenitus* and imperial patron of learning *par excellence*, Constantine VII, was the addressee of the little book. This identification seemed so obvious that without further discussion it was universally accepted and Theophanes was even promoted to the rank of personal physician of the ailing emperor.[53] In view of the complete lack of external evidence for this identification it seems useful to look in the texts themselves for any indications that might confirm it. In this repsect it is of interest to pay attention to the historical perspective into which Theophanes' works and his manual on therapy in particular are placed. The preface to this work begins with the phrase Τὰς προσταχθείσας ἐπιτομὰς παρὰ τῆς σῆς θειότητος, ἐκ Θεοῦ αὐτοκράτορ. . . . These are exactly the same words with which the preface to Oribasius' *Collectiones medicae* begin, only the address is, of course, different there: αὐτοκράτορ Ἰουλιανέ. Since Theophanes' treatise is not based on Oribasius' *Collectiones* at all, this is not simply the first of many borrowings from a plagiarized source. These words are quoted in order to highlight the parallel situation: Theophanes is writing on commission of His Most Christian Majesty as the great Oribasius had been doing on commission of Julian.[54] Theophanes is the new Oribasius. On commission of the ruler he writes what—by virtue of this commission—constitutes, so to speak, the official contribution to medical literature of his time.

The immense discrepancy in size and substance which exists between his modest treatise and Oribasius' vast work cannot have escaped Theophanes. So the claim implied in this quotation could seem foolishly arrogant or simply in bad taste. But it is not impossible that this program did not originate with Theophanes but was thought up by his patron, who saw in Julian's patronage over the celebrated work of Oribasius an example worth imitating in his own patronage of letters. One must admit that of all *porphyrogeniti* Constantine VII would be the most likely to have devised such an ambitious concept.[55]

The fact that none of the three treatises shows influences from the Islamic orient may also be significant. To be sure, much is still to be investigated in the field of Islamic influence on Byzantine medicine. But as far as we can see at the moment, the large-scale importation of Islamic material by the way of translations did not begin before the end of the tenth century.[56] Of course, this cannot be but an argument *ex silentio*. Still the absence of any Islamic influences may be a slight indication that our texts were compiled prior to that period.

A final consideration regards the first name of the author. As we have seen in the case of Νόννος, given names have their history. For the period from 500 A.D. to the middle of the fifteenth century I know from various sources—seals, manuscripts, archival documents—of fifty-two men named Theophanes whose time of life is more or less certain. Of these, thirty-six lived before, sixteen after the year 1000. The years from about 650 to 900 form the period of greatest popularity of the name: twenty-eight of the fifty-two people bearing it lived in these centuries.

In addition to sheer frequency, it is important to consider the social position of these men. Of the thirty-six namesakes of our author who lived before the year 1000, twenty-four were government officials, two bishops and six monks (four cannot be assigned to any specific group). Of the sixteen people attested for the centuries after the year 1000, only two were government officials, two seem to have belonged to the secular clergy, four were bishops, and five monks (three cannot be assigned). So it looks like "Theophanes" was a generally popular, indeed very popular, given name in the late seventh, eighth, and ninth centuries. Its popularity

---

[53] See e.g., Théodoridès (note 1 above), G. K. Pournaropoulos, Θεοφάνης ὁ Νόννος, ὁ ἀρχίατρος τοῦ αὐτοκράτορος Κωνσταντίνου Ζ΄ τοῦ Πορφυρογεννήτου, Πρακτικὰ τῆς Ἑλληνικῆς Ἑταιρείας Ἱστορίας τῆς Ἰατρικῆς, and simultaneously in the monthly Ἀκαδημαϊκὴ Ἰατρική, 28 (1964; accessible to me only in an offprint without the original pagination) and, more cautiously, Felici (note 1 above), 59, who, however, in turn declares him to have been "massima autorità in campo medico."

[54] This is emphasized also by the echo of the title of Oribasius' main work—Ἰατρικαὶ συναγωγαί—in the words with which Theophanes continues his preface: περὶ τῆς τῶν ἰατρικῶν θεωρημάτων συναγωγῆς. Note that the phrase ἐκ Θεοῦ αὐτοκράτορ is perhaps not only a standard expression but may be used in order to put emphasis on the fact that the present work is not flawed by an unacceptable religious persuasion like that of Julian and Oribasius.

[55] The phrase τὸ ὑπερφυὲς τῆς τοῦ αὐτοκράτορος ἡμῶν λογιότητος, which occurs in the preface to the dispensatory (Felici, [note 1 above] 63, line 8 f. of the Greek text) may refer to the actual learnedness of the addressee, in which case Constantine VII again would be the most likely *porphyrogenitus* to be referred to in this way. But as λογιότης from about the fourth century A.D. on can also be used as a mere amplification in addressing or referring to people politely (see e.g., Basil the Great, *ep. 1* [PG 32, 221B]; Isidore of Pelusium, *ep. V 125* [PG 78, 1396D]) is too weak to be used even as an indicium.

[56] The first major work to be translated seems to have been Abū Ǧaʿfar's Ἐφόδια τοῦ ἀποδημοῦντος, cf. Hunger, "Medizin," 306. (Constantine of Rhegion, who produced the Greek version, and Constantine the African, who translated the work into Latin, are not, however, one and the same person.)

declined in the tenth century and after the year 1000 it very quickly became exclusively a religious name. Again this is but an indication that our Theophanes is more likely to have lived in the tenth century, in which this name was still relatively common, than in the eleventh. All the more so since, if Constantine VII was not his patron, the next possible candidate for this role[57] would in theory be Constantine, the son of Michael VII Ducas and fiancé of Anna Comnena. But the fact that, even allowing for Byzantine rhetorical exuberance, it is hardly conceivable that a prince who may not have

reached even the age of twenty-one could have been addressed in the way the *porphyrogenitus* of our texts is, rules out this possibility as well. The further down we go, however, the less probable becomes the figure of a layman named Theophanes.

These are the only indicia at our disposal for narrowing down the lifetime of the author. None of them provides a cogent proof. Still, they point in the same direction: that Θεοφάνης Χρυσοβαλάντης/Χρυσοβαλαντίτης indeed lived in the tenth century. We may, therefore, with reasonable confidence continue to consider his writings as the contribution to medical literature from the circle of Constantine VII Porphyrogenitus.

Freie Universität, Berlin

---

[57] It is totally improbable that Constantine VIII, who of course was a *porphyrogenitus*, could have initiated these works.

THE IMAGE OF THE MEDICAL DOCTOR IN BYZANTINE LITERATURE OF THE TENTH TO TWELFTH CENTURIES

A. Kazhdan

One Late Roman emperor, Theodosius II, and two Byzantine *basileis*, Basil I and John II, died from hunting accidents.[1] Since it is so early, I will leave aside the story of Theodosius' death and concentrate on the two cases that took place in 886 and 1143 respectively. Both are minutely described in contemporary (or almost contemporary) sources that do not differ substantially from each other. Basil is said to have been lifted up by a huge deer that pushed his antlers under the emperor's belt and carried him off; once he had been released by a servant who managed to cut the belt, the emperor ordered the man to be arrested, as if he had drawn his sword to murder the prince. "After suffering severe internal pains and hemorrhage of the stomach, nine days later he paid our common debt . . . leaving his scepter to his sons." Such is the version of the Life of Patriarch Euthymius. It is generally supported by both the so-called *Logothetes-Sippe* and the anonymous chronicler widely known as Joseph Genesius.[2]

Two Byzantine historians, John Cinnamus and Nicetas Choniates, relate Emperor John's end. The emperor was out hunting in Cilicia; he encoun-

tered a boar, wielded a spear, but awkwardly touched a quiver full of poisoned arrows and wounded his wrist, which became inflamed. The doctors who were called in discussed what should be done and decided to lance the swelling. The treatment failed and John died.[3]

There is a substantial difference between the two stories: the authors of the tenth century make no mention of physicians. None of the chroniclers speaks even briefly of doctors who tended the dying emperor, although they describe the fatal hemmorhage of the stomach. The twelfth-century authors, on the other hand, are very explicit as to the role of the *paides iatron* (Cinnamus) or *iatroi, asklepiadai* (Choniates). "To some it seemed best to lance the swelling, but its unripeness disquieted the others, and they preferred that it be relieved in some other way. But as it seems that he had to fare ill, the opinion for surgery carried the day." And so forth.

Now we face the problem. Is this difference between the two stories a random phenomenon, a reflection of personal and incidental tendencies only, or are we entitled to suggest that the place of the doctor in Byzantine society changed between the first half of the tenth century, when the chroniclers were able to ignore the doctors' call to Basil's deathbed, and the end of the twelfth century, when Choniates and Cinnamus centered the story of John's demise on the doctors' attitude? Let us con-

---

[The reader is referred to the list of abbreviations at the end of the volume.]

[1] R. Guilland, *Etudes byzantines* (Paris, 1959), 11 f.

[2] *Vita Euthymii Patriarchae CP*, ed. and trans. P. Karlin-Hayter (Brussels, 1970), 2–5; Leo Grammaticus, *Chronographia*, ed. I. Bekker (Bonn, 1842), 262.1–11; Josephus Genesius, *Regum libri quattuor*, ed. A. Lesmüller-Werner and I. Thurn (Berlin and New York, 1978), 91.29–32. The name "Genesius" has been added by a later hand in the single manuscript; "Joseph" is the result of arbitrary identifications. The episode is completely disregarded by the Life of St. Theophano, which asserts that Basil died from "ailment and old age" (*BHG*, 1794: E. Kurtz, *Zwei griechische Texte über die hl. Theophano* [St. Petersburg, 1898], 12.20–21, 14.4).

[3] Ioannes Cinnamus, *Epitome*, ed. A. Meineke (Bonn, 1836), 24 f. (see John Kinnamos, *Deeds of John and Manuel Comnenus*, trans. Ch. M. Brand [New York, 1976], 27–29); Nicetas Choniates, *Historia*, ed. I. A. van Dieten (Berlin, New York, 1975), 40 f. Both authors have, probably, used a common source. On this episode, R. Browning, "The Death of John II Comnenus," *Byzantion*, 21 (1961), 236.

trol our observation by shifting to a different type of source—to Byzantine epistolography.

Among the relatively vast correspondence of Photius (the second half of the ninth century), containing more than two hundred letters, only two were addressed to an *iatros*, the monk Acacius.[4] But was this monk really a doctor, or rather a doctor of moral pains, as some saints used to be called? At any rate, Photius speaks here of a cure for the passions, not of the healing of physical illnesses.

Even fewer traces of the medical profession are to be found in tenth-century collections of letters: none of about two hundred letters dispatched by Nicholas Mysticus[5] was addressed to a physician, nor are there physicians among the addressees of Leo Choirosphactes, Theodore Daphnopates or Nicetas the Magistros.[6] No letter to a doctor was written by an anonymous teacher of the tenth century;[7] and in the tenth-century epistolaria containing several hundreds of letters sent by various persons, none was addressed to a physician.[8] We do not know to what extent the epistolary corpus would coincide with, or represent proportionally, the social structure of addressees in actually dispatched letters; but if we assume that some individuals of the tenth century did write to doctors, we have to recognize that they preferred not to include those letters in their collections. The situation changes drastically as we move towards the twelfth century.

Theophylact of Ochrid sent several letters to Michael Pantechnes, the *iatros* of Emperor Alexius I.[9] According to one of the lemmata (PG, 126, col. 464C), Michael was Theophylact's pupil. Michael Pantechnes is mentioned in the *Alexiad* of Anna Comnena as one of the doctors who attended the dying Alexius in 1117–18.[10] The lead seal of a certain *proedros* or *protoproedros* Michael Pantechnes is

preserved, but the identification of both personages is not assured.[11] It is also debatable whether the *proedros* and *proximos* Pantechnes, the addressee of two other letters of Theophylact, was our Michael or another person, namely John Pantechnes, also a correspondent of Theophylact.[12] Michael was not the only medical friend of Theophylact: a series of letters was also sent to Nicholas Callicles, who is designated as *archiatros* in a lemma (PG, 126, col. 440D). Again, the "senior physician" Callicles is known from other sources: Anna Comnena includes him in the list of the three "best doctors" (*koryphaioi ton iatron*), side by side with Michael Pantechnes and a certain eunuch Michael (*Alexiad* 3.236.20–24); Callicles was a court poet,[13] and he is considered as one of the possible candidates for the authorship of the anonymous dialogue *Timarion*.[14] The third medical addressee of Theophylact was the emperor's *iatros* Nicetas.[15]

The collection of letters of Michael Italicus is not large: it contains about thirty-five missives. Even so, two of them were addressed to physicians. One of these men is mere called *aktouarios* in the lemma, but P. Gautier is inclined to identify him with the above-mentioned Michael Pantechnes.[16] The second letter was sent to an *iatros*, Leipsiotes by name, who is otherwise unknown; according to Michael Italicus, he was the most "philosophical" and the most literate (*grammatikotatos*) among physicians, and we can hypothesize that Leipsiotes, like Callicles, was a writer as well.[17]

Three of the 107 letters of John Tzetzes' epistolographic collection are intended for physicians: the *archiatros* Michael, a "long-armed" person who provided Tzetzes with partridges from Adrianople; the imperial doctor Basil Megistus, Tzetzes' "lord and brother," who was not only versed, according to Tzetzes, in the skill of the *asklepiadai*, not only brilliant in general scholarship, not only distinguished by pleasant bearing, by reliability and prudence, but—what counted particularly for a

[4] Photius, *Epistolae*, ed. I. N. Barlettas (London, 1864), 428, nos. 106–7. There are no medical addressees in the collection published by A. I. Papadopulos-Kerameus, *Svjatejšego patriarcha Fotija XLV neizdannych pisem* (St. Petersburg, 1896).

[5] Nicholas I Patriarch of Constantinople, *Letters*, ed. R. J. H. Jenkins and L. G. Westerink (Washington, 1973); two more letters are included in Nicholas' *Miscellaneous Writings*, ed. L. G. Westerink (Washington, 1981), nos. 193 and 198.

[6] *Léon Choerosphactès . . . Biographie—Correspondance*, ed. G. Kolias (Athens, 1939); *Nicétas Magistros, Lettres d'un exilé*, ed. L. G. Westerink (Paris, 1973); *Théodore Daphnopatès, Correspondance*, ed. J. Darrouzès and L. G. Westerink (Paris, 1978).

[7] R. Browning and B. Laourdas, "To keimenon ton epistolon tou kodikos BM 36749," 'Επ.'Ετ.Βυζ.Σπ., 27 (1957), 151–212.

[8] J. Darrouzès, *Epistoliers byzantins du Xe siècle* (Paris, 1960).

[9] S. Maslev in *Fontes Graeci Historiae Bulgariae* IX, 1 (Sofia, 1974), 28–32.

[10] Anne Comnène, *Alexiade*, ed. and trans. B. Leib (Paris, 1945), 231.2, 236.22.

[11] G. Schlumberger, *Sigillographie de l'empire byzantin* (Paris, 1884), 687; Ch. Diehl, "De la signification du titre de 'proêdre' à Byzance," *Mélanges G. Schlumberger*, 1 (Paris, 1924), 116.

[12] J. Darrouzès, in Georges et Dèmètrios Tornikès, *Lettres et discours* (Paris, 1970), 50, n. 32, identifies him with John Pantechnes.

[13] His poems have been published by R. Romano: Nicola Callicle, *Carmi* (Naples, 1980).

[14] R. Romano in Pseudo-Luciano, *Timarione* (Naples, 1974), 25–31.

[15] PG, 126, col. 472C. See Maslev in *Fontes*, 69.

[16] Michel Italikos, *Lettres et discours*, ed. P. Gautier (Paris, 1972), 209. See Gautier's comment, 46–48.

[17] Michel Italikos, 204 f.

Byzantine—he was known to the emperor and was dubbed "the eye of the Senate." The third letter is addressed to the *nosokomos* of the hospital of the Pantocrator monastery, whose name is, unfortunately, omitted from the lemma; the letter reveals nothing about this obscure director of a very famous hospital; what Tzetzes is discussing here is the time of Galen's life.[18]

The last collection of letters I wish to consider is that of Michael Choniates, the archbishop of Athens at the time of the Fourth Crusade: among the 180 letters of his collection, one is addressed to the *archiatros* George Callistus and three to the *iatros* or *archiatros* Nicholas Calloduces.[19] Callistus is described as a dexterous doctor of the body, as a representative of the "philanthropic vocation," but Choniates puts the emphasis on his quality as a healer of souls, whose letters are remedies and antidotes for those who suffer. The letters to Caloduces are less rhetorical and more specific. Choniates thanks his correspondent—not without irony—for his care of the exiled archbishop, the old man who found refuge on a small island: in fact, Caloduces, in answering Choniates' complaints, had sent him a book of Galen's about diet, drink and exercise, but it turned out that the archbishop was unable to apply the medical advice to his situation. For instance, he says, there is no bathhouse on the island; the inhabitants would wash themselves in a small booth, the door of which could not be closed; some parts of the body were suffering from fire, while others froze as if in an open field. The people choked from the smoke of the hearth and peeped their heads outdoors. The local bishop, continues Choniates, would always cover his head lest he catch cold, and wash his hair outside the booth.[20] Even more relevant is another letter to Caloduces, in which Choniates formulates two moral rules for an honest doctor: first, you should not raise your fees too high (*me baryneis tous misthous tes therapeias*), and secondly, you should not be negligent and indifferent to the pain of your patients, especially those who combine grave illness with severe poverty (p. 264.9–14).

Certainly, not all the major epistolographic collections of the twelfth century contain letters ad-

dressed to medical doctors; thus, to my knowledge, neither Eustathius of Thessalonica nor Euthymius Malaces left letters of this kind. So far as other epistolographers are concerned, the very insignificant number of epistles they have left us allows us to dispense with them.

More complex is the question of the treatment of the medical profession in Byzantine hagiography. Saints' Lives of the sixth and seventh centuries, as H. J. Magoulias has demonstrated,[21] present a series of Late Roman physicians who are loaded with ignorance and avarice and who are unable to vie with healer-saints. Then the doctor disappears from hagiography (we might say with hagiography, since we do not possess hagiographic texts of the eighth century):[22] when the genre was reintroduced, the writers practically ignored the medical profession, as it was the case of the Life of Philaretus the Merciful (*BHG*, 1511z–1512). The lives of the ninth-century saints are vague in their attitude towards medical doctors and lenient to their vices, so colorfully described by earlier hagiographers. Saints are presented as capable of miraculous healings, but their secular rivals are just left in the shadow, and their incapacity is rather silenced than not. Thus St. Evariste is praised as "the best physician and the guide of the greatest salvation," and many sinners are said to have received cures and healing from him.[23] This passage doubtlessly refers to the spiritual healing of sins, but Evariste served as a doctor of bodily illnesses as well: he cured a woman by sending her a ring from the iron chain he wore to tame his flesh (van de Vorst, p. 314.28–36; also p. 315.1–7); another woman was healed by olive oil (p. 319.15–20); and the hagiographer registered many cases of cures on the tomb of the saint (p. 314.20–24, 323.10–11, 20–22). He teaches that the divine energy and grace is much

---

[18] Ioannes Tzetzes, *Epistulae*, ed. P. A. M. Leone (Leipzig, 1972), nos. 48, 74, 81. On Galen's tradition in Tzetzes, J. Scarborough, "The Galenic Question," *SA*, 65 (1981), 20. On Byzantine hospitals, see T. Miller's paper by that title, in this volume.

[19] Michael Akominates, *Ta sozomena*, ed. S. Lampros, 2 (Athens, 1880), nos. 92, 107, 115, 131.

[20] On this letter, A. Berger, *Das Bad in der byzantinischen Zeit* (Munich, 1982), 71.

[21] H. J. Magoulias, "The Lives of the Saints as Sources of Data for the History of Byzantine Medicine in the Sixth and Seventh Centuries," *BZ*, 57 (1964), 128–33. To the *Vitae* used by Magoulias we can add now the pre-Metaphrastic Life of St. Sampson written, according to F. Halkin ("Saint Sampson le xénodoque de Constantinople [VIᵉ siècle]," *RSBN*, 14–16 [1977–79], 6), "sans doute" in the seventh or at the very beginning of the eighth centuries. To the best of my knowledge, Magoulias' work has not been continued. Some remarks, however, are to be found in A. P. Rudakov, *Očerki vizantijskoj kul'tury po dannym grečeskoj agiografii* (Moscow, 1917), 96–98.

[22] I. Ševčenko, "Hagiography of the Iconoclast Period," in his *Ideology, Letters and Culture in the Byzantine World* (London, 1982), 1–3 (first published in *Iconoclasm* [Birmingham, 1977], 113 f.); less clearly in A. Papadakis, "Hagiography in Relation to Iconoclasm," *The Greek Orthodox Theological Review*, 14 (1969), 161–63.

[23] *BHG*, 2153: C. van de Vorst in *AnalBoll*, 41 (1923), 314.3–10. See also p. 315.11–12, 316.8–9.

more powerful than "human medical service" (p. 315.29–30); Evariste was able to cure the very diseases that doctors proclaimed incurable (p. 316.6–8, 19–23). However, there is no sharp animosity against doctors in this Life. Typically, for this Life, the hagiographer describes the illness of Evariste's spiritual teacher, Nicholas of Studius (d. 868), without any hint of doctors' assistance (p. 307.28–32)—he does not care about them.

The author of the Life of Theophano, the wife of the Emperor Leo VI (886–912), mentions his own and his brother's illnesses: in both cases many of the best doctors were called. They tried various means and medications (Kurtz, *Zwei griechische Texte*, 19.34–35, 22.24–26), and even though their treatments turned out to be of no avail, the Life shows no flouting of them. Again, the Life of Nicholas of Studius recorded several cases of doctors' helplessness before grave diseases (*BHG*, 1365: PG, 105, col. 913D, 916C, 924BC) which the saint was able to cure, but the hagiographer does not scoff at the poor *iatroi*. In the same indirect way the Life of Thomais of Lesbos expresses the author's attitude towards the medical profession: a certain Eutychianus spent his whole life with the *asklepiadai* longing for his physical health, but it was a miracle that finally cured his paralysis (*BHG*, 2454; *ActaSS*, Novembris IV, 240CD).

Even more evocative is the Life of Peter of Argos, who acted, according to his biographer, with more experience than the *asklepiadai*, since he was a doctor of the soul and they doctors of the body.[24] The saint was the genuine doctor, indeed,[25] but his secular colleagues retained their medical functions, albeit on a reduced scale.

Nicetas Paphlago is a very controversial figure: we do not know whether this name covers one or two different writers, and to which of them, in this case, we should ascribe the authorship of the Life of the Patriarch Ignatius (847–58, 867–77), a notorious work that combines eulogy of the saint and the pasquinade on his enemy, the Patriarch Photius (858–67, 877–86). Nicetas describes several miraculous healings achieved by applying the holy relics of Ignatius. One of these cases refers to obstetrics, and in this connection Nicetas mentions *iatroi*: the delivery was troubled because of the baby's wrong position, so the doctors suggested using surgery and extracting the child piece by piece. The saint's intervention, however, saved the baby (PG, 105, col. 564B). Again, the physicians are less effective than the piece of Ignatius' cloak applied to the body of the suffering mother, but they are in no way villains. Nicetas even produced a Life of a medical doctor, St. Diomedes of Tarse, a healer of bodies and souls who tended the poor for free and visited Christian martyrs in prisons.[26]

Some of the Saints' Lives produced during this span of time ignored the medical topic completely (for instance, that of Irene of Chrysobalantus, *BHG*, 952), or briefly related the saint's miraculous healings without mentioning doctors (among others, that of Euthymius the Younger, *BHG*, 655). But towards the end of the tenth century, the medical doctor of hagiographical texts ceases to be a nebulous name functioning somewhere at the background as a kind of foil to the saint: the saint met his match, who was doomed to be mocked, despised and rejected. Symeon Metaphrastes inserted in his reworked version of the Life of St. Sampson a long passage about a hospital in tenth-century Constantinople during the reign of Emperor Romanus II (959–63): Metaphrastes does not disparage the quality of medical service, but he complains that the hospital would run out of olive oil, and that its employees acted with such negligence that Sampson felt obliged to appear from the other world and punish the culprits (*BHG*, 1615: PG, 115, col. 300B–304B).

The Life of the tenth-century saint Luke the Stylite is especially abundant in tales that illustrate the preference for the saint over his secular rival. Cyrus, an official of the postal service (*dromos*), fell sick and suffered from acute pain, but was treated in vain by *iatron paides*.[27] A woman who had experienced intermittent fever and chills for three years wasted her fortune looking for medical help but did not recover (Delehaye, p. 227.32–36). The eunuch Sergius was severely beaten at the Hippodrome of Constantinople and brought to the hospital (*nosokomeion*) of Eubulus for treatment. The people so versed in medical skill, says the hagiographer ironically, tried to cure him but without any result. His head was so swollen that one could not see his eyes or nose or ears. The poor victim had a

---

[24] *BHG*, 1504: Ch. Papaoikonomou, *Ho poliouchos tou Argou Petros episkopos* (Athens, 1908), 64.28–29.

[25] See, for instance, the Lives of St. Blasius (*BHG*, 273: *ActaSS*, Novembris IV, 667E) and St. Theocletus (*BHG*, 2420: ed. A. Sgouritzes in *Theologia*, 27 [1956], 592.15–16). On St. Evariste see note 23 above.

[26] *BHG*, 551: L. G. Westerink, "Trois textes inédits sur s. Diomède de Nicée," *AnalBoll*, 84 (1966), 170, par. 4.

[27] *BHG*, 2239: H. Delehaye, *Les saints stylites* (Brussels, 1923), 224.24–26.

vision, after which he asked for surgery. An *iatros* was summoned, but frightened by the terrible swelling he refused to operate until Sergius, in desperation, grasped the lancet (*siderion*)[28] and handed it over to the doctor (p. 219.29–37). If doctors appeared timid and awkward, St. Luke healed patients confidently and quickly: when the wife of "illustrious" John Iubes could not give birth to her baby for twenty days, Luke immediately helped her by giving her some holy bread and water (p. 229.13–21); after physicians had lost hope of curing Euthymius, a *clericus* of the New Church, Luke healed him (p. 222.30–37, 223.24); he sent holy bread to a certain Anna who dwelt near the Brazen Gate and was hopelessly ill, and she recovered right away (p. 229.33–230.5); in seven days he healed Phlorus Sarantopeches from leprosy with holy water and the "drastic remedy" (the hagiographer uses the words of the *Geoponica* 13:14.5) of his prayers (p. 225.24–226.3). The hagiographer cites many other examples of Luke's medical successes, and calls him a universal doctor (p. 224.16–17), a distinguished doctor of the soul and body (p. 210.25–26), whose usual means of healing were prayers and holy bread and water. The hagiographer even makes the medical professionals acknowledge Luke's triumph: a certain Stephen, "a man experienced in the medical art," is said to have had a miraculous vision, in which he saw Luke's soul ascending into heaven (p. 234.4–9).

In another *Vita*, that of St. Luke the Younger, or Steiriotes, we are transported to a different world: unlike the Stylite, his namesake was acting in a remote province, but the image of the doctor remains the same. A certain Nicholas is said to have had cholera. He turned to doctors for help; to some of them he paid a lot of gold, to some he promised to pay, if they could cure him of his grave illness. When his purse was empty, the doctors proclaimed his illness incurable, and so Nicholas lost both money and hope.[29] The wife of a nobleman from Thebes was ill (no definition of her ailment is given), and

her husband spent a great deal of money on doctors, ruined his fortune but got no help (Martini, 106.34–107.1). And again, in the cases in which secular physicians stood helpless, Luke the Younger performed miracles. A Boeotian woman suffered from an eye illness, and the doctors' science and hands were of no avail. However, she was cured immediately at Luke's tomb (Martini, 109.28–110.4). A certain John from the island of Terbenia had an unbearable pain in his legs; again, the illness was declared incurable, and again, he was immediately cured after having addressed his prayers to St. Luke (Martini, 112.36–113.13). The *clericus* Nicholas of Dauleia had dropsy; he visited doctors but they were evil and negligent, and only water from Luke's tomb brought recovery (Martini, 117.1–15). An unnamed woman suffered from the illness that the *paides iatron* call *phagedaina* (cancerous sore) and no physician could help her; but in eight days she was healed at the tomb of Luke (Martini, 109.11–25). Many other healings are recorded in the *Vita* as performed by Luke both during and after his earthly existence, but even though his tomb is called "the free hospital (*amisthon iatreion*)" (Martini, 108.31), and though he appeared in a dream to the monk Gregory as an *iatros*, holding in his hands a *kauter*, a branding iron, to apply to Gregory's sick stomach (Martini, 106.17–18), he modestly refused to be regarded as a physician and announced that there was one and only one doctor of the soul and body, God Himself (Martini, 101.15–17). He differs from his Constantinopolitan namesake also in that his favorite remedy was not holy bread and water but olive oil from a *photagogos* ("lamp"; Lampe, *s.v.*, gives only the meaning of window) (Martini, 109.20–25, 110.3–4 and others).

Olive oil from a *photagogos* is also the favorite remedy of another contemporary provincial saint, Paul of Latros,[30] who by these means healed even leprosy. He too used prayers defined as "the very drastic remedy" (Delehaye, p. 144.11). And like his colleagues he triumphed over "all the *iatroi*," who were powerless before the strange and distressing disease of a certain Leo-Luke, an inhabitant of a site called Thebes near Miletus (p. 143.13–144.11).

The incompetence of physicians is strongly emphasized in the *Vita* of Nicon Metanoeite. A *strategos* of the Peloponnese named Gregory suddenly fell sick and, although he was carefully tended by local doctors, did not recover; even the bishop of

---

[28] See L. Bliquez, "Two Lists of Greek Surgical Instruments and the State of Surgery in Byzantine Times," in this volume.

[29] *BHG*, 994. The *Vita* is published in PG, 111, col. 441–80, with important additions by E. Martini, "Supplementa ad acta S. Lucae junioris," *AnalBoll*, 13 (1894). Here p. 118.3–119.3. Some unique evidence to the amount of doctors' fee is preserved in the Life of Anthony the Younger (d. 865): the saint, at that time still a governor of the *theme* of Cibyrraeotes, disguised himself as a physician; a rich proprietor promised him a third of his estate if Anthony cured his wife of barrenness; the saint-governor-doctor required ten war stallions instead, and the agreement was concluded (*BHG*, 142: A. I. Papadopulos-Kerameus in *Pravoslavnyj Palestinskij sbornik*, 57 [1907], 196.1–7).

[30] *BHG*, 1474: H. Delehaye in *AnalBoll*, 11 (1892), 173.2–6, 175.5–6.

Sparta tried to help him, the man who was, according to the hagiographer, at the very acme of medical science.[31] Of course, Nicon's prayers cured Gregory at once. Medical skill was of no avail when a servant of Basil Apocaucus was found paralyzed in his bed (Lampros, p. 184.31–185.3) and in the case of a kind boy named Manuel who had illness of the testicles (p. 204.22–31). Neither the skill of *asklepiadai* nor the cures suggested by neighbors helped Vitalius of Aquileia (p. 215.16–28). No human help was successful, repeats the hagiographer in several other cases, but Nicon managed to heal, applying various remedies—anointment, olive oil, vision. A certain George, the son of Stephen, whose illness resisted all medical skill and science, was healed by Nicon's image (p. 204.13–20).

The *iatron paides* in the Life of Michael Maleinus turn out to be helpless in the face of the tremendous swelling that covered the ears, eyes, nose and mouth of Theophanes, Michael's disciple. They managed only to pry open the sick man's mouth and pour in some water; in desperation, they decided to cut open his face and neck, even though they guessed that Theophanes would not survive surgery. Of course, the saint's intervention healed the poor wretch.[32]

We can observe the same change in Greek Saints' Lives from South Italy. The Life of Elias the Younger (d. 903) records sundry cases of healing performed by this saint.[33] Even the Saracens called him "doctor and savior sent by God" (1.298–99), although he was first and foremost "the doctor of souls" (1.610–11). But there is no contempt for the medical profession in this Life. Quite a different attitude is disclosed in the Lives written about a century later.

The Life of Elias Speleotis, who belonged to the next generation,[34] describes an inexperienced physician: in his boyhood, Elias fell from a high place and damaged his fingers; "an ignorant and inexperienced *iatros*" put on a splint (*narthex*), with the

result that in eight days Elias lost all his fingers (*ActaSS*, Septembris III, 852DE). Elias, on the other hand, functioned as a doctor with a great success: his skill consisted predominantly in extracting strange objects from the ill body. Thus, in a dream he approached a certain Christopher, cut his belly open, and extracted a goose egg (p. 883B). He drove a raven out of the mouth of the ill priest Epiphanius (p. 871B). Further details are related about the illness of the noble *archon* Gaudiosus, who was frustrated by visiting various temples of saints and made up his mind to sail to Palermo and consult the doctors there. On the boat, however, he had a vision: "the great doctor Elias" approached him, opened his mouth and extracted from his stomach a suckling piglet that he tossed into the sea (p. 871C–872D).

St. Sabas the Younger, another holy man from Byzantine South Italy, was very successful in curing all sorts of illnesses. His Life, written by Orestes of Jerusalem (d. 1005), comprises all the essential features of the hagiographical pattern: medical doctors who cannot help the sick,[35] money squandered on doctors without result (Cozza-Luzzi, p. 56.34–36, 61.8–11), and innumerable cures of the saint himself, who is called "the great doctor who requires no fee" (p. 56.39–40). More specific about medical rivals of the saint is the Life of Nilus of Rossano: he met a Jewish doctor, Domnulus by name,[36] who is characterized as a man of profound knowledge and medical experience. Domnulus proposed a medication to St. Nilus and boasted that after taking it Nilus would never know sickness, but the saint rejected the proposal. He wanted nothing to do with human drugs since, as he put it, his only physician was God Jesus Christ. Domnulus reappears once more in the Life—as an eyewitness and admirer of Nilus' victory over a high Byzantine official (*BHG*, 1370: *ActaSS*, Septembris VII, 290F–291A, 293C).

The opposition of saint and doctor is a typical phenomenon of Byzantine hagiography, and this opposition acquires a particular sharpness towards the end of the tenth century. Eventually it was softened, and we do not meet any trace of animosity against the physician in the richest eleventh-century hagiographical text, the Life of Lazarus Galesiotes, even though the hagiographer, Lazarus' disciple Gregory, records several cases of miraculous heal-

[31]*BHG*, 1366: S. Lampros in Νέος Ἑλλ., 3 (1906), 173.7–11.
[32]*BHG*, 1295: L. Petit in *ROChr*, 7 (1902), 566.23–567.14.
[33]*BHG*, 580: G. R. Taibbi, *Vita di sant'Elia il Giovane* (Palermo, 1962), 11.287–89, 582–85, 515–22, 806–9, 1127–33, 1311–30, 1620–23.
[34]Elias Speleotis was still young when Elias the Younger foretold his own death (*BHG*, 581: *ActaSS*, Septembris III, 861B). A certain Elias "spileot" was a scribe of a manuscript (Paris. 375) completed in 1021, but G. Schirò, "Testimonianza innografica dell'attività scriptoria di S. Elia lo Speleota," *ByzF*, 2 (1967), 316 f., denies the identity of the two namesakes. At any rate, the hagiographer seems to have lived some considerable span of time after Speleotis' death.

[35]*BHG*, 1611: I. Cozza-Luzzi, *Historia et laudes SS. Sabae et Macarii junioris* (Rome, 1893), 48.1–7, 52.10–13.
[36]On Domnulus, E. Lieber, "Asaf's *Book of Medicines*," in this volume.

ings. Moreover, Gregory did not care much about bodily recovery: according to him, Lazarus admonished those who were afflicted by ailments or tortured by demons not to lose their spirit but praise God and live in anticipation of future rewards (*BHG*, 979: *ActaSS*, Novembris III, 563B). The Life of Lazarus is "neutral." Two rare cases in which the hagiographers tried to overcome traditional adversity against the medical profession deserve attention. The first case is relatively late and belongs to the area of South Italy. Cyprian of Calamizzi[37] was born into a doctor's family and was taught medicine by his father; after his father's death he inherited his wealth, glory and estates. Cyprian built "a holy house" on one of his paternal estates and would heal the sick—as the hagiographer emphasizes—without taking money.[38] This exceptional case could be explained as referring to the outlying areas of Byzantium; similarly, the Kievan *Paterik* appreciates rather positively the doctor Agapit (probably a Greek, Agapetus) who acted at the court of Vladimir Monomach (1113–25).[39] More complicated is the case of the Life of Athanasius of Athos.

I am not going to dwell here on the controversy over the priority of the versions of this *Vita*. Let us assume that both versions were produced almost simultaneously, in the beginning of the eleventh century, soon after Athanasius' death (ca. 1001). One of these versions, that of the Lavra, contains many traditional elements of the medical image: Athanasius is called the wisest physician (*BHG*, 188: L. Petit in *AnalBoll*, 25 [1906], 60.16–17), his tomb, "the free hospital" (p. 82.15); the *apothecarius* Athanasius had dropsy and doctors had lost all hope of healing him, but the saint touched his belly and drove the illness away (p. 74.27–75.4). The monk Eustratius had blood in his urine; the saint recommended that he set off for Constantinople and address himself to first-class doctors who, however, gave him no relief and even did him substantial damage. At last Athanasius helped him by prescribing water drunk with roses (p. 80.7–81.6). Incidentally or not, there are no such invectives against doctors in the other version of the Life produced in Constantinople. Even more curious is the story

about the incurable disease of a monk, in which the author of the Constantinopolitan version stresses that the nature of this disease remained obscure both to "the wise doctor" (i.e., Athanasius) and to all other people,[40] whereas the phrase about Athanasius' ignorance is lacking in the Lavra version (Petit, 68.29–31). Perhaps the clue to the reserve of the Constantinopolitan version is the existence of the Lavra hospital founded by Athanasius, in which he tended severe wounds (Petit, 53.24–33, Noret, par. 141.6–12). The hagiographer mentions a *nosokomos* who was one of the distinguished monks of the Lavra (Petit, 53.25–26, Noret, par. 154.1–5), and the Lavra doctor Timotheus is also mentioned (the words "of the Lavra" are lacking in the Lavra version), even though quite naturally he could not compete with "the great physician" Athanasius (Petit, 69.24–33, Noret, par. 204.13–30).

To a certain extent, Byzantine moralists of the eleventh century retained the hagiographers' negative attitude towards the medical profession. Christopher of Mitylene left at least two epigrams dedicated to medical problems. One of them was written on hospitals and the patients who stay in them, but unfortunately the text is so corrupted that we cannot glean much information from this poem. The second epigram is addressed to an anonymous doctor, and it is typical of a transitional period, since it reflects both old and new attitudes. "You should not be proud of your profession," says Christopher. "You rather ought to despise yourself, for you get your living from urine and excrement."[41] The doctors of the eleventh century were already proud of their activity, but they had not yet acquired the high esteem of those elements of society whose opinions were reflected by Christopher. Cecaumenus, in his *Admonitions*, written in the 1070s, dedicated a long paragraph to a vicious doctor.[42] There he stresses—in full accord with hagiography—the doctor's tendency to pump out the patient's entire fortune. But Cecaumenus' physician acts this way not out of lack of experience; rather, he is "very knowing" (*sphodra epistemon*), and deliberately revives the illness in search of profit. Symeon the Theologian follows the traditional pattern, and speaks of an inexperienced doctor who frequently misused both surgery and cauteriz-

---

[37] He lived in the second half of the twelfth century, according to D. Stiernon, "Saint Cyprien de Calamizzi († vers 1210–1215)," *REB*, 32 (1974), 247–52.

[38] *BHG*, 2089: G. Schirò in *BGrottaf*, 4 (1950), 88.1–29, 90.37–38.

[39] *Das Paterikon des Kiever Höhlenklosters*, ed. D. Tschiževskij (Munich, 1964), 128–33, *slovo* 27: "On Holy and Saint Agapit, the Doctor who Performed Cures without Payment."

[40] *BHG*, 187: J. Noret, *Vitae duae antiquae S. Athanasii Athonitae* (Turnhout, Leuven, Brepols, 1982), par. 197.1–7.

[41] *Die Gedichte des Christophoros Mitylenaios*, ed. E. Kurtz (Leipzig, 1903), nos. 130 and 85.

[42] *Sovety i rasskazy Kekavmena*, ed. G. G. Litavrin (Moscow, 1972), 224.12–226.6.

ing.[43] Accordingly, in Symeon's *Vita* by Nicetas Stethatus, we read a story about a certain Manasses, whom doctors thought incurable but who was healed by the oil from a lamp at Symeon's icon.[44] But quite unexpectedly, Symeon, a religious writer of the beginning of the eleventh century, draws a parallel between the spiritual doctor and the surgeon who performs an autopsy in order to understand the structure of the human body and apply the knowledge acquired to the healing of patients.[45]

The twelfth-century authors paid special attention to the medical profession: one of them is the court poet of John II, Theodore Prodromus; the second, the anonymous author of the *Timarion*, has been identified either with Nicholas Callicles, Alexius I's physician (see above), or with Prodromus himself. Among other works, Prodromus wrote the Life of St. Meletius the Younger; another Life of the same saint came from the pen of the contemporary theologian Nicholas of Methone.[46] While Nicholas does not mention medical doctors in his version of the *Vita*, Prodromus does. He accepts the traditional pattern, and tells us of *asklepiadai* summoned to cure a young relative of Leo Nicerites: they acted, he says, like vultures and harvested a fortune (p. 60.26–27). Prodromus plainly contrasted "the unadorned medical science of the Savior" with the sophisticated but inefficient methods borrowed from Galen's books or Hippocrates' aphorisms (p. 53.31–33). Traditional though he was, Prodromus had, at least, the hearsay of Galen and Hippocrates. Moreover, he dared to acknowledge that a certain Theodosius of Athens was a man of marvellous medical skill (p. 61.11–12). Yet Prodromus took another step. He produced a new genre—a funny and tragicomic scene entitled *Executioner or Doctor* and describing his own visit to a dentist, a runt who immediately fetched a gigantic tool, fit to extract an elephant's tusk. But the poor doctor could not manage it and succeeded only in breaking off a part of the aching tooth.[47] The wan-

dering plot of the clumsy dentist finally wound up in one of the most famous short stories of Chekhov. In Prodromus' story the event is not only secularized and the medical profession mocked, but the author opposes good physicians to ignorant and boorish *asklepiadai*: at the end of the scene he addresses two praiseworthy doctors and gives their names—one of them is his close friend Michael Lizix, and another one, Nicholas Callicles, whom we have already mentioned (Podestà, 21.17–21). In the monody on the death of Stephen Scylitzes, Prodromus relates the arrival of his dying friend from Trebizond at Constantinople: the goal of this last journey was Stephen's desire to be treated "by the most experienced doctors."[48]

Even more paradoxical is the *Timarion*'s approach to medicine. Like the *Executioner or Doctor*, the anonymous dialogue is written as satire. The external plot is as follows: a certain Timarion, while visiting a fair in Thessalonica, was affected with a serious infirmity. According to the demons' judgment pronounced at his bed, he had lost all his bile, and since Asclepius and Hippocrates state that the human being cannot exist if deprived of one of his major elements, Timarion was condemned to be transferred to the nether world. There he met various people, including his own teacher Theodore of Smyrna, a famous rhetorician, who was also knowledgeable about ancient medicine. The image is thoroughly ironical, even though the lion's share of allusions escape the perception of the twentieth-century reader. In the first place, if the earthly Theodore had been sturdy, the man whom Timarion met in the nether world was tremendously skinny; the change is explained in terms of diet: Theodore has tamed his gluttonous stomach, lost unnecessary flesh, and by so doing healed himself of the gout he suffered in the days when he served the emperor. Dietary self-restraint is a mandatory element of every hagiographical legend, and accordingly, in the *Timarion*, Theodore is said to "cure the soul and the body" (ed. Romano, 71.611). But what was utterly serious in the *Vitae* acquires a nuance of play in the *Timarion*: Theodore displays only the parody of Christian temperance, and what this faster discusses with Timarion is a present from above of the one thing he is longing for, his favor-

[43] K. Holl, *Enthusiasmus und Bussgewalt* (Leipzig, 1898), 117.9–10.

[44] *BHG*, 1692: I. Hausherr, "Un grand mystique byzantin," *OrChr*, 12 (1928), par. 144.4–20.

[45] Syméon le Nouveau Théologien, *Traités théologiques et éthiques*, ed. J. Darrouzès, 2 (Paris, 1967), 138.269–140.278.

[46] *BHG*, 1247–48: V. G. Vasil'evskij in *Pravoslavnyj Palestinskij sbornik*, VI, 2 (1886).

[47] G. Podestà, "Le satire Lucianesche di Teodoro Prodromo," *Aevum*, 21 (1947), 17 f. On an "ignorant *iatros*," see also Prodromus' letter to the metropolitan of Trebizond (PG, 133, col. 1256A). The equation of the doctor and the executioner was a

topos of the Late Roman literature—see B. Baldwin, "Beyond the House Call," in this volume.

[48] L. Petit, "Monodie de Théodore Prodrome sur Etienne Skylitzes métropolitain de Trébizonde," *IRAIK*, 8 (1902), 13.211–34.

ite food (p. 74.673). Secondly, Theodore is presented as a braggart, who promises—by his cleverness—to liberate Timarion, to release him from the nether world, and to win over the famous ancient gods and healers. But his criticism of Hippocrates and Erasistratus is philological rather than medical, limited to ridiculing their stylistic and grammatical shortcomings, whereas Galen is for Theodore no more than a man concealed in a remote corner of Hell and hastily filling gaps in his book *On Various Kinds of Fever*. The central scene of the dialogue, the trial of Timarion and the speech pronounced by Theodore on behalf of Timarion, are consummate parodies: Timarion's fate is entrusted to the council of doctors, who act as judges rather than physicians and whose chairman, Hippocrates, is clad in a funny Arab costume.

The relentless rejection of secular medicine so typical of the hagiographical literature, especially of the second half of the tenth century, was replaced in the twelfth century by satirical nicety, and it was hard to distinguish who was more the butt of ridicule, the awkward and verbose doctor or his garrulous victim. At the same time, sincere respect for the medical profession was emerging. George Tornices was, perhaps, the most eloquent defender of physicians: in his letter to Alexius Ducas Bryennius he argues against the image of the doctor-executioner (*demios*) that was reflected, as we have seen, in Prodromus satire. Tornices contrasts the two figures: he speaks of the cup of medication passed over by the human-loving palms of the physician that are opposed to the rash hands of the executioner. Again, the actions of executioners and malicious cooks are contrasted with those of doctors (Darrouzès, *Georges et Dèmètrius*, 164.5–7, 165.9–10). The topic was touched upon by another twelfth-century writer, Nicetas Choniates (*Historia*, 298.14), who overtly differentiated the doctor and the poisoner. Several times Tornices re-

turns to the subject of medicine in his panegyric of Anna Comnena: even though he retains the traditional contrast between the limitations of "the best *iatroï*" and God's almightiness (Darrouzès, p. 313.2–4), he asserts that "the hand of the *iatros*" cleans the wound and heals "with minimal pain" (p. 293.27–28) and marvels at the skill of the "wise among doctors" who use wonderful and fitting tools in operating on people and cutting open corpses (p. 225.13–14). And his lady-patroness Anna was also very attentive to doctors, whose activity she describes and whose names she mentions. We can come back to the letters I quoted at the beginning: again, the letters of the twelfth century are mostly full of respect towards doctors who were friends of epistolographers.

I would like to formulate a hypothesis by way of conclusion: it seems to me that we have indications—however slight they may appear—that after the seventh century the medical profession in Byzantium temporarily lost its social standing; in any case the society became lukewarm and negligent towards medical doctors, hagiography ignored them, and intellectuals did not consider them as their peers. The situation began to change, probably, at the end of the tenth century: hagiography of about *l'an mil* wages a sharp war against secular physicians and scolds greediness and incompetence of the medical doctor who dares to match the omnipotent healing power of the saint; in other words, the doctor had become too influential to be neglected. But the anti-doctoral attack was no success: by the twelfth century, the physician enters as equal the establishment of functionaries and literati (one of whom he, indeed, was); he becomes respected, although mocked time and again by a society that started to care for its health more than for its salvation.

Dumbarton Oaks

BYZANTINE HOSPITALS

Timothy S. Miller

Byzantine hospitals for the sick drew support from powerful groups within East Roman society. The emperors both as public officials and private philanthropists, the bishops of the official church, monastic leaders, lay aristocrats, and for many centuries the medical men, sought to secure institutions for the sick which could provide both men and women with bed, board, nursing care, and the expertise of highly qualified physicians. Byzantine hospitals were designed with one purpose—restoring their patients to health. To explore fully the history of these remarkable medical facilities would require a careful study of most major facets of Byzantine society, a task too great for a single monograph, to say nothing of a short study such as this.[1] But it is both possible and useful in such a brief account to address a few key questions about public medical institutions in the East Roman Empire.

Consideration of the following questions should help, on the one hand, to introduce East Roman hospitals to students of Byzantine and medieval society in general and, on the other hand, to underscore their central role in the development of Byzantine medicine—the subject of this symposium. First, when were Byzantine hospitals organized? Second, where were they usually located? Third, who sought them out as patients? Fourth, what sort of staff did these institutions maintain? And, finally, why did Byzantine physicians choose to work in hospitals? These questions will apply only to those philanthropic agencies which functioned as modern hosptials do—as institutions which set as their goal healing their patients by rational medical therapy while they fed, sheltered, and nursed them.[2] Such a definition excludes agencies which served as hospices, old-age homes, or almshouses, as well as shrines renowned for miraculous cures.

When were hospitals first organized in the provinces of the East Roman Empire? Of the four questions this one poses the greatest difficulty for two reasons. First, Byzantine sources employed many different terms to describe philanthropic institutions, terms which only gradually acquired precise meanings. Thus, words such as *xenon* or *nosokomeion* which came to designate hospitals exclusively might have had more general meanings in the formative stages of Byzantine philanthropic institutions. As a result, it is impossible to argue that a given institution, mentioned by a Byzantine source, functioned as a hospital unless the passage includes some information on the kind of services which the facility offered.[3] Second, philanthropic

---

[The reader is referred to the list of abbreviations at the end of the volume.]

[1] Byzantine hospitals have not been treated by most general histories of the Eastern Roman Empire. For example, the standard account of Byzantine history—G. Ostrogorsky, *The History of the Byzantine State* (New Brunswick, N. J., 1969)—ignores them along with other philanthropic institutions. Even the recent work by A. Kazhdan and G. Constable, *People and Power in Byzantium* (Washington, D. C., 1982) mentions them only rarely. H. Hunger (*Reich der neuen Mitte* [Graz, 1965], 173–81), however, does incorporate hospitals and other charitable agencies into a general account of the empire's religious life. In the 1960s two works appeared which concentrated on the hospitals: A. Philipsborn, "Der Fortschritt in der Entwicklung des byzantinischen Krankenhauswesens," *BZ*, 54 (1961), 338–65 and D. Constantelos, *Byzantine Philanthropy and Social Welfare* (New Brunswick, N. J., 1968), esp. 152–221. In his study Constantelos has tried to identify as many Byzantine *xenones* and *nosokomeia* as possible. For the study of Byzantine hospitals two primary sources are of special importance. I list them here with the abbreviations used hereafter.

Miracula Artemii: *Miracula S. Artemii*, ed. A. Papadopoulos-Kerameus, *Varia graeca sacra* (St. Petersburg, 1909), 1–75.
PantTyp: "Le typicon du Christ Sauveur Pantocrator," ed. P. Gautier, *REB*, 32 (1974), 1–145.

[2] Cf. the definition in *The New Encyclopedia Britannica* (Chicago, 1978), Micropaedia, vol. 5, 147: "an institution staffed and equipped for the diagnosis and treatment of the sick or injured, for their housing during treatment, for health examinations, and for the management of childbirth."
[3] See E. Patlagean's *Pauvreté économique et pauvreté sociale à Byzance, 4ᵉ–7ᵉ siècles* (Paris, 1977), 193–94.

institutions of the Latin West developed far more slowly than did those of the Byzantine East and did not begin to offer anything resembling hospital care until the thirteenth century. Basing their assertions only on these Western institutions, some scholars have even claimed that true hospitals did not emerge as distinct agencies for medical therapy until the nineteenth century.[4] These researchers, as well as most of those who would concede an earlier date for the inauguration of hospital services, simply ignore the Byzantine medical institutions of the late antique era and the early middle ages or class them together with the more primitive hospices and almshouses of the medieval Latin West.[5] A careful consideration of the Greek sources from the fourth through the seventh centuries, however, should overcome both of these difficulties.

No sources refer to permanent charitable foundations of any kind before the fourth century of the Christian era. Although classical Greco-Roman society had provided material benefits for citizens of the local *polis*, it had no permanent institutions to relieve the misery of the very poor or of those migrants to the towns who had no political standing in the city community.[6] The early Christian Church, on the other hand, stressed the virtue of charity toward society's most unfortunate members, but local congregations were not yet sufficiently large or well organized to institute permanent agencies to succor the poor, the hungry, and the sick.[7] The first evidence that the churches of the Roman Empire had begun to open permanent philanthropic institutions comes from the cities of

the Greek provinces in the fourth century, just as Christianity was emerging as the dominant religion in the urban areas of the eastern Mediterranean. At Antioch Bishop Leontios (344–58) founded a number of hostels for the poor and the strangers in his city, institutions which a later source, the *Chronicon paschale*, described as both *xenodocheia* and *xenones*. Neither the terms themselves nor the references to Leontios' foundations in this chronicle give any indication that they served the sick.[8] Archaeological evidence, however, reveals that one of Leontios' *xenodocheia* was built at Daphne, a fashionable spa outside Antioch to which the wealthy repaired when in bad health.[9] Perhaps Leontios located a hospice there so that the sick among the poor could enjoy the advantages of Daphne's salubrious air and water alongside of the rich.

Sometime between 357 and 377, Eustathios, bishop of Sabasteia in Asia Minor, built a renowned *ptochotropheion* (a house to nourish the poor) for his city. Although the fourth-century author Epiphanios describes this institution as one designed for those crippled with disease, he does not mention any physicians working in it, nor does he indicate in any other way that Eustathios' *ptochotropheion* had advanced beyond providing food and shelter for these sick. In other words, his account does not offer any evidence that the bishop had founded a hospital.[10]

The first indications that Christian philanthropic institutions were taking special measures to aid the sick surface in the last third of the fourth century. In a letter addressed to the governor of Cappadocia, Bishop Basil of Caesarea (370–79) referred to several lodges or inns (*katagogia*) which he had built outside of his city. He emphasized that these were to serve strangers, both those passing through and those who were in need of care because of some illness. To assist these people Basil had hired nurses for the sick and doctors as well as pack animals and escorts. The pack animals and escorts were surely for the strangers who were passing through, but the nurses and physicians must

[4] Such indeed is the standard view among historians of modern medicine. See K. J. Williams, "Hospitals," *Encyclopedia of Bioethics*, ed. W. Reich (New York, 1978), 2, 677–83; P. Starr, *The Social Transformation of American Medicine* (New York, 1982), 145–47.

[5] H. Sigerist, "An Outline of the Development of the Hospital," *BHM*, 4 (1936), 573–81. K. Sudhoff, "Aus der Geschichte des Krankenhauswesens im früheren Mittelalter in Morgenland und Abendland," *SA*, 21 (1929), 164–203, recognizes the difference in the quality of Byzantine hospitals (176), but he does not trace the evolution of these institutions. The classic work on Christian philanthropy, G. Uhlhorn, *Die christliche Liebestätigkeit* (Stuttgart, 1882–90) does not pursue Byzantine philanthropic institutions beyond their origins at the end of the fourth century.

[6] A. R. Hands, *Charities and Social Aid in Greece and Rome* (Ithaca, New York, 1968), ch. 9: "Health and Hygiene." G. E. Gask and J. Todd, "The Origin of Hospitals," in E. A. Underwood, ed., *Science, Medicine and History: Essays . . . in honour of Charles Singer* (London, 1953; 2 vols.), I, 122–30. G. Harig, "Zum Problem ‚Krankenhaus' in der Antike," *Klio*, 53 (1971), 179–95. J. Scarborough, "Roman Medicine and Public Health," in T. Ogawa, ed., *Public Health* (Tokyo, 1981), 33–74.

[7] Uhlhorn (note 5 above), 241–42, 316–18; E. Troeltsch, *The Social Teaching of the Christian Churches* (New York, 1931), 47–50.

[8] *Chronicon paschale*, ed. G. Dindorf, Bonn ed. (1832), 1, 535–36. Both *xenodocheion* and *xenon* are derived from the Greek word *xenos* which means simply stranger or guest. Although *xenon* later came to mean a hospital for the sick, before the end of the sixth century it still could refer to a simple inn or hostel: for example, Procopius, *De aedificiis* I.11, 23–27.

[9] R. Devreesse, *Le patriarcat d'Antioche* (Paris, 1945), 111, note 11.

[10] Epiphanios, *Panarion* 75.1, ed. K. Holl, GCS, 37 (Leipzig, 1933), 3, 333.

have offered some kind of hospital care to the sick strangers—probably those from among the immigrants to Caesarea who had no homes or families in the town. The presence of doctors suggests that Basil had founded a facility which included medical treatment for the sick, certainly to alleviate their suffering, but perhaps also to find a cure for their ailments.[11]

At the very end of the fourth century, John Chrysostom, bishop of Constantinople (398–404), opened similar institutions in the capital of the East Roman Empire. His biographer Palladios called these philanthropic houses nosokomeia (places to care for the sick). To staff them John appointed two priests as directors and hired physicians, cooks, and servants who were recruited from among celibate ascetics in Constantinople. Although Palladios adds that these institutions served both those stricken with disease and the strangers (xenoi), the term nosokomeion, derived from nosos (disease), suggests that the care of the sick predominated in these foundations. Again, the presence of physicians implies that rational medical procedure played a central role in ministering to the patients.[12]

A student of Bishop John, the ascetical writer Neilos of Ankyra, offers another glimpse inside institutions such as those of Chrysostom and Basil. In an extended metaphor illustrating Christ's care for sinful men, Neilos compares the world and its sinners to a great nosokomeion filled with patients and Christ the physician of souls to the staff doctor. Christ does not give all sinners the same remedy for their spiritual diseases. Rather He adjusts His cures to fit the individual problems of each soul just as the staff physician carefully examines each patient in the nosokomeion to determine the proper medicines and diet to restore health. In this metaphor Neilos assumes that the physician or physicians of early fifth-century nosokomeia were seeking to cure the patients, not simply trying to relieve their discomforts until they died. Neilos' account thus implies that these institutions did indeed offer hospital care, at least to the poor and homeless.[13]

Historians of modern institutions, however, might still object on several grounds to designating as hospitals the charitable facilities which Neilos pictured. First, these institutions treated only the very poor—the homeless immigrants who were collecting in the larger cities of the East Roman Empire during the fourth and fifth centuries. Second, they did not maintain a professional nursing staff; indeed, Chrysostom engaged urban ascetics to tend the patients of his nosokomeia. Finally, they offered only rudimentary medical services, access to a physician; a hospital implies a complex hierarchy of medical professionals.[14] A valuable hagiographical text of the seventh century reveals that later Byzantine philanthropic institutions for the sick fit even this much more limited definition of a hospital, and should banish any doubts about the true nature of East Roman xenones or nosokomeia.

Written shortly after 650, the Miracula Sancti Artemii includes two miracle tales which describe seventh-century hospitals in some detail. The first recounts the story of Stephen, a deacon of Hagia Sophia, who was afflicted with a malady of the groin. When home remedies failed, his parents advised him to commit himself to the surgeons of the Sampson Xenon. During his brief stay, Stephen was assigned a bed near the section for ophthalmic patients. After undergoing cold-cautery treatments for three days, Stephen went into surgery. Having suffered these painful therapies, he was released apparently cured. This tale reveals first that xenones of seventh-century Constantinople admitted patients above the poverty line—in this case a deacon of the principal church of the city who must have received a substantial income and also had family support. Nevertheless, when he fell ill, he sought a hospital for surgery just as a person today would do. Second, it indicates that the xenon staff included specialists—surgeons certainly and perhaps doctors who specialized in eye problems. In any case, ophthalmic patients had a separate station in the xenon.[15]

The second tale describes the ordeal of a cantor who likewise suffered from a disease affecting his groin. During his long stay at the Christodotes Xenon, he was treated by physicians styled archiatroi, the successors to the chief physicians of the Antonine Age who had led the medical profession in the Greek cities of the East. Medics or trained nurses called hypourgoi assisted these doctors. The hypourgoi, in turn, had at their command servants (hyperetai) who carried out non-medical nursing chores about the institution. The story suggests that the hypourgoi, just like the physicians, were career

[11] Ep. 94: Saint Basil, Letters, trans. R. J. Deferrari and M. R. McGuire, Loeb (1961), 2, 150.

[12] Palladii dialogus de vita S. Joannis Chrysostomi, ed. P. R. Coleman-Norton (Cambridge, 1928), 32.

[13] S. Nili epistolarum liber II, epp. 109–11, PG, 79, 248–49.

[14] See the comments on hospitals before the nineteenth century in Starr (note 4 above), 145–62.

[15] Miracula Artemii, mir. 21, 25–28.

professionals, a suggestion supported by a contemporary Egyptian papyrus which lists an association of hospital *hypourgoi* together with other lay guilds.[16] This tale, thus, confirms the presence of specialized staff positions in Byzantine *xenones*. At the Christodotes, the *archiatroi* supervised therapy, assisted by trained *hypourgoi* and the servants. Second, it demonstrates that nursing had become a profession in the hands of specialists, no longer a pious exercise for ascetics. In sum, these two stories from the *Miracula Sancti Artemii* prove that seventh-century *xenones* functioned in almost every respect as do hospitals of the twentieth century.

Clearly these seventh-century *xenones* offered more elaborate services than did their predecessors of the late fourth century. It is likely that a gradual growth in services took place in the intervening two hundred years. There is evidence, however, that a major improvement in the status of hospitals as medical centers took place in the sixth century. The emperor Justinian supposedly terminated the state subsidies to the local leaders of the medical profession, the *archiatroi* of the cities.[17] Several sources, including the *Miracula Sancti Artemii*, however, prove that physicians called *archiatroi* were still functioning in the late sixth century and long afterwards, but now as *xenon* doctors. It appears, therefore, that Justinian did not abolish the city *archiatroi*; rather, he transferred them to the wards of Christian hospitals where they were now subject to the hospital administrator instead of the curial council of the city.[18] When the premier practitioners of Greek medical science entered the *xenones*, they no doubt encouraged greater professionalism among other employees directly engaged in patient care.

To summarize, philanthropic institutions offering hospital services were certainly assisting the poor by the end of the fourth century; most students of ancient and medieval society will feel comfortable in calling these *nosokomeia* and *xenones* hospitals. By the end of Justinian's reign, however, some *xenones* in Constantinople and probably in other large towns as well had developed into elaborate medical facil-

ities with highly specialized classes of what today are called health professionals.

Where were Byzantine hospitals located? In nineteenth-century America, hospitals first appeared in larger cities, especially in centers of commerce where people who had left their homes collected in search of employment.[19] In the East Roman Empire, too, the surviving sources first mention *xenones* for the sick in trading and political centers. Basil opened his medical facility near Caesarea, the economic, political, and ecclesiastical center of the large Cappadocian province.[20] Chrysostom built his *nosokomeia* in the imperial capital. Between 400 and 600, several *xenones* were built in Constantinople. The Sampson, the Euboulos, and the St. Irene in Perama were established before 500.[21] The St. Panteleemon and probably the Christodotes were added before 600.[22] Many other *xenones* whose names the surviving sources fail to record no doubt also served the capital. The great commercial cities of Antioch and Alexandria possessed a number of hospitals by the sixth century.[23] Even smaller towns had them. An inscription from the fifth or sixth century, found near the city of Dervisos in Asia Minor, marks the grave of a doctor who had worked in the *nosokomeion*.[24] Indeed, *xenones* seem to have

[16] *Ibid.*, *mir.* 22, 28–31; *Greek Papyri in the British Museum*, ed. F. G. Kenyon and H. I. Bell, vol. 3 (London, 1907), 276–77, no. 1028.

[17] Procopius, *Anecdota* 26.5.

[18] *Miracula Artemii*, *mir.* 22, 28–31; no. 67151, in *Catalogue général des antiquités égyptiennes du musée du Caire: Papyrus grecs d'époque byzantine*, ed. M. J. Maspero (rep. Osnabrück, 1973); *Theodori Studitae epistolae*, PG, 99, 1509.

[19] Starr (note 4 above), 151.

[20] A. H. M. Jones, *The Cities of the Eastern Roman Provinces* (New York, 1937), 175–82.

[21] To establish when these hospitals were opened it is necessary to examine the tenth-century *De cerimoniis* of Constantine Porphyrogenitus, I:32: Bonn ed. (1828), 1, 173 (= *Le livre des Cérémonies*, ed. A. Vogt [Paris, 1967], 1, 161). This section describes the entrance of the heads of five *xenones*: the Sampson, the Euboulos, the Irene in Perama, the Narses, and the Irene. The order of their entrance is based on the age of the *xenones* they administer, with the director of the most recent foundation entering last. The last *xenon* in the list was founded by the empress Irene, 797–802 (*Scriptores originum Constantinopolitanarum*, ed. T. Preger [Leipzig, 1907], 246); the fourth in the list in the reign of the emperor Maurice, 582–602 (Zonaras, *Epitomae historiarum libri*, Bonn ed. [1897], 3, 199); the Irene in Perama in the reign of the emperor Marcian, 450–57 (*Scriptores originum Constantinopolitanarum*, 234; *Vita S. Marciani oeconomi*, A. Papadopoulos-Kerameus, *Analekta hierosol. Stachyologias*, 4 [Petersburg, 1897], 258–70). The Sampson and the Euboulos were opened sometime before the Irene in Perama; i.e. before ca. 450.

[22] For the Panteleemon see Zonaras, Bonn ed. (1897), 3, 199. The *Miracula Artemii*, *mir.* 22, 28–31 reveals that the Christodotes was established by the mid seventh century. Since the time from 600 to 650 had been one of constant military effort, it is more likely that civilian foundations like the Christodotes Xenon date from the prosperous years before 600.

[23] For Antioch see Procopius, *De aedificiis* II.10, 25; for Alexandria the guild of hospital *hypourgoi* organized by the seventh century is evidence of a well-established *xenon* system (*Greek Papyri* [note 16 above], 276–77, no. 1028).

[24] *CIG*, no. 9256.

become one of the features of the late antique *polis*, the Christian city of God. Thus, when the emperor Maurikios (582–602) decided to beautify his native Arabissi, a town of Cappadocia, he first constructed a magnificent church there and then a large hospital.[25]

The prosperous era of the early Byzantine Empire (395–602) came to an end with the calamities of the seventh century—invasions, internal upheavals, and dramatic demographic decline which resulted in greatly diminishing the prosperity of the Byzantine capital on the Bosporos and radically altering the quality of provincial city life. At Constantinople, however, at least four *xenones* survived the catastrophic seventh century—the Sampson, the Euboulos, the St. Irene in Perama, and the St. Panteleemon.[26] Moreover, at the end of the eighth century, the empress Irene founded a new hospital.[27] Following her example, the emperor Theophilos (829–42) opened a famous *xenon* which he designed to afford patients both a healthy exposure to the breezes and a beautiful view. He apparently considered endowing this hospital together with improving the city's walls among his principal benefactions to the people of Constantinople.[28] Thereafter, prominent emperors often expressed their beneficence by building new hospitals, a tradition which culminated in the twelfth-century Pantokrator Xenon which the emperor John II Komnenos founded.[29]

The disasters of the seventh century produced their most striking effects beyond the great walls of Constantinople. Archaeological evidence from the famous urban sites of Asia Minor, Thrace, and Greece suggests that most Byzantine cities rapidly declined after 600; some almost vanished.[30] Despite the decline of ancient city life, there are enough scattered references to hospitals in provincial towns to demonstrate that these institutions did not disappear outside Constantinople. Metropoli-

tan Andrew of Crete built a *xenon* in the eighth century for the people of Gortyna.[31] Bishop Theophylakt founded a medical facility for the citizens of Nikomedeia in the ninth century.[32] Eleventh-century Antioch had at least two hospitals, while twelfth-century Thessalonica had at least one.[33] In the thirteenth century Nicea claimed several.[34] At the same time Philadelphia's bishop Phokas built a new *xenon* for that vigorous town at the head of the Meander Valley in Asia Minor.[35] From the fourteenth century, on the other hand, no references to hospitals in cities other than the capital have so far come to light. It is especially curious that Mistra in the Peloponnesus does not seem to have had a *xenon* for its citizens.

Byzantine sources indicate that *xenones* were usually associated with cities. In fact, they took their place alongside of other buildings as representative features of Byzantine urban life. In praising the efforts of Michael VIII Palaiologos to restore Constantinople to its former brilliance, Gregory of Cyprus first describes how the emperor replaced the splendid crown of the city's walls to her brow. Second, he mentions the churches he restored, and third, the hospitals and other philanthropic institutions he had reopened.[36] The thirteenth-century intellectual and statesman, Theodore Metochites, considered the two hospitals of Nicea better evidence of the city's high cultural level than its baths or its fortifications.[37] Indeed, as early as the reign of Justinian, *xenones* for the sick had been hallmarks of the new Christian *polis*.[38]

Despite their association with city life, monastic leaders occasionally included hospitals as part of rural religious houses. One of the most famous examples is the Lavra monastery on Mount Athos

[25] *Iohannis Ephesini historiae ecclesiasticae pars tertia* V.22, ed. E. W. Brooks, Scriptores Syri, 85: CSCO, 106 (Louvin, 1952), 206–7. John of Ephesus describes Maurice's foundation with the Syriac word for *xenodocheion*. II.4, *ibid.*, p. 41, however, shows that he used this same term in describing a hospital for the sick at Constantinople.

[26] *De cerimoniis* I.32, 173 (Vogt, 1, 161–62).

[27] *Scriptores originum Constantinopolitanarum* (note 21 above), 246.

[28] Theophanes Continuatus, *Chronographia*, Bonn ed. (1838), 94–95.

[29] *PantTyp*, intro., 21.

[30] R. Browning, *The Byzantine Empire* (New York, 1980), 62–64.

[31] *Vita S. Andreae*, ed. A. Papadopoulos-Kerameus, *Analekta hierosol. stachyologias*, 5 (Petersburg, 1888), 176.

[32] *Vita S. Theophylacti*, ed. A. Vogt, *AnalBoll*, 50 (1932), 75.

[33] For Antioch see J. Schacht and M. Meyerhof, *The Medico-Philosophical Controversy between Ibn Butlan of Baghdad and Ibn Ridwan of Cairo* (Cairo, 1937), 56 and 65. For Thessalonica, Eustazio di Tessalonica, *La espugnazione di Tessalonica*, ed. S. Kyriakides (Palermo, 1961), 146.

[34] *Theodori Metochitis Nikaeus*, ed. C. Sathas, *Bibliotheca graeca medii aevi*, 1 (Venice, 1872), 145.

[35] *Theodori Ducae Lascaris epistulae* CCXVII, ed. N. Festa (Florence, 1898), *ep.* 118, 164–65.

[36] *Gregorii Cyprii laudatio Michaelis Paleologi*, PG, 142, 377.

[37] *Theodori Metochitis Nikaeus* (note 34 above), 144–45.

[38] Procopius, *De aedificiis* II.10, 1–25 describes Justinian's restoration of Antioch after its sack by the Persians in 540. He closes his account with a reference to the emperor's rebuilding a hospital for the sick. This hospital is listed together with other urban amenities.

which the renowned holy man, Athanasios the Athonite, established in the reign of Nikephoros II (963–69). One of the oldest versions of Athanasios' *vita* mentions that he built a *nosokomeion* as part of this community, a facility which was to serve both monks of the monastic community and people from the outside world.[39] By the fourteenth century, however, this hospital accepted only monks.[40]

Who went to Byzantine hospitals for help? To what classes in society did patients belong? Since no patient register from any *xenon* survives, it is possible only to collect casual references to the people whom hospitals helped. All the sources agree that the late fourth-century medical facilities were designed to serve the poor—and especially the homeless migrants described as *xenoi*. Less than a hundred years later, however, the monastic leader Theodosios the Cenobearch opened a separate *xenon* designed to treat people above the poverty level.[41] Already Byzantine hospitals were becoming institutions to dispense medical services, rather than shelters for the homeless which included doctors and nurses for those who happened to suffer from disease. The *Miracula Sancti Artemii* prove that people of some status in seventh-century Constantinople were prepared to go to *xenon* physicians and even spend days, weeks, or months in a hospital bed.[42] The twelfth-century Pantokrator Xenon did not permit staff physicians to accept tips from patients, a rule which assumes that some of the sick had money.[43] The fourteenth-century poet, Manuel Philes, was treated for some illness at a hospital founded by Michael Glabras. Though not a wealthy man, Philes was surely not one of the desperately poor or a wandering pilgrim—the only sort who would have sought aid from the hospice-hospital in the medieval or early modern West.[44]

That both the poverty-stricken and men of the middle class patronized Byzantine hospitals like the Pantokrator doubtless helped to win for the *xenones* society's respect. They never came to symbol-

ize despair and degradation as did Latin institutions for medical care. Indeed, Western hospitals acquired a bad reputation which managed to survive into the nineteenth century.[45] Byzantine *xenones*, on the other hand, seem to have become the normal *loci* for the practice of medicine, at least in twelfth-century Constantinople. When the emperor Manuel I developed some new drugs, his court historian, John Kinnamos, assumed that most people would see these compounds on their visits to the city's *xenones*.[46]

Not only did members of the middle class occupy hospital beds, but there is some evidence that the emperors themselves sought out the advantages of a *xenon* when they fell ill. A fourteenth-century manuscript (Vaticanus graecus 299, fols., 368–393ᵛ) contains a remedy list from the Mangana Xenon, a hospital located on the very tip of the Constantinopolitan peninsula. One of the remedies (on fol. 374) the list attributes to the emperor's personal physician, Abraam the *aktouarios* of the Mangana Xenon. Since the twelfth century, physicians with the rank of *aktouarios* had served as the doctors to the imperial family. Apparently, this post was also linked with the Mangana Xenon. In fact, in 1118, when the emperor Alexios fell desperately ill, the *aktouarios* and two other doctors transferred him from the old palace to the Mangana complex, according to the historian Zonaras so that Alexios would be close to the hospital there.[47] Since niether the *Typikon* of the Mangana monastery and hospital survive nor any descriptions of this *xenon* in action, it is impossible to determine exactly what provisions were made at the hospital for treating the emperor and his family.

Who worked in Byzantine hospitals in the service of the sick? The most important group of *xenon* employees were surely the *iatroi*, the staff physicians. In this, Byzantine medical centers resemble far more closely the hospitals of the modern world than they do the hospice-hospitals of the medieval West. Moreover, the role of physicians in East Roman *xenones* continually expanded until the twelfth century, when they seem to have controlled almost all aspects of these institutions.

The earliest medical facilities—the proto-hospitals of Basil and John Chrysostom—hired *iatroi* to treat

[39] *Vita S. Athanasii Athonitae B*, chap. 41, *Vitae duae antiquae sancti Athanasii Athonitae*, ed. J. Noret, Corpus Christianorum: Series graeca, 9 (Turnhout, 1982), 173.

[40] Doc. 123, in *Actes de Lavre: III. De 1329 à 1500*, ed. P. Lemerle et al., Archives de l'Athos, 10 (Paris, 1979), 25.

[41] *Lobrede auf den heiligen Theodosios von Theodoros Bischof von Patrai*, in *Der heilige Theodosios*, ed. H. Usener (Leipzig, 1890), 40.

[42] E.g., Deacon Stephen in *Miracula Artemii*, mir. 21, 25–26.

[43] *PantTyp*, 107 lines 1307–8.

[44] *Manuelis Philae carmina*, ed. E. Miller, vol. 1 (Paris, 1855), no. 98, 280–81.

[45] Starr (note 4 above), 151.

[46] *Ioannis Cinnami epitome rerum ab Ioanne et Alexio Comnenis gestarum*, Bonn ed. (1836), 190.

[47] Zonaras (note 22 above), 3, 759.

their sick guests.[48] In the hospital which Neilos of Ankyra described, a physician examined the patients and ordered appropriate therapies.[49] By the sixth century, the leading representatives of Greek medicine—the municipal *archiatroi*—were conducting daily rounds in the *xenones* of Constantinople.[50] Despite their prestige as the most experienced physicians, however, these *archiatroi* did not manage the hospitals where they worked. They did not even exercise complete control over admissions. When the cantor of the *Miracula Sancti Artemii* fell seriously ill in his apartment, the *xenodochos*—the hospital administrator and member of the patriarch's clergy—made the decision to assign him a hospital bed. The medical staff labored in vain for ten months to cure the man. When one of the *archiatroi* observed the extent of the malady after such treatment, he declared the case incurable. Nevertheless, he did not remove the patient from the hospital area. Rather, he prescribed some medicines to soothe the pain and allowed the cantor to remain in a *xenon* bed.[51]

The hospital administrators, whom Byzantine sources call *xenodochoi* or *nosokomoi*, were originally members of the clergy, deacons or priests. When John Chrysostom established new *nosokomeia* in Constantinople, he assigned two pious priests to supervise them.[52] A sixth-century *xenodochos* of the Sampson Xenon named Eugenios held the rank of deacon.[53] These clerical administrators had to manage the material resources of the hospitals, a task which required expertise in the Roman Law and the rules governing ecclesiastical property. As the miracle tale of the cantor illustrates, they also retained considerable influence over the medical aspects of *xenones* as well.

By the tenth century, however, physicians had gained greater control over the therapeutic side of hospital business. After having suffered severe head injuries, a subdeacon named Sergios was committed to the Euboulos Xenon of Constantinople. The staff physicians worked on Sergios for seven days with absolutely no success. They then decided that his case was hopeless and ceased to treat him. They turned him over to the nursing staff who transferred him out of the *xenon* proper to a hospice of some sort where they could try to make his last days as comfortable as possible.[54] The physicians reached the decision whether or not to treat Sergios in the *xenon* not under the orders of an administrator, but on the basis of the ancient rules of their profession, in this case the Hippocratic injunction not to treat hopeless cases.[55] Discharging Sergios was a medical decision, and thus out of the hands of the administrator.

The twelfth-century rules governing the Pantokrator Xenon demonstrate that by that time the physicians controlled the admission of all new cases. The chief physicians of the hospital's medical staff—now called *primmikerioi*—were normally responsible for receiving patients into the institution. Most of the sick first entered the hospital through the outpatient clinic. Here two junior physicians were on duty to examine those who walked in or were carried to the door. If these doctors felt a case was serious enough for hospital care, they notified the *primmikerios* on duty who then dispatched a senior physician to decide on admission.[56] If a resident of the old-age home adjoining the Pantokrator fell ill, the priest of the home notified the hospital administrator who then sent a physician or medic to conduct a medical examination and determine whether the case warranted hospitalization.[57]

Not only had doctors gained control of all aspects of medical care at the Pantokrator, but the directors themselves were now chosen from among the physicians. In a letter to the *nosokomos* of the Pantokrator Xenon, John Tzetzes hailed the man as a leader of the medical profession.[58] So, too, the poet Prodromos described a *nosokomos* of an unnamed hospital as a physician who performed surgery.[59] At some time after the seventh century, then, physicians had replaced legal experts from among the clergy in the top administrative posts, at least in the sophisticated hospitals of Constantinople. That in the eleventh century the renowned Arab Christian physician Ibn Butlan was asked to organize a hospital in Antioch would seem to indicate

[48] Basil, *ep*. 94 (note 11 above), 2, 150; *Palladii dialogus* (note 12 above), 32.

[49] *S. Nili epistolarum liber II*, *epp*. 109–11, PG, 79, 248–49.

[50] *Miracula Artemii*, *mir*. 22, 31.

[51] *Ibid.*, 28–31.

[52] *Palladii dialogus* (note 12 above), 32.

[53] Nov. 59.3, *Corpus iuris civilis: III. Novellae*, ed. R. Schoell and W. Kroll (Berlin, 1895), 319.

[54] *Vita S. Lucae Stylitae*, in *Les saints stylites*, ed. H. Delehaye, SubsHag, 14 (Paris-Brussels, 1923), 218.

[55] Hippocrates, *The Art* 3.

[56] *PantTyp*, 87 lines 975–79.

[57] *PantTyp*, 111 lines 1370–78.

[58] *Ep*. 81, *Ioannis Tzetzae epistulae*, ed. P. Leone (Leipzig, 1972), 121.

[59] Theodore Prodromos, *Historische Gedichte*, ed. W. Hörandner (Vienna, 1974), poem. 46, p. 432.

that physicians had won a dominant role in hospitals outside Constantinople as well.[60]

The relationship between the *xenones* of the Byzantine Empire and the medical profession was extremely close. In this respect, too, the facilities for the sick in the East Roman state resemble more the hospitals of the modern era than they do Western philanthropic institutions of the Middle Ages. Only in the nineteenth century did hospital service have a major impact on the organization of the Western medical profession. Here in the United States, as hospitals gained in status after 1800, physicians eagerly sought to associate with them and vied with one another for senior staff positions. The ascending ranks of hospital jobs gradually imposed a hierarchical structure on the medical profession in general. Those who held the highest rank on a hospital staff were also considered the leaders of the local profession.[61] One can trace the same development in Byzantine hospitals.

The small committees of *archiatroi* serving the cities of the Late Roman Empire already possessed an order of precedence. In 370 the emperor Valentinian I required that the *archiatroi* of Rome be ranked according to years in office.[62] The same system must have existed at Constantinople and in other cities throughout the Empire.[63] When the *archiatroi* took over hospital responsibilities under Justinian, they introduced this hierarchy of service into the *xenon* medical staff. The seventh and eighth centuries witnessed new developments in ranking hospital physicians, for a letter of Saint Theodore the Studite sketches a novel set of titles for hospital physicians. Doctors called *protarchoi* led the staff, followed by *archiatroi*; then came the middle physicians (*mesoi*) and the last physicians (*teleutaioi*)— no doubt the most recent to join the staff.[64] In the tenth century, the title *protomenites* (leader of the month) first appears among *xenon* dignitaries, probably replacing *archiatros*.[65] The twelfth-century Pantokrator Xenon had a staff led by two *primmi-*

kerioi (the old *protarchoi*), followed by two *protomenitai* and two senior surgeons; then came the four *iatroi* of the general wards, and at the bottom of the regular staff, the doctors of the women's ward. Four doctors described as extra (*perissoi*) treated the sick in the outpatient clinic.[66] These *perissoi* doctors received a salary, but there were apparently other *perissoi* physicians at the hospital who did not have posts with pay. These junior physicians may have been studying the practice of medicine as interns do in modern hospitals.[67]

Although the staff doctors of the Pantokrator had to come to the *xenon* all seven days of the week, they still had time for private practice. The entire staff of physicians was divided into two shifts with each shift working at the hospital only six months a year.[68] This practice was at least as old as the seventh century, for the *archiatroi* of the Christodotes Xenon alternated hospital duties in a similar fashion.[69] Such a system left six months a year entirely free for private practice. While treating hospital patients during the other six months, physicians received very low salaries—equal to or lower than the bare minimum income of day laborers.[70] These doctors, however, received some additional reward for their hospital service. The reward probably came from the great prestige which a hospital appointment or a higher-ranking *xenon* post brought with it—prestige which increased the earning potential of private practice. This, indeed, was the system in the highly regarded voluntary hospitals of nineteenth-century America, where the leading physicians of the community labored for the hospitals, collecting neither fees from the patients nor stipends from the institutions. These doctors were satisfied with the fame hospital service merited and the concomitant increase in the profits of private practice.[71] Both the low salaries and the part-time schedules of Byzantine *xenon* physicians suggest a similar system obtained in the East Roman Empire.

The method of training Byzantine physicians

[60] Schacht and Meyerhof (note 33 above), 65.

[61] Starr (note 4 above), 162–69.

[62] *CTh* 13.3, 9.

[63] *Cod.* 1.27, 41: *CIC, CI*, 79 probably refers to the municipal *archiatroi*, though it appears in a list of salaries for the praetorian prefect's offices. The number of doctors is set at five, which corresponds to the number of municipal doctors fixed by Antoninus Pius (*Digest* 27.1, 6, 2: *CIC, Dig*, 391) for each city. Moreover, *Cod.* 1.27, 41 lists the physicians together with grammarians and rhetors just as Antoninus Pius did. *Cod.* 1.27, 41 was issued for Africa in 534 by Justinian. It probably reflects the arrangement in the Eastern provinces.

[64] *Theodori Studitae epistolae*, PG, 99, 1509.

[65] Hunger, "Medizin," 307.

[66] *PantTyp*, 85 line 937–87 line 979.

[67] *PantTyp*, 87 lines 948–49 and 93 lines 1063–73.

[68] *PantTyp*, 87 lines 955–64.

[69] *Miracula Artemii, mir.* 22, 30.

[70] The salaries of the Pantokrator physicians are listed by Gautier, *PantTyp*, intro., 13. The highest-ranking physician, the *primmikerios*, received a salary of only 11.75 *noumismata* a year (8 *noumismata* and forty-five *modioi* of wheat). A living wage has been reckoned at roughly a *noumisma* a month (G. Ostrogorsky, "Löhne and Preise in Byzanz," *BZ*, 32 [1932], 297). The regular ward doctors received approximately 10 *noumismata*—less than a minimum wage.

[71] Starr (note 4 above), 162–63.

surely strengthened the bonds between the *xenones* and the medical profession. In the classical world each established physician had gathered apprentices about him.[72] After the legislation of Antoninus Pius defined a small group of privileged doctors in each city, the *archiatroi*, these men came to predominate in training new physicians.[73] By Justinian's reign (527–65), they were the ordinary teachers of medicine.[74] When these *archiatroi* entered *xenon* service, they simply continued to teach their science as they had before. There is, however, no direct evidence of medical instruction in Byzantine *xenones* before the end of the tenth century, although teaching medicine dominated the early Moslem hospitals, which surely derived from the *xenones* of the East Roman Empire.[75] When sometime in the tenth century the surgeon Niketas illustrated a manuscript both for reference and teaching in Constantinopolitan *xenones*, he provided the first indication that medical schooling formed a regular part of hospital routine.[76] In the twelfth century the Pantokrator Xenon hired a physician of the highest status to teach medical theory to the children of staff doctors.[77] Moreover, the group of *perissoi* doctors at the hospital was involved in some kind of student program.[78] Most probably they accompanied the *primmikerioi* on their daily rounds to observe the actual practice of the medical art. The most famous of the fourteenth-century physicians, John Zachariah, began his career in this fashion as a *xenon* intern somewhere in Constantinople.[79] Hospitals still functioned as medical schools as late as the fifteenth century. The illustrious physician and philosopher John Argyropoulos was lecturing at the Krales Xenon just before the Turks conquered the Byzantine capital in 1453.[80] An illumination in an Oxford Aristotle manuscript (Baroccianus 87, fol. 35) represents Argyropoulos teaching from a lofty *cathedra* with the *xenon* buildings in the background.

The physicians, of course, were not the only employees of the Byzantine hospitals. As the discussion of the *Miracula Sancti Artemii* illustrated, professional medical assistants or nurses called *hypourgoi* aided the doctors in caring for the sick. These *hypourgoi* applied medicines and frequently checked the patients' progress.[81] Some of them apparently could perform minor surgery as well.[82] They also were required to supervise the wards when the physicians were not present—a responsibility which made night duty mandatory.[83]

The rules governing the Pantokrator Xenon provide the most information on the *hypourgoi*. Each of the five wards at this hospital had three ordained (*embathmoi*) *hypourgoi* and two extra (*perissoi*) *hypourgoi*. The outpatient clinic had four of each rank. The medical assistants of the women's ward were themselves women (*hypourgissai*).[84] The extra *hypourgoi* were certainly full staff members since they received salaries only slightly less than the ordained assistants.[85] The status of *perissos* seems to have reflected a lower grade of competence. The *perissoi* doctors and medical assistants had not reached a certain level of experience and/or knowledge. Perhaps *perissos* connotes some rank in a guild organization. The term *bathmos* (ordained) was used to describe full membership in the guild of Byzantine notaries, and the closely related *embathmos* probably had the same meaning for the medical profession.[86] If this is true, then its opposite—*perissos*—would imply non-guild or apprentice status.

The *hypourgoi* were very poorly paid at the Pantokrator. The ordained medical assistants received only 2.5 *noumismata* a year from the hospital when a *noumisma* a month was considered a living wage. They also were given an *annona* allotment of twenty *modioi* of wheat, valued at approximately 1.66

[72] Aeschines, *Contra Timarchum* 40; *Historia Apollonii regis Tyrii* 26.

[73] For the office of *archiatros* see V. Nutton, "Archiatri and the Medical Profession in Antiquity," *PBSR*, 45 (1977), 191–226.

[74] *Cod.* 10.53, 6 (note 63 above), 422; Justinian reissued the earlier law of the emperor Constantine (*CTh*, 13.3, 3), adding that *archiatroi* normally taught.

[75] *The Encyclopaedia of Islam*, new edition, vol. 1 (Leiden and London, 1960), 1222–25.

[76] This ms. (Laurentianus gr. 74.7) includes three poems of thanks dedicated to the copyist, Niketas (on folio 7ᵛ). These poems are published in A. M. Bandini, *Catalogus codicum graecorum Bibliothecae Laurentianae* (Florence, 1770), cols. 80–83. Bandini dates the ms. to the eleventh century (col. 55), but J. Kollesch and F. Kudlien, *Apollonios von Kition: Kommentar zu Hippokrates über das Einrenken der Gelenke*, (Berlin, 1965), *CMG* XI.1, 1, p. 5 prefer the tenth century.

[77] *PantTyp*, 107 lines 1313–24.

[78] They were seen as advancing toward the status of *embathmos* (ordained). See *PantTyp* 93 lines 1063–73. Cf. V. Grumel, "La profession médicale à Byzance a l'époque des Comnènes," *REB*, 7 (1949), 42–46.

[79] *Georgii Lacapeni epistulae x priores cum epimerismis editae*, ed. S. Lindstam (Upsala, 1910), *ep.* 10, 21 *scholium* to line 26.

[80] F. Fuchs, *Die höheren Schulen von Konstantinopel* (Leipzig, 1926), 71.

[81] *Miracula Artemii, mir.* 22, 28–31.

[82] Bandini (note 76 above), poem. I, col. 81.

[83] *Miracula Artemii, mir.* 22, 30; *PantTyp*, 85 lines 939–41.

[84] *PantTyp*, 85 line 937–87 line 954.

[85] *PantTyp*, intro., 13.

[86] *Liber Prefecti* I.2 and 3, reprinted with introduction by I. Dujčev (London, 1970).

noumismata, and some small additional donatives. Moreover, these trained *hypourgoi* earned only half as much as did the simple servants (*hyperetai*).[87] The medical assistants, like their superiors the physicians, must have had some opportunity for private practice as paramedics to augment their meager incomes. The Pantokrator rules, however, do not state that they worked in monthly shifts as the doctors did.

Besides the *hypourgoi*, the Pantokrator Xenon employed a staff of eleven servants (*hyperetai*), five laundresses, two cooks, two backers, one usher, one keeper of the cauldrons, one groom for the doctors' horses, one gate keeper, one purser, four pall bearers, one miller, one latrine cleaner, and one employee to polish and sharpen the surgical instruments.[88] There is absolutely no evidence that the patients at the Pantokrator or at any other Byzantine hospital performed physical tasks on behalf of the *xenon*. In this, the *xenones* of the East Roman state differed radically from the typical institution of the West, where the patient-residents had many duties about the facility.[89] Even as late as the eighteenth century, a progressive foundation such as the Pennsylvania Hospital of Benjamin Franklin required the stronger patients to wash linens and assist in cleaning chores.[90] At the Pantokrator, on the other hand, paid professionals were responsible for all tasks in the hospital. Just as in modern hospitals, the only obligation on the patient was responding to treatment.

Although far from complete, the answers to the questions above should serve to introduce the hospitals of the Byzantine Empire and to dispel the notion that they were not essentially medical institutions. There remains, however, one final question to discuss. Why did Byzantine physicians choose to devote a substantial portion of their time and energy to hospital work? One reason, of course, was the imperial will. At some point early in his reign, the emperor Justinian required the *archiatroi* to become hospital staff physicians. By the mid sixth century, however, East Roman physicians had thoroughly accepted hospitals as the proper theaters of their labors. When finding themselves in the service of Shah Khusro I ca. 560, a group of them requested that the Persian ruler establish a *xenon* where they could fittingly practice their science.[91] Is it possible that these Byzantine doctors had developed some technology which demanded a hospital setting—new surgical equipment perhaps or more complex pharmacological treatment which required constant monitoring? The results of this symposium may help to answer these two questions. Or did Byzantine physicians feel that hospital work enhanced the prestige of their profession? Certainly, the Christian philanthropic institutions which originated in the fourth century were extremely popular—indeed, they won the Christian Church many new converts in the cities of the Eastern Roman provinces.[92] Although some doctors resisted Justinian's hospital system, most no doubt saw advantages in an alliance with stable institutions enjoying the full support of the Church, the State, and popular opinion.[93] Finally, a change in the ratio of the number of physicians to the size of the population as a whole might have stimulated hospital organization as a method which enabled fewer physicians to care for more patients. Perhaps the rapid population increase of the fifth and early sixth centuries forced a limited number of physicians to realign the profession around the hospitals. On the other hand, the radical upheavals of the seventh and eighth centuries might have drastically reduced the percentage of trained doctors in the population. In both cases, hospitals would have allowed Byzantine society to provide better medical care to more of its citizens, to both the very poor and to men and women of some substance.

From the reign of Justinian, hospitals stood at the center of the medical profession in the Byzantine Empire. Among the beds of these *xenones*, the best doctors spent half of their professional lives; in their lecture rooms and wards future physicians studied both the theory and practice of medicine. Indeed, the organization of the East Roman medical profession resembles in many ways the clinical medicine of Revolutionary France which recentered medical research and instruction in the hospitals of Paris. In the early nineteenth century, this

---

[87] *PantTyp*, intro., 13. Cf. Ostrogorsky (note 70 above), 297.

[88] *PantTyp*, 85 lines 937–43; 89 lines 996–1006; 105 lines 1271–79.

[89] S. Reicke, *Das deutsche Spital und sein Recht im Mittelalter* (Stuttgart, 1932), 2, 231–33; Starr (note 4 above), 159.

[90] Starr (note 4 above), 159.

[91] *The Syriac Chronicle Known as that of Zachariah of Mitylene* XIII.7, trans. F. S. Hamilton and E. W. Brooks (London, 1899), 331–32.

[92] *Ep.* 22: *The Works of the Emperor Julian* (Loeb), 3, 68; Theodoros Anagnostes, *Kirchengeschichte*, ed. G. C. Hansen, GCS, 54 (Berlin, 1971), 59 lines 4–6, accuses Julian of desiring to win back the urban populace—the *demoi*—to paganism by imitating the Christian philanthropic institutions.

[93] Some physicians joined a pagan plot against Justinian. See F. Nau, "Analyse de la seconde partie inédite de l'histoire ecclésiastique de Jean d'Asie," *ROChr*, 2 (1897), 481–82.

clinical movement made great progress in improving hospital care, in describing accurately the symptoms of diseases, in compiling statistical records regarding these same symptoms and the outcome of similar cases, and in pursuing pathological anatomy through repeated autopsies.[94] Is it possible that the *xenones* led Byzantine physicians along the same paths? East Roman physicians displayed an indifference to medical theories as did early nineteenth-century clinicians. Like the doctors of the clinical movement, they designed hospitals to promote hygiene and the comfort of patients. But did they pursue new anatomical studies or conduct autopsies frequently? Were they interested in careful records of individual cases with detailed descriptions of the symptoms? So far, no evidence has surfaced that they had such interests. Careful consideration of Byzantine medical science, however, is only beginning, and the study and publication of medieval Greek medical treatises will surely reveal more clearly the achievements and failings of Byzantine medicine and the contribution of hospitals to its development.[95]

[94] For a history of the clinical movement in France, see E. Ackerknecht, *Medicine at the Paris Hospital, 1794–1848* (Baltimore, 1967). See also the difficult study of M. Foucault, *The Birth of the Clinic*, trans. from the French by A. M. Sheridan (New York, 1973).

[95] A postscript. At this symposium on Byzantine medicine, Professor Alexander Kazhdan announced that he had found evidence in an ethical treatise of Symeon the New Theologian that Byzantine physicians of the eleventh century did indeed practice autopsies on human cadavers (see *Syméon le nouveau théologien: Traités théologiques et éthiques.*, ed. and trans. J. Darrouzès, SC, 129 [Paris, 1967], 2, 138–39).

ART, MEDICINE, AND MAGIC IN EARLY BYZANTIUM*

GARY VIKAN

In Byzantium the world of art touched that of medicine in a variety of ways and with varying intensity. Among the material remains of the Byzantine physician's trade are finely crafted surgical implements and richly carved ivory medicine boxes—and at least one silver stamp belonging to a certain *iatros* named Ishmael.[1] Aesthetically more impressive are the handful of deluxe medical manuscripts which have survived from Byzantium, including the famous copy of Dioscorides' *De materia medica* in Vienna, and the luxurious medical compendium in Florence (Plut. LXXIV, 7) which contains Soranus of Ephesus' treatise on bandaging, and that by Apollonius of Kitium on the set-

ting of dislocated bones.[2] Unfortunately, however, their miniatures like their texts usually reveal less about contemporary Byzantine medicine than about Antique prototypes. The opposite is true of portraits of such popular healing saints as Cosmas and Damian, Abbacyrus, and Panteleimon who, because they were holy doctors, were portrayed with the paraphernalia of practicing physicians of the time.[3] Yet even here, the relationship between Byz-

[The reader is referred to the list of abbreviations at the end of the volume.]

*This article is adapted from my paper "Medicine, Magic, and Pilgrims," delivered as part of the 1983 Dumbarton Oaks Spring Symposium.

[1] See L. Bliquez's article in this volume. That so few Byzantine surgical implements have survived suggests that they may customarily have been made of iron. Among the *miracula* of St. Artemius is one wherein physicians are ridiculed with the observation that their scalpels were "being consumed by rust." See A. Papadopoulos-Kerameus, *Varia graeca sacra* (St. Petersburg, 1909), *mir.* 25. It is noteworthy that while approximately 60,000 lead sealings survive from Byzantium, only half a dozen of the iron *bulloteria* with which they were made are extant. For ivory medicine boxes, see W. F. Volbach, *Elfenbeinarbeiten der Spätantike und frühen Mittelalters*, Romisch-Germanisches Zentralmuseum zu Mainz: Kataloge, vor- und frühgeschichtlicher Altertümer, 7 (3rd ed.) (Mainz, 1976), nos. 83–85. For a wooden medicine box from Early Byzantine Egypt with what may be medicine tablets still inside, see F. Petrie, *Objects of Daily Use*, British School of Archaeology in Egypt, 42 (London, 1927), pl. LVIII, 52. In the Yale University Art Museum is a doctor's leather instrument case with attached *pyx* (acc. no. 57.48.1). Apparently from Early Byzantine Egypt, it bears an *orans* portrait of a little-known doctor-saint, Antiochus of Sebaste, what appears to be a set of tables for mixing medicines, and, along its upper edge, the phrase "Use in good health" (*Hygienon chro*; cf. *IGLSyr*, no. 370). See also note 3 below for depictions of Byzantine medicine boxes. The silver doctor's stamp is unpublished, and in the Limbourg Collection, Cologne. It is mid-Byzantine in date and bears the following inscription: "Lord, help Ishmael [the] doctor."

[2] H. Gerstinger, Kommentarband to the sumptuous, full-color reproduction, *Dioscurides. Codex Vindobonensis med. gr. 1 der Osterreichischen Nationalbibliothek* (Graz, 1970). A shorter commentary, with selected plates (again in full color) is available: O. Mazal, *Pflanzen, Wurzeln, Säfte, Samen: Antike Heilkunst. Miniaturen des Wiener Dioskurides* (Graz, 1981). The best Greek text remains that edited by M. Wellmann. Soranus' *Bandages* is part of the collected Greek texts of Soranus (ed. Ilberg [*CMG* IV], 159 ff., with black and white reproductions of cod. Laur. LXXIV, 7 as plates I–XV). Apollonius of Kitium (*fl.* c. 50 B.C.) composed a *Commentary on Hippocrates' Joints*, and the best surviving texts are those from the tenth and eleventh century in Byzantium, perhaps compiled and re-edited by Nicetas (early tenth century). The illuminations of the cod. Laur. LXXIV, 7 seem to be contemporary with the Greek text of Apollonius' *Commentary*. Sarton, *Introduction*, I, 608. The best modern edition is J. Kollesch and F. Kudlien, eds., with translation (German) by J. Kollesch and D. Nickel, *Apollonii Citiensis In Hippocratis De articulis commentarius* (Berlin, 1965 [*CMG* XI 1, 1]), with thirty plates (black and white) of cod. Laur. LXXIV, 7 as an accompanying pamphlet. See also L. MacKinney, *Medical Illustrations in Medieval Manuscripts* (Berkeley, 1965), 89–91, with plate 91A (color: cod. Laur. LXXIV, 7, fol. 200). For the dependence of these picture cycles on Antique archetypes, see K. Weitzmann, *Ancient Book Illumination*, Martin Classical Lectures, 16 (Cambridge, Mass., 1959), 11 ff.

[3] Such hagiographic portraiture provides an especially rich typology of medical boxes. See P. J. Nordhagen, "The Frescoes of John VII (A.D. 705–707) in S. Maria Antiqua in Rome," *ActaIRNorv*, 3 (1968), 58. For two later boxes quite different from those cited by Nordhagen, see S. Pelekanides, *Kastoria*, I (in Greek) (Thessaloniki, 1953), pl. 26 (St. Panteleimon, Church of the Holy Anargyroi); and K. Weitzmann, "The Selection of Texts for Cyclic Illustration in Byzantine Manuscripts," *Byzantine Books and Bookmen*, Dumbarton Oaks Colloquium, 1971 (Washington, D.C., 1975), fig. 23 (St. Panteleimon; icon at Mt. Sinai). Occasionally, as in the icon just cited, a doctor-saint is shown in the act of healing one of his patients. Usually these "healings" are of a generic sort, morphologically dependent on Christ healing scenes from illustrated Gospels. However, some representations

antine art and Byzantine medicine remained distant. Much more interesting and illuminating for both are those rarer cases, specifically within the realm of supernatural healing, where the vehicle of the cure (whether pill or amulet) was itself an art object—where, in other words, art and medicine were one and the same. And nowhere was this phenomenon more pervasive or richer in its complexity than within the world of Early Byzantine pilgrimage.[4]

Pilgrimage played a central role in the life and culture of early Byzantium.[5] Indeed, within a few decades of the foundation of the Empire the east Mediterranean had come alive with pious travelers. Among the first was Constantine's own mother, Helena, who journeyed to the Holy Land at her son's request to dedicate his newly built churches located at the sites identified with the Birth and Ascension of Christ: Bethlehem and the Mount of Olives. Thousands were to follow in a mass mobilization of body and spirit which grew uninterrupted until the Arab conquests of the seventh century.

Ultimately, each pilgrim was driven by the same basic conviction; namely, that the sanctity of holy people, holy objects, and holy places was somehow transferable through physical contact.[6] They came not simply to see but to touch, to be close to the power of sanctity. For some, the hope was simply that this proximity would serve to intensify their faith. St. Jerome, for example, writes that when

Paula first came before the wood of the cross "she fell down and worshipped . . . as if she could see the Lord hanging on it."[7] For many others, however, pilgrimage was undertaken with the more specific goal of finding a miraculous cure at journey's end. Among them were the sick who filled the rows of beds in the hospice beside the Basilica of St. Mary in Jerusalem, and the infirm who for months would sleep on mats in the sanctuary of Sts. Cyrus and John in Menuthis, each night hoping for a miracle-working visitation from the shrine's holy doctors so that they could finally return home again, cured.[8] A description of the shrine of St. Thekla at Seleucia, as it functioned at mid fifth century, suggests an atmosphere somewhere between that of the Mayo Clinic and the Shrine of the Immaculate Conception:

> One never found her church without pilgrims, who streamed there from all sides; one group on account of the grandeur of the place in order to pray and to bring their offerings, and the other in order to receive healing and help against sickness, pain, and demons.[9]

That "healing and help" were indeed readily forthcoming was manifest to all who might enter the shrine; one need only have paused to listen for the recitation of the patron saint's most impressive *miracula* or have looked for the scores of precious *ex votos* which had been left behind to acknowledge them.[10] Perhaps the most explicitly "medical" of the many pilgrim votives to have survived from early Byzantium is a series of tiny silver reliefs of eyes found in northern Syria and now preserved in the Walters Art Gallery, Baltimore. Some among them bear the inscription, "Lord help, amen," while others (e.g., fig. 1)[11] show the words, "In fulfillment of a vow"; all, however, have basically the same set of large staring eyes. Like their modern counterparts in the Orthodox churches of Greece, and their ancient counterparts excavated at pagan healing

---

seem to show patients with identifiable disorders. See, for example, Mt. Athos, Panteleimon cod. 2, fol. 197r: "Sts. Cosmas and Damian heal a man with dropsy" (S. M. Pelekanidis, P. C. Christou, C. Tsioumis, and S. N. Kadas, *The Treasures of Mount Athos*, 2 [Athens, 1975], no. 278). For a rare glimpse into a Byzantine doctor's office, see folio 10v of the fourteenth-century Nicholas Myrespus manuscript in Paris (BN gr. 2243) (T. Velmans, "Le Parisinus grecus 135 et quelques autres peintures de style gothique dans les manuscrits grecs à l'époque des Paléologues," *CahArch*, 17 [1967], fig. 26).

[4] For a more general discussion of art and Early Byzantine pilgrimage, see G. Vikan, *Byzantine Pilgrimage Art*, Dumbarton Oaks Byzantine Collection Publications, 5 (Washington, D.C., 1982).

[5] For an excellent introduction to Early Byzantine pilgrimage, see J. Wilkinson, *Jerusalem Pilgrims Before the Crusades* (Warminster, 1977), "Introduction." See also, B. Kötting, *Peregrinatio religiosa.* (Regensberg, 1950), *passim*; and E. D. Hunt, *Holy Land Pilgrimage in the Later Roman Empire, A.D. 312–460* (New York, 1982), *passim*.

[6] John of Damascus writes of the True Cross (*Orth. Faith*, 4.11; *Fathers of the Church*, 37 [Washington, D.C., 1958], 165 ff.): ". . . that honorable and most truly venerable tree upon which Christ offered Himself as a sacrifice for us is itself to be adored, because it has been sanctified by contact with the sacred body and blood."

[7] Wilkinson, *Jerusalem Pilgrims*, 49.

[8] *Ibid.*, 84 (the anonymous pilgrim from Piacenza describing the Jerusalem hospice). For the sick sleeping on mats in the shrine (i.e., "incubation"), see H. Delehaye, "Les recueils antiques de miracles des saints," *AnalBoll*, 43 (1925), 11 f., 24 f., 64 f., and Kötting, *Peregrinatio*, 395.

[9] Basil of Seleucia, *Vita S. Teclae* (PG, 85, cols. 473ff. [vit., 1]).

[10] Delehaye, "Les recueils," 17 (for recitation of miracles in the shrine). Sophronius, *SS. Cyri et Ioannis, Miracula* (PG, 87.3, cols. 3423 ff.), *mir.* 69, describes a votive plaque at the entrance to the healing shrine of Sts. Cyrus and John at Menuthis, in northern Egypt: "I, John from Rome, have come here and have been healed by Sts. Cyrus and John of eight years of blindness, after I had suffered here unmoving." For votives at healing shrines, see Kötting, *Peregrinatio*, 399 f.

[11] Acc. no. 57.1865.560; illustrated 1:1. See Vikan, *Byzantine Pilgrimage*, fig. 38, for the "Lord help" type.

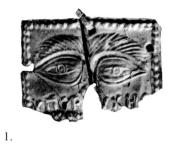

1.

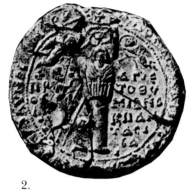

2.

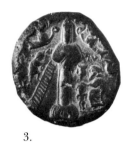

3.

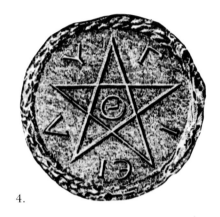

4.

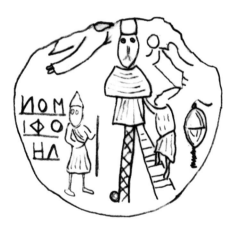

5.

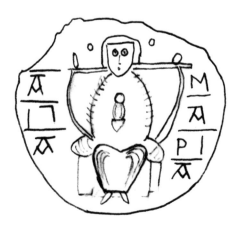

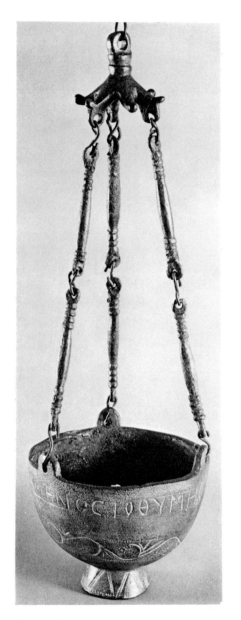

6.

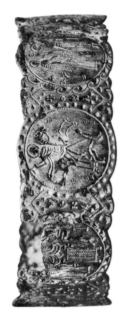
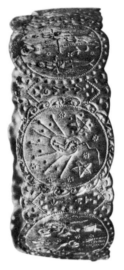

9.

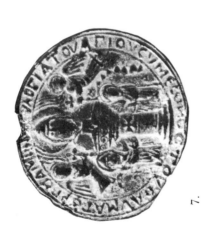

7.

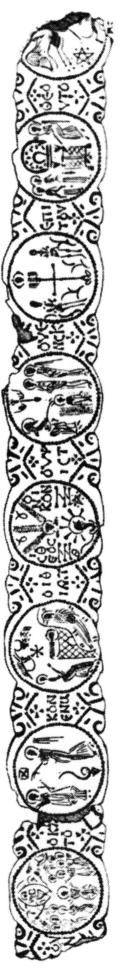

8.

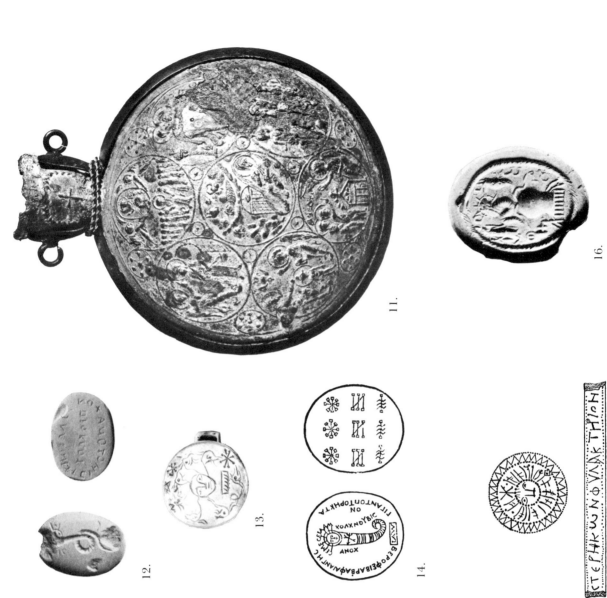

11.

16.

12.

13.

14.

15.

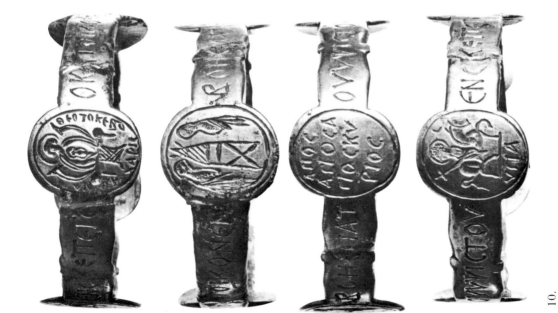

10.

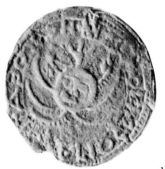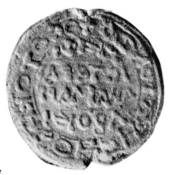

17.

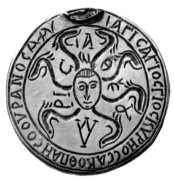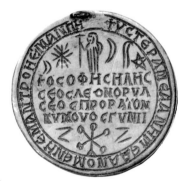

18.

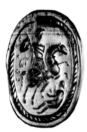

19.

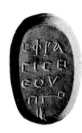

20.

22.

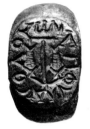

21.

23.

24.

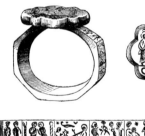

25.

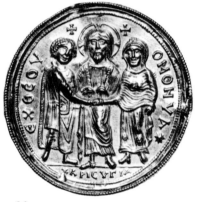

26.

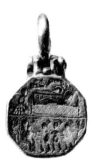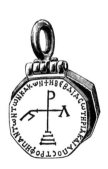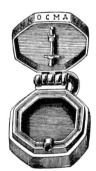

27.

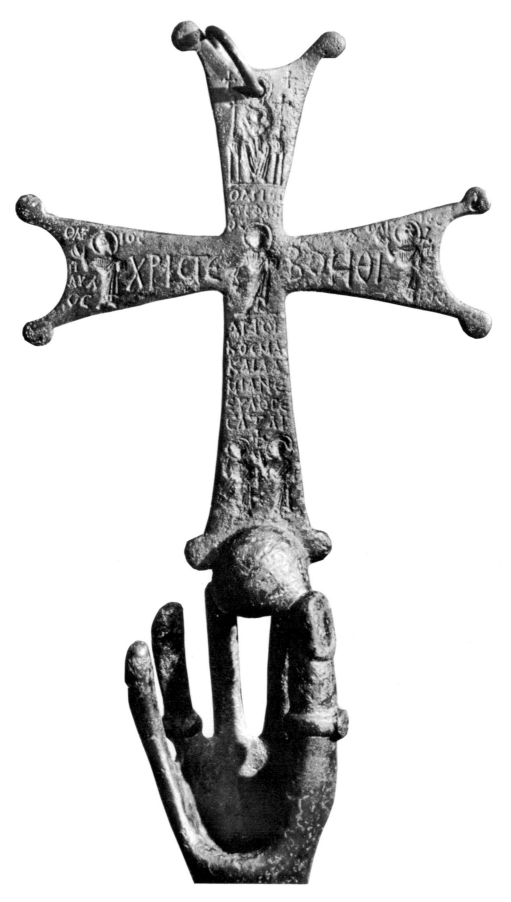

28.

shrines around the Mediterranean (e.g., at the Asklepieion in Corinth), these simple, anonymous votives acknowledge a successful healing by showing that part of the body which was formerly diseased.[12] And to judge from the words of Theodoret, the practice was not at all unusual in early Byzantium:

> Christians come to the martyrs to implore them to be their intercessors. That they obtained what they so earnestly prayed for is clearly proven by their votive gifts, which proclaim the healing. Some bring images of eyes, others feet, others hands, which sometimes are made of gold, sometimes of wood. . . .[13]

How and with what were such cures accomplished? These questions have been asked and answered by scholars of the caliber of Delehaye and Kötting.[14] Yet typically, each relied on textual evidence to the virtual exclusion of material remains, and in so doing failed to appreciate the integral role that art once played in effecting miraculous cures, and the instrumental role that it can still play in explicating the circumstances under which such cures were accomplished.[15] In order to help establish a more balanced interpretation, I now propose to examine in detail miraculous healing as it was practiced at the shrine of St. Symeon the Younger, because for no other Early Byzantine pilgrim site is our textual evidence (the saint's *Vita*) so effectively complemented by our material evidence ("Symeon tokens")—the how by the what.[16] This

examination will in turn serve as the basis for a reinterpretation of several categories of Early Byzantine amulets, which will be shown to be not merely apotropaic, but specifically medicinal.

The ruins of Symeon the Younger's shrine may still be seen atop his "Miraculous Mountain" (*Kutchuk Djebel Semaan*), which rises above the Mediterranean some sixteen kilometers southwest of Antioch. Included in the complex were a cruciform church, a monastery, and a column, for this famous Symeon, who died in 592, had chosen the life of a stylite in imitation of his equally famous, homonymous predecessor of the fifth century.[17] Evidence of what transpired on the Miraculous Mountain during Symeon's lifetime and in the decades immediately after his death consists of a long, contemporary *Vita* comprising more than 250 miracles, and, as their material complement, several dozen clay Symeon tokens of the sort illustrated in figure 2.[18] Most, like this example, are between the size of a quarter and a half-dollar, and most show basically the same composition. At the center is Symeon's column topped by his bust-length portrait. To the left a monk climbs a ladder toward the saint, with a censer in his raised hands, while just below a second monk kneels in supplication, reaching forward to touch the column. Finally, above and to the right and left of the saint are a pair of flying angels bearing leafy victory crowns.

In a sense, the token identifies itself through the inscription which fills its circumference: "Blessing [i.e., *eulogia*] of St. Symeon of the Miraculous Mountain." "Of the Miraculous Mountain" is simply

---

[12] Unfortunately, there is nothing in the design of the reliefs to suggest the nature of the disease. Centers for the miraculous healing of the eyes were as well known in Early Byzantine times as they had been in antiquity. That closest to the findspot of these reliefs would likely have been the St. Thekla shrine at Seleucia (Kötting, *Peregrinatio*, 154).

[13] Theodoret, *Graecarum affectionum curatio* 8.64 (I. Raeder, *Theodoreti graecarum affectionum curatio* [Leipzig, 1904; rpt. Stuttgart 1969], 1 ff.).

[14] Delehaye, "Les recueils," *passim*; and Kötting, *Peregrinatio*, 400 ff.

[15] Similarly, those few art historians who have been attracted to pilgrimage art have paid far too little attention to textual evidence, and thus have usually missed the medico-amuletic essence of the genre. Instead, there has been a tendency to view the sort of pilgrim tokens and ampullae discussed below as little more than tourist souvenirs. They are thought to be cheap imitations of (lost) prototypes in precious metal whose iconography derives from (lost) mural archetypes at the shrine. For a recent review of received opinion among art historians, see R. J. Grigg, "The Images on the Palestinian Flasks as Possible Evidence of the Monumental Decoration of Palestinian Martyria," (diss., University of Minnesota, 1974).

[16] P. van den Ven, *La vie ancienne de S. Syméon Stylite le Jeune (521–592)*, SubsHag, 32 (Brussels, 1962 [I], 1970 [II]). For Symeon tokens, see J. Lafontaine-Dosogne, *Itinéraires archéologiques dans la région d'Antioche*, Bibliothèque de *Byzantion*, 4 (Brussels, 1967), 140 ff. (and *passim*, for the shrine in general).

[17] For additions to Lafontaine-Dosogne's list, see *idem*, "Une eulogie inédite de St. Syméon Stylite le Jeune," *Byzantion*, 51 (1981), 631 ff., and notes 3 and 7; R. Camber, "A Hoard of Terracotta Amulets from the Holy Land," *Actes du XVe Congrès International d'Études Byzantine*, Athens, September 1976, II, A (Athens, 1981), 104, fig. 15; and Vikan, *Byzantine Pilgrimage*, figs. 22, 25, 29. Four additional specimens are in the J. Spier Collection, New York City.

[17] For the Elder's shrine, see G. Tchalenko, *Villages antiques de la Syrie du Nord*, I (Paris, 1953), 223 ff.; and for the Younger's, see van den Ven, *La vie ancienne*, I, 191 ff.; and J. Mécérian, "Les inscriptions du Mont Admirable," *Mélanges offerts au Père René Mouterde, MélUSJ*, 38 (1962), II, 298 ff.

[18] Bobbio, Museo di S. Colombano; illustrated 1:1. See G. Celi, "Cimeli Bobbiesi," *La civiltà cattolica*, 74 (1923), III, 429 ff. And for the others, see note 16 above.

It was van den Ven's view that Symeon's *Vita* was written by a contemporary; more recently (in his paper "The Gate of Chalke: The Bulletin Board of the Palace," delivered at the 1984 Dumbarton Oaks Spring Symposium), Paul Speck has suggested a dating for it to the second half of the seventh century. If Speck is correct, the "center of gravity" of the phenomena and objects discussed in this article (and, more generally, of the rise of the cult of images) would shift from the decades around A.D. 600 to the decades around and soon after the Arab Conquests.

the epithet which, for the Byzantines, distinguished the Younger from the Elder Symeon. Specifically, it identifies this Symeon's hill as literally being a source of miracles, since its soil had been sanctified via the column through contact with the saint. Such "sanctified hills" seem not to have been unusual; Theodoret, for example, describes one upon which a certain ascetic named James had stood—a hill which ". . . according to general belief received so powerful a blessing that people come from all sides and carry away [pieces of] earth in order to take them home as *prophylactica*."[19] Significantly, Theodoret uses the word "blessing"—the same as that on the token—to describe the prophylactic quality which the earth of the hill had received from contact with the saint. Among the Jews of the Old Testament, the concept of "blessing" evoked by the word *eulogia* was thoroughly abstract, as in the pietistic acclamation, "Blessed be the Lord God, the God of Israel. . . ."[20] For early Christians, however, *eulogia* gradually came to be applied to blessed objects, such as bread, and eventually even to unblessed objects exchanged as gifts among the faithful. In the fifth century, for example, Akakios of Melitene sent a letter to Firmus of Caesarea and along with it, as a "blessing," a large fish.[21] For the pilgrim the word *eulogia* held a special meaning somewhere between that common in the Old Testament, and the gift of the fish.[22] It was the blessing conveyed—or more precisely, received—by contact with a holy place, a holy object, or a holy person. It could either be received directly and immaterially (through action), as by kissing the wood of the True Cross, or it could be conveyed indirectly and materially. In the latter case it would customarily come by way of a substance of neutral origin which itself had been blessed by direct contact—as, for example, through oil which had passed over the bones of a martyr. Theodoret's hill receives the immaterial blessing contact of the ascetic James, and once having received that contact itself becomes a material blessing which, in pieces, pilgrims can carry away as *prophylactica*.

That the same truth applies to Symeon's Miraculous Mountain and to the token in figure 2 is clear from the saint's *Vita*. The word *eulogia* (in the pil-grim sense) appears nearly a dozen times among the text's 259 chapters, and in each instance it refers to a substance rather than to an action-variety of blessing. One time (chap. 100) it is water from the cistern near the column; another (chap. 116), bread blessed by the saint; and in still another instance (chap. 130), a bit of hair from Symeon's head. But most often, St. Symeon's *eulogia* came in the form of the reddish earth or "dust" collected from near the base of his column. This was "the *eulogia* made from dust blessed by him" (chap. 163), or "the dust of his *eulogia*" (chap. 232). And this, of course, is at once the material of his tokens and the stuff of his Miraculous Mountain.

Knowing what these tokens are made of raises the much more interesting question of their function. And here, the testimony of *Vita* and token is identical and unequivocal: they were medicinal. First, consider the evidence of the *Vita*: In two places, chapters 41 and 255, Symeon's biographer lists in clinical fashion the half-dozen different ways whereby the saint customarily exercised his healing powers. In chapter 255 the author is nearing the end of his narrative and so attempts an overview of Symeon in his role as holy doctor:

> We shall not be tempted to list the innumerable healings that have been effected by the intermediation of St. Symeon, being weak and incapable of reporting them [all]; for sought cures were obtained as if they were pouring forth from an inexhaustible fountain. For many [the healing] was [accomplished] by [Symeon's] words; for certain others, by the mere invocation of his name; for others, by the imposition of his saintly staff; for others, by visions; and for others again, by the application of his holy dust.

Other passages in Symeon's *Vita* provide specific accounts of the medicinal application of the saint's holy dust. Chapter 115, for example, records the cure of a certain three-year-old boy in the village of Charandamas who suffered from severe constipation. Eventually the child's abdomen became distended to the point of bursting, which prompted his parents to invoke the name of St. Symeon and smear him with holy dust. Immediately, of course, the child found relief. In a similar vein, chapter 163 relates the story of a certain poor cripple in Antioch who is returned to health after having been rubbed with "the *eulogia* made from [Symeon's] blessed dust." In chapter 194 Symeon himself gives the following prescription to a man who has not a strand of hair on his entire body:

> Take my dust and rub it all over your body, and as soon as you do, the Lord, through my humble service,

---

[19] Theodoret, *Historia religiosa* c. 21 (PG, 82, cols. 1431 ff.).
[20] A. Stuiber, "Eulogia," *RAC*, VI (1966), cols. 900 ff.
[21] Firmus, *Epistolae* 30 (PG, 77, cols. 1481 ff.).
[22] For an excellent survey of the various *eulogiai* current among sixth-century pilgrims, see the account of the anonymous pilgrim from Piacenza (Wilkinson, *Jerusalem Pilgrims*, 79 ff.). See also, Vikan, *Byzantine Pilgrimage*, 10 ff.

will make hair grow [on you] appropriate to the condition of [someone] your age.

These are three typical stories of cures effected through the agency of Symeon's dust. Almost invariably, the dust was applied externally—most often, it seems, dry, but occasionally (e.g., chap. 214) mixed with water or saliva to form a reddish paste. Moreover, the prescription was as consistent and conservative as it was simple, for unlike the well-known doctor-saints of the period—Cosmas and Damian, Cyrus and John, and Artemius—Symeon did not normally make individual diagnoses or recommend such exotic remedies as roasted crocodile, camel dung or Bithynian cheese mixed with wax.[23] The same reddish earth was used year in and year out to cure any number of disparate human afflictions, from deformities and broken bones, to fevers. In fact, the same agent was used to bring an ailing donkey back to life (chap. 148), to restore a vat of sour wine to its former sweetness (chap. 230), and even, on one occasion, to calm a storm at sea (chap. 235). There could be no doubt, in other words, that Symeon's *eulogia* was, from the pharmaceutical point of view, the pilgrim's cure-all.

That Symeon's *eulogia* tokens were specifically medicinal, and that their medical qualities were generic, are both explicitly stated in the inscriptions which some of these objects bear. Within the circular field of the token in figure 2, for example, are the words, "Receive, O Saint, the incense, and heal all," while another type of Symeon token, illustrated in figure 3, bears the word "health" (*hygieia*) across its face.[24] This token, like the first, shows Symeon's column topped by his bust portrait, a pair of flying angels above, and a monk with censer on a ladder at the left. On this token, however, the circular *eulogia* inscription does not appear, and the "heal-all" invocation has been supplanted by a tiny representation of the Baptism of Christ—a scene which, because it bears more on Symeon's theology than on his pharmacology, will not figure in this paper.[25] Rather, the point of most immediate interest is the word *hygieia*, which is spelled backwards and split by the column, slightly above the token's mid-level. That its letters are reversed, and that John incorrectly places his left hand on the head of Christ

instead of his right, simply result from the mechanical process whereby all such tokens were produced. Symeon himself, in chapter 231, uses the word *sphragis* or "seal" to describe a token's image because he understands that it was made with a stamp; the letters of *hygieia* are reversed in the impression simply because the die cutter failed to reverse them on the stamp.

But what of the word itself? Initially, one might assume that it was added simply to invoke that all-important state of renewed health which the possessor of the token would hope to achieve. But its original significance may well have been more profound. The word *hygieia* is found frequently among the minor arts of early Byzantium, and especially on objects of personal adornment, like rings and belts; it appears, for example, on the clasps of the well-known gold marriage belt at Dumbarton Oaks, which is roughly contemporary in date with the token (fig. 26).[26] There, Christ acting as officiating priest oversees the *dextrarum iunctio*, the joining of the right hands of the bridal couple. Surrounding the group is the inscription, "From God, concord, grace, health." These words are as essential to the meaning of the belt as is the image, since they serve to invoke from God a threefold blessing on the marriage. By analogy, the word *hygieia* on the token serves to invoke from Symeon the blessing of health on the suppliant. But it may have done even more than that. After all, the token differs fundamentally from the belt clasp insofar as its very substance is instrumental to the realization of the blessing. In this respect, it—or rather, the stamp that produced it—belongs to the same tradition as a Late Antique doctor's stamp published more than fifty years ago by Franz Joseph Dölger (fig. 4).[27] Running clockwise around its circumference is the word *hygieia*, while at its center is a *theta* which, according to Dölger's persuasive argument, stands for *thanatos*. Between health and death, literally enclosing and trapping death, is the *pentalpha*, one of the most powerful amuletic signs in the Late Antique lexicon of magic. The *pentalpha* was the de-

[23] For an entertaining survey of such exotic cures, see H. J. Magoulias, "The Lives of Saints as Sources of Data for the History of Byzantine Medicine in the Sixth and Seventh Centuries," *BZ*, 57 (1964), 144 ff.

[24] Houston, Menil Foundation Collection, II.J1; illustrated 1:1. See Vikan, *Byzantine Pilgrimage*, 34 f., fig. 25.

[25] For a discussion of this scene, see *ibid.*, 35.

[26] M. C. Ross, *Catalogue of the Byzantine and Early Mediaeval Antiquities in the Dumbarton Oaks Collection, Volume II: Jewelry, Enamels, and Art of the Migration Period* (Washington, D.C., 1965), no. 38.

[27] Basel, History Museum; illustrated ca. 1:1. See F. J. Dölger, *Antike und Christentum*, I (Münster, 1929), 47 ff. Note that the letters on the stamp have not been cut in reverse. The failure to reverse letters and/or words is a common, random phenomenon among Byzantine stamping and sealing implements—with the exception of the more "legalistic" and "official" lead sealings.

vice of the legendary Solomonic seal; it was engraved on the signet ring given by God to King
Solomon in order that he might seal and thereby
control the power of demons.[28] On the stamp, *hygieia* and *pentalpha* together seal and control *thanatos*; more importantly, their impression conveyed
that same magical power to the doctor's pill. The
analogy to our Symeon token, both in means of
manufacture and in medicinal use, seems inescap-
able, although for the Symeon pill the impressed
word only served to complement the healing power
already inherent in Symeon's blessed earth.[29]

As for extant Symeon stamps—the functional
descendants of the doctor's stamp illustrated in our
figure 4—at least two may be cited: One, published
in 1962 by Jean Mécérian, was found on the Miraculous Mountain itself, in the ruins of the gate-
house.[30] Approximately ten centimeters in diameter and made of basalt, it bears inscriptions on both
of its faces: "Seal [*sphragis*] of the Holy Thauma-
turge, Symeon," and (much abbreviated), "Jesus
Christ, Son of God."[31] The second implement, preserved in the Cabinet des Médailles, Paris, is also
made of stone, and although it is not inscribed with
Symeon's name or epithet, it too should probably
be assigned to the Miraculous Mountain, since its
iconography closely matches that of extant clay *eulogiai* issued there (fig. 5).[32] One surface shows a
monk climbing a ladder toward the saint, who appears *en buste* at the top of his column with victory
angels flying in from left and right. At the base of
the ladder is a large censer, while on the opposite
side is a frontal standing figure—assumedly Symeon's disciple, Konon—in a pointed hat and cape,
holding a staff and labeled "sole friend" (*MONO-
PHILE*).[33] The other side of the stamp shows a

crude iconic portrait of the Virgin with the Christ
Child on her lap; its inscription, "Holy Mary," indicates for it an Early Byzantine dating.[34] This device, too, is matched on at least a few extant clay
tokens from the Miraculous Mountain.[35] Indeed,
that an image of "Holy Mary" should occasionally
complement (or even supplant) that of Symeon on
his medicinal *eulogiai* is hardly surprising, since her
powers were invoked along with his (and Christ's)
in the performance of miraculous cures—including that whereby Konon was brought back from
the dead.[36]

The inscriptions on both variant token types (figs.
2, 3) corroborate the evidence of the *Vita*; namely,
that Symeon's blessed earth was medicinal in its intent and general in its applicability. Yet, the words
that these objects bear have something additional
to reveal of the specific circumstances under which
their generic medicinal powers were brought to bear.
Recall the invocation that appears on the token illustrated in figure 2: "Receive, O Saint, the incense, and heal all." Incense—or more specifically,
the offering of incense to the saint—is as prominent textually in this invocation as it is visually in
the iconography of this and of most other Symeon
tokens. Here, we see a man climbing toward the
saint with an upright censer in both hands, while
in figure 3 an analogously placed suppliant holds
a swinging censer in his right hand. Obviously, invocation and iconography mirror one another, and
just as obviously, the significance they share for these
tokens depends on how we interpret incense, a
substance and process which in Early Byzantine
Christianity had several variant meanings reflec-
tive of its several variant uses. In private piety one
of its main uses was as a propitiatory sacrifice offered in conjunction with intense prayer. To cite
one typical illustration close in time and place to
St. Symeon: Evagrius tells the story of a certain holy
man named Zosimas, who happened to be in Caesarea in 526 when a terrible earthquake struck Antioch:

> Zosimas, at the very moment of the overthrow of An-
> tioch, suddenly became troubled, uttered lamenta-

---

[28] C. C. McCown, *The Testament of Solomon* (Leipzig, 1922), 10*.
See also note 67, below.

[29] The supposed efficacy of "consumable words" is no more
clearly documented than in Julius Africanus' prescription for
keeping wine from turning sour: write the words of Psalm 34.8
("O taste and see that the Lord is good") on an apple and throw
it into the cask (see Dölger, *Antike*, 21).

[30] Mécérian, "Les inscriptions," 304, pl. II, 1.

[31] In fact, the raised matrix of the side bearing the *sphragis*
inscription is only about 5 cm. across, making it only slightly
larger than the token from Bobbio illustrated in figure 2.

[32] Unpublished; my line drawing is reproduced ca. 1:1. The
piece is about 1.5 cm. thick, and is made of a hard, dark stone
(basalt?).

[33] For such a censer, see O. Wulff, *Altchristliche Bildwerke*, Kön-
igliche Museen zu Berlin, Beschreibung der Bildwerke der
christlichen Epochen, 2, 1 (Berlin, 1909), no. 977. "Sole friend"
is otherwise unattested on Symeon (or any other) *eulogiai*. Konon's miraculous resurrection, one of Symeon's most famous
miracles, is described in chapter 129 of the *Vita*. Konon appears,

usually labeled *KONON*, on many of the extant mid-Byzantine
"*eulogiai*" of St. Symeon the Younger (e.g., our fig. 7).

[34] The chronology of epithets accompanying portraits of the
Virgin will be discussed by Anna Kartsonis in her forthcoming
book, *Anastasis: The Making of an Image*. "Holy Mary," as distinct
from "Mother of God" or "Theotokos," is confined to the pre-
Iconoclastic period.

[35] Lafontaine-Dosogne, *Itinéraires archéologiques*, figs. 98 ff.

[36] *Vita* chaps. 129, 141, 226; and Mécérian, "Les insciptions,"
318 ff.

tions and deep sighs, and then shedding such a pro-fusion of tears as to bedew the ground, called for a censer, and having fumed the whole place where they were standing, throws himself upon the ground, pro-pitiating God with prayers and supplications.[37]

Both in a literal and in a symbolic sense, smoke and prayer were conjoined for Zosimas as they rose toward heaven; one an offering to intensify and fa-cilitate the request conveyed in the other.

That incense shares the same meaning for these tokens as for Zosimas, and that both reflect a real aspect of contemporary piety, are corroborated by a small but important group of inscribed bronze censers from Early Byzantine Sicily (fig. 6).[38] Most show slight variations on the inscription, "God, who received the incense of the Holy Prophet Zachar-ias, receive this [incense]." The allusion, of course, is to the story of the father of John the Baptist, who, according to the first chapter of Luke, en-tered the Temple to burn incense before the altar. As he did he prayed, and at that moment an angel appeared before him with the words: "Fear not, Zacharias, for thy prayer is heard. . . ."

The iconography of these tokens, their inscrip-tions, Evagrius, and extant censers together seem to be painting a single coherent image—one wherein ailing pilgrims would offer Symeon in-cense in propitiation as they invoked his interces-sory aid and the healing power of his *eulogia*. We imagine lines of pathetic suppliants, each waiting his turn to climb the ladder and, with censer in hand, to put his case before the holy doctor. How-ever, to judge from the evidence of Symeon's *Vita*, our imagination would seem to be deceiving us, for while there are a number of references to the burning of incense in the *Vita*, only once is it being offered directly to the saint at the top of the col-umn (chap. 222), and in that one case the offering is expressly refused. In other words, Symeon's biographer neither states nor implies that the saint customarily or even occasionally gave audience to suppliants with censers—which seems to leave us with a fundamental conflict between our material evidence on one hand and our textual evidence on the other, between token and *Vita*. But in fact, this is only an apparent conflict, since it is not inherent in the evidence at all, but lies rather in an assump-

tion which we enforce on that evidence; namely, that the scene on the token is to be understood as reflecting the experienced reality at the shrine. To reconcile the two, we need only discard that as-sumption and look away from Symeon's column; we need only suppose, in other words, that the censing suppliant is not at the shrine at all, but that he is offering up his incense prayer from another location.

And here, through this unlikely but in fact nec-essary supposition, token and *Vita* fall into har-mony with one another. Consider the following three cures. Chapter 53 relates the story of a youth from Daphne who is suddenly struck blind; discov-ering this, his parents light lamps and throw on incense, imploring the help of Emmanuel in the name of St. Symeon. Chapter 70 describes an un-named victim of an unspecified disease; he lights a lamp in his house and throws on incense, praying quietly and saying, "Christ, God of Your Servant Symeon of the Miraculous Mountain, have pity on me." And finally, chapter 231 relates the story of a priest from the village of Basileia; his third son, near death with a fever, begs his father to take him to St. Symeon. His father replies, "St. Symeon, my son, has the power to come to visit you here, and you will be healed, and you will live." With these words of the priest, the young man cries out, "St. Symeon, have pity on me," and then tells his father to get up quickly, throw on incense, and pray, for the Servant of God, St. Symeon, is before him. In each instance the scenario is basically the same: a devotee of St. Symeon falls ill while away from the shrine, but instead of traveling to the saint, he in-duces the saint to come to him—to perform "bi-location"—by burning incense, lighting lamps, and by offering a fervent prayer for healing.[39]

It seems, then, that the words and images on these tokens should be taken neither in a strictly literal sense nor in a strictly symbolic sense. There was a real suppliant, he did pray for healing, and he did offer incense to the saint; but this in all probability took place away from the Miraculous Mountain, as part of a private healing ritual. Thus the suppliant is a participant in the iconography, but only at one

---

[37] *Ecclesiastical History* 4.7 (Bohn's Ecclesiastical Library [Lon-don, 1854], 255 ff.).

[38] Syracuse, Museo Archeologica (P. Orsi, *Sicilia bizantina*, I [Rome, 1942], 171 ff., pl. XIIc). See, more recently, A. M. Fal-lico, "Recenti ritrovamenti di bronzetti bizantini," *Siculorum gymnasium*, 21 (1968), 70 ff.

[39] For a bi-location healing performed by Sts. Cosmas and Damian (*mir.* 13), see Delehaye, "Les recueils," 16, and note 45 below. Symeon's *Vita* describes the process of healing as it ex-isted during his lifetime; the shrine, however, continued to function long after his death in 592. Perhaps lights and incense were then used at the shrine to induce Symeon's healing pres-ence much as they had formerly been used away from the shrine for the same purpose.

remove, since his identity is subsumed by anonymous counterparts who act out the spiritual and, in part, the physical reality of his piety. His supplicatory relationship to his intercessor, St. Symeon, is visualized in the figure kneeling beside the column,[40] his incense offering is presented quite graphically (though in symbolic terms) on the ladder above, and the prayer itself is spelled out to the right of the column.

Suppliant, censer, and saint, entities which did not customarily converge in the experienced reality of the public shrine, here meet in a sort of private, liturgical reality on the face of a Symeon *eulogia*.[41] Moreover, it is clear that the very substance of that imagery, the *eulogia* itself, had an instrumental role to play in the consummation of the healing rite portrayed on it.[42] This only makes sense, and, in fact, is at least implicit in the list of healing techniques enumerated in chapters 41 and 255 of the *Vita*. Were the pilgrim actually at the shrine, he would have had the option of receiving the saint's blessing words or his healing touch, but away from the shrine the pilgrim must necessarily rely on some blessed intermediary to accomplish the same effect. In essence, this was the medicine he was obliged to take when he couldn't reach (or remain with) the doctor. Recall the story of the constipated three-year-old who was smeared with medicinal dust in his native village of Charandamas, and the paralytic who was dusted and healed in Antioch. In fact, there is not one miracle in the entire *Vita* of the saint where a medicinal *eulogia* is described as being used at the shrine itself; rather, they were given out there to accomplish their cures somewhere else. Consider the scenario evoked by chapter 231. A priest brings his second-born son to St. Symeon to be cured of a terrible disease. Symeon blesses the young man, but then sends him home to await his miraculous healing. The father is troubled and suggests that they stay near the saint a bit longer, since, "the presence at your side assures us a more complete cure." At this Symeon becomes annoyed,

scolds the priest for his lack of faith, and sends him on his way with these words: "The power of God . . . is efficacious everywhere. Therefore, take this *eulogia* made of my dust and depart. . . ."[43]

The images on these tokens, their inscriptions, and the healing miracles recounted in Symeon's *Vita* converge in a single coherent medico-religious phenomenon wherein each has a complimentary role to play—with the exception, perhaps, of the image itself. After all, that the iconography found on these tokens is explicable does not explain why it was put there in the first place. Certainly blessed earth could effect miraculous cures all by itself; why, then, the image?

Recall the miracle narrated in chapter 231 of the *Vita*. A priest brings his second son to Symeon to be healed; the saint blesses the boy but then sends him home to await the cure. A sceptical father does not wish to leave, but is persuaded to do so by the following statement from Symeon, the first half of which was quoted above:

[40] Compare analogous suppliants as they appear beside the True Cross on the well-known ampullae in Monza and Bobbio (A. Grabar, *Ampoules de Terre Sainte* [Paris, 1958], *passim*); for "vicarious" participation in pilgrimage iconography, see Vikan, *Byzantine Pilgrimage*, 24 f.

[41] These tokens clearly contradict conventional art-historical wisdom which would trace pilgrimage iconography back to lost mural models at the shrines. And in any event, no evidence exists that the shrine of Symeon the Younger (among others) ever had figurative mural decoration.

[42] That clay is the object's raison d'être obviously contradicts the notion that this medium was chosen for reasons of economy.

[43] No sooner do father and son arrive home than Symeon appears, disguised, in a vision. He puts this question to the priest: "What do you prefer, this *eulogia* that Symeon has sent you, or his right hand?" To which the priest responds, "Don't be angry, Lord, for great is the power of his *eulogia*, but I was seeking his right hand." At this point Symeon extends his right hand and gives the priest his clay *eulogia*, then, revealing his true identity, scolds him once again for his lack of faith. This desire for "the right hand" may explain why palm prints appear so frequently and so clearly on the back sides of Early Byzantine clay tokens (see Vikan, *Byzantine Pilgrimage*, 38 f., figs. 29a, b). There is additional evidence of how Symeon's earthen *eulogiai* were dispersed. Chapter 163 of the *Vita* describes Symeon's practice of giving blessed dust as "a favor . . . to the poor, for their subsistance." The poor in turn give out the *eulogiai* (here, specifically, in Antioch) and thereby the Lord "heals the world." According to chapter 181, a woman places in her bag "the *eulogia* that she got from the saint," while chapter 196 describes a specific building at the shrine for the storage of *eulogiai* (of Symeon's hair). According to chapter 232, a monk attached to the shrine who is traveling to Constantinople on business carries with him pieces of Symeon's hair and "the dust of his *eulogia*," with which he heals the praetorian prefect. Finally, miracle 54 of St. Martha (see note 45 below) describes a Georgian monk as leaving the shrine of St. Symeon with several image-bearing clay tokens. The stamps for the manufacture of clay *eulogiai* were likely made for and controlled by the monastic community which operated the shrine. At the shrine of Sts. Cosmas and Damian, for example, blessed wax was distributed to those undergoing incubation in the church during the all-night Saturday vigil (L. Deubner, *Kosmas und Damian* [Leipzig/Berlin, 1907], *mir.* 30). Molds (in fact, an entire worshop) for the production of clay ampullae for blessed water have been discovered at the Menas shrine in Egypt (see K. M. Kaufman, *Die heilige Stadt der Wüste* [Munich, 1924], 195 ff). Not surprisingly, those *eulogiai* bearing words or images are almost invariably "impersonal," and thus generically applicable to any suppliant and any disease. (For a unique pair of tokens made expressly for a certain Constantine, see Vikan, *Byzantine Pilgrimage*, figs. 22 and 29a.) Multiple surviving specimens from the same mold are not uncommon (cf. Lafontaine-Dosogne, *Itinéraires archéologiques*, figs. 82, 83).

The power of God ... is efficacious everywhere. Therefore, take this *eulogia* made of my dust, depart, and when you look at the imprint of our image, it is us that you will see.

Symeon is here offering the priest two quite different kinds of assurance that his son's cure will indeed eventually be accomplished. One, of course, is the blessed dust, which assumedly the priest will recognize as the saint's typical, highly efficacious curative agent. The other, however, is the saint's image impressed on that dust; somehow the anxiety of the priest should be lessened by knowing that when he and his son get home and look at that impression, they will, in effect, be confronted with a vision of the saint himself. But how can this be reassuring?

The answer comes later in the same chapter, when the priest's third son falls ill. Naturally, he asks that he be taken to the Miraculous Mountain, but his father recalls the words of the saint and replies, "St. Symeon, my son, has the power to come to visit you here, and you will be healed, and you will live." With this the young man gasps, then calls out, "St. Symeon, have pity on me." He then turns to his father and cries, "Get up quickly, throw on incense, and pray, for the servant of God, St. Symeon, is before me. . . ." With these words Symeon appears to the boy in a vision, battles with the demon that possesses him, and soon restores the youth to good health. Other miracles, though in less detail, suggest the same scenario; namely, that a vision of the saint was instrumental to the miraculous cure, and that this vision might be induced by a man-made representation of the saint. In chapter 118, for example, a hemorrhaging woman from Cilicia invokes Symeon's aid with the words, "If only I see your image I will be saved," while chapter 163 describes a healing accomplished in Antioch by means of blessed dust:

Instantly the paralytic was healed . . . by the intermediation of his saintly servant Symeon, whom he saw with his own eyes under the aspect of a long-haired monk, who extended his hand and put him upright. . . .

It is clear that for these people seeing was essential to healing, to making real and effective Symeon's miraculous, healing presence at their side.[44] And

chapter 231 of the *Vita* leaves no doubt that the image stamped on the earthen *eulogia* was itself instrumental to the "seeing" of the saint. In Symeon's own words, "When you regard the imprint of our image, it is us that you will see."[45]

The saint's image, the pilgrim's invocation, the pair of suppliants, the censer, the red clay, the concepts of *eulogia*, bi-location, and visitation, and the magic of *hygieia*; these were all multiple facets of a single medico-religious phenomenon through which one segment of the population of early Byzantium believed that it was effectively treating its diseases. Pilgrim tokens like those illustrated in figures 2 and 3 were at once the distillation of and the catalyst for that phenomenon. Indeed, there is no clearer indication of the subtle cohesion with which they responded to their medico-religious function than to contrast them with their "imitations" of later centuries. Image-bearing, earthen *eulogia* reached their peak of popularity in the later sixth and seventh centuries; a fairly rapid decline seems to have set in soon thereafter. Yet, like many another product of Early Byzantine culture, the Symeon *eulogia* was destined to be exhumed and revived centuries later, during the mid-Byzantine period. For with the reoccupation of the region of Antioch in the later tenth century, the Miraculous Mountain and its pilgrim trade were revitalized, and pilgrim token designs popularized before the Arab Conquest were consciously imitated (fig. 7).[46]

---

[44] As incubation was instrumental to healing at the most famous of early Byzantium's holy doctor shrines (e.g., those of Cosmas and Damian, Cyrus and John, and Artemius), so a dream-vision was instrumental to successful incubation. And the fact that the healing saint is said to appear "in his customary manner" (e.g., Cosmas and Damian, *mir.* 1), strongly suggests that representations of the saint (whether on tokens, or as icons or murals) were instrumental to the evocation and confirmation of that vision. See Delehaye, "Les recueils," 16; and Kötting, *Peregrinatio*, 217 f.

[45] References to image-bearing, consumable *eulogiai* are not confined to the *Vita* of St. Symeon. Miracle 16 of St. Artemius (Papadopoulos-Kerameus, *Varia graeca sacra*) relates the story of a suppliant undergoing incubation who wakes up with a wax seal in his hand bearing the saint's portrait. The previous night the holy doctor had appeared to him in a dream, and had given him the seal "to drink." The patient is cured through the application of the melted wax. Miracles 54, 55 in the *Vita* of St. Martha (van den Ven, *La vie ancienne*) narrate the story of a certain Georgian monk who leaves the shrine of St. Symeon with several image-bearing clay tokens. On the way home he begins to doubt the saintliness of Symeon, and throws all but one token (which escapes his attention) into a fire. Suddenly, his arms become white from leprosy; he asks forgiveness of the saint, rubs his arms with the blessed earth, and is healed. Miracle 13 of Sts. Cosmas and Damian (Deubner, *Kosmas und Damian*) tells the story of a member of the military who is sent to Laodicea, taking with him an "icon," which is apparently identical with the blessed wax later used to treat his sick wife. See E. Kitzinger, "The Cult of Images in the Age Before Iconoclasm," *DOP*, 8 (1954), 148.

[46] For the revitalization of the Miraculous Mountain in the mid-Byzantine period, see van den Ven, *La vie ancienne*, 214* ff. Figure 7: Houston, Menil Foundation Collection, II.J4; illustrated 1:1. See Vikan, *Byzantine Pilgrimage*, fig. 30, 39 f. It is

Superficially, this typical mid-Byzantine descendant shares much in common with its Early Byzantine ancestor (fig. 2); its iconography appears to be much the same and its inscription is virtually identical. Yet over the centuries, much had changed: gone are the kneeling suppliant, the man on the ladder, the censer, and the invocation—gone, in other words, is the "incense prayer" and the concept of bi-location it evoked. We see instead Symeon's disciple Konon on the left and his mother Martha on the right, each turning toward Symeon's column as though an intercessor in a Deësis; they have, in effect, not only physically supplanted the suppliants, they have interposed themselves spiritually between suppliant and stylite. Above, the angels still appear but they have been altered in a most telling way. By the well-established canons of Late Antique victory iconography, they ought to be carrying either crowns (figs. 2, 3) or palm fronds to the victorious "athlete of Christ," St. Symeon. But instead, each carries a small martyr's cross, as if about to hand it to the saint. Yet, iconographic substitutions such as these are only symptoms of what was a very profound transformation in the function of the object, and thereby in its very genre. For in fact, what appears in figure 7 is not a clay token at all, but rather a cast lead pendant whose suspension loop has broken away.[47] It is, in other words, an object which by its very nature cannot possibly convey the medicinal earthen "blessing" of the Miraculous Mountain.

What these mid-Byzantine lead medallions still had to offer, however, was the inherent power of their image—the same power which Theodoret ascribed to representations of Symeon Stylites the Elder († 459) more than five hundred years earlier:

> Of [pilgrimage from] Italy it is unnecessary to speak, since they say that this man [Symeon the Elder] has become so famous in Rome, the greatest city, that they have set up small images of him in the vestibules of all the workshops for the warding off of danger and as a means of protection.[48]

Indeed, it was this belief in the power of images which made it inevitable that pilgrimage iconography, popularized and disseminated through the idiom of the *eulogia*, should come to enjoy its own existence and evolution independent of blessed substance.[49] And it is hardly surprising to discover that some of these pilgrimage-generated images were thought to possess specifically medicinal powers. In chapter 118 of the *Vita*, for example, is the story of a woman from Cilicia who, after having been purged of a demon by St. Symeon, returns home and there sets up an icon of the saint. This image, even though it was never blessed by Symeon, performs a variety of miracles, including cures, "because the Holy Spirit which inhabits Symeon covers it with its shadow"; thus, a hemorrhaging woman can invoke Symeon's power with the words, "If only I see your image I will be saved."[50] Similarly, there is recorded among the *miracula* of Cosmas and Damian one (no. 15) wherein a pious woman is cured of colic simply by consuming plaster fragments scraped from the frescoed portraits of those holy doctors which had been painted on the walls of her house.[51]

Yet, it is one thing to know that some pilgrimage-generated imagery could sometimes be medicinal, even without the aid of accompanying blessed substance, and quite another to identify specific, extant objects which by their imagery may be said to have been medicinal in intent at their point of manufacture. Most simply stated, the problem is to identify implements of supernatural healing among the much larger categories of pilgrimage-related amulets and votives.[52]

One such implement—a true "medical amulet"—is represented by our figures 8 to 10.[53] These

---

inscribed: "Blessing of St. Symeon of the Miraculous [Mountain], Amen."

[47] For the genre, see P. Verdier, "A Medallion of Saint Symeon the Younger," *The Bulletin of the Cleveland Museum of Art*, 67, 1 (1980), 17 ff. For a mid-Byzantine mold for the casting of lead Symeon pendants, see J. Lassus, "Un moule à eulogies de Saint Syméon le Jeune," *MonPiot*, 51 (1960), 149 f., fig. 6.

[48] *Historia religiosa*, 26.11 (H. Leitzmann, *Das Leben des heiligen Symeon Stylites*, *TU*, 32, 4 [Leipzig, 1908], 1 ff.).

[49] For some examples, see Vikan, *Byzantine Pilgrimage*, 40 ff.

[50] On the implications of this passage for the icon cult, see Kitzinger, "The Cult of Images," 117 f., 144 f.

[51] Deubner, *Kosmas und Damian*; and Kitzinger, "The Cult of Images," 107, 148.

[52] Ever since Gustave Schlumberger's pioneering study of 1892, "Amulettes byzantins anciens destinés à combattre les maléfices et maladies" (*REG*, 5, [1892], 73 ff.), Byzantinists have tended to blur the distinction between amulets that were intended to be only generally efficacious, and those among them which were intended to act specifically against, for example, the Evil Eye, stomach pains or infertility. Students of Greco-Egyptian amulets have evolved a much richer and far more precise typology, in part of course, because of the greater number and variety of objects with which they deal. See C. Bonner, *Studies in Magical Amulets, Chiefly Graeco-Egyptian* (Ann Arbor, 1950); and A. Delatte and P. Derchain, *Les intailles magiques gréco-égyptiennes* (Paris, 1964).

[53] Figure 8: Fouquet Collection, Cairo; illustrated 1:1. Found in Egypt. Inscriptions: Psalm 90; *Heis Theos*. Iconography: As-

are three of more than a dozen surviving examples of a type of amuletic armband produced in the east Mediterranean (i.e., Syria-Palestine and/or Egypt) in the sixth and seventh centuries.[54] The group is distinguished by recurrent inscriptions and images, and by a ribbon-like design highlighted by incised, figurative medallions; finer specimens, like the three here illustrated, are of silver. That the iconographic roots of these armbands lie in the pilgrim trade is clear from: (1) the fact that their version of the Women at the Tomb (figs. 8–10) includes architectural elements of the Holy Sepulchre Shrine (e.g., the "grills"); and (2), the striking similarity that exists between the choice and configuration of their scenes and those that appear on the well-known Palestinian metal ampullae preserved in Monza and Bobbio.[55] For example, six of the eight medallions on the Fouquet armband (fig. 8: Ascension, Annunciation, Nativity, Baptism, Crucifixion, and the Women at the Tomb) closely match those found on the reverse of Monza ampulla 2 (fig. 11).[56] Similarly, that these armbands were intended to be at least generally amuletic is clear from

their recurrent use of the apotropaic verse from Psalm 90, "He that dwells in the help of the Highest . . . ," and from their inclusion of the so-called holy rider and of such patently magical symbols as the *pentalpha* (figs. 8, 9).[57] Yet, what has thus far escaped notice is that the magic they were supposed to convey was specifically medicinal.[58] The evidence is of two sorts. First, there is the recent addition to the group of an armband bearing the word *Hygieia* on its holy rider medallion (fig. 10).[59] And second, there is the fact, somehow hitherto unnoticed, that several of the best-known members of the group, including our figures 8 and 9, show the Chnoubis, one of Antiquity's most popular medical "gem amulets"—and one long recognized as specifically effective in the cure of abdominal disorders.[60] The *Peri lithon* of Socrates and Dionysius, for example, gives the following instruction:

> Engrave on it [a kind of onyx] a serpent coil with the upper part or head of a lion, with rays. Worn thus it

---

cension, Annunciation, Nativity, Chnoubis, Baptism, Crucifixion, Women at the Tomb, Holy Rider. See J. Maspero, "Bracelets-amulettes d'époque byzantine," *Annales du service des antiquités de l'Égypte*, 9 (1908), 246 ff., fig. 1. Figure 9: Egyptian Museum, Cairo; illustrated ca. 1:1. Found in Egypt. Inscription: Psalm 90. Iconography: Annunciation, Nativity, Trinity (?), Baptism, Chnoubis, Crucifixion, Women at the Tomb, Holy Rider. See *ibid.*, 250 ff., figs. 2–5, pls. at end of volume. Figure 10: New York, J. Spier Collection; illustrated ca. 1:1. Inscriptions: Psalm 90; *Trisagion*; *Theotoke Boethei Anna, Charis*. Iconography: Women at the Tomb, Virgin and Child, Holy Rider. Unpublished. I would like to thank Mr. Spier for these photographs, and for permission to publish them.

[54] For the group in general, see Maspero, "Bracelets-amulettes," 246 ff.; and M. Piccirillo, "Un braccialetto cristiano della regione di Betlem," *Liber Annuus*, 29 (1979), 244 ff. (with illustrations of several specimens). For additional, related examples, see J. Strzygowski, *Koptische Kunst*, Catalogue général des antiquités Égyptienne du Musée du Caire (Vienna, 1904), 331 f.; Wulff, *Altchristliche Bildwerke*, no. 1109; and Bonner, *Magical Amulets*, no. 321.

[55] For the Holy Sepulchre, see J. Wilkinson, "The Tomb of Christ: An Outline of its Structural History," *Levant*, 1 (1969), 83 ff.; and for the ampullae, see Grabar, *Ampoules, passim*, and the following note.

[56] Monza, Treasury of the Cathedral of St. John the Baptist; illustrated 1:1. Tin-lead ampulla for sanctified oil. See *ibid.*, pl. V. The only scene without a match is the Visitation, at the upper right of the ampulla. For the dating, localization, iconography, and function of these ampullae, see, in addition to Grabar, J. Engemann, "Palästinische Pilgerampullen im F. J. Dölger Institut in Bonn," *JbAChr*, 16 (1973), 5 ff.; Vikan, *Byzantine Pilgrimage*, 20 ff.; and, most recently, L. Kötzsche-Breitenbruch, "Pilgerandenken aus dem heiligen Land," *Vivarium: Festschrift Theodor Klauser zum 90. Geburtstag, JbAChr*, Ergänzungsband, 11 (1984), 229 ff.

[57] For Psalm 90.1 and the holy rider, see Bonner, *Magical Amulets*, 5, nos. 294 ff. The holy rider in figure 10 differs from the more common sort illustrated in Bonner (and appearing, for example, in the central medallion in the front view of fig. 9) insofar as he does not impale an evil, prostrate figure or beast. This more stately version likely derives from traditional *adventus* iconography as it was adapted for Christ in the Entry into Jerusalem—a scene which appears with remarkable frequency on Early Byzantine amulets (e.g., Wulff, *Altchristliche Bildwerke*, no. 825). This was the one biblical episode wherein Christ was, in effect, a "holy rider"; moreover, the victorious nature of the event was itself fully appropriate to amulets, which necessarily relied on the invocation of Christ's power. Usually, as here, the iconography is reduced to a single figure (holding a large cross) and the animal that carries him; often, though not here, that animal is characterized as a donkey by its long ears (cf. our fig. 23). Both types of holy rider appear on one armband in our group; see W. Froehner, *Collection de la comtesse R. de Béarn* (Paris, 1905), 10.

[58] For the most recent statement of received opinion, see E. Kitzinger, "Christian Imagery: Growth and Impact," *Age of Spirituality: A Symposium*, ed. K. Weitzmann (New York, 1980), 151 f. (illustrating the armbands in our figures 8 and 9).

[59] Remarkably similar in general design and apparent function is a bronze medico-amuletic *tabella ansata* (?) in the British Museum which shows a stately rider (not Christ) and his attendant, three snakes, and the inscriptions: *Heis Theos* and *Hygieia*. Dalton assigned the piece, which came from Tyre, to the sixth century, and suggested that it was made "to bring health or luck." See O. M. Dalton, *Catalogue of Early Christian Antiquities and Objects from the Christian East in the . . . British Museum* (London, 1901), no. 543.

[60] On the Chnoubis, see Bonner, *Magical Amulets*, 54 ff.; and Delatte and Derchain, *Intailles magiques*, 54 ff. There is an unpublished armband with the Chnoubis in the Benaki Museum, Athens (no. 11472). This was kindly brought to my attention by L. Bouras.

prevents pain in the stomach; you will easily digest every kind of food.[61]

Most often the Chnoubis takes the form it has at the bottom center of the central medallion in figure 8; namely, as stipulated above, that of a lion-headed snake with nimbus and rays—either seven for the planets or twelve for the signs of the zodiac. Indeed, this Chnoubis closely matches that of a jasper intaglio in the Cabinet des Médailles, on whose back side are the words, "Guard in health the stomach of Proclus" (fig. 12).[62] On the other hand, the Chnoubis which fills the central medallion of our figure 9, second view, is of a more unusual, highly abstract sort; although its seven rays are immediately recognizable, its tail is now much withered and its lion head, within a bean-shaped nimbus, seems almost more human than leonine. Nevertheless, its iconographic identity and functional significance remain unmistakable: not only were these armbands specifically medicinal, they were very likely designed specifically to treat distress in the abdomen.

This group of medico-amuletic armbands, once recognized for what it is, holds the key to the identification of several other related types of implements for supernatural healing among the arts of early Byzantium. Consider, for example, the octagonal silver ring, of seventh- or eighth-century date, illustrated in figure 13.[63] It appears to have been designed as a condensed, "finger-sized" version of an armband, for not only are its technique and medium the same, its hoop bears the familiar words from Psalm 90, while its (single) incised medallion shows—in even more degenerate form—the armband's Chnoubis. Actually, this ring's Chnoubis bears closer comparison with the "mummified," human-headed form that the creature takes on some earlier amuletic gems (fig. 14).[64] Besides the face and

seven rays,[65] note that on both amulets the creature is set over a rectangular base (inscribed *Iaw* on the gem), and that it is accompanied by much the same assortment of complementary magical characters or "ring signs."[66] Two of the three characters on the ring—the stars and the "Z"—are matched on the back of the gem, while the third—the *pentalpha*—accompanies the Chnoubis in the medallions of our two illustrated armbands.[67] Notice that the "Z" also appears with the Chnoubis on the Fouquet armband (fig. 8); significantly, this specific character is known to have had a long and close association with Chnoubis (i.e. abdominal) amulets.[68] In fact, it is this character that Alexander of Tralles instructs be placed "on the head" (bezel?) of medico-amuletic rings used to treat colic—rings which, like this one, were to have eight-sided hoops.[69] Thus it seems that in both iconography and function this ring may legitimately be charac-

---

[61] F. de Mély and C. E. Ruelle, *Les lapidaires de l'antiquité et du moyen age, II: Les lapidaires grecs* (Paris, 1896–1902), II, 177 (quoted in Bonner, *Magical Amulets*, 55).

[62] Paris, Cabinet des Médailles, no. 2189; illustrated 1.5:1. See Delatte and Derchain, *Intailles magiques*, no. 80. Another such gem is in the Benaki Museum, Athens (no. 13537).

[63] Houston, Menil Foundation Collection, II.B24; illustrated 1:1. Said to have come from Asia Minor. Inscription: Psalm 90. Iconography: Chnoubis head with *pentalpha* and ring signs. See G. Vikan and J. Nesbitt, *Security in Byzantium: Locking, Sealing, and Weighing*, Dumbarton Oaks Byzantine Collection Publications, 2 (Washington, D.C., 1980), 20. A dating to the seventh or eighth century is indicated by the form of the *beta* ("R" with a bar across the bottom).

[64] Formerly in a private collection, Paris; illustrated ca. 1:1. For the iconography and inscriptions of this intaglio, see Bonner, *Magical Amulets*, 59; and E. R. Goodenough, *Jewish Symbols*

in the Greco-Roman Period, Bollingen Series, 37 (New York, 1953), II, 263 f., fig. 1137.

[65] One "ray," detached and at the bottom of the bezel, may well be an echo of the creature's lost serpent's tail. The rays on the Paris gem terminate in the letters for the semitic formula *semes eilam*, "eternal sun" (*ibid.*, 263).

[66] This "base" may well have developed from the *cista* which sometimes appears below the Chnoubis (cf. Delatte and Derchain, *Intailles magiques*, nos. 70, 79). On magical characters or "ring signs" (so-called because they often terminate in tiny rings), see Bonner, *Magical Amulets*, 58 f., 194 f.; Delatte and Derchain, *Intailles magiques*, 360; and A. A. Barb, "*Diva matrix*," *JWarb*, 16 (1953), note 48. Such symbols appear frequently on Greco-Egyptian medico-magical gems.

[67] These armbands and the stamp illustrated in our figure 4 suggest that the *pentalpha* may have been a specifically "medical" character. Among the Pythagoricians it was recognized as the symbol of health and was, in fact, named *hygieia*. See P. Perdrizet, *Negotium perambulans in tenebris*, Publication de la Faculté des Lettres de l'Université de Strasbourg, 6 (Strasbourg, 1922), 35 ff.

[68] See Bonner, *Magical Amulets*, 59. The bottom character on the reverse of the gem in figure 14 is also distinctive to Chnoubis amulets.

[69] Alexander of Tralles VIII, 2 (= *On Colic*): Grk. text, ed. Puschmann, *Alexander*, II, 377; Fr. trans., Brunet, IV, 81:

> Take an iron ring and make its hoop eight-sided, and write thus on the octagon: "Flee, flee, O bile, the lark is pursuing you." Then engrave the following character on the head of the ring: N. I have used this method many times, and I thought it inappropriate not to draw your attention to it, since it has a power against the illness. But I urge you not to communicate it to people you happen to meet, but to reserve it to those who are virtuous and capable of guarding it.

The "Z" (or "N") symbol Alexander recommends has qualities of that of the Fouquet armband (fig. 8) and that of the Menil ring (fig. 13): the terminations of the bars are marked by small rings, and two more tiny rings appear to each side of the transverse stroke. No ring with precisely the above characteristics is known to have survived, which is hardly surprising considering the metal that Alexander stipulates. However, the Menil Foundation Collection does include an octagonal iron ring (no. II.B23)

terized as the Byzantine descendant of Greco-Egyptian ancestors like those illustrated in our figures 12 and 14. True, the medium and format have changed, the inscription is now biblical, and the Chnoubis itself has turned into a creature very much like Gorgon—it's tail, once compressed (fig. 8), desiccated (fig. 9), and detached (fig. 13), has been all but forgotten, and its seven "rays," now fully circumscribed by their traditional solar disc, have acquired monster heads. Yet, through all of this, the basic function of this object type remained the same and, even today, the genealogical thread that binds its distinctive imagery over centuries and cultures is unmistakable.[70]

The Menil ring (fig. 13) is one of a group of Byzantine amuletic rings of similar design and decoration, some of which bear inscriptions shedding additional light on their medical use.[71] One silver specimen in the British Museum shows a bezel much like the Menil ring, with a human head and seven monster-headed rays; its octagonal hoop, however, is inscribed with the words, "Lord, help the wearer."[72] Now significantly, the gerund used for "wearer" bears a feminine case ending, which sug-

gests the possibility that the abdominal distress against which this Chnoubis' powers were invoked was of a specifically womanly sort[73]—a possibility which is substantially strengthened if not confirmed by yet another silver ring in the group, excavated at Corinth (fig. 15).[74] Again, the bezel takes the form of a solar disc, at the center of which is the rayed Chnoubis/Gorgon, though this time without the monster terminations. The point of special interest, however, is the inscription on the hoop, which reads, "Womb amulet" ([Hy]sterikon Phylakterion). For not only does the uterus fall naturally within the Chnoubis' abdominal domain,[75] the Chnoubis was one of just a few magical creatures—all "masters of the womb"—who were specifically charged with control over the uterus on Greco-Egyptian gem amulets. The Chnoubis will, for example, often appear atop a bell-shaped representation of the womb, at the lower orifice of which will be the great key by which the organ is "closed" and thereby controlled (fig. 16).[76]

As silver armbands led naturally into this group of rings, so these rings draw us into a much larger, generally much later group of uterine pendant amulets which have long been recognized as medico-amuletic, because the inscriptions that many of them bear address the womb (Hystera) directly, as though it were a living creature.[77] They usually apply to it the double epithet "dark and black one," and often accuse it of "coiling like a serpent, hissing like a dragon, and roaring like a lion"—and then admonish it to "lie down like a lamb."[78] Most

---

with a large square bezel bearing the opening words of Psalm 90.

[70] It is unmistakable, thanks to the silver armbands illustrated in figures 8 and 9, which show clearly the process whereby the rayed Chnoubis head, in its human form, came to dominate and then eliminate the creature's snake tail—even while the distinctive number of rays and associate magical characters remained constant. For the Byzantines, the rayed Chnoubis head thus acquired the character of a Gorgon-like emblem. Indeed, there is evidence that Gorgon and the Chnoubis may fairly early on have been confused with one another: a gem amulet published three decades ago by Campbell Bonner shows on one of its faces a very classical Gorgon head; on its other side a later inscription addresses that creature as "Gorgon" at its beginning and "Chnoubis" at it closing. See C. Bonner, "A Miscellany of Engraved Stones," *Hesperia*, 23:2 (1954), no. 42. The adaptation of the Chnoubis to ring bezels and pendants (cf. our fig. 18), and its seeming identification with (and partial transformation into) Gorgon, was probably facilitated by the fact that Late Antiquity already knew a tradition of Gorgon (Medusa) pendants. Compare, for example, M. Hewig, *A Corpus of Roman Engraved Gemstones from British Sites*, BAR British Series 8, 2nd ed. (Oxford, 1978), nos. 750 ff.

[71] The group is characterized by large, thin bezels with flat, usually octagonal hoops, and by Chnoubis heads and magical ring signs; like the armbands, most of these rings are silver. See Dalton, *Early Christian Antiquities*, no. 142; Orsi, *Sicilia bizantina*, fig. 68; and G. R. Davidson, *Corinth, XII: The Minor Objects* (Princeton, 1952), 231, nos. 1947–1953. There are two unpublished members of this group in the Clemens Collection, Cologne (Kunstgewerbemuseum nos. H 937 and G 848). Both are from Sicily, and are close to those published by Orsi. One (G 848) shows a six-rayed Chnoubis head set upon shoulders. I would like to thank B. Chadour for bringing them to my attention.

[72] Dalton, *Early Christian Antiquities*, no. 142.

[73] It is worth noting here that the Spier armband (fig. 10) carries an invocation naming a certain "Anna."

[74] Davidson, *Corinth*, no. 1947 ("not later than the tenth century"); illustrated 1:1.

[75] This is true whether considered simply as a potentially troublesome organ, as the process of healthy childbirth (or birth control), or as the generic womanly organ whose "wanderings" might cause any number of physical or emotional problems. See Bonner, *Magical Amulets*, 90; and Barb, "*Diva matrix*," 193 ff. Cf. *PGM*, VII, 260–71.

[76] Paris, Cabinet des Médailles, no. B1 14; illustrated 1.5:1. See Delatte and Derchain, *Intailles magiques*, no. 345. To the left and right of the Chnoubis are Isis and a dog-headed mummy; enclosing the group is the Ouroboros, the snake with its tail in its mouth.

[77] For the most recent treatment of the group, and references to most of the extensive earlier bibliography, see V. N. Zalesskaja, "Amulettes byzantines magiques et leur liens avec le littérature apocryphe," *Actes du XIVe Congrès International des Etudes Byzantines, Bucharest, 6–12 Septembre, 1971*, III (Bucharest, 1976), 243 ff. See also Bonner, *Magical Amulets*, 90 f.; and notes 78 and 86 below. Cf. *PGM*, VII, 260–71.

[78] For the inscriptions, see W. Drexler, "Alte Beschwörungsformeln," *Philologus*, 58 (1899), 594 ff.; and V. Laurent, "Amulettes byzantines et formulaires magiques," *BZ*, 36 (1936), 303 ff.

members of this group carry some such uterine charm and an appropriate invocation addressed to the Virgin, while all show a form of the Gorgon-like head familiar from our group of rings. Only relatively few of these amulets are of the period of the earlier extant rings (i.e., seventh to eighth century), and none appears to be contemporary with the armbands (sixth to seventh century). Among the earliest members of the group is a cast lead specimen in the Hermitage (fig. 17),[79] whose apotropaic device is remarkably like that of the Corinth ring; around its circumference is a garbled version of the *Trisagion*, while on its back side the uterus is named, and the help of Holy Mary and the Theotokos are invoked against it. On the other hand, a slightly later—perhaps ninth century—silver pendant in the Menil Foundation Collection (fig. 18)[80] is closer in general design to the Menil ring; moreover on both, the creature's seven rays individually take a form surprisingly close to that of the more traditional lion-snake Chnoubis.[81] The many errors in transcription on this pendant betray the hand of a craftsman basically ignorant of the rich medico-magical tradition that lies behind it. Between the creature's serpentine solar rays are the letters for "Grace of God" (without the initial *chi*) and *Iaw*,[82] while around its circumference is, again, the *Trisagion* (with *alphas* for *lamdas* and a *kappa* for a *beta*).[83] On the pendant's back side is a complete but confused rendition of the *Hystera* charm common to the group: (around the circum-

ference) "Womb, dark [and] black, eat blood [and] drink blood";[84] (within the field) "As a serpent you coil; as a lion you roar; as a sheep, lie down; as a woman. . . ." Framing the inscription is a series of traditional but again confused magical characters and symbols: above are the *pentalpha*, two crescent moons, a star, an erect snake(?), and a figure—perhaps a misunderstood archangel—holding a long cross staff, while below are a pair of "Z"s and a ring-sign star lacking two of its normal eight points. All of these symbols appear frequently on Late Antique gem amulets and, as we have already seen, the "Z," the star, and the *pentalpha* have strong traditional ties with Chnoubis abdominal amulets—and now through them, with the uterus.[85] Indeed, that these pendants bear charms which admonish the uterus to "lie down," and here, moreover, to consume blood—presumably the blood that it would otherwise discharge—suggest that they may have functioned specifically to enhance fertility; that is, a tranquil, bloodless womb will avoid miscarriage and favor healthy parturition.[86]

Those for whom our silver armbands were made need not have relied solely on the magic of the

---

[79] Leningrad, State Hermitage Museum, *omega* 1159; illustrated 1:1. The suspension loop has broken away. See Zalesskaja, "Amulettes," 244, fig. 3; and for an identical specimen, Laurent, "Amulettes," 308, fig. 2 (who renders and discusses the inscription). Note that the rays again number seven, and that above the head of the creature is a three-pronged fork motif which recalls the central, Chnoubis medallion of the Fouquet armband (fig. 8).

[80] Houston, Menil Foundation Collection, no. 824; illustrated ca. 1:1. The suspension loop has broken away. Said to have come from Asia Minor. Unpublished. I wish to thank Nicolas Oikonomides and Werner Seibt for help in reading and dating this inscription. A nearly-illegible bronze pendant much like this one is preserved in the Benaki Museum, Athens.

[81] Characteristics, besides the serpentine body, include the rearing head, long snout, open mouth, and projecting tufts of mane behind the head. Compare, in addition to our figures 8, 12 and 16, Bonner, *Magical Amulets*, nos. 81, 82; and Delatte and Derchain, *Intailles Magiques*, no. 62. The device on the Menil pendant is formed as if of a single human-headed Chnoubis which itself sprouts seven lion-snake Chnoubis rays.

[82] Compare our figure 14. On *Iaw* as an amuletic expression of divine power, see Bonner, *Magical Amulets*, 134 f.

[83] That a *K* could be substituted for a *B* (in *Sabaoth* of the *Trisagion*) suggests that the form of the *beta* in the craftsman's model was that characteristic of the seventh and eighth centuries (and found on the hoop of the Menil ring), which looks like a Latin "R" with an (easily overlooked) bar across the bottom.

[84] I take this as an injunction addressed to the uterus. Although references to the consumption of blood have not hitherto been documented among this particular group of pendant uterine charms, they do appear on earlier amulets of similar function. See Bonner, *Magical Amulets*, 88, 217 f.; and A. A. Barb, "Bois du sang, Tantale," *Syria*, 19 (1952), 271 ff.

[85] For the stars, moons, "snake," and "Z," see Bonner, *Magical Amulets*, nos. 75, 108, 163, 222, 280, 339, etc. For the figure with the long staff, see M. C. Ross, *Catalogue of the Byzantine and Early Mediaeval Antiquities in the Dumbarton Oaks Collection, Volume I: Metalwork, Ceramics, Glass, Glyptics, Painting* (Washington, D.C., 1962), no. 117 (one of many of this type).

[86] Barb ("Bois du sang," 279) offers a similar interpretation for an amulet bearing Tantalus, a representation of the uterus, and the injunction that Tantalus "drink blood." The origin and meaning of the Gorgon-like device that dominates the pendants in this group has intrigued and puzzled scholars for more than a century. (For a brief review of scholarship, see Zalesskaja, "Amulettes," 243 f.; and add to it: Bonner, *Magical Amulets*, 90; and Barb, "*Diva matrix*," 210 f.) That no satisfactory solution was ever offered is due in large measure to the fact that these pendants were never studied within the broader context of Early Byzantine medical amulets, for it is only by way of related rings and armbands that their imagery (and function) may be traced back to Antique Chnoubis gems. Most recently Zalesskaja, taking up Sokolov's arguments of 1889, rightly rejected all prevailing theories with the observation that none accounted for the fact that the creature's serpentine rays usually number seven (on earlier specimens) or twelve (on later examples). Yet, when he chose to disregard Greco-Egyptian gem amulets and instead to explain the "seven" textually, by way of the "seven female spirits" from the *Testament of Solomon* (McCown, *Testament*, 31* ff.) who have control over (e.g.) "deception, strife, jealousy, and error," Zalesskaja failed to account for the pendants' uterine connection, much less for their rich iconographic tradition, and that of their accompanying magical characters.

Chnoubis, for there were two other iconographic "charms"—the holy rider and the Palestinian christological cycle—whose powers converged toward the same end. Indeed, two of the earliest members of our uterine pendant group show a holy rider on their reverse side.[87] Surely this rider and the Chnoubis on the obverse were thought to act in concert against a common evil, and surely that evil is to be recognized in the bare-breasted female who, beneath the hooves of the horse, is about to be impaled by the rider's lance (cf. figs. 9, 19, 20).[88] But who is she? As many scholars have already concluded in discussing the same iconography on other, contemporary amulets, this can only be antiquity's female archdemon: Lilith among the Jews, Alabasdria in Early Byzantine Egypt (and so labelled in the well-known fresco at Bawit), Gyllou to the Byzantines, and Abyzou in the *Testament of Solomon.*[89] The evil intent of this creature, who went by as many as forty names and took nearly as many shapes, is spelled out in the *Testament of Solomon*:

I am Abyzou [or Obizuth]; and by night I sleep not, but go my rounds over all the world, and visit women in childbirth. And . . . if I am lucky, I strangle the child.[90]

Obviously, in attacking this archenemy of parturient women the holy rider was serving one and the same goal as that implicit in the very presence of the Chnoubis/Gorgon (as "master of the womb") and explicit in uterine charms like "lie down," and "drink blood"; namely, the goal of healthy, successful childbirth.[91]

The holy rider was one of Late Antiquity's most popular amuletic motifs; indeed, in this statistical sense alone it may be said to have taken over the role once played by the Chnoubis.[92] One of its most characteristic appearances is on the obverse of a distinctive genre of intaglio haematite amulet; the rider is labelled "Solomon" and the gem's back side usually bears the words: *Sphragis Theou,* "Seal of God" (figs. 19, 20).[93] Although Solomon was not, in fact, a mounted warrior, he was renowned as the most powerful of the Kings of Israel; endowed with exceptional wisdom, he was believed by Jews and Christians alike to wield power over evil spirits. According to the *Testament of Solomon,* which was probably the most popular magic treatise in early Byzantium, King Solomon was able to control and exploit the forces of evil, and thereby build the Temple, only because God had given him a "little

---

[87] See Schlumberger, "Amulettes," 79; and H. Möbius, "Griechisch-orientalische Bleimedaillons aus Ionien," *AA,* 56 (1941), 26. On the armbands the Chnoubis and the holy rider seem to have been interchangeable as well as complementary. A few of the more elaborate examples in the group (e.g., Froehner, *Collection,* 7) add the apotropaic acclamation *Heis Theos O Nikon Ta Kaka* over the rider; significantly, that same acclamation is coupled instead with the Chnoubis on the Fouquet armband (our fig. 8).

[88] That the figure beneath the horse is indeed female and bare-breasted is clear on a few of the finer armbands, (e.g., *ibid.,* 7; and O. M. Dalton, "A Gold Pectoral Cross and an Amuletic Bracelet of the Sixth Century," *Mélanges offerts à M. Gustave Schlumberger* [Paris, 1924], II, pl. XVII,3).

[89] See Perdrizet, *Negotium,* 15 ff.; A. A. Barb, "*Antaura*: The Mermaid and the Devil's Grandmother," *JWarb,* 29 (1966), 4 ff.; and C. Detleff and G. Müller, "Von Teufel, Mittagsdämon und Amuletten," *JbAChr,* 17 (1974), 99 ff. On Early Byzantine amulets this she-devil is frequently coupled with the "much-suffering" Evil Eye—the destructive eye of envy—which was her *modus operandi.* See Perdrizet, *Negotium,* 30; and, for some examples, Bonner, *Magical Amulets,* nos. 298–303. For the Bawit frescoes, see J. Clédat, *Le monastère et la nécropole de Baoît,* MémInstCaire, 12 (Cairo, 1904), pl. LVI. There is an interesting Early Byzantine rock crystal cone seal in the Malcove Collection, University of Toronto, which shows above the holy rider three letters, *gamma, iota* (?), and *lamda,* which were probably intended to label "Gilou" (Gyllou), which here takes a very snakelike form. On variant spellings of this demon's name, see Perdrizet, *Negotium,* 20; and on the Byzantine cone seal as a genre, see Vikan and Nesbitt, *Security,* 20 ff., fig. 46. In the Benaki Museum in Athens is a gold belt(?) clasp of sixth- or seventh-century date with a monogram which may resolve as *Gelou.* See B. Segall, *Museum Benaki, Athens: Katalog der Goldschmiede-Arbeiten* (Athens, 1938), no. 267. Thanks for this reference are due to L. Bouras.

[90] McCowan, *Testament,* 43* ff.; and F. C. Conybeare, "The Testament of Solomon," *JQR,* 11 (1899), 30.

[91] In the *Testament of Solomon (loc. cit.)* Abyzou is described as having: a woman's form, a head without limbs, dishevelled hair tossed wildly, and a body in darkness. This Gorgon-like description, plus the close medico-magical association of Abyzou and the Chnoubis (one the demon and the other the antidote) may well have contributed to the latter's iconographic transmutation in medieval Byzantium—where, after all, the Greco-Egyptian Chnoubis would have been little understood. Yet, it would be a mistake to identify Abyzou with Gorgon and, in turn, both with the device on our uterine rings and pendants—as A. A. Barb has done ("*Antaura*," 9). For then left unexplained would be the recurrent choice of precisely seven "rays," the solar disc, the associated Chnoubis magical characters, and the close relationship of the pendants and rings to the armbands, where the Chnoubis is unmistakable. Furthermore, it should be recalled that Abyzou (as a bare-breasted female) does appear occasionally on one and the same object with the Gorgon-like uterine device (note 87 above). And finally, Gorgon-Medusa, when it does appear in early Byzantium (e.g., on Athena bust weights) in fact looks nothing like our pendants' apotropaic device (cf. G.F. Bass, "Underwater Excavations at Yassi Ada: A Byzantine Shipwreck," *AA,* 77 [1962], 560). Contrast also the earlier Gorgon-head pendants cited in note 70 above.

[92] See Bonner, *Magical Amulets,* 208 ff., nos. 294 ff.; B. Begatti, "Altre medaglie di Salomone cavaliere e loro origine," *RACr,* 47 (1971), 331 ff.; and J. Russell, "The Evil Eye in Early Byzantine Society," *XVI. Internationaler Byzantinistenkongress, Akten* II/3, *JÖBG,* 32:3 (1982), 540 ff.

[93] Figure 19: Columbia, University of Missouri Museum of Art and Archaeology, Robinson no. 35; illustrated 1:1. See Bonner, *Magical Amulets,* no. 296. Figure 20: Ann Arbor, University of Michigan, no. 26092; illustrated 1:1. See *ibid.,* no. 294. For the genre as a whole, see P. Perdrizet, "*Sphragis Solomonis,*" *REG,* 16 (1903), 49 f.; Bonner, *Magical Amulets,* 208 ff., nos. 294 ff.; and Delatte and Derchain, *Intailles magiques,* nos. 369 ff.

seal ring" with which he could "lock up all the de-mons."[94] Solomon's identification on the obverse of these amulets with the holy rider—a generic emblem of victory—evokes in a graphic but symbolic way his victory over demons, while the inscription on the reverse simply identifies the vehicle of that victory, the "Seal of God."

From the beginning, Solomon's supernatural powers were thought to have a specifically medical dimension.[95] According to Josephus:

> God granted him knowledge of the art used against demons for the benefit and healing of men. He also composed incantations by which illnesses are relieved, and left behind forms of exorcisms with which those possessed by demons drive them out, never to return.[96]

Similarly, the *Testament of Solomon* includes a number of purely medical encounters between this Old Testament king and sickness-inducing spirits, each of whom Solomon forces—with God's seal ring—to reveal his name and the magical influence to which his powers are subject. Solomon's interrogation of the "Thirty-Six Elements of the Cosmic Ruler of Darkness," for example, provides a veritable litany of human afflictions and of supernatural antidotes:

> And the ninth [Element] said: "I am called Kurtael. I send colics in the bowels. I induce pains. If I hear the words, Iaoth, imprison Kurtael, I at once retreat." And the tenth said: "I am called Metathiax. I cause the reins to ache. If I hear the words, Adonael, imprison Metathiax, I at once retreat." And the eleventh said. . . .[97]

Against this background it is hardly surprising to discover that at least some Solomonic amulets were intended to be specifically medicinal from their point of manufacture. For example, a bronze amuletic ring from Early Byzantine Egypt bears around the circumference of its bezel the words, "Solomon, guard [i.e., preserve] health," while at its center is an anchor-cross with fish, one of the most frequently-employed devices on Early Christian signet rings (fig. 21).[98] In both design and effect

this ring shares much in common with the Chnoubis gem amulet illustrated in our figure 12, on the back side of which are the words: "[Chnoubis], guard in health the stomach of Proclus."[99]

Returning now to the holy rider/Abyzou, and specifically to our group of haematite amulets, several points are worthy of note. First, some of these amulets bear magic characters beneath the inscription on their back side, and the one that appears most frequently—the "barred-triple-S" (fig. 19)—was, even more than the "Z," specifically associated with the Chnoubis (cf. fig. 14).[100] Second, at least a few specimens within this series of intaglios show, instead of the "barred-triple-S," what is unmistakably a key beneath the inscription on their back side (fig. 20). And while it is certainly true that the key was, in early Byzantium (and especially in the *Testament of Solomon*), functionally equivalent to, and interchangeable with, the seal,[101] it is also true that the key had its own special meaning within the tradition of Antique gem amulets: it was the "key to the womb" (note again our figure 16).[102] This brings us to the third and most interesting point: the vast majority of surviving Greco-Egyptian "clé de matrice" amulets are of the same size, shape, and *material* as our group of Solomon amulets—which suggests, of course, that they were part of the same

---

abbreviated. The beginning of the inscription is marked by what appears to be a simple cross. For another Solomon amulet with similar inscription, see Perdrizet, "*Sphragis*," 46; and for this verb on amulets, see Bonner, *Magical Amulets*, 179 f. A "neutral" subject already popular among pagans, the anchor-with-fish motif was one of the most readily accepted devices for Early Christian signets. Specifically sanctioned by Clement of Alexandria (*Paed.* 3.11), the anchor evoked the cross and the hope of the faithful for salvation (Hebrews, 6.19). The fish, on the other hand, may have been intended to evoke the *ICHTHYS* acrostic for Christ, the souls of the faithful, or it may have been nothing more than a compositional carryover from pagan prototypes.

[99] Another Solomonic *phylakterion*, though of a less permanent sort, is described to Pseudo-Pliny (3.15: *ad quartanas*): ". . . *in charta virgine scribis quod in dextro brachio ligatum portet ille qui patitur: recede ab illo Gaio Seio, tertiana, Solomon te sequitur.*" V. Rose, ed., *Plinii secundi quae fertur una cum Gargilii Martialis Medicina* (Leipzig, 1875), 89 = A. Önnerfors, ed., *Plinii secundi iunioris: De medicina* (Berlin, 1964 [*CML* III]), III, 15.7–8 (p. 78). Similarly, a papyrus amulet of the fifth or sixth century (PO, 18, 415 ff.) bears the Lord's Prayer followed by "the exorcism of Solomon against all impure spirits"; it concludes with these words: "guard those who carry this amulet from fever, from all sorts of maladies, and bad wounds. Thus be it."

[100] Bonner, *Magical Amulets*, 58 f., nos. 296, 297; Delatte and Derchain, *Intailles magiques*, 56 f., nos. 371, 376.

[101] Thus Solomon was able to "lock up all the demons." See G. Vikan, "Security in Byzantium: Keys," *XVI. Internationaler Byzantinistenkongress, Akten* II/3, *JÖBG*, 32:3 (1982), 503 ff. (esp. 506).

[102] Bonner, *Magical Amulets*, 85 ff.; and Delatte and Derchain, *Intailles magiques*, 245 ff.

---

[94] It was this ring which, according to some variants of the text, bore the *pentalpha* as its device. See McCown, *Testament*, 10*. For the composition, text tradition, and scholarship of the *Testament of Solomon*, see A.-M. Denis, *Introduction aux pseudépigraphes grecs d'Ancien Testament* (Leiden, 1970), 67.

[95] Perdrizet, "*Sphragis*," 44 ff.

[96] *Jewish Antiquities* 8.45 (Loeb, V [Cambridge, Mass./London, 1935]).

[97] McCown, *Testament*, 53*; and Conybeare, "Testament," 35.

[98] Illustrated ca. 1:1. This ring, which should probably be dated from the fourth to the sixth century, was kindly brought to my attention by its owner, who lives in California. Although "Solomon" is spelled out in full, *Hy*[*ieia*] and *Phyla*[*xon*?] are much

medico-magical tradition and fulfilled basically the same function.[103] And it seems likely that the most important "constant" in that tradition was neither format nor iconography, but rather the material itself: haematite ("bloodstone").[104] For among the many virtues attributed to haematite over the centuries in treatises on stone, the most important was its ability to stop the flow of blood.[105] And naturally, with this styptic function we are drawn back again to those uterine charms which adjure the consumption of blood and the calming of the womb, and to the impaled Abyzou (with her designs on infants), and to the Chnoubis (as "master of the womb"), and, finally, to that lonely key in figure 20, whose magical function was surely that of closing and controlling the womb.[106]

Complementing the Chnoubis and holy rider medallions on the more elaborate of our armbands is a third inconographic "charm": the Palestinian

christological cycle (figs. 8–10).[107] And it seems likely that this charm, too, was thought to convey a measure of supernatural healing power. After all, on the pilgrim ampullae (fig. 11) it was coupled with *eulogia* oil of the sort often used, like blessed earth, to perform miraculous cures; this, for example, was the practice at the shrine of St. Menas, near Alexandria:

> The pilgrim suspended a lamp before the grave [of St. Menas]. . . . It burned day and night, and was filled with fragrant oil. And when anyone took oil of this lamp . . . and rubbed a sick person with it, the sick person was healed of the evil of which he suffered.[108]

Moreover, there have recently appeared two hoards comprising more than ninety tiny image-bearing clay tokens (figs. 22–24) which in design and fabric are much like small Symeon tokens, but which iconographically match up instead with the ampullae and armbands.[109] Some bear scenes like the

---

[103] Barb ("Bois du sang," 279) was the first to note this; it had escaped the notice of both Bonner and Delatte.

[104] Haematite is a black iron ore which, when powdered or rubbed against a rough surface, becomes red (cf. Pliny, *Nat. Hist.* 36.147). In the case of the armbands, rings, and pendants, the genealogical thread leading back to Greco-Egyptian gems was iconographic; medium and format had changed radically. Here, on the other hand, medium and format were maintained while the main (though not the secondary) iconographic motifs were changed radically.

[105] See Barb, "Bois du sang," 279.

[106] Both Perdrizet ("*Sphragis*," 50) and Barb ("Bois du sang," 279) recognized the power for "blood control" in haematite amulets. Moreover, Perdrizet drew this conclusion specifically in relation to these Solomon haematites—though, unaware of their links to earlier uterine amulets, he did not see their significance for the womb and for procreation.

That the demon Gyllou, Solomon, and childbirth were closely linked in the Byzantine mind (at least in later centuries), is indicated by a passage in Michael Psellus (K. Sathas, *Bibliotheca graeca medii aevi*, V [Paris, 1876], 572 f.) wherein the latter two are introduced in his short discussion of the former. Late antiquity knew another, specifically Christian blood-control (by implication, "birth") amulet: the healing of the woman with the issue of blood (Mark 5.25 ff.). A rock crystal pendant with that iconography is preserved in the J. Spier Collection, N.Y.C., while one in green jasper is in the Benaki Museum, Athens (no. 13527; with a Crucifixion on its back side). Both are likely of east Mediterranean origin and of sixth- to seventh-century date; a later specimen in haematite is in the Metropolitan Museum (*Age of Spirituality: Late Antique and Early Christian Art, Third to Seventh Century*, ed. K. Weitzmann, Exhibition: Metropolitan Museum of Art, New York [1977–1978; published 1979], no. 398). Pliny notes that "the people of the East" wear green jaspers as amulets (*Nat. Hist.* 36.118); Dioscorides, on the other hand, notes that jaspers in general are effective as amulets for childbirth (*De mat. medica* 5.142). In a well-known passage from his *Church History* (7.16.2) Eusebius describes at Paneas the following sculptural ensemble, which was taken in his day to represent (i.e., commemorate) the miracle of the woman with the issue of blood (*The Nicene and Post-Nicene Fathers*, 2nd series, 1 [Grand Rapids, Mich., 1952], 304):

For there stands upon an elevated stone, by the gates of her house, a brazen image of a woman kneeling, with her hands stretched out, as if she were praying. Opposite this is another upright image of a man, made of the same material, clothed decently in a double cloak, and extending his hand toward the woman. At his feet, beside the statue itself, is a certain strange plant, which climbs up to the hem of the brazen cloak, and is a remedy for all kinds of diseases.

[107] See Kitzinger, "Christian Imagery," 151 f. Contrary to Kitzinger, this "cycle" need not have been complete to convey its magic; only a few scenes (our figures 10 and 27) or just one (Wulff, *Altchristliche Bildwerke*, no. 885) might be excerpted and applied to an amulet.

[108] Kötting, *Peregrinatio*, 198. In fact, both the inscriptional and the iconographic evidence provided by the Monza-Bobbio group of ampullae suggests that they were used as travel amulets—though not necessarily to the exclusion of other magical functions. See Vikan, *Byzantine Pilgrimage*, 24. Cyril of Skythopolis writes that St. Saba used oil of the True Cross—which, according to their inscriptions, the Monza-Bobbio ampullae contained—to exorcise evil spirits, at least some of which must have been sickness-inducing (*Vit. Saba* 26).

[109] One hoard, perhaps of Syrian origin, was acquired by the British Museum in 1973 (acc. nos. 1973,5–1, 1–80); it consists of seventy-nine specimens (plus one Symeon token), and has been published by Richard Camber ("A Hoard," *passim*). The second hoard, as yet unpublished, was purchased in 1980 through H. Drouot by Professor Robert-Henri Bautier, Paris; it consists of fourteen specimens, including our figures 22–24 (slightly enlarged). I would like to thank Professor Bautier for a set of photographs of his tokens, and for permission to published them. Together, these two hoards form a homogeneous group of ninety-three clay tokens measuring between .5 and 1.5 cm. in diameter (making them roughly half the size of most Symeon tokens). A preliminary survey indicates that these ninety-three specimens derive from just twenty-two molds representing twelve iconographic themes:

*1.	Adoration of the Magi	21 specimens (3 molds)
2.	"Solomon" (fig. 24)	16 specimens (2 molds)
*3.	Baptism	11 specimens (2 molds)
*4.	Bust of Christ	9 specimens (1 mold)
*5.	Nativity	7 specimens (3 molds)

Women at the Tomb (fig. 22), which depend on a specific *locus sanctus*,[110] while others show the Entry into Jerusalem (fig. 23) which, though biblical, is substantially amuletic;[111] and finally, there are a number of purely magical tokens which bear the name "Solomon" (backwards) and show what appears to be (at least on the better-preserved specimens) a coiled serpent (fig. 24).[112] That these tokens functioned as medicine—deriving their

*6.	Women at the Tomb (fig. 22)	6 specimens (2 molds)
*7.	Annunciation	5 specimens (3 molds)
8.	Transfiguration (?)	5 specimens (1 mold)
*9.	Entry into Jerusalem (fig. 23)	5 specimens (1 mold)
*10.	Adoration of the Cross	5 specimens (2 molds)
11.	Tempest Calmed	2 specimens (1 mold)
12.	Miracle of Cana	1 specimen (1 mold)

*Indicates those themes paralleled on the ampullae or the armbands.

The genre represented by these two hoards was not unknown. Indeed, nearly two dozen iconographically related clay tokens have been published from various museum collections; some may actually derive from the matrices attested within our two hoards, though most specimens tend to be larger. See Dalton, *Early Christian Antiquities*, nos. 966–68; Wulff, *Altchristliche Bildwerke*, no. 1149 (limestone?); Tchalenko, *Villages antiques*, III (1958), 62, figs. 27, 28; Lafontaine-Dosogne, *Itinéraires archéologiques*, 159 ff., nos. 20–26 (27–31?); H. Buschhausen, *Die spätrömischen Metallscrinia und früchristlichen Reliquiare, 1. Teil: Katalog*, Wiener Byzantinistische Studien, IX (Vienna, 1971), no. C10; L.Y. Rahmani, "The Adoration of the Magi on Two Sixth-Century C.E. Eulogia Tokens," *IEJ*, 29 (1979), 34 ff., pl. 8, B-D; idem, "A Representation of the Baptism on an *Eulogia* Token," '*Atiqot: English Series*, 14 (1980), 109 ff.; and Camber, "A Hoard," notes 6 and 9. Just one additional iconographic theme, the frontally-seated Virgin and Child, is attested in this series (Lafontaine-Dosogne); as in our two hoards, the Adoration of the Magi is by far the most frequently attested subject (see also note 116 below).

[110] Compare our figures 10 and 11. Here, the two Marys have been deleted for lack of space. Note again the "grill" of the pilgrim accounts (see note 55 above).

[111] Compare our figure 10. For this scene of "Christ as Holy Rider," see note 57 above. Here, the animal is clearly identifiable as a donkey. And here, as in several other holy rider compositions of the period (e.g., Dalton, *Early Christian Antiquities*, no. 543; and Bonner, *Magical Amulets*, no. 324), the *propempontos* (escort) of traditional *adventus* iconography appears—even though he is not called for by the Gospel account of the Entry into Jerusalem. See K. G. Holum and G. Vikan, "The Trier Ivory, *Adventus* Ceremonial, and the Relics of St. Stephen," *DOP*, 33 (1979), 118 f.

[112] This reading of these Solomon tokens is corroborated by a bronze amulet from Early Byzantine Egypt published by Wulff (*Altchristliche Bildwerke*, no. 825). Its obverse shows the Entry into Jerusalem, while its reverse bears the words *Sphragis Solomonos*, a standing figure (Solomon?), a small cross in a nimbus, and a coiled serpent-like monster. This same form appears between personifications of the sun and moon on a group of closely-interrelated bronze amulets, all but one of which bear an inscription invoking the *Spragis Solomonos*. They are apparently Syro-Palestinian in origin and of sixth- to seventh-century date. See Schlumberger, "Amulettes," nos. 2 and 3; and *Byzantine Art*

curative powers from their "blessed" earth and amuletic imagery[113]—is suggested by their inherently "consumable" nature, by their inclusion of Solomon,[114] and by their obvious similarity to medicinal Symeon tokens (cf. figs. 2, 3); indeed, the larger of the two hoards included a Symeon token.[115] And just as a Symeon pendant (fig. 7) was capable of conveying that saint's healing power, independent of blessed substance, so also these scenes

in the Collection of the U.S.S.R. (in Russian), Exhibition: The Hermitage, Leningrad; The Pushkin Museum, Moscow (1975–1977), no. 62 (with earlier bibliography, wherein Zalasskaja suggests that the form is Golgotha). An excellent representative of the type is preserved in the Benaki Museum, Athens. For yet another, slightly different rendition of the same creature (with the inscription "Christ, help") see G. Tchalenko, *Villages antique de la Syrie du Nord*, III (Paris, 1958), 62, fig. 29.

[113] The homogeneity of the tokens within this series, plus the fact that some of them (e.g., those with "Solomon") are topographically "anonymous," suggest that they came from a single blessed source and not from so many *loca sancta*. Indeed, there can be no doubt that christological tokens of this sort were being produced from the *eulogia* clay of the Miraculous Mountain: there is the evidence of the two-faced stamp reproduced in our figure 5, and the fact that many non-Symeon clay tokens (among those cited in the second part of note 109 above) have been discovered in the region of Antioch (Lafontaine-Dosogne, *Itinéraires archéologiques*, nos. 20–26; and Tchalenko, *Villages antiques*, III [1958], 62, figs. 27, 28). Several specimens in the Antioch Museum show a frontal Virgin and Child much like that on the reverse of the stamp (cf. fig. 5 and Lafontaine-Dosogne, *Itinéraires archéologiques*, pl. XLVI, no. 20). The possibility that a single blessed hill could be the source of a variety of iconographically heterogeneous tokens obviously runs counter to prevailing art-historical opinion, which would trace each *eulogia* scene back to its own *locus sanctus* and, in specific, to a mural at that shrine (cf. Rahmani, "The Adoration," 35 f.).

[114] The snake may be symbolic of evil (e.g., of the uterus, which "coils like a serpent") or, more likely, of good (e.g., the Chnoubis snake or the snake of Asklepios and Hygieia [cf. Volbach, *Elfenbeinarbeiten*, nos. 84, 84a, 85]). In the latter case especially, a medicinal function is strongly suggested. Three snakes and the word *Hygieia* appear on the medico-amuletic *tabella ansata* in the British Museum cited in note 59 above.

[115] Camber, "A Hoard," fig. 15. One wonders how these two hoards—which may originally have been one—came to be formed. That so many tokens so much alike should have come from a pilgrim's purse seems unlikely. Perhaps instead they were found in the remains of a storeroom or workshop at some holy site (see note 43 above), or perhaps they represent the contents of a doctor's or churchman's medicine box. They look very much like the dozens of clay/resin pellets preserved in (what certainly must be) a Late Roman medicine box found by Petrie in Egypt (*Objects*, pl. XXXIII, 3). Moreover, we know that churchmen could be doctors (cf. Magoulias, "Lives of Saints," 128), and that doctors were not above putting "blessed" ingredients in their remedies (cf. F. Cabrol, "Amulettes," *DACL*, II, 2 [Paris, 1907], 1855). If a medicine box like that preserved in the Vatican (Volbach, *Elfenbeinarbeiten*, no. 138) can bear a Christ miracle scene on its cover, why should not the pills inside be impressed with comparable imagery? It is worth noting here that a clay token with the Adoration of the Magi was discovered in a reliquary in the Chur Cathedral along with an (earlier) ivory medicine box (Buschhausen, *Metallscrinia*, no. C10).

must have had that ability when transferred from their *eulogia* clay (figs. 22, 23) to a silver armband (fig. 10)—or vice versa.[116]

The Palestinian christological cycle shared by the ampullae and armbands appears in its more or less complete form once again during this period, on a series of well-known octagonal gold rings in Baltimore, London (fig. 25), Palermo, and Washington, D.C.[117] These rings are clearly amuletic, and seem to have been designed to exercise their magical powers specifically for married couples. This is suggested by the fact that three of four show husband and wife on their bezel, and by the somewhat unusual quote from Psalm 5.12 which appears on the Palermo ring, "Thou hast crowned us with a shield of favor."[118] To judge from the three rele-

vant bezel compositions, the "us" should be understood as the bridal couple, and the "crowning"—at once metaphorical and literal—as that which takes place as part of the marriage ceremony (over which, in this case, Christ and the Virgin preside).[119] But what is the nature of the "shield"—the amuletic protection or benefit—with which the wedding couple should thereby be provided? Assumedly, it is a protection that applies to them collectively, as does *Omonia* ("[Marital] Harmony"), which is inscribed below the couple on the bezel of the British Museum ring (fig. 25).[120] But if the arguments put forward in this paper are correct, the octagonal shape of the hoop and the Palestinian christological cycle incised on it would seem to imply (if not require) that the benefit to the couple be somehow medical—if not more specifically abdominal or even uterine. And indeed, to judge from the inscription on the Dumbarton Oaks marriage belt (fig. 26; detail), "Health" was a benefit which, along with "Harmony" and "Grace," the bridal couple might legitimately invoke "from God" on their wedding day.[121] And how else can marital health be understood than in terms of healthy and successful procreation?[122]

---

[116] Here must be added a caveat which applies to all the "medicinal" amulets and *eulogiai* discussed in this paper. Although their primary purpose seems to have been the inducement of supernatural healing, they were almost certainly not confined to that single function. Consider, for example, these two hoards of "medicinal" tokens: the pair of tokens which show the Tempest Calmed clearly betray concerns of the seafaring pilgrim (cf. Vikan, *Byzantine Pilgrimage*, 24), while the one specimen with the Miracle of Cana probably had something to do with the consumption or preservation of wine (cf. other such wine amulets in *Papyrus Erzherzog Rainer: Führer durch die Ausstellung* [Vienna, 1894], 124 f.; and note 29 above). It should also be recalled that among the many *eulogia*-induced cures narrated in the *Vita* of Symeon the Younger, there is one miracle (chap. 235) wherein Symeon's dust is used to calm a storm at sea, and one (chap. 230) wherein it is used to restore spoiled wine.

Individual scenes very much like those appearing on these clay tokens were used, often in the form of press-gold medallions, on amuletic fibulae and pendants. See E. B. Smith, "A Lost Encolpium and Some Notes on Early Christian Iconography," *BZ*, 23 (1920), 217 ff.; W. F. Volbach, "Zwei frühchristliche Gold medaillons," *Berliner Museen*, 34 (1922), 80 ff.; *idem*, "Un medaglione d'oro con l'immagine di S. Teodoro nel Museo di Reggio Calabria," *AStCal*, 13 (1943–1944), 65 ff.; J. H. Iliffe, "A Byzantine Gold Enkolpion from Palestine (About Sixth Century A.D.)," *QDAP*, 14 (1950), 97 ff.; Ross, *Catalogue* (1962), no. 86; *idem*, *Catalogue* (1965), no. 37; and J. Engel, "Une decouverte enigmatique: La fibule chretienne d'Attalens," *Dossiers histoire et archéologie*, 62 (1982), 88 ff. The famous Strzygowski gold medallion at Dumbarton Oaks (Ross, *Catalogue* [1965], no. 36) is basically a deluxe pendant amulet bearing three typical scenes from the Palestinian christological cycle.

[117] London, British Museum; illustrated ca. 1.25:1. See Dalton, *Early Christian Antiquities*, no. 129. Iconography: Annunciation, Visitation, Nativity, Baptism, Adoration of the Magi (out of order), Crucifixion, Women at the Tomb. For the other three rings, see P. Verdier, "An Early Christian Ring with a Cycle of the Life of Christ," *The Bulletin of the Walters Art Gallery*, 11:3 (1958); C. Cecchelli, "L'anello bizantino del Museo di Palermo," *Miscellanea Guillaume de Jerphanion*, *OCP*, 13 (1947), 40 ff.; and Ross, *Catalogue* (1965), no. 69. For the group, see Engemann, "Palästinische Pilgerampullen," 20 f.; *Age of Spirituality* no. 446 (G. Vikan); and Kitzinger, "Christian Imagery," 151.

[118] For another Byzantine marriage ring with this inscription, see A. Banck, *Byzantine Art in the Collections of the USSR* (Leningrad/Moscow, n.d.), no. 106c.

[119] Some Byzantine rings of the period show crowns hovering over the heads of the bride and groom (e.g., Ross, *Catalogue* [1965], no. 67); on this bezel and on that of the Dumbarton Oaks ring, Christ and the Virgin appear to be putting the crowns in place. See P. A. Drossoyianni, "A Pair of Byzantine Crowns," *XVI. Internationaler Byzantinistenkongress, Akten* II/3, *JÖBG*, 32:3 (1982), 531 f.

[120] This word appears on many Early Byzantine marriage rings. See Ross, *Catalogue* (1965), nos. 67 and 69; and *Age of Spirituality*, no. 263.

[121] Acc. no. 37.33; illustrated 1:1. See Ross, *Catalogue* (1965), no. 38. "Health" is also invoked on the de Clercq gold marriage belt (A. de Ridder, *Collection de Clercq, catalogue: VII, les bijoux et les pierres gravées, 1, les bijoux* [Paris, 1911], no. 1212), and on at least a few bronze marriage rings of the period, including one in the Cabinet des Médailles (Seyrig Coll.), and one in the Menil Foundation Collection (II.B26).

[122] For the Byzantine marriage ceremony, see P. N. Trempela, "*Hē akolouthia tōn mnēstrōn kai tou gamou*," *Theologia*, 18 (1940), 101 ff. (based on manuscripts dating from the mid- to post-Byzantine period). In addition to "Harmony" and "Grace," there are repeated references to childbearing in the form of a formula based on biblical "models": (e.g.) "Bless us, O Lord our God, as you blessed Zacharias and Elisabeth" (*ibid.*, 149). One is reminded of the inscribed censers from Sicily of the sort illustrated in our figure 6 (cf. note 38 above), which bear the phrase, "Fear not, Zacharias, for thy prayer is heard. . . ." Perhaps the prayers this censer was intended to accompany were those specifically directed toward conception—as were those of Zacharias. It is noteworthy that Symeon the Younger's mother, Martha, went to the Church of St. John the Baptist in Antioch to pray for the conception of a child; after successful incubation, she awoke with a ball of incense in her hand, with which she censed the entire church (*Vita*, chaps. 2 and 3).

That the function of these marriage rings was not merely amuletic, but more specifically medicinal, is corroborated by a closely-related gold and niello "reliquary" locket in the British Museum (fig. 27).[123] Not only are medium and technique the same, this locket, like the rings, is octagonal in outline, and it bears on its obverse two scenes from the Palestinian christological cycle: the Nativity and the Adoration of the Magi. The locket's back side shows a cross-on-steps whose arms terminate in what are probably the letters of a magical number, name or phrase;[124] around its circumference are the words: "Secure deliverance and aversion [from] all evil," while into the edge of its octagon is inscribed: "of Sts. Cosmas and Damian." That these famous holy doctors are named leaves little doubt that this was a medical amulet—that the "evil" from which its wearer should be "delivered" was first and foremost that of ill health. And of course, the power for that deliverance came from the locket's very shape, from its imagery, and from its words, but more than any of these, it must have come from that sanctified bit of material "of Sts. Cosmas and Damian" that this capsule once contained. Most scholars have assumed that this was a tiny relic but, by analogy with the Monza-Bobbio ampullae, it could as well have been a *eulogia*.[125] And indeed, to judge from the *miracula* of these saints, that would seem to be the more likely conclusion: miracle 30, for example, describes the (customary) distribution of blessed wax in the church-shrine during the all-night Saturday vigil, while miracle 13 evokes the practice, already familiar from Symeon's *Vita*, of taking *eulogiai* to be employed in the event of illness away from the shrine.[126] In that instance, the holy medicine—which was ultimately melted and applied to the body—was carried "under the armpit," but it could just as well have been transported in a locket. This would require, of course, that the

locket be easily opened (as this one can be), and would imply that its contents might be periodically consumed and replenished. But if such were true of this gold and niello locket, the net effect would be to make of it much less a "reliquary" than an "amuletic pill box."[127]

Cosmas and Damian, and the problem of how one might ensure one's health while away from their shrine, draw us toward one final genre of Early Byzantine medical artifact: the invocational votive. In our figure 1 is reproduced a tiny silver plaque with a pair of eyes and the words, "In fulfillment of a vow." This object might legitimately be labelled an "acknowledgment votive," since it was almost certainly designed and dedicated to acknowledge a healing received. But if so, it would seem to presuppose a *proactive* counterpart; that is, a votive designed and dedicated to invoke future healing. Yet, as logical as this seems, and as abundant as surviving Early Byzantine votives are,[128] those among them that are demonstrably "medical" in this invocational sense are extremely rare.

One such object, a richly-incised bronze cross supported by a hand, was recently acquired by the Metropolitan Museum (fig. 28).[129] Likely of sixth- to seventh-century date and east Mediterranean manufacture, it shows on its four arms: the Virgin and Child enthroned (top), Sts. Peter and Paul (right and left, inscribed), and Sts. Cosmas and Damian (bottom), while at its center appears St. Stephen (inscribed), with a censer in one hand and an incense box in the other.[130] There are, in addition, two invocations: that in large letters on the horizontal cross arm, "Christ, help [me]," is at once

[123] London, British Museum; illustrated ca. 1:1. See Dalton, *Early Christian Antiquities*, no. 284. Acquired in Constantinople. See M. Rosenberg, *Geschichte der Goldschmiedekunst auf technischer Grundlage: Niello, bis zum Jahre 1000 nach Chr.* (Frankfurt am Main, 1924), 51; and M. Hadzidakis (Chatzidakis), "Un anneau Byzantin du Musée Benaki," *BNJbb*, 17 (1939–1943), 178 ff. (for its correct dating, along with the rings, to the seventh century).

[124] For the argument that these letters provide a date, see Hadzidakis, "Un anneau," 178 ff. The Cologne ring (G 848) cited in note 71 above, and the Benaki bronze pendant cited in note 112 above show the same "number."

[125] To judge from its inscriptions, the well-known Demetrius locket at Dumbarton Oaks held both a relic (of blood) and a *eulogia* (of *myron*). See Ross, *Catalogue* (1965), no. 160.

[126] See Deubner, *Kosmas und Damian*; and Kitzinger, "The Cult of Images," note 89.

[127] Rosenberg (*Geschichte der Goldschmiedekunst*, 51) had, without reference to the *miracula*, come to much the same conclusion. The Malcove Collection at the University of Toronto preserves a very unusual—and as yet unpublished—belt or harness fitting which, like this pendant locket, may have functioned as an "amuletic pill box." In place of the belt plate is a small rectangular box with a sliding lid bearing a large cross. The three sides of the box are inscribed with the same phrase as that appearing on the Yale doctor's case cited in note 1 above. Functioning as a belt, this box would perhaps have been found over that part of the body where its powers were thought most effective (cf. Bonner, *Magical Amulets*, 80). It is bronze and likely dates to the later sixth or seventh century. That its lid can be easily slid open suggests that a consummable *eulogia* and not a relic was preserved inside. This box is like a miniature version of those in wood which were used to hold medicine (cf. note 1 above).

[128] For those in the pilgrim trade, see Vikan, *Byzantine Pilgrimage*, 44 ff.

[129] The Cloisters Collection, 1974; 1974.150; reduced. See *Age of Spirituality*, no. 557 (M. Frazer). This votive is now attached to a chandelier, to which it does not belong.

[130] On this as an incense box, see J. Duffy and G. Vikan, "A Small Box in John Moschus," *GRBS*, 24:1 (1983), 97 f.

common and generic, while that on the lower arm, "Sts. Cosmas and Damian, grant [me] your blessing,"[131] is both less common, and more specific in its request. For what else can the "blessing" of these holy doctors be than the blessing of good health? And indeed, that this object was created with precisely that goal in mind is substantially confirmed by two peculiarities, one in its design and the other in its decoration. First, like only a few other Early Byzantine crosses, this one is supported by a hand, a striking conception which has been shown to derive from apotropaic votive hands of Jupiter Heliopolitanus and of Sabazios.[132] And second, St. Stephen is interjected in a position of prominence among an otherwise predictable pantheon of saints for the simple reason that he, like Zacharias, was traditionally associated with incense—and we have already seen how essential censing was to the ritual invocation of supernatural healing.[133]

CONCLUSIONS

A votive cross (fig. 28) and votive eyes (fig. 1) bracket this survey of "Art, Medicine, and Magic in Early Byzantium" both literally and conceptually; one invoked supernatural healing and one acknowledged it, and everything illustrated and discussed in between—*eulogiai* and amulets—palpably induced it. These are the objects which could satisfy our criterion of being, at one and the same time, "art" (albeit usually of a plebeian sort) and "medicine" (albeit always of an unscientific sort). As a group they evoke a world of supernatural medicine as pervasive as it was multifaceted: they span the Mediterranean, from Sicily through Greece and Asia Minor to Syria-Palestine and Egypt; they span society, from anonymous lead and bronze through silver to personalized gold.[134] And although fewer than two dozen pieces were illustrated, they can be taken to speak for a significant portion of early Byzantium's "minor arts," since many were items of mass production (from stamps or molds), while those that were not (e.g., the armbands, rings, and intaglios) represent extensive, substantially undifferentiated series. The significant point is that behind most of our illustrations stands a large, often well-known object type or genre. Moreover, those "object types" constitute, *in toto*, an affectively complete medicine chest, whose remedies were as varied in their mode of application as they were in their medical applicability: there are clays to be powdered and drunk or, as paste, rubbed on the body—and oils and waxes to be used in the same way; there are amuletic lockets and ampullae in which to carry these pills and potions, stamps with which to make them, and censers to swing while they're being used; there are large medico-magical silver bands for the arm, smaller ones for the finger, and single silver discs to be hung around the neck—or, for those of lesser means, bronze and lead equivalents; there are styptic gemstones for the purse and "health" jewelry for newlyweds; and there are, finally, votives to ask for the preservation of health, and votives to give thanks when lost health has been restored.

Harnessed in our hypothetical Early Byzantine medicine chest are the pharmaceutical powers of a truly democratic pantheon which, at once Judeo-Christian and Greco-Egyptian, can accommodate the coexistence of Christ and the Chnoubis, St. Symeon and King Solomon, and the cross and the *pentalpha*. When applied to consumable *eulogiai* their powers seem to have been essentially generic; Symeon clay, for example, could cure anything from baldness to leprosy. On the other hand, a surprising number of our amulets seem to have been designed to govern female ailments, and perhaps specifically infertility.[135] Yet these objects, too, pre-

[131] Or, "Sts. Cosmas and Damian, bless [me]."

[132] See M. C. Ross, "Byzantine Bronze Hands Holding Crosses," *Archaeology*, 17 (1964), 101 ff.; V. N. Zalesskaja, "Un monument byzantin à l'Ermitage et ces prototypes," (in Russian) *Palestinsky Sbornik*, 17(80) (1967), 84 ff. As with the Chnoubis, there is every reason to believe that this formal continuity carried with it a continuity of meaning and function. Yet even independent of its origins, this hand has qualities which corroborate its "medical" inscription, including an implication of power and prerogative (via the *globus cruciger*), of magic (note the two rings), and of healing (as in the "healing hand"—cf. Vikan, *Byzantine Pilgrimage*, 38 f.; and note 43, above). There is a formal, and perhaps contentual, parallelism between the hand that supports the cross and the (healing) hand that each of the two holy doctors raises toward the suppliant before the cross. There is an Early Byzantine bronze ring in the Clemens Collection, Cologne, which shows an open hand surrounded by *Sphragis Solomonos*. See E. Moses, *Der Schmuck der Sammlung W. Clemens* (Cologne, 1925), 10 f., fig. 17.

[133] Peter and Paul, of course, frequently accompany the cross, while the Virgin and Child and the holy doctors are called for by their respective invocations. I know of no other Early Byzantine appearance of St. Stephen on a cross (those incised, hinged crosses in bronze upon which Stephen appears with some regularity are mid-Byzantine or later). Stephen carries his censer as the protodeacon. It must be for this medico-liturgical reason also that St. Stephen appears in the company of holy doctors in the so-called Chapel of the Physicians in S. Maria Antiqua. See Nordhagen, "S. Maria Antiqua," 55 ff.

[134] For an archeologist's view of the pervasiveness of Early Byzantine magic, see Russell, "The Evil Eye," 543 f.

[135] A similar observation was made by L. Bouras in her paper on "Security in Byzantium" delivered at the 1983 Birmingham Spring Symposium.

cisely because they invoke a variety of healing powers, could probably be counted on to do much more.

The roots of early Byzantium's supernatural
medicine lie in the hellenized east Mediterranean,
in Syria-Palestine and Egypt, the same region which
saw its flowering during the sixth and seventh centuries. There the Chnoubis, apotropaic hands,
haematite, and ring signs all enjoyed (in their various stages of mutation) a Byzantine afterlife, but
only in the shadow of the pilgrim's experience, and
in the objects and images that were developed to
serve it. For it was holy sites and healing shrines—
and the curative powers thought to reside there—
which gave the artifacts of Early Byzantine med-
ico-magic their distinctive flavor. The Chnoubis,
after all, entered Byzantium's medicine chest in the
company of a pilgrimage-generated christological
cycle, and even the Jewish magician-doctor Solomon was on the pilgrim's agenda, for it was in the
Church of the Holy Sepulchre that his famous seal
ring was to be revered as a relic, beside the wood
of the True Cross.[136]

One final point is worthy of note. Our survey has
revealed a continuous spectrum in early Byzantium's world of miraculous healing, between rem-

edies and implements thoroughly Christian and
those patently magical. Why? Because while one's
local bishop, town doctor, and neighborhood sor-
ceress were almost certainly at odds over how best
to evict the demon that possessed one,[137] the possessed did not indulge in the luxury of subtle differentiations. If need be, he called upon Christ,
Solomon, and the Chnoubis in one breath; this is
the truth that our objects reveal with incontrovert-
ible clarity. They reveal a world thoroughly and
openly committed to supernatural healing, and one
wherein, for the sake of health, Christianity and
sorcery had been forced into open partnership.

Dumbarton Oaks

---

[136] See Wilkinson, *Jerusalem Pilgrims*, 59 (*Breviarius*).

[137] The antipathy that existed between doctors and healing
shrines is well known. See Magoulias, "The Lives of Saints," 129
ff. As for the attitude of doctors and churchmen to healing magic,
the following two examples may be cited from the sixth century:
Severus of Antioch, in his Homily CXX (PO, 29, 1, 583 f.), alludes to the practice of wearing medico-amuletic jewelry when
he urges Christians to avoid those who propose "the suspension
and attachment to necks or arms, or to other members [of those
objects] called *phylacteria*, or protective amulets, even if they have
an appearance of piety, for fear that, seeking the health of the
body, we might not become even more sick of the soul. . . ." On
the other hand, Alexander of Tralles (Puschmann, *Alexander*, II,
579) naively confesses that he finds himself obliged to recommend amulets for the treatment of colic, but only because some
patients will not follow a strict regimen or endure drugs.

PHYSICIANS AND ASCETICS IN JOHN OF EPHESUS: AN EXPEDIENT ALLIANCE*

SUSAN ASHBROOK HARVEY

It is commonly agreed that hagiography has much to tell us about Byzantine health, illness, and medicine.[1] The problem for historians lies in the task itself: that is, how to get at whatever it is that hagiography has to tell us. The present study is, I hope, a suggestion on ways of doing the task. Although a small contribution, perhaps the issues raised here will open larger possibilities.

John of Ephesus is a Syriac writer well known to historians of the sixth-century Byzantine Empire.[2] A native of Mesopotamia, John's varied career led him to travel widely in the empire of his day, as monk, missionary, bishop, and monophysite spokesman in the imperial court under both Justinian and Justin II. A writer whose zeal exceeds his elegance, John has left us two major works of serious importance for our understanding of the time in which he lived: his *Ecclesiastical History*, extending from Julius Caesar to the late 580s;[3] and his

hagiographical collection, the *Lives of the Eastern Saints*, fifty-eight short biographies of monks and nuns he himself knew, written in the late 560s.[4] By their very nature, histories and saints' Lives concern themselves with differing aspects of people, events, and experiences,[5] and John, too, perceives his task differently in each of these works. Cautious of the many pitfalls in handling hagiography as an historical source, scholars have turned to John's *Ecclesiastical History* far more quickly and far more often than to his *Lives* in their efforts to untangle the sixth-century empire.

But John's *Lives* have just as much to offer in this regard, particularly in the glimpses they provide us of the daily world in which John lived. Indeed, John's motivation as a writer of both molds is to portray faithfully the experiences of the crisis-ridden populace of his day, especially of the monophysites of the eastern empire. Persecuted by the Chalcedonian government, stricken with the hardships of war, bubonic plague, famine, and earthquakes, these people suffered repeated calamities throughout John's lifetime.[6] In his effort to be hon-

[The reader is referred to the list of abbreviations at the end of the volume.]

*I am indebted to Dr. Kenneth L. Caneva for his advice and help with sources.

[1] E.g., H. J. Magoulias, "The Lives of the Saints as Sources of Data for the History of Byzantine Medicine in the Sixth and Seventh Centuries," *BZ*, 57 (1964), 127–50; E. Patlagean, *Pauvreté économique et pauvreté sociale à Byzance 4e–7e siècles* (Paris/La Haye, 1977), 101–12.

[2] On John of Ephesus see the summary biography in E. Honigmann, *Évêques et évêchés Monophysites d'Asie antérieure au VIe siècle*, CSCO Subsidia 2 (Louvain, 1951), 207–15.

[3] John's *Ecclesiastical History* consists of three parts. Part I, covering from Julius Caesar to the death of Theodosius II has been lost, apart from a few fragments preserved in Michael the Syrian's *Chronicle*. Part II, continuing to 571, survives in fragments; some were collected in J. P. N. Land, *Anecdota Syriaca* (Leiden, 1868), II, 289–330, 385–92. Large sections are preserved in ps.-Dionysius of Tell-Mahre; these are gathered and annotated by F. Nau, "Etudes sur les parties inédites de la chronique ecclésiastique attribuée à Denys de Tellmahré," and "Analyse de la seconde partie inédite de l'Histoire Ecclésiastique de Jean d'Asie, Patriarche Jacobite de Constantinople," *ROChr*, 2 (1897), 41–68, 455–93. The best text for these fragments is now ed. I.-B.

Chabot, *Incerti Auctoris Chronicon Pseudo-Dionysianum vulgo dictum* II, CSCO 104/53 (Louvain, 1952). More fragments of Part II were edited by E. W. Brooks, *Accedunt Iohannis Ephesini Fragmenta*, also in CSCO 104/53, pp. 402–20. Part III survives almost intact; the best edition is edited and translated by E. W. Brooks, *Iohannis Ephesini Historiae Ecclesiasticae Pars Tertia*, CSCO 105/54 and 106/55 (Paris, 1935–36). On re-dating Part III so that John's death can be placed in 589, see P. Allen, "A New Date for the Last Recorded Events in John of Ephesus' *Historia Ecclesiastica*," *Orientalia Lovaniensia Periodica*, 10 (1979), 251–54.

[4] John of Ephesus, *Lives of the Eastern Saints*, ed. and trans. E. W. Brooks, PO 17–19 (Paris 1923–25).

[5] Cf., e.g., H. Delehaye, *The Legends of the Saints*, trans. D. Attwater (New York, 1962); E. Patlagean, "A Byzance: ancienne hagiographie et histoire sociale," *Annales: écon. soc. civ.*, 23 (1968), 106–26; P. Brown, "The Rise and Function of the Holy Man in Late Antiquity," *JRS*, 61 (1971), 80–101.

[6] For a survey of this situation see S. Ashbrook, "Asceticism in Adversity: An Early Byzantine Experience," *BMGS*, 6 (1980), 1–11.

est to their experiences, John writes his hagiographical collection—as much a celebration of holy presence in the midst of human suffering as it is an exhortation to hearten a battered people. The results of his efforts are sometimes surprising.

Tucked away in the *Lives of the Eastern Saints*, there is a brief but striking account of one of John's co-workers, the presbyter Aaron.[7] An Armenian by birth, and an ascetic since his youth, Aaron had long excelled both physically and spiritually in the taxing labors of his chosen vocation. John of Ephesus lived and worked with Aaron for thirty years, sometimes in the exile suffered by the eastern monastic community, but mostly working together in the monophysite settlements and refugee camps of Constantinople. Aaron distinguished himself by the severity of his ascetic practices, and also by the vigor with which he performed the menial tasks of the monasteries where he lived and the care he exerted for those in need. Admirable, then, on these two accounts—private and public labors for God— Aaron fulfilled the ascetic model dearest to John's own heart.[8] However, the remarkable point of Aaron's story lies not in what John tells us he did, but in what John tells us Aaron survived. Here is John's account:

> Once [Aaron] fell under a serious disease of gangrene in his loins; and he bore this affliction with great discretion, until his loin was eaten up and mutilated and had vanished down to its root, and his disease began to enter his inner organs. But seeing that he was afflicted by a harsh malady and was cruelly rent in private, we besought him to tell what his illness was. But he for his part, until his wound had worsened severely, held fast—constant in prayer and filling his mouth with praise and thanksgiving to God. Finally, when he could no longer pass water he was forced and so persuaded to reveal and make known his disease. Then the whole of his loin was found eaten away and consumed, so that the physicians contrived to make a tube of lead (*'abūbtā' d'abārā'*) and placed it for the passing of his water, while also applying bandages and drugs to him. And so the ulcer was healed. Furthermore, Aaron lived eighteen years after the crisis of this test, praising God, and having that lead tube in place for the necessity of passing water.[9]

A compelling tale, indeed! But if one's heart goes out to Aaron for what he endured, one's mind sa-

lutes the ingenuity and skill of the physicians involved. These, to be sure, displayed their art at its best—something we see all too rarely in our ancient sources.[10] Their efforts were in keeping with the fullest medical knowledge of their times, a factor not to be divorced, surely, from the setting of the incident in Constantinople. Gangrene was a common, and commonly horrifying, problem;[11] and not least amongst ascetics, whose lifestyles often invited the danger.[12] The technique of surgically removing only the dead tissue was well known.[13] The problem in Aaron's case would be the healing of an area so widely ulcerated: gangrene in the genitals was the most serious of this type of infection.[14] Indeed, it is this accomplishment in Aaron's situation that is most impressive. The surgical procedures involved were within the competence of the time: the excision of the diseased flesh, as noted, and the use of tubing for the removal of bodily waste, a technique employed in relieving the buildup of pus or other fluids in various parts of the body,[15] but also practised in cases of complete castration— a circumstance perhaps more relevant.[16] Aaron's emasculation by disease presented its gravest challenge by the extent of infection involved.[17] That he lived not only to tell the tale, but to tell it for eighteen more years is high tribute to the work of these doctors.

But the most striking element of Aaron's experience is not the illness or its cure, although we gain here more data for substantiating the state of medical skill in the early Byzantine Empire. It is not the content of this passage, but its context that is so surprising. For John's manner of telling the incident is markedly discordant with hagiographical style and form. This holy man, as John tells the

[7] Jo. Eph., *Lives*, 38 (PO 18, pp. 641–45).

[8] Cf. S. Ashbrook Harvey, "The Politicisation of the Byzantine Saint," *The Byzantine Saint*, ed. S. Hackel, Studies Supplementary to Sobornost 5 (1981), 37–43; and *idem, Asceticism and Society in the Sixth Century Byzantine East* (forthcoming).

[9] Jo. Eph., *Lives*, 38 (PO 18, pp. 643–44); my translation.

[10] See Magoulias, "Lives of the Saints"; cf. G. Majno. *The Healing Hand: Man and Wound in the Ancient World* (Cambridge, Mass., 1975), 395–422 on Galen and his legacy.

[11] Majno, *op. cit.*, 4–6.

[12] Patlagean, *Pauvreté*, 106.

[13] Majno, *op. cit.*, 191–92; L. H. Toledo-Pereya, "Galen's Contribution to Surgery," *JHM*, 28 (1973), 357–75, esp. at 366–67; L. J. Bliquez, "The Tools of Asclepius: The Surgical Gear of the Greeks and Romans," *Veterinary Surgery*, 2.iv (Oct.–Dec. 1982), 150–57, esp. at 155.

[14] D. Brothwell and A. T. Sandison, *Diseases in Antiquity: A Survey of Diseases, Injuries and Surgery of Early Populations* (Springfield, Ill., 1967), 241, 515.

[15] Majno, *op. cit*, 156–58; cf. Toledo-Pereya, *art. cit.*, 371–74, and L. J. Bliquez, *art. cit.*, 156–57.

[16] Majno, *op. cit.*, 253–54; Brothwell and Sandison, *op. cit.*, 514–15; and cf. N. M. Penzer, *The Harem* (Philadelphia, 1937), 140–44.

[17] Majno, *op. cit.*, 183–88; 417–20.

story, suffers a fully human illness and a fully human cure. Physicians are summoned, rather than saints living (e.g., a priest-physician) or saints dead (as the miracle healers Cosmas and Damian); and the physicians are effective not because of divine intervention, of which John makes no mention, but because of their own expertise. Moreover, the story is told without allegorical or moralizing embellishment. It is altogether a most curious account to be found in hagiography.

To see the peculiarities of John's method, we need only compare Aaron's story with parallel passages in other hagiographical collections of the same genre—Palladius' *Lausiac History*, Theodoret of Cyrrhus' *Historia Religiosa*, and John Moschus' *Pratum Spirituale*.[18] The contrasts are at once clear, and on various levels.

It is apparent that Aaron himself did not share John's attitude toward his illness. John tells us that Aaron accepted the infection without acknowledging its presence to others; despite his suffering, Aaron was "constant in prayer, filling his mouth with praise and thanksgiving for God." Although John was aware that Aaron was ill, he was unable to extract any information on Aaron's condition for a long time, until the disease had progressed to a critical state.

Aaron's attitude was common amongst ascetics of late antiquity. The care of others was a significant part of the ascetic's career, particularly care for the sick. In hospitals as trained physicians,[19] in hospices as lay nurses,[20] and above all in their own sanctuaries as miracle workers,[21] the holy men and

women of late antiquity reenacted Christ's ministry to the afflicted with various efficacious skills.[22] Some ministered with medical training from the Christianized Galenic teaching, some by the folk wisdom of herbal lore, some by common sense and cooperative arrangement with hospital establishments. But in each case the treatment was given with the added aura for all concerned of healing by holy hands.[23] However, the ascetic's care for the illnesses of others was precisely that; rarely would holy men or women, however sick, allow themselves medical treatment.

Nor was the attitude surprising. To the ascetic, illness was simply one more form of suffering to endure in the imitation of Christ.[24] Indeed, illness worked for the ascetic as another means of bodily discipline, not unlike the severe physical exertion of ascetic exercises. Palladius had once chastised Dorotheus for his harsh treatment of his body—to which the Egyptian anchorite had flatly replied, "[My body] kills me, I will kill it."[25] But when Palladius found the hermit Benjamin gravely ill with excessive swelling, he found exactly the same attitude: "Pray, my children, that the inner man may not contract dropsy; for this body did not help me when it was well, nor has it caused me harm when faring badly."[26] Indeed, Benjamin continued healing others while his own condition worsened, until he died eight months later. John Moschus records a similar view. The Palestinian anchorite Barnabas, refusing treatment for an infected foot, declared, "As much as a man suffers outside, so much does he bloom within."[27]

The ascetic's suffering of illness was a means both of discipline by endurance and of carrying out the literal symbolism characteristic of early Christian asceticism: to suffer an illness without treatment while carrying on with one's daily activities was to deny the physical for the spiritual, to declare one's commitment to the divine by divorcing oneself from the temporal realm. It was a virtual requirement on the part of the ascetic, even as the heal-

---

[18] Palladius, *Historia Lausiaca*, ed. and trans. C. Butler, *The Lausiac History of Palladius* (Cambridge, 1898–1904) 2 Vols.; English trans. by R. T. Meyer, Ancient Christian Writers 34 (London, 1965). Theodoret of Cyrrhus, *Historia Religiosa*, ed. and tr. P. Canivet and A. Leroy-Molinghen, *Théodoret de Cyr, Histoire des moines de Syrie*, SC 234 and 257 (Paris 1977–79). John Moschus, *Pratum Spirituale*, ed. J.-P. Migne, PG 87, iii, cols. 2851–3112; trans. M.-J. Rouët de Journel, *Jean Moschus, Le Pré Spirituel*, SC (Paris, 1946).

[19] Cf. D. J. Constantelos, *Byzantine Philanthropy and Social Welfare* (Rutgers, 1968), 152–84 for the general setting. The first notable effort of this kind was the welfare complex established by Basil of Caesarea in the 370s, consisting of a poor house, hostel, and hospital noted especially for its treatment of leprosy. The complex also served as headquarters for the distribution of wealth and possessions bequeathed to the church for use among the needy. Gregory of Nazianzus, *Or.* XLIII, 63 (where he describes the complex as a "new city"); Basil of Caesarea, *Ep.* 94, and 142–154; Sozomen, *HE*, VI, 34.

[20] Majno, *The Healing Hand*, 393–94; Constantelos, *op. cit.*, 185 ff. Cf. John of Ephesus, *Lives*, 12, 33, 45, 46.

[21] E.g., Magoulias, "Lives of the Saints"; and cf. Theodoret, *HR*, 6, 9, 11, 13, 16, 21, 26; Jo. Eph., *Lives*, 2, 3, 4, 6, 26, 35; John Moschus, *Pratum*, 28, 56, 206.

[22] H. E. Sigerist, *Civilization and Disease* (New York, 1944), 69 ff.

[23] *Ibid.*, 131–47; D. J. Constantelos, "Physician-Priests in the Medieval Greek Church," *Greek Orthodox Theological Review*, 12 (1966–67), 141–53.

[24] Sigerist, *op. cit.*, 69 ff.

[25] Palladius, *HL*, 2 (trans. Meyer, 33); cf. the awesome Macarius of Alexandria, Pall., *HL*, 18.

[26] Pall., *HL*, 12 (trans. Meyer, 48); cf. John Moschus, *Pratum*, 8.

[27] Jo. Mos., *Pratum*, 10 (my trans.).

ing of the lay populace was itself a requirement.

Such a perspective on sickness allowed the perception of ascetic suffering a further development as a source of literary imagery. The metaphorical dimensions of illness provided the hagiographer a wealth of parallels with which to play off the spiritual and physical health of the ascetic. Soul and body mirrored one another, but, as noted in the passages just cited, they did so in reverse: bodily health indicated sickness of soul, bodily disease spiritual well-being, in a direct quantitative relation—the more of one, the greater the other.[28] It was but a short step from this relationship to its moralistic counterpart.

The body represented the soul's demise, because it tempted the ascetic with desire. The early Church's ambiguous and indecisive stance regarding castration in pursuit of Christian perfection indicates the uncertainty that prevailed as to what physical longing was about. If desire was the symbol of evil, and of the evil of the material world as a whole, then castration was to be valued as a means of severing oneself altogether from a life of sin—a view most comfortable in gnostic circles. But if sin is the result of human weakness rather than the product of an evil creation, then celibacy rather than castration proves the higher virtue: Adam's sin was an act of will, and so to be corrected by such. The mitigating moderation of the latter, orthodox view did not, however, override the tenacity with which popular Christianity clung to dualistic ideas.[29] The dilemma about castration survives hagiographically for centuries, long after the practice itself was condemned by the mainstream church.

At its most allegorical level, castration in hagiography happens "spiritually"—that is, in a vision. So Palladius and John Moschus speak of instances where holy men who are counsellors to women are unable to bear the temptation they suffer. In both cases their "cure" is worked in a dream, and heals them as completely as if it were physical.[30] But the mysticism of these incidents is played out more luridly by both writers through the metaphor of bodily illness as a sign of spiritual health. Both tell of holy men unable to withstand the temptation of desire, who seek relief in sexual promiscuity. In Palladius' story of Heron, this sinful ascetic suffers a severe ulceration that causes the loss of his genitals, and so brings salvation to the monk ("unwillingly," we are told), who returns to the ascetic life thus cleansed.[31] Moschus' account, similarly, describes how the fallen monk in question was covered by leprosy as soon as he entered a brothel, and thence returned to his monastery praising God for sending illness to his body in order to save his soul.[32] The stories in fact are thematic to hagiography.[33]

In these instances, disease represents a thinly disguised metaphor for sin; if the disease of the soul can be transferred to the body, itself the source of sin, salvation is possible. Further, the condition of sin is reduced, as so often in early Christian literature, to the question of sexuality. And if the mainstream Church would not allow the radical cure of castration, then the Divine Physician himself would accomplish it through disease. The conflation of body, sexuality, and sin is inextricably worked into the mind-set of late antiquity, despite the protests of theologians (like John Chrysostom) to the contrary.[34] Against such a backdrop, John of Ephesus' story about Aaron stands out starkly on two accounts: first, because although emasculation by disease becomes a *topos* in hagiography to escape its otherwise heretical connotations, John presents us with its occurrence in real rather than thematic terms. The illness happens, but no hint of allegorical overtone is read into the event; Aaron's ascetic career hides no skeletons in its closet. Secondly, John's concern is that Aaron's sickness be healed. He does not follow the pattern of using illness of the body to heal the illness of the soul.

Where Palladius and John Moschus present ill-

---

[28] As an example, consider the impassioned speech by John the Nazarite in Jo. Eph., *Lives*, 3 (PO 17, at pp. 51–53).

[29] Cf. E. Patlagean, "L'Histoire de la femme déguisée en moine et l'évolution de la sainteté féminine à Byzance," *StM*, 17 (1976), 597–623, at pp. 610–11; Penzer, *The Harem*, 135–40. Cyril of Skythopolis noted the general alarm about the presence of eunuchs in Palestinian monasteries: *Vita Euth.*, 16, 31; *Vita Saba*, 7, 29, 69; *Vita Kyr.*, 4. Compare the similar attitude in Egypt, as discussed in D. Chitty, *The Desert a City* (Oxford, 1966; repr. London, 1977), 66–67; and in the Syrian Orient in A. Vööbus, *History of Asceticism in the Syrian Orient* II, CSCO 197/Sub. 17 (Louvain, 1958), 257. On the body as the source of sin, see in general J. Bugge, *Virginitas: An Essay in the History of a Medieval Ideal* (The Hague, 1975).

[30] Pall., *HL*, 29; Jo. Mos., *Pratum*, 3.

[31] Pall., *HL*, 26.

[32] Jo. Mos., *Pratum*, 14.

[33] Patlagean, *Pauvreté*, 106.

[34] E.g., Bugge, *op. cit.*; but especially Patlagean, *Pauvreté*, 113–55; *idem*, "La femme déguisée"; *idem*, "Sur la limitation de la fécondité dans la haute époque byzantine," *Annales: écon. soc. civ.*, 24 (1969), 1353–69 (= "Birth Control in the Early Byzantine Empire," in *Biology of Man in History*, ed. R. Forster and O. Ranum [Baltimore, 1975], 1–22). Cf. W. D. Hand, "Deformity, Disease, and Physical Ailment as Divine Retribution," *Festschrift Mattias Zender: Studien Volkskultur, Sprache und Landesgeschichte*, ed. E. Ennen and G. Wiegelmann (Bonn, 1975) I, 519–25.

ness in an ascetic as a means of spiritual and moral testing, Theodoret of Cyrrhus views it more as an instrument of spiritual instruction.[35] In the cases of the paramount holy men Julian Saba and Symeon the Stylite, Theodoret tells us they suffered serious illness or infection so that people would realize they, too, were human. Disease was proof that these living martyrs of the flesh were not spiritual beings in the form of men, and thus not to be worshipped as such.[36]

But if Theodoret gives the sense that illness in the ascetic serves an admonitory purpose for the public, he implies, too, that illness serves the ascetic in similar manner—to warn the holy man or woman against hubris, excessive spiritual pride. For Theodoret there is divine purpose in illness, not in the sense of moral chastisement for the body's sinful nature, but for the use or necessity of deepening our awareness of the relation between the human and the divine. Theodoret perceives these realms as separated by an insurmountable gulf, crossed only by the will of divine grace. Illness in an ascetic provides a framework in which the mystery of that grace is witnessed. Theodoret's personal involvement in what he describes underscores his point. As bishop of Cyrrhus, he assumes responsibility for the ascetics of his region—not in the sense of spiritual mentor, but as a kind of attendant overseer, keeping watch that all is well and looking out for problems. In this capacity, Theodoret wields his ecclesiastical authority out of duty, while viewing the ascetics themselves as persons of holy vocation whose spiritual authority exceeds his own. Illness is a place where the interconnection of grace, authority, and spirituality is found. In the case of infection, ill health, or sickness, Theodoret will intervene with an ascetic's practice, at least to the extent that the holy one allows some acquiescence to the affliction: nursing by Theodoret himself, or a lightening of ascetic exercises for the duration of the problem.[37]

But Theodoret's concern that the ascetic should not suffer sickness and the dangers of infection—matters beyond the ascetic's capacity for regulation—is not the end of these stories. Having described the illness, the ascetic's suffering, and his

own compassionate involvement, he bears witness that these holy ones effect their own cures miraculously. The human lesson having been learned, and appropriate humility summoned, the divine is suddenly manifest in the ascetic's healing, wrought by prayer and the sign of the cross. The very locus which reveals human weakness becomes the place where God's grace is displayed: the ascetic's body is the point where human and divine intersect. The metaphorical parallel to the mystery of the incarnation is not far off.

Here again, in the fundamental understanding of illness, the contrasts between John of Ephesus and Theodoret are greater than the similarities. Like Theodoret, John is an ecclesiastical leader whose duties involve overseeing the general welfare of ascetics. Throughout his career, John felt compelled to intercede with an ascetic's practice if issues of physical health were involved. He invariably appears as the voice of moderation when confronting the harshness of the Syrian ascetic's traditional activities.[38] Nonetheless, John's narrations of such episodes are once again devoid of didactic undertones, even of the kind Theodoret interjects. So, for example, John describes his alarm at the occurrence of sickness in ascetics, and particularly of untended sores.[39] Festering ulcerations of the skin were common amongst holy men and women, the product of their obsessive lack of hygiene, made worse by the indifference to personal attention that characterized the ascetic lifestyle.

John's descriptions of these episodes are uneasy. The ascetic's suffering and endurance are duly acknowledged, but when John or others sharing his views are ineffectual in urging that proper care be taken, his frustration, too, is apparent. The message in these accounts holds no moral or spiritual allegory; John draws no divine purpose into his telling of these occasions. Instead, his attention in each case is focused on how the illness or infection affects the ascetic's work. His concerns are pragmatic. He offers no packaging here of divine control, or purpose to the situation; these are problems to be dealt with commonsensically. The ascetics carry on, with or without attending to their infirmities; no miracles are wrought to wipe away their discomfort or sickness. If, as in the case of Aaron, the situation becomes critical, John's practicality is rapidly employed: medically knowledgeable and

[35] Cf. A. Adnes and P. Canivet, "Guérisons miraculeuses et exorcismes dans l'Histoire Philothée de Théodoret de Cyr," *RHR*, 171 (1967), 53–82, 149–79.
[36] Theo., *HR*, 2, 26.
[37] Esp. *HR*, 21, 22, 24; cf. 26.

[38] Jo. Eph., *Lives, passim.*
[39] E.g., *Lives*, 12, 13, 21, 27.

skilled practitioners are summoned. If there is any moral to John's depiction of illness for the ascetic, it is in his reminder that the commandment charges us to love not only our neighbour, but ourselves also.[40] His story of Aaron, then, is consistent with the attitude towards illness and its requirements that John displays throughout the *Lives of the Eastern Saints.*

But what is this attitude? If the story as it stands were a part of John's *Ecclesiastical History*, there would be nothing surprising (though perhaps something heartening) in his account. But as we have seen, when comparable situations are found in hagiography similar to John's, literary protocol reigns supreme. If the healing is described at all; if, indeed, the healing is allowed, it happens by the holy hands of a saint, in person or in a vision, and in all events miraculously. Further, description of this type of gangrene and its consequent effects on the body's organs ought to be portrayed with the symbolic admonishment implied. John tells Aaron's story with no such adornment and without stylization, and he tells it in his *Lives of the Eastern Saints* rather than elsewhere.

In looking at parallel accounts, we have gained some sense of the understanding of illness for various hagiographers. It is clear that the use of hagiography for the study of medicine must depend upon ascertaining the hagiographer's own perception of illness and health in terms of the individual's spiritual well-being. But our comparisons have shown up no ulterior religious design to John of Ephesus' portrayal of disease and its appropriate treatment. What, then, does this curious paradox of content and context tell us about John?

We must return to John himself. John was a monophysite, at the very time when the dispute over Chalcedonian orthodoxy was splitting into a framework of two distinct and independent churches, each viewing the other as heretical.[41] Himself from Mesopotamia, John writes in the *Lives* primarily of his compatriots from the predominantly monophysite eastern provinces, though often, as in Aaron's case, persecutions have forced these people into exile elsewhere. John's "saints" are for the most part otherwise unknown to us. He writes about ascetics whose works have been of special meaning for their communities; celebrities

of the day are only occasionally included. John's selection is instructive. His people suffered relentlessly ongoing tragedy during the sixth century: violent if sporadic persecutions, war against Persia, chronic famine and blight, the Great Bubonic Plague and its lingering aftermath. The "saints" John commemorates are not solitaries in the wilderness, separated from this suffering world. They are those who worked their ministry and service within it, manifesting the grace of holy presence in the midst of continual calamity.

It was not a world that encouraged an unrealistic attitude, especially amongst the monophysites.[42] Survival both physical and spiritual was of critical import. Although their language and thought relies heavily on the miraculous,[43] these people have not seen much of miracles in the glorious sense. Nor, although they see a great deal of divine wrath in the events of their times,[44] do they see much clear correlation between sin and divine retribution. The suffering of the monophysites, those of the true faith, evoked instead the re-charged imagery of the martyr's crown. Nonetheless, as John's *Lives* proclaim, these people have seen something of the holy, and they have seen it amongst themselves, through the work of the ascetics John glorifies.

For John is truly a monophysite.[45] He understands no division between the human and divine realms: the unity of Christ human and divine meant a unity of God's presence and action in His created world. Ever pragmatic, John has his own understanding of what that means, as Aaron's story shows. Indeed, the key to Aaron's story lies in the result of the action taken: Aaron lived *and worked* another eighteen years after "the crisis of this test." Aaron's work is the real issue. Aaron is a holy man: he is how the divine is present in the midst of such unholy times. Throughout the *Lives of the Eastern Saints,* John shows little interest in supernatural miracles, little concern for didactic moralizing (either on his own part or on that of his subjects), and little time for sugarcoated portraits. There is much that needs

---

[40] E.g., *Lives*, 11, 12, 13, 21, 36.

[41] Honigmann, *Évêques et évêchés*; W. A. Wigram, *The Separation of the Monophysites* (London, 1923; repr. New York, 1978).

[42] The *Plerophories* of John Rufus were written in 512, at the height of monophysite ascendency; they reflect that optimism. John Rufus, *Plérophories, témoignages et révélations contre le Concile de Chalcédoine*, ed. and tr. F. Nau, PO 8 (1912), 5–208.

[43] Cf. N. Baynes, "The Thought-World of the East Roman Empire," *Byzantine Studies and Other Essays* (London, 1955), 24–47.

[44] Cf. A. A. Vasiliev, "Medieval Ideas of the End of the World: East and West," *Byzantion*, 16 (1944), 462–502.

[45] See esp. J. Lebon, *Le Monophysisme Sévérien* (Louvain, 1909); and Wigram, *op. cit.*

doing, and those who can do God's work are preciously vital. For Aaron, as for others, John shows a thorough expediency: there is no time, in the midst of such hardship, for anything less honest. John's alliance with doctors is born of necessity—as he would be the first to admit. And so it happens that there is one hagiographer who reveals to us not simply the thought-world of his time, but something of its reality as well.

University of Rochester

BYZANTINE COMMENTARIES ON DIOSCORIDES

John M. Riddle

In the mid-first century, Dioscorides had written "And some have recorded that if someone were to bury rams' horns broken into small pieces, asparagus grows,"[1] but a Byzantine scribe, living no later than the fourteenth century, simply could not accept this assertion. Reacting strongly, he wrote, "it seems incredible to me" (ἐμοὶ δὲ ἀπίθανον).[2] Thereafter the texts of at least ten Dioscorides Greek manuscripts incorporated the phrase into the chapter on this common vegetable.[3] This added comment must have appeared strange to later readers, confronted by "Dioscorides" expressing skepticism about what he had just written, and doing so in the first person.

Having interrupted Dioscorides with his own doubt, the scholiast decided to add new material to Dioscorides' pharmaceutical descriptions of asparagus. Dioscorides had set down the following about the plant:

[The reader is referred to the list of abbreviations at the end of the volume.]

Growing in rocky soil, asparagus or "spiky-mushroom,"[4] which some term a sage,[5] has a stalk which boiled and eaten softens the bowels and is also a diuretic. When drunk, the decoction of its roots is helpful for those having difficulty micturating, and for those afflicted by jaundice or sciatica; when decocted with wine, the roots are helpful for those bitten by a poisonous spider (φαλάγγιον),[6] and those suffering from toothache are benefited when the decoction is applied to the painful tooth. Also asparagus seeds made into a drink provide the same effects [as the root decoction]. And also they say that dogs die after they have drunk the decoction of asparagus.[7] And some have recorded that if someone were to bury rams' horns broken into small pieces, asparagus grows.[8]

The commentator added, "it seems incredible to me," even though the tenth-century Byzantine compilation of agricultural lore, the *Geoponica*, had honored the same tradition as follows:

If one wants to produce an abundance of asparagus, chop up (κόψας) wild rams' horns into small pieces, throw them onto the [asparagus] beds, and water. Some say even more incredibly (παραδοξότερον) that if whole rams' horns are bored and laid down, they will bear asparagus.[9]

---

[1] Dioscorides II, 125 (ed. Wellmann, Vol. I, p. 198).

[2] *Ibid.*, *apparatus criticus* to line 2.

[3] I have noted the commentary in the following manuscripts (an asterisk indicates the manuscripts used by Wellmann): Leiden, Bibl. Univ., MS Voss Gr. F. 58, 14th cent.; *Vatican, MS Palatinus gr. 77, 14th cent.; Paris, B.N., MS gr. 2182, anno 1481; *Paris, B.N., MS gr. 2183, 15th cent.; Salamanca, Bibl. univ. MS 2659 (formerly *Madrid, MS palat. Reg. 44), 15th cent.; *Venice, San Marco, MS Gr. Z 271, 15th cent.; Venice, San Marco, MS Gr. Z. 272, 15th cent.—Michael Apostoles, scribe; Venice, San Marco, MS Gr. Z. 597, 15th cent.; El Escorial, MS T–II–12, 16th cent. Generally throughout I shall not give foliation. While I have seen all these manuscripts, I normally follow Wellmann's critical apparatus and list the manuscripts which have the commentary and were not included by Wellmann. My expanded list includes those I studied and in which I observed the particular scholium; therefore, the actual number of texts with the scholium under discussion will probably be larger than what is recorded in this article. Still, the number of manuscripts will be greater than known by Wellmann.

[4] This translation of μυάκανθος is offered as an approximation of what appears to be the meaning suggested by Dioscorides' sources. The literal roots of the term suggest both a "mouse" and a "mushroom." R. Strömberg, *Griechische Pflanzennamen* (Göteborg, 1940), 28; Alexander of Tralles IX, 1 (ed. Puschmann, Vol. II, p. 395), and Dioscorides III, 151, and IV, 143.2 (ed. Wellmann, Vol. II, pp. 159 and 287), show that this name (μυάκανθος) was given to the shoots of butcher's broom (*Ruscus aculeatus* L.), which explains why Dioscorides would say some call it a "sage"—even though ὅρμινον is definitely another plant.

[5] Ὅρμινον is probably red-topped sage (*Salvia horminum* L.), considered separately by Dioscorides (III, 129). The plant certainly does not resemble asparagus.

[6] For a discussion of the identities of this venomous spider, see Scarborough, "Nicander II," 7–14.

[7] According to Pliny, *Natural History* XX, 43.111, the assertion that asparagus will kill dogs was made by Chrysippus (4th cent. B.C.). See *RE*, Vol. III, pt. 2 (Stuttgart, 1899), cols. 2509–10.

[8] Dioscorides II, 125 (ed. Wellmann, Vol. I, pp. 197–98).

[9] *Geoponica* XII, 18.2–3 (ed. Beckh, p. 365).

It is quite probable that the Byzantine scholiast was well aware of this venerable "rams' horns" custom for cultivators of asparagus—quite similar to modern gardeners in their adding bone meal to certain vegetable plots—but the commentator has chosen to supplement Dioscorides with a botanical morphology very much in keeping with the pattern of description laid down by Theophrastus,[10] and then to add further pharmacological details about asparagus:

> Be that as it may (μέντοι), this asparagus shrub is multibranched, has many leaves, and is large, and is similar to fennel.[11] The roots are rounded off, are large, and have a knob, and their stalks, made soft with white wine, abate phrenitis.[12] Taken either boiled or baked, they slake strangury, difficulty in micturation, and dysentery. Boiled down in vinegar or wine, the roots alleviate sprains; taken boiled with figs and chickpea,[13] they cure jaundice and alleviate sciatica and strangury. Hung as an amulet and drunk as a decoction, the root causes barrenness (ἀτοκία) and sterility (ἄγονος).[14]

The Byzantine commentator has added a botanical description, frequently omitted by Dioscorides, especially for common plants. Unlike the scribe's classical model Theophrastus, Dioscorides normally provided topical habitats, information probably helpful for finding it in the wild. The commentator properly terms asparagus a "shrub" because it grows to a height of one and one-half meters. He says that it is multibranched, and calls the leaves "large," somewhat inaccurate by modern botanical morphology: technically, according to modern botany, asparagus has no leaves, simply modified branchlets which serve that morphological function. The scribe, however, likens asparagus leaves to fennel leaves. The modern botanist would state that fennel (*Foeniculum vulgare* Miller) has true

leaves, much divided and feathery, but the casual observer could easily compare fennel leaves with those of asparagus.

The commentator's purpose in supplementing Dioscorides' text was therapeutic, not botanical, and one may assume that he was attempting to explicate the medical and pharmacological properties of asparagus, as contrasted to their fusion with farm lore, seen both in Dioscorides and the abridgment of Didymus in the *Geoponica*. The scholiast adds medicinal employment for phrenitis, dysentery, and sprains, and the use of asparagus as an antifertility agent. There is repetition: he repeats Dioscorides and he repeats himself. Dioscorides had said that the root was good for those with difficulty in micturation, and the Byzantine commentator repeats this twice and adds the affliction called strangury, a painful and interrupted urination in drops, produced by spasmodic muscular contraction of the ureter and bladder. Asparagus remains a strongly recommended diuretic in folkmedicine.[15] Dioscorides had prescribed a boiling of the root, and the scholiast has added "or baking." Lest one conclude too quickly from the skepticism about ram's horn growing into asparagus that the Byzantine scribe was more "rational" than Dioscorides, one should note his statement of asparagus' use as an amulet: the scholiast has included the amuletic asparagus without Dioscorides' manner of disclaiming folklore with such phrases as "they say" and "it is reported."

The final aspect of the scribe's additions is the use of asparagus as an antifertility agent. Curiously, a Hippocratic work suggests that asparagus seeds are to be used in a pessary to promote conception, not contraception.[16] In 1952, Russian investigators reported that a decoction of asparagus (*A. acutifolius officinalis*) was used in folkmedicine for its contraceptive effect.[17] While asparagus has asparagin, an amino acid, its use for the regulation of fertility cannot be verified.[18] In 1975, however, the *Journal of Pharmaceutical Sciences* published an article which suggested asparagus as a future can-

---

[10] Schol. Dioscorides II, 125 (ed. Wellmann, Vol. I, p. 198: *app. crit.* to line 2, lines 1–2). Cf. Theophrastus, *HP* I, 3.1.

[11] *Foeniculum vulgare* Miller. Cf. Theophrastus, *HP* I, 11.2.

[12] φρενῖτις. LSJ, *s.v.* wrongly defines this as "inflammation of the brain," whereas the cited texts show an inflammation of the diaphragm. Berendes, in translating Dioscorides (p. 222), included the commentary as part of Dioscorides' text, and interpreted the meaning as an affliction of the bladder or spleen. A long discussion of phrenitis is given by Caelius Aurelianus, *On Acute Diseases* Bk. I (ed. and trans. Drabkin), who certainly included febrile delirium and several psychotic states within the meaning of phrenitis. One of the better discussions on the φρένες among the Greeks is R. B. Onians, *The Origins of European Thought* (Cambridge, 1951), esp. 13–15, 23–28, 29–32, 37–40, and 116–17.

[13] *Cicer arietinum* L.

[14] Schol. Dioscorides II, 125 (ed. Wellmann, Vol. I, p. 198: *app. crit.* to line 2, lines 1–8).

[15] W. Schneider, *Lexikon zur Arzneimittelgeschichte* (Frankfurt, 1974; 7 vols.), Vol. V, pt. 1, 147–49.

[16] The Hippocratic *Diseases of Women* I, 75 (ed. Littré, Vol. VIII, p. 166). Cf. J. H. Dierbach, *Die Arzneimittel des Hippokrates* (Heidelberg, 1824; rptd. Hildesheim, 1969), 20.

[17] V. J. Brondegaard, "Contraceptive Plant Drugs," *Planta Medica*, 23, 2 (1973), 169.

[18] P. G. Stecher, *et al.*, eds., *The Merck Index*, 8th ed. (Rahway, New Jersey, 1968), 106–7; J. E. Driver and G. E. Trease, *The Chemistry of Crude Drugs* (London, 1928), 8.

didate for the testing of antifertility agents in natural products.[19] Aside from the possible effectiveness of asparagus as a contraceptive, it is important to note that the Byzantine commentator has recorded data otherwise unknown to us, either from earlier authorities now lost, or as testimony of contemporary late Byzantine medical pharmacognosy.

Commentaries and scholia on Dioscorides are rather common in the manuscript traditions. The famous alphabetical Greek codex of c. A.D. 512, the so-called Anicia Juliana, contains numerous scholia and commentaries, but the Anicia Juliana is excluded from consideration in this study because there exists a good scholarly literature on the commentaries to the Vienna codex.[20] The concentration in this study is on later manuscripts, since many preserve Dioscorides' original (non-alphabetical) order and have fewer alterations than found in the Anicia Juliana and the later Greek texts which descend from it. Wellmann, in the critical apparatus to his edition of the Greek text of Dioscorides' *Materia medica*, faithfully recorded most of the scholia and commentaries in the manuscripts he employed to establish his text, but Wellmann used less than half of the Greek manuscripts of Dioscorides now known to be extant. For example, the earliest manuscript employed by Wellmann for the asparagus scholium is Vatican Palatinus MS graec. 77 (fourteenth century). One other manuscript is at least as early as the Palatine, and it was not known to Wellmann: the marvellously illustrated manuscript at Padua's seminary library (MS 194).[21] The scribe or scribes of the Padua manuscript use the text and iconographical tradition of the Anicia Juliana, but when the plants beginning with the letter *Omega* are reached, the scribes show awareness of another Dioscorides text with its own set of illuminations. Thus, the scribes start over with *Alpha* and go again through *Omega*. In this second text, the copyists include plants omitted in the initial manu-

script, and the second text contains substantially different readings in many instances. It is in the second copying that the scribes of the Paduan manuscript include the additional material on asparagus, significantly by using a Greek text far less corrupted than that represented by the Anicia Juliana and its descendants. Since the Paduan manuscript did not employ the non-illustrated Palatine text, it is clear that both of these fourteenth-century manuscripts had a common source for the scholia on asparagus.

Wellmann's stemma stands in need of revision, but until this arduous task is performed, one may make general assumptions concerning the commentaries and scholia to Dioscorides by observing when they appear in the manuscripts. Since there are a variety of styles, forms, and quality of comments in the scholia, and since the commentaries are in various combinations of manuscript families, one may assume that there were certain scribes who hoped to supply addenda or corrections to the Greek texts of Dioscorides. Both the Byzantine Greek vocabulary and the dates of the manuscripts which contain commentaries show that most scholia were appended after the tenth century but not later than the fourteenth. Consequently, these Byzantine commentaries and scholia indicate numerous facets about the nature and quality of Byzantine medicine.

Generally, the commentaries were attached at the conclusions of Dioscorides' chapters, and most of them consider therapeutics. In one instance, Dioscorides had written about a plant called γιγγίδιον, probably a species of wild carrot, *Daucus gingidium* L.,[22] as follows:

It grows plentifully in both Cilicia and Syria, a little herb like the wild carrot (σταφυλῖνος = *Daucus carota* L. [*D. guttatus* Sibthorp])[23] but thinner and more bitter; its root is somewhat white, pungent. It is grown as a pot herb, eaten raw, and boiled and pickled. It is good for the upper digestive tract, and is diuretic.[24]

To which a copyist adds:

boiled down and drunk with wine, it is useful for the bladder.[25]

At least eight manuscripts subsequently integrated

[19] N. R. Farnsworth, *et al.*, "Potential Value of Plants as Sources of New Antifertility Agents. I," *Journal of Pharmaceutical Sciences*, 64, 4 (1975), 544.

[20] There are two facsimile printings, each with lengthy commentaries: J. de Karabacek, ed., *De codicis Dioscuridei Aniciae Iulianae, nunc Vindobonensis Med. Gr. I* (Leiden, 1906; 4 vols.); and H. Gerstinger [Kommentarband zur Faksimileausgabe (1970)], *Dioscurides Codex Vindobonensis med. gr. 1 der Österreichischen Nationalbibliothek* (Graz, 1965–1970; 5 vols.). See also O. Mazal, *Pflanzen, Wurzeln, Säfte, Samen: Antike Heilkunst in Miniaturen des Wiener Dioskurides* (Graz, 1981). For a partial bibliography, see J. Riddle, "Dioscorides," in *Catalogus*, 14–15.

[21] See E. Mioni, "Un novo erbario greco di Dioscoride," *Ressegna Medica. Convivum Sanitatis* [Milan], 36 (1959), 169–84.

[22] Berendes, trans., *Dioskurides*, p. 228; Carnoy, 130; LSJ, *s.v.*

[23] Berendes, trans., *Dioskurides*, p. 299; Carnoy, 252.

[24] Dioscorides II, 137 (ed. Wellmann, Vol. I, pp. 208–9).

[25] Schol. Dioscorides II, 137 (ed. Wellmann, Vol. I, p. 209: *app. crit.* to line 3).

the new line into Dioscorides' chapter.[26] From the view of pharmacological chemistry, the carrot is not known to have an effect on the bladder,[27] except as a diuretic through the kidneys. Possibly the scholiast intended his addition as an elaboration, but this seems implausible, since the appended data is superfluous. Another reason is more likely. In a chapter on the plant called λεπίδιον, Dioscorides gives γιγγίδιον as its synonymn.[28] Identified either as dittander (*Lepidium latifolium* L.) or broad-leaved pepperwort (*L. sativum* L.) in the family Cruciferae, these pepperworts are in distinct contrast to a carrot in the Diapensiaceae family.[29] It is likely that the Byzantine scholiast thought that γιγγίδιον was pepperwort, and added the line to correct Dioscorides' omission. In the Latin West during the Middle Ages, *lepidium* and *gingidion* were often presumed to be the same plant, a pepperwort,[30] and through the nineteenth century folkmedicine used pepperwort in the treatment of bladder ailments.[31]

In almost half of the manuscripts that contain the scholium on pepperwort,[32] there is an interesting commentary added to Dioscorides' chapter on plantain (*Plantago* spp.):

> The Syrians say that the broth [of plantain], and of the catmint (καλαμίνθη: prob. *Nepeta cataria* L.), with honey, cures the fevers; the broth is given for a quotidian, a quartan, just in a preparation; accept this as some secret talisman (μυστήριον).[33] For this is very true, even through experiences.[34]

These comments are quite distinct from other scholia, since they may be connected with Hermetic literature or other magical texts.[35]

In other instances, Byzantine scholiasts give a classical source as the authority. In his original, Dioscorides had referred to at least two species of plants—by our system of taxonomy—with a single Greek name, ἀσφόδελος, which would include both *Asphodelus ramosus* L., and *A. albus* Miller (a St. Bernard's lily, and white asphodel) in Liliaceae. The following appears in a number of manuscripts:[36]

> Another kind flowers at harvest time. It is necessary to cut the white asphodel during the spring equinox before its fruit increases. It is said that its root taken in a drink creates an appetite for sexual activity.[37] And Crateuas the Rhizotomist said the same thing, and also that the root drunk with wine successfully treats the pain in those who suffer from gout.[38]

These comments are important because if we knew their origin we then would know when a "true" cure for gout was first discovered. Our natural product drug of choice for gout is colchicine, which breaks the chemical chain of excessive uric acid deposits on joint tissue and tophoi.[39] Colchicine is present in asphodel.[40] One needs more data than what ancient, medieval, and Byzantine sources tell us, before there is assurance that this is a cure for gout, and such information would include the concentration of colchicine, particular species, preparation method, and dosages and frequency of administration. Lacking these details, one suspects that pre-modern use of the drug would have been less spectacular than the modern synthesized drug, which gives a clinical response within twenty-four hours. Nevertheless, in all probability, the ancient and Byzantine asphodel preparation for gout would have been effective.

The earliest test of this scholium ends with "an appetite for sexual activity."[41] Later manuscripts add the fragment attributed to Crateuas, who had written a medical tract on root medicine in the second

[26] Leiden, Bibl. Univ. MS Voss G. F. 58, 14th cent.; *Vatican, MS Pal. gr. 77, 14th cent.; *Venice, San Marco, MS Gr. Z. 271, 15th cent.; Salamanca, Bibl. univ. MS 2659, 15th cent.; *Paris, B.N., MS gr. 2183, 15th cent.; Paris, B.N., MS gr. 2182, anno 1481, fol. 62; El Escorial, MS T–II–12, 16th cent.; Paris, B.N., MS gr. 2185, 16th cent., fol. 64.

[27] Carrot juice, however, is sometimes substituted for coffee as a stimulating beverage. Lewis and Elvin-Lewis, 387.

[28] Dioscorides II, 174 (ed. Wellmann, Vol. I, pp. 241–42).

[29] Schneider, *Lexikon* (n. 15 above), Vol. V, pt. 2, 17–19 and 246–48.

[30] H. Fischer, *Mittelalterliche Pflanzenkunde* (Munich, 1929), 273; Schneider, *Lexikon* (n. 15 above), Vol. V, pt. 2, 246–47.

[31] Schneider, *Lexikon* (n. 15 above), Vol. II, 73.

[32] To the three manuscripts identified by Wellmann (Paris 2183, Salamanca 2659, and Venice Z. 272), one adds another in which the scholium also appears (Paris, B.N., MS gr. 2182, fol. 50), but it is not in other codices in which there are scholia already mentioned, e.g. Leiden, MS Voss. Fr. F. 58 (fols. 266ᵛ–67 have plantain), El Escorial MS T–II–12, and Venice, San Marco MS Gr. Z. 597.

[33] *PGM*, XII, 331–34 [talisman]. This is also the name of a particular drug, "The Secret," or "The Talisman," as recorded by Galen (ed. Kühn), XIII, 96, quoting Niceratus; cf. Alexander of Tralles V, 4 (ed. Puschmann, Vol. II, p. 161), and Oribasius, *For Eunapius* IV, 135 (ed. Raeder, p. 496).

[34] Schol. Dioscorides II, 126.4 (ed. Wellmann, Vol. I. p. 200: *app. crit.* to line 15).

[35] J. M. Riddle, *Marbode of Rennes' De lapidibus* (Wiesbaden, 1977 [*SA* Beiheft 20]), 3–5, 10, and 28–30.

[36] Leiden, Bibl. univ., MS Voss. Gr. F. 58; *Vatican, MS Pal. gr. 77; Paris, B.N., MS gr. 2182; *Paris, B.N., MS gr. 2183; Paris, B.N., MS gr. 2185; El Escorial MS T–II–12.

[37] Vatican, MS Pal. gr. 77 ends here.

[38] Schol. Dioscorides II, 169.3 (ed. Wellmann, Vol. I, p. 236: *app. crit.* to line 8).

[39] A. Goth, *Medical Pharmacology*, 9th ed. (St. Louis, 1978), 533–34. Lewis and Elvin-Lewis, 199 and 219.

[40] J. A. Duke, "Phytotoxin Tables," *Critical Reviews in Toxicology* (Nov. 1977), 215.

[41] Schol. Dioscorides II, 169.3 (ed. Wellmann, Vol. I, p. 236: *app. crit.* to line 8 [line 4]).

century B.C.[42] An extensive fragment on asphodel from Crateuas' treatise is preserved in the Anicia Juliana, and the text is separate from that of Dioscorides; the use of asphodel for gout appears in this fragment.[43] The extant texts suggest the following: Crateuas was the first known writer on herbal medicine to recommend an effective remedy for gout, but the drug was not employed by his successors, including Dioscorides.[44] The copyist of the Anicia Juliana manuscript in the early sixth century recognized that Dioscorides' account could be augmented, and so he added the quotation from Crateuas, but in a separate section, clearly identified as a different source. After the citation of the Anicia manuscript, there is no evidence before the fourteenth century that asphodel was used against gout, even by the Byzantine commentator who provides information about its collection and employment as an aphrodisiac. The old Latin translation of Dioscorides (c. sixth century) does not include asphodel as a remedy for gout.[45] It first reappears in extant texts of the late fourteenth century by a Byzantine scholiast who again recognized asphodel as a treatment for gout, and he appended it to a previous commentary on this section of Dioscorides' text. Credit for this rediscovery should be given to this unknown Byzantine scribe, who perceived important data inexplicably lost for 800 years, and added the information to the text of Dioscorides.

In a similar manner, new information is appended to the description of another plant, emerging partially from Crateuas and Galen, but with a possible major innovation. In the chapter on the birthwort (ἀριστολοχεία), Dioscorides had written that there was a third kind (κληματῖτις) with the same pharmaceutical properties as the other two (probably *Aristolochia pallida* Willd., and *A. sempervirens* L.), but this third kind was not as strong.[46] Some Byzantine scholiasts were not satisfied by this terse description, and chose to elaborate on what is probably our *Aristolochia clematitis* L.:

[The *klēmatitis*] is called by some *arariza*, as well as *melekaproum, erestios, lestitis, pyxionyx, dardanon,* and *iontitis*; the Gauls call it *theximon,* the Egyptians *sophoeph,* the Sicilians *chamaimēlon,* the Italians *terra mala,* the Dacians *apsinthion chōrikon.* It grows in mountainous country, in warm and flat places or rough and rocky areas. It "works" in the treatment of an oppressive fever in this way: [have the patient] with fever [breathe the odors] from a charcoal fumigator with birthwort [on it], and the fever will subside. And applied as a plaster, birthwort cures wounds. With nut grass (*Cyperus rotundus* L., possibly a galingale, *C. longus* L.) and the tuber of the dragon arum (*Dracunculus vulgaris* Schott)[47] and honey, it helps [Paris, Venice, and Salamanca MSS: "cures" Vienna 16 MS and Vatican MS] those with carcinomas of the skin. Boiled in oil, or pig's fat, and rubbed on, it is a treatment for periodic shivering fevers [Paris, Venice, and Salamanca MSS end here]. And Crateuas the Rhizotomist and Galen [or Galos] have said the same things [El Escorial MS ends], and it also helps those with gout.[48]

This commentary is more complete than many others on Dioscorides: it has synonyms, plant habitat, and medicinal usages. Wellmann thought that this scholium had come from the Pseudo-Apuleius *Herbarius.*[49] While there are similarities, the Byzantine commentator's source is not the *Herbarius,* a work in Latin composed perhaps in the fourth century, and not, as previously believed, based on an original Greek work.[50] The list of synonyms resembles that in the *Herbarius,* but there are notable differences.[51] Pseudo-Apuleius has no recommendation for gout, and prescribes *clematitis*-birthwort for nasal carcinoma[52]—probably a polyp of the

[42] M. Wellmann, *Krateuas* (Berlin, 1897 [AbhGöttingen, Phil.-hist.Kl., n.f. 2, no. 1]).

[43] Vienna, Nationalbibliothek MS med. gr. 1 (= Anicia Juliana MS), fol. 27ʳ, published as Crateuas fragment No. 5 in Wellmann, ed., Dioscorides, Vol. III, p. 145.

[44] E.g., the discussion of asphodel in Galen, *Properties of Foods* II, 55, and *Mixtures and Properties of Simples* VI, 77 (ed. Kühn, VI, 651–52, and XI, 842), and the fragment of Galen in the Vienna Anicia Juliana MS, fol. 27. Cf. Paul of Aegina VII, 3 (ed. Heiberg, Vol. II, p. 198). For Hippocratic works, see Dierbach (n. 16 above), 99–100.

[45] Munich, MS lat. 337, fol. 66ᵛ–7, published by H. Stadler, "Dioscorides Langobardus," *Romanische Forschungen,* 10 (1897), 238–39.

[46] Dioscorides III, 4.5 (ed. Wellmann, Vol. II, p. 8).

[47] The scholiast's δρακοντίου σπέρματος is probably to be rendered "tuber," given the manner of reproduction of the dragon arum.

[48] Schol. Dioscorides III, 4.5 (ed. Wellmann, Vol. II, p. 8: *app. crit.* to line 10). This is appended in at least the following MSS: *Vatican MS Pal. gr. 77; Vienna, N.B., MS gr. 16, 15th cent.; *Paris, B.N., MS gr. 2183; *Salamanca, MS 2659; *Venice, San Marco, MS Gr. Z 271; El Escorial, MS T–II–12.

[49] Ed. Wellmann, Vol. II, p. 8: *app. crit.* to line 10 init.

[50] H. E. Sigerist, "Zum Herbarius Pseudo-Apulei," *SA,* 23 (1930), 197–204, esp. 200.

[51] Pseudo-Apuleius, *Herbarius* 19 (ed. Sigerist, p. 57, lines 24–27), has the following synonyms not found in the Greek scholium: *feuxicterus, erectitis, Itali opetes.* The Greek scholium has ἰοντῖτις and θέξιμον, not found in the Latin *Herbarius.* Also variant is *Dardani sopitis,* cf. χαμαίμηλον. Both the Byzantine scribe and the author of the *Herbarius* apparently employed the same source. For an early study of plant synonyms, especially those appearing in the Anicia Dioscorides manuscript, see M. Wellmann, "Die Pflanzennamen des Dioskurides," *Hermes,* 33 (1898), 360–422.

[52] *Herbarius* 19.7 (ed. Sigerist, p. 57, lines 20–22): *Ad carcinomata, quae in naribus nascuntur. Herba aristolochia cum cipero et draconteae semen cum melle inpositum emendat.*

nares, usually a benign tumor in the nasal passage, displaying a pedicle, especially on the mucous membrane. Most of the medicinal suggestions in the commentary originated in the Crateuas fragment found in the Anicia Juliana on two separate folios,[53] and from Galen who clearly borrowed from Crateuas for the description of birthwort.[54] The major difference in the Byzantine scholium is the use of the herb for skin carcinomas (ἐν ῥινὶ καρ-κινώμασι). Byzantine diagnostics certainly did not include malignant neoplastic lesions as in modern oncology, but there is little doubt that they suffered from various kinds of malignant cancers,[55] and one of several terms to describe them was καρκίνωμα.[56] Recently, aristolochic acid, found in *Aristolochia baetica* and *A. clematitis*, was discovered to have anti-tumor properties,[57] and currently it is employed in chemotherapy for cancer.[58] It seems that a Byzantine physician, in or before the fourteenth century, had discovered *clematitis*-birthwort's pharmaceutical properties in use against skin cancers, and the scribe thereby modified the Greek text derived from Crateuas and added the scholium to Dioscorides' account, writing that *klēmatitis* "helps" skin cancer. Significantly, another copyist strengthens the claim by changing the verb from "helps" to "cures." This last alteration is correct, as judged in 1983, a fact we have had to rediscover. In early modern employment of the plant in Europe, it was apparently not used against cancer, but its history requires further research.[59]

There is a similar scholium attached to Dioscorides' account of βολβὸς ἐδώδιμος, one of the grape hyacinths, and most likely tassel hyacinth (*Muscari comosum* [L] Miller).[60] At the end of *Materia medica* II, 170.2, the scribes of three manuscripts have appended:

> [tassel hyacinth] boiled with barley meal[61] and pig's fat causes οἰδήματα and φύματα quickly to suppurate and break up.[62]

Oidēmata and *phymata* are two other Greek terms for tumorous growths or lumps, the lexical range of which include our "malignancies," "carcinoma," and "sarcoma."[63] An extract from the bulb of tassel hyacinth is currently used in chemotherapy for cancer.[64]

Not all commentaries and scholia attached to Dioscorides are rational or even empirical. Appended to the same group of manuscripts which include the tassel hyacinth scholium is a short text at the end of Dioscorides' clipped description of the herb called *mōly* (prob. *Allium* spp.):[65]

> The roots being cut and gathered up and carried next to the body, *mōly* helps against drugs [or poisons: φάρ-μακα] and frees one from his enemies.[66]

In this case, the Byzantine scholiast may have borrowed from the anonymous first- or second-century work called *Carminis de viribus herbarum*,[67] a collection of poems retailing quasi-magical properties of certain herbs. Even if the scholium can be traced to an ultimate source in Greek from the early Roman Empire, the data has been filtered and changed through centuries of transmission.

In other instances, the contents of the commentaries are apparently new, and one may also judge them rational. The same manuscripts that have the scholium on *mōly*, as well as the Anicia Juliana, also

[53] Vienna, Nationalbibliothek, MS med. gr. 1, fols. 18 and 19ᵛ; printed as Crateuas, Frgs. Nos. 1 and 2 in Wellmann, ed., Dioscorides, Vol. III, p. 144. A Galen fragment on *klēmatitis* is in fol. 19ᵛ of the Vienna MS, but it also does not include the statement on *karkinōma*.

[54] Galen, *Simples* VI, 56 (ed. Kühn, XI, 835–36).

[55] D. Brothwell, "The Evidence for Neoplasms," in D. Brothwell and A. T. Sandison, eds., *Diseases in Antiquity* (Springfield, Illinois, 1967), 320–45, using the findings of paleopathology. See also J. Reedy, "Galen on Cancer and Related Diseases," *Clio Medica*, 10 (1975), 227–38.

[56] L. J. Rather, *The Genesis of Cancer* (Baltimore, 1978), 9.

[57] G. E. Trease and W. C. Evans, *Pharmacognosy*, 11th ed. (London, 1978), 98 and 577; S. Munavalli and C. Viel, "Etude chimique, taxonomique et pharmacologique des Aristolochi-acées," *Annales pharmaceutiques français*, 27 (1969), 449–64 [463]; *Chemical Abstracts*, 80 (1974), 24780g for *A. baetica*, and 81 (1974), 111458z for *A. clematitis*. Cf. earlier uses as listed in *Dispensatory of the United States*, 25th ed. (Philadelphia, 1955), 1841.

[58] Lewis and Elvin-Lewis, 134.

[59] Schneider, *Lexikon* (n. 25 above), Vol. V, pt. 1, 124–29.

[60] Dioscorides II, 170 (ed. Wellmann, Vol. I, pp. 236–37); Berendes, trans., *Dioskurides*, p. 247; Carnoy, 51.

[61] ἄλφιτον.

[62] Schol. Dioscorides II, 170.2 (ed. Wellmann, Vol. I, p. 237: *app. crit.* to line 14).

[63] Rather, *Genesis of Cancer* (n. 56 above), 9–13.

[64] Lewis and Elvin-Lewis, 135.

[65] J. Stannard, "The Plant Called Moly," *Osiris*, 14 (1962), 254–307, traces the remarkable history of plants called by this name in Greek. Cf. Schneider, *Lexikon* (n. 15 above), Vol. V, pt. 1, 65, and B. Langkavel, *Botanik der spaeteren Griechen* (Berlin, 1866; rptd. Amsterdam, 1964), 12.

[66] Schol. Dioscorides III, 47 (ed. Wellmann, Vol. II, p. 61: *app. crit.* to line 2).

[67] E. Heitsch, ed., *Carminis de viribus herbarum fragmentum*, 179–91 (esp. 190–91) in *Die griechischen Dichterfragmente der römischen Kaiserzeit*, Vol. II (Göttingen, 1964), pp. 35–36; Stannard, "Moly" (n. 65 above), 286; Wellmann, ed., Dioscorides, Vol. II, p. 61: *app. crit.* to line 2 (accepting the *Carminis de viribus*—known in Wellmann's day as *Carmen de herbis*—as the source).

have added details on κρόμυον) or onion (prob. *Allium cepa* L.).

> Thus boiled and laid on in a plaster with stavesacre (*Delphinium staphisagria* L.) or fig, onion softens and breaks up tumors (φύματα) very quickly.[68]

Modern Chinese medicine employs the onion for its anti-tumor properties,[69] and western folkmedicine uses it as a stimulant for the nervous system.[70] The scholium also suggests stavesacre, which contains a strong alkaloid which may have anti-tumor properties as do many alkaloids, but no ancient author on pharmacy recommends the onion for treatment of tumors.[71] Therefore, this discovery can be assumed to be early Byzantine, since the addendum on onion for tumors is first found in the Anicia Juliana manuscript.[72]

Some of the scholia are botanical, but clearly with a medicinal purpose. Dioscorides had written that the stem of the reedmace, a kind of cattail (prob. *Typha latifolia* L., possibly *T. angustifolia* L.) was smooth and uniform;[73] a Byzantine scribe added "the stem white, uniform."[74] Modern botanical manuals describe two types of spikes for *T. latifolia*, a female which turns brown, and a male which forms a yellow spike but which later falls off to leave a slender, colorless terminal axis,[75] so that the Byz-

antine addition of "white" probably aided identification.

Some of these manuscripts[76] have added a habitat description to Dioscorides' ἄκανθα 'Αραβική, with "It grows in rugged places." Sprengel believed that Dioscorides' "Arabian acanthus" was *Onopordon arabicum* [= *acanthium* L.], but Berendes thought it was no particular species, simply "acanthus" from Arabia.[77] Dioscorides says only that "Arabian acanthus" is similar to "white acanthus," identified as a thistle,[78] and several other plants.[79] A larger number of species passed under the name of "acanthus," as recorded in Theophrastus.[80] The illumination of the "Arabian acanthus" in the Anicia family of Dioscorides manuscripts, as well as the textual description are, however, more appropriate for *Onopordon acanthium*, Scotch thistle, sometimes also called cotton thistle from its fluffy purple flowers.[81] Scotch thistle grows on waste ground, which is in keeping with the "rugged places" in the scholium. Whatever might have been Dioscorides' intent regarding the plant, the Byzantine commentator most likely understood the description as that of Scotch thistle, and so described its habitat, since this was omitted in Dioscorides' text. In a modern herbal, Scotch thistle is recommended as an astringent,[82] the same use as given by Dioscorides, which makes the identification of Scotch thistle appropriate in its pharmacognosy. Not surprisingly, the Byzantine scribe is seeking clarity in the confusing nomenclature of plants called "acanthus," and his appended remark would be helpful.

In correcting Dioscorides' description of "wild isatis," a Byzantine scholiast shows remarkable botanical observation, surpassing by far Dioscorides. In this instance, moreover, the scribe says that Dioscorides is wrong. From a modern perspective, Dioscorides is not incorrect as the Byzantine scho-

---

[68] Schol. Dioscorides II, 151.2 (ed. Wellmann, Vol. I, p. 217: *app. crit.* to line 7).

[69] Bin Hsu, "Use of Herbs as Anti-Cancer Agents," *American Journal of Chinese Medicine*, 8 (1980), 305.

[70] *Dispensatory* (n. 57 above), 1538. Cf. V. E. Tyler, Lynn R. Brady, and J. E. Robbers, *Pharmacognosy*, 8th ed. (Philadelphia, 1981), 482, who write: "Further chemical and pharmacologic research is needed to determine the real value of garlic and onion for the many conditions in which they are reputed to be effective."

[71] No such recommendation appears in the Hippocratic corpus, Galen, Aetius of Amida, and Theophrastus, among the Greek sources, and none appears in Latin in the tracts by Pliny, Gargilius Martialis, Pseudo-Apuleius, and Scribonius Largus.

[72] The copyists of the early sixth-century Anicia Juliana MS, or an earlier prototype (the text is also in Naples, N.B., MS suppl. gr. 28, 7th cent.), were apparently of the opinion that Dioscorides had not given enough attention to plants of the genus *delphinium*, of which stavesacre is one species. After δαῦκος (Dioscorides III, 72) in the original order, the Anicia Juliana and the Naples MSS add two more plants, called δελφίνιον and δελφίνιον ἕτερον, along with descriptions. Venice, San Marco, MS Gr. Z 273 (12th cent.) is a fragmentary Dioscorides in the regular order, and this allowed Wellmann to discern the chapter's proper position in Dioscorides' work. Book III in the Venice MS begins on folio 21.

[73] Dioscorides III, 118 (ed. Wellmann, Vol. II, p. 129); Berendes, trans., *Dioskurides*, p. 342; Carnoy, 271.

[74] Schol. Dioscorides III, 118 (ed. Wellmann, Vol. II, p. 129: *app. crit.* to line 3).

[75] Polunin, *Flowers of Europe*, nos. 1827–28.

[76] Schol. Dioscorides III, 13 (ed. Wellmann, Vol. II, p. 20: *app. crit.* to line 11). *Vatican, MS Pal. gr. 77; *Paris, B.N., MS gr. 2183; *Venice, San Marco, MS gr. Z 271; Vienna, Nationalbibliothek, MS gr. 16; and El Escorial, MS III–R–3. The first three MSS also have the scholium to Dioscorides III, 118.

[77] Berendes, trans., *Dioskurides*, 271.

[78] *Ibid. Cnicius ferox* L; Langkavel, *Botanik* (n. 65 above), 74.

[79] E.g. *Acacia albida* Delile; *Cnicius arvensis* Hoffm. = *Cirsium arvense* (L.) Scop.; Carnoy, 3.

[80] Theophrastus, *HP* IV, 2.8 (tree); IV, 10.6 (creeping thistle, prob. *Carduus* [= *Cirsium*] *arvense* [L.] Scop.); IX, 12.1 (pine thistle, *Atractylis gummifera* L.), etc.

[81] Polunin, *Flowers of Europe*, no. 1494.

[82] M. Grieve, *A Modern Herbal* (New York, 1931; 2 vols.; rptd. 1971), Vol. II, 798.

liast alleges, but the scribe apparently believes that Dioscorides was describing a plant other than the one we now think he intended. Knowing it to be wrong, the Byzantine commentator hoped to correct the description with details so exact that we can be virtually certain which plant he intended.

Dioscorides devotes one chapter to woad (ἰσάτις [*Isatis tinctoria* L.]) and another to "wild woad" (ἰσάτις ἀγρία),[83] which modern authorities agree is another species of woad, while disagreeing on the exact nomenclature.[84] He writes that the plant is similar to ordinary woad except that it has larger leaves, like lettuce, but with slender stems which are reddish and multi-branched, on the end of which hang many tongue-like pods containing the seeds, the flowers being yellowish and small.[85] Modern descriptions add only that woad has petals up to twice as long as the sepals.[86] The Byzantine scribe believes he is correcting Dioscorides as he writes:

> One must consider faulty the information on woads. The cultivar (ἡ ἥμερος) bears a quince-yellow flower, thinner and greatly subdivided branches, and little pods from the top which are like tongues, in which are the seeds; but there is enclosed in these a black seed like black cummin (μελάνθιον, *Nigella sativa* L.),[87] and its stalk grows to a height of over two πήχεις (c. 3 ft./95 cm.), not to a height of a πῆχυς (c. 1½ ft./47 cm.). The wild kind, however, bears blacker leaves than the cultivar, and the wild kind has a shorter and thicker stalk, a purple or blue flower, and a prickly fruit shaped like a cross, in which the seed is as if divided into five equal small leaflets.[88]

The scholiast's description compares well with technical, modern depictions of cow basil (*Vaccaria pyramidata* Medicus) and its flowers, stalk, ovary, and seeds.[89] The Byzantine commentator observes that the seed pod has five small equal leaflets, and the

Hortus Third, a modern botanical reference, says "epicalyx absent, calyx 5-lobed, 5-winged, inflated petals 5 . . . seeds nearly globose."[90] By contrast, woad's seed is black, but flat and pendulous, and does not compare to the seed of black cummin in the manner of cow basil's seed. In summary, this scholium reveals excellent attention to botanical detail rarely equaled in ancient or medieval herbals. Although the scholiast probably has mistaken Dioscorides' intended plant, he has boldly and explicitly written that Dioscorides was wrong and proceeded with his corrections. The unknown Byzantine commentator has trusted his observation of the plant in nature in a way that his western counterpart would not have done.

Byzantine commentaries on Dioscorides are apparently carefully pondered, and their contents are rationally constructed corrections and supplements to the text. A certain number of them are clearly derived from classical authorities, but most seem to be the results of Byzantine medicine's experience with the drugs mentioned in Dioscorides' *Materia medica*. By comparison, the manuscripts of the Old Latin Translation of Dioscorides reveal clumsy copyist errors by scribes who knew little about the material they were handling. It was not until the late eleventh century, when Constantine the African (or someone from his school) rearranged the Old Latin Translation in alphabetical order, that a large scale,[91] rationally designed set of commentaries were attached to Dioscorides' Latin text. By contrast, the Byzantine commentaries were more modest, but generally of a high medical and botanical quality. These Byzantine scholia show the purpose toward which Dioscorides' works were directed: medicine. The texts were not exclusively warehoused in isolated monastic libraries awaiting a Renaissance dusting. They must have been used by physicians.

North Carolina State University

[83] Dioscorides II, 184 and 185 (ed. Wellmann, Vol. I, pp. 253–54).

[84] Berendes, trans., *Dioskurides*, 258, with list of suggested spp.

[85] Dioscorides II, 185 (ed. Wellmann, Vol. I, p. 254).

[86] Polunin, *Flowers of Europe*, no. 292. *Hortus Third*, 606.

[87] Cf. Dioscorides III, 79 (ed. Wellmann, Vol. II, pp. 92–93).

[88] Schol. Dioscorides II, 185 (ed. Wellmann, Vol. I, p. 254: *app. crit.* to line 11). *Vatican, MS Pal. gr. 77, and Paris, B.N., MS gr. 2182 end with οἰονεὶ διειλημμένον (line 8 of scholium); but three earlier MSS add five further lines (as printed by Wellmann).

[89] Polunin, *Flowers of Europe*, no. 182; *Hortus Third*, 1142.

[90] *Hortus Third*, 1142.

[91] J. M. Riddle, "The Latin Alphabetical Dioscorides," *Proceedings of XIIIth International Congress of the History of Science, Moscow, August 18–24, 1971* Sections III & IV (Moscow, 1974), 204–9, and Riddle, "Dioscorides," *Catalogus*, 23–27.

PHILOSOPHY AND MEDICINE IN JOHN PHILOPONUS' COMMENTARY ON ARISTOTLE'S *DE ANIMA*

ROBERT B. TODD

John Philoponus' commentary on Aristotle's *De anima* was probably written in Alexandria in the first quarter of the sixth century, and was paraphrased seven centuries later by Sophonias.[1] It is allegedly an edition of the lectures of the neoplatonic philosopher Ammonius, a pupil of Proclus, on Books I and II of the *De anima* (that on Book III is no longer extant in Greek).[2] At least the title in one manuscript indicates this and refers to supplements by Philoponus himself, but it is difficult to determine whether the medical material to be discussed here could be part of such an accretion. I shall follow convention and refer to the author of the whole commentary as "Philoponus,"[3] and

comment later on the possible sources of his and Ammonius' medical knowledge. This work deserves the attention of historians of ancient and Byzantine medicine as the best extant example of a Greek philosophical commentary employing medical ideas. Although this characteristic must in some way be connected with the status of medicine in the educational system of the fifth and sixth centuries, I have not been able to establish any firm links between my evidence and that wider context; I shall therefore concentrate for the most part on an analysis of the relevant texts as perhaps a preliminary to further research.

I. PHILOPONUS AND THE RELATION BETWEEN PHILOSOPHY AND MEDICINE IN GREEK ARISTOTELIANISM

Our text is one of numerous Greek and Byzantine Aristotelian commentaries. The Aristotelian treatises that received most attention in this exegetical tradition were those on logic, physics, metaphysics, and psychology, and references to medical writers and medical ideas can be detected in many of them.[4] As Westerink's studies of sixth-century exegesis have also shown, such references can be used to demonstrate a growing professional overlap between philosophy and medicine.[5] But where

[The reader is referred to the list of abbreviations at the end of the volume.]

Note on References: The Greek Aristotelian commentators are cited by the page and line number of the *Commentaria in Aristotelem Graeca* (Berlin, 1883–1907), hereafter CAG, and the title of the relevant *Aristotelian* work. References to Galen will usually be to Kühn's edition (Leipzig, 1821–1833), with later editions cited as appropriate.

[1] Philoponus' commentary is at CAG XV, ed. M. Hayduck (Berlin, 1897); Sophonias' paraphrase at CAG XXIII:1, ed. M. Hayduck (Berlin, 1883). This commentary had also been used by Michael Psellus (see Hayduck's edition of Philoponus at pp. xiv–xix) while Gennadius Scholarius claimed that St. Thomas' commentary on Aristotle's *De anima* was dependent on Philoponus; see *Oeuvres complètes de Gennade Scholarios* (Paris, 1933), VI, 327.

[2] Book III of the Philoponus commentary is attributed to Stephanus of Alexandria; on its relation to the commentary on the preceding books see H. Blumenthal, "John Philoponus and Stephanus of Alexandria: Two Neoplatonic Christian Commentators on Aristotle?," chap. 6 of *Neoplatonism and Christian Thought*, ed. D. J. O'Meara, Studies in Neoplatonism Ancient and Modern, III (Norfolk, Virginia, 1982). This article also contains references to further secondary literature on this commentary. The medieval Latin translation of Philoponus' commentary on *De anima* III.4–8 is edited by G. Verbeke at *Corpus Latinum Commentariorum in Aristotelem Graecorum III* (Louvain/Paris, 1966).

[3] On the relation between Philoponus and Ammonius see the literature cited at p. 152, notes 5–8 of my article, "Some Concepts in Physical Theory in John Philoponus' Aristotelian Commentaries," *Archiv für Begriffsgeschichte*, 24 (1980), 151–70. The

reference to Ammonius' lectures occurs in the titles of Par. Gr. 1914 (s. xii), and of the first edition of 1535. The question is whether this evidence can outweigh a Byzantine tradition (cf. note 1 above) regarding Philoponus as the sole author.

[4] See my "Galenic Medical Ideas in the Greek Aristotelian Commentators," *SOsl*, 52 (1976), 117–34 (hereafter "Galenic Medical Ideas").

[5] See L. G. Westerink, "Philosophy and Medicine in Late Antiquity," *Janus*, 51 (1964), 169–77 (= *Texts and Studies in Neoplatonism and Byzantine Literature* [Amsterdam, 1980], 83–99). See also his *Pseudo-Elias (Pseudo-David), Lectures on Porphyry's Isagoge* (Amsterdam, 1967), pp. xiii–xv, and *The Greek Commentaries on Plato's Phaedo*, Vol. I, *Olympiodorus* (Amsterdam, 1976), 27.

Aristotle's *De anima* and parts of his *De generatione et corruptione* are concerned, a commentator's knowledge of medical ideas can significantly affect the actual content of interpretation when it touches on such issues as the theory of nutrition, the operation of the senses, or indeed on the general theory of the soul.[6] Although Aristotle's more medically relevant biological and zoological treatises were known in antiquity, they were not made the subject of commentaries until Michael of Ephesus' work in the eleventh century; but while this Byzantine scholar had some knowledge of Galen, he did not examine medical ideas very closely, nor did he use them to reconstruct Aristotelian thought.[7]

It is, however, just this kind of exercise that occupies John Philoponus in parts of his commentary on the *De anima*. In comparison with the treatment of the same work by his predecessors Alexander of Aphrodisias, who had a fairly extensive knowledge of Galen's works,[8] and Themistius,[9] and by his contemporary Simplicius,[10] Philo-

ponus' commentary shows greater knowledge of medical thought and greater sensitivity to its philosophical implications. This is partly because it is written from a neoplatonic perspective.[11] Plato and Galen could therefore, for example, be followed in their accounts of the primacy of the brain over the heart, and the Galenic anatomy of the brain and doctrine of psychic pneuma could, as we shall see, be introduced to redescribe Aristotlelian accounts of sensation (see Part II below). At the same time, neoplatonic philosophy could be contrasted with a materialistic explanation of the soul and its faculties offered by medical thought, and of this too we shall see some striking examples (Part III below).

But we can also ask whether Philoponus' interest in medicine arose solely within neoplatonism, or whether it depended on the external sustenance of a system of medical education. Unfortunately, we know very little about the neoplatonists' knowledge of Galen in the fifth century; we do not have Proclus' commentary on the biological parts of the *Timaeus*,[12] and the medical references in the commentaries assigned exclusively to Ammonius are too scanty to be decisive.[13] As for Philoponus', or Ammonius', links with contemporary medical teaching, these are difficult to establish, particularly since the Arabic tradition that Philoponus was a medical commentator is so questionable.[14] Also, professionally he was not a doctor, or philospher, but a γραμματικός, and his philosophical commentaries show none of the stylized form that marks both medical and philosophical exegesis later in the sixth century, including indeed the commentary on Book III of the *De anima* by a Stephanus (possibly himself a medical author) that completes Philoponus' commentary in the Greek manuscripts.[15]

If we turn to the evidence of the text, we find

[6] See "Galenic Medical Ideas," *passim.*

[7] Michael's commentaries on the *De partibus animalium, De motu animalium,* and *De incessu animalium* are at CAG XII:2, ed. M. Hayduck (Berlin, 1904). His commentary on the *De generatione animalium,* falsely attributed to Philoponus, is at CAG XIV:3, ed. M. Hayduck (Berlin, 1903). On the historical context of these commentaries see R. Browning, "An Unpublished Funeral Oration on Anna Comnena," *Proceedings of the Cambridge Philological Society,* n.s. 8 (1962), 1–12, and more recently A. Preus, *Aristotle and Michael of Ephesus on the Movement and Progression of Animals* (Hildesheim and New York, 1981). I have discussed some of Michael's Galenic references at "Galenic Medical Ideas," 117–18, and 126–27. As evidence of Michael's orthodoxy, cf. *De gen. an.* 223.12–17, *De part. an.* 44.20 ff. and *De mot. an.* 123.6–14, all of which accept the heart as the central organ (ἡγεμονικόν) of the soul; in the case of the latter, reference is made to Alexander of Aphrodisias' discussion of this topic, an indication of Michael's dependency on orthodoxy. On the latter see further P. L. Donini, "Il *de anima* di Alessandro di Afrodisia e Michele Efesio," *Rivista di Filologia e Istruzione Classica,* 96 (1968), 316–23.

[8] See "Galenic Medical Ideas," 121–23. Extant in Arabic, for example, is Alexander's polemic against Galen on motion: see N. Rescher and M. Marmura, *The Refutation by Alexander of Aphrodisias of Galen's Treatise on the Theory of Motion* (Islamabad, 1965). Alexander's commentary on Aristotle's *De anima* is not extant, only his interpretative essay *de anima,* at *Supplementum Aristotelicum,* II.2, ed. I. Bruns (Berlin, 1892).

[9] I have not been able to identify any specifically medical ideas in Themistius' commentary, at CAG V:3, ed. R. Heinze (Berlin, 1899). He does, however, refer to Galen regarding points of physical theory; cf. *Phys.,* CAG V:2, ed. H. Schenkl (Berlin, 1900), 114.9–115.12, 144.24–145.2, 149.4.

[10] Simplicius' commentary is at CAG XI, ed. M. Hayduck (Berlin, 1882). Its authorship has been questioned; on this and the general doctrine of the work see H. J. Blumenthal, "The Psychology of (?) Simplicius' Commentary on the *De anima,*" at 73–93 of *Soul and the Structure of Being in Late Neoplatonism,* ed. H. J. Blumenthal and A. C. Lloyd (Liverpool, 1982).

[11] See Blumenthal's article cited in note 1 above, and on the general issue of the neoplatonists' reading of Aristotle see the same author's "Neoplatonic Elements in the *De Anima* Commentaries," *Phronesis,* 19 (1976), 64–87.

[12] The commentary ends at *Timaeus* 44d. On Proclus' one reference to Galen see note 70 below. Marinus, *Vita Procli* (p. 14 Boissonade) mentions that Proclus had some medical skill.

[13] See note 26 below for one example. Otherwise he just makes the standard complaint about Galen's prolixity at *In Porph. Isag.,* CAG IV:3, ed. A. Busse (Berlin, 1891), 38.15.

[14] On his identification with John of Alexandria see the discussion, and catalogue of manuscripts, in Ullmann, *Medizin,* 89–91, with the literature cited there.

[15] See Westerink (note 5 above), 171. On such methods in medical commentaries see O. Temkin, "Studies on Late Alexandrian Medicine, I. Alexandrian Commentaries on Galen's *De Sectis ad introducendos,*" *BHM,* 3 (1935), 405–30 (= Temkin, *Double Face of Janus,* 178–97). On the complex question of this Stephanus' identity see R. Vancourt, *Les Derniers Commentateurs d'Aristote* (Lille, 1944), 26–33.

that Philoponus is generally more interested in the principles behind medical ideas and theories than in their specific details. Though this is what we might expect from a philosopher, we are on safer ground in probing this evidence as it stands than in trying to speculate about the immediate sources of his medical knowledge. The situation can be well illustrated by noting that while the medical references in Philoponus' commentary on the *De anima* are certainly Galenic, this commentator never refers in that work to Galen by name; elsewhere, in his treatise *De aeternitate mundi*, he mentions briefly the works *De locis affectis* and *On Demonstration*.[16] If he bothers to preface his introduction of medical ideas at all, it is with a generic reference to "the doctors" (οἱ ἰατροί).[17] It is in fact in this way that he introduces references to the titles of two Galenic treatises, mentioning the doctors' view "that the faculties of the soul follow the temperaments of the body,"[18] and their "discourses concerning the use of parts."[19] This type of reference, coupled with the simplicity shown in anatomical descriptions when compared with the relevant Galenic precedents,[20] makes it difficult to speculate constructively about whether Philoponus has epitomized medical literature himself, or whether he is drawing on some tradition that had fashioned Galenic ideas into the doxographical form in which we encounter them in this commentary. This is the philological analogue to the difficulties already noted

in establishing any historical context for Philoponus' knowledge of medicine.

Philoponus does, however, allow us to approach his medical interests from another perspective by his occasional programmatic statements about the role of the doctor, or the status of the medical art. In discussing various Aristotelian passages dealing directly with this subject, or, as in the *Posterior Analytics*, with the relationship between different sciences, Philoponus regularly categorizes medicine as an applied art, often said to be drawing its principles from φυσιολογία. It is said, for example, to be concerned with the balance between the elements and not with the forms of the elements.[21] Indeed in some passages from the commentary on the *Physics* the doctor, *qua* doctor, is explicitly denied any philosophical identity and is represented as unconcerned with the concepts of primary matter and form, or with teleology.[22] If this evidence were taken as a projection of a professional reality then it would seem that Philoponus regarded medicine and philosophy as radically distinct disciplines. But it is best to use this account of medicine simply as a guide to his use of medical ideas, and in this respect it can be said in broad terms to underwrite his procedure. His anatomical and physiological supplements to the Aristotelian text use essentially factual material, the evidence of a first-order discipline, while it is just such material that is elsewhere set in the wider context of neoplatonic philosophy. These two aspects of his use of medical ideas will concern us in the rest of this paper.

The first reflects the purely exegetical goal of the commentary, in which neoplatonism is a general influence licensing the introduction of Galenic material that restates, and even supports, Aristotelian ideas without radically altering them. The second aspect represents the deeper effect of neoplatonism on Philoponus' commentary, and involves its confrontation with medical ideas occasioned by the Aristotelian text. The two overlap, of course, but it will be useful for us to keep them apart.

---

[16] *De aet. mund.* 319.5–8 Rabe: the reference is specifically to a view expressed ἐν τῇ διαγνωστικῇ; as John Duffy has pointed out, I was wrong (at "Galenic Medical Ideas," 134, note 2: Addendum) to claim that this title was in any way vague. This formula is typical in Alexandrian medicine; Duffy cites Palladius, *On Epidemics Bk. VI*, 14.30, 129.6, 186.8 Dietz. The reference to the ἀποδεικτικὴ πραγματεία in laudatory terms is at *De aet. mund.* 600.2 Rabe; cf. O. Temkin, "Byzantine Medicine: Tradition and Empiricism," *DOP*, 16 (1962), 97–115 (= *Double Face of Janus*, chap. 14), at 105 note 58. Hippocrates, it should also be noted, is not mentioned by name, though cf. 284.11–12 and 112.26 for references to his works.

[17] To the nine references given in the index for the commentary on Bks. I and II, add 33.2.

[18] *De an.* 50.30–31: ἔνθεν οἱ ἰατροί φασιν ἔπεσθαι ταῖς κράσεσι τοῦ σώματος τὰς τῆς ψυχῆς δυνάμεις. Cf. 51.13–14, 51.30–31; at 51.16, 21, 28 and 33 ὁρμή or ὁρμαί is substituted for δυνάμεις. πάθη (mentioned in the Aristotelian text being discussed, 403a 16) are also referred to in this context. The Galenic treatise is ὅτι ταῖς τοῦ σώματος κράσεσιν αἱ τῆς ψυχῆς δυνάμεις ἕπονται (*Quod animi mores corporis temperamenta sequantur*) at IV 767–822K; ed. I. Muller (Leipzig, 1891) (= *Galeni Scripta Minora*, II). Cf. Pt. III below for further discussion of this topic.

[19] *De an.* 274.8–9: δηλοῦσι δὲ καὶ αἱ περὶ χρείας μορίων τῶν ἰατρῶν πραγματεῖαι ὅτι οὐδὲ τὸ ἐλάχιστον ἔργον τῆς φύσεως μάτην ἐστίν, ἀλλ' ἕνεκά του. The καί links this with a general reference to Aristotle's *Physics*.

[20] Cf. Pt. II below for examples of this.

[21] E.g., *De an.* 23.21–23, 57.9–11; *Anal. post.*, at CAG XIII:3, ed. M. Wallies (Berlin, 1909), 34.24–35.1, 146.17–25; cf. 100.25–31. Cf. earlier, and more briefly, Themistius, *Anal. post.*, CAG V:1, ed. M. Wallies (Berlin, 1900), 25.25. Aristotle, however, envisages a certain type of doctor being a φυσικός; cf. *De sensu*, 436a 17–436b 1 and *De resp.*, 480b 23–30.

[22] *Phys.*, at CAG XVI, ed. H. Vitelli (Berlin, 1887), 232.27–30, 240.11–15. Cf. Galen, *Anat. adm.*, II.2, II.286K (= Galen, *Procedures* [trans. Singer], 31–32), for a classification of different approaches to the study of nature in terms of their theoretical or practical aspects. As with Philoponus, the study of nature in order to show that it has a purpose is distinguished from the applied art of medicine.

II. Philoponus, Aristotle, and Medical Ideas

We can introduce the first group of examples with a case reflecting a common philosophical ground between Philoponus, Aristotle, and Galen. The ubiquitous Aristotelian principle that nature does nothing in vain naturally met with a neoplatonic commentator's approval, and it was with reference to it that he cited the doctors' discussion of the use of parts mentioned earlier.[23] In other contexts he goes further and introduces Galenic anatomical detail as evidence of the natural teleology that Aristotle identifies. He thus praises nature's protection of the ear and eye by giving (non-Aristotelian) accounts of the acoustic nerve, and of the lens, aqueous humor, and cornea.[24] Again, in the course of elaborating Aristotle's claim[25] that breath exists both to maintain internal heat, and for the purpose of speech, which involves "living well" (εὖ ζῆν), he identifies the pharynx, larynx, trachea, and the three associated cartilages.[26] This can be regarded as a simplified version of Galen's account at *De usu partium* VII.11,[27] but set in a context dominated, like that treatise, by a philosophical concern with natural teleology.

In our other examples medical data accord with the more strictly factual matters that Philoponus saw as the concern of the medical art. They mostly involve the operation of the faculties associated with the brain, heart, and liver. The liver is identified, contrary to Aristotle but following Galen, as the source of blood; indeed in passages from the commentary on the *De generatione et corruptione* that I have examined elsewhere we find Philoponus assimilating the principles of Galen's account of digestion and nutrition as a supplement to Aristotle's account of nutrition in Book I chapter 5 of that treatise.[28] Since the heart is not of great significance in the psychology of Aristotle's *De anima* it is not discussed much in Philoponus' commentary, and

it is only in another work that he shows knowledge of the Galenic vital pneuma being generated in the heart.[29] As the locus of the sensory faculties the brain was regarded as the central organ of the body, and Philoponus quotes medical evidence in support of this view that recalls some Galenic texts. He refers to the application to the brain of the instrument called the μηνιγγοφύλαξ that was used in trepanning, and its having the effect of rendering an animal immobile and without sensation,[30] but notes that where the spine was injured or "bound" only the lower part of the body was affected while the upper part continued to function.[31] The latter case may be a distant reference to Galen's descriptions of transverse incisions of the spine.[32]

Close attention is given to the anatomy of the eye and the mechanism of vision.[33] Of the tunics of the eye the cornea (ὁ κερατοειδής), and the iris and choroid membrane (ὁ ῥαγοειδής) are named along with the crystalline moisture (τὸ κρυσταλλοειδές—the lens) and the aqueous humor (τὸ φοειδές).[34] Vision is said to occur through the optical pneuma passing along the optic nerve and reaching the crystalline body (the lens) where, as Philoponus says, "it has its terminations" and where "the discrimination of sense objects occurs."[35] This account differs in one important respect from Galen's, in that there is no extramission of the optical pneuma into the surrounding air.[36] This is rejected partly on the grounds that such a theory of vision would involve material light rays, an explanation that Philoponus

[23] Cf. note 19 above.

[24] *De an.* 364.15–32 (on the ear), and 364.32–365.2 (on the eye); the discussion is apropos Aristotle, *De anima* II.8, 420a 3–4.

[25] *De anima* II.8, 420b 16–22.

[26] *De an.* 381.22–382.3. Ammonius, *De int.*, at CAG IV:4, ed. A. Busse (Berlin, 1897), 24.33–25.6 gives a much briefer description of the organs of speech in referring to the views of οἱ ἰατροί (24.33).

[27] At 381.22–26 Philoponus distinguishes between ἡ φάρυγξ, pharynx proper, and ὁ φάρυγξ, or the larynx. I have not established a Galenic antecedent for this distinction in gender. From V. Nutton's note on Galen, *On Prognosis*, 5 XIV.628K, at CMG V, 8, 1, on p. 96.27–98.4, I would suspect that there is none.

[28] See "Galenic Medical Ideas," 118–20. To the reference there add Philop. *De an.* 119.33–34, where the liver is identified as τὸ τοῦ αἵματος ἐργαστήριον.

[29] *De aet. mund.* 396.27–397.2 Rabe. Cf. also note 58 below.

[30] *De an.* 19.8–11. The closest parallel is Galen, *De Plac. Hippocr. et Plat.*, I. 6, V.186K (= Galen, *Doctrines* [ed. De Lacy], 78.33 to 80.3). Cf. also *De loc. affect.* IV.3, VIII.232K, or II.10, VIII.128K. On this instrument see Puschmann at *Alexander*, I, 534, note 1.

[31] *De an.* 19.11–15.

[32] Cf. *De loc. affect.*, III.14, VIII.290K; and *Anat. adm.*, VIII.9, II.696–698K. (Singer, *Procedures*, 221–22).

[33] I omit discussion of passages showing knowledge of the anatomy and process of hearing and smelling; e.g., 364.15–32 (cf. 353.32–33), 433.32–33.

[34] Note especially the gloss on τὸ ἐπὶ τῇ κόρῃ δέρμα (Aristot., *De an.* II.8, 420a 14–15) at Philop., *De an.* 368.1–3: ἢ καὶ ἁπλούστερον κόρην ἀκουστέον κατὰ τὸ σύνηθες αὐτὸ τὸ τρῆμα τοῦ ῥαγοειδοῦς, τὸ δὲ ἐπὶ ταύτῃ δέρμα τὸν κερατοειδῆ . . . χιτῶνα. Cf. also Simplic., *De an.* 144.29. For the humors mentioned see e.g., 336.34–35 (κρυσταλλοειδές) and 350.24–33 (on the relation between the κρυσταλλοειδές and φοειδές).

[35] *De an.* 336.33–35; cf. 337.13–16, 350.24–26.

[36] Thus at *De Plac. Hippocr. et Plat.* VII.5, V.623K (= Galen, *Doctrines* [ed. DeLacy], 460.2–3) Galen refers to the air becoming an ὄργανον πρὸς τὴν τῶν αἰσθητῶν οἰκείαν διάγνωσιν. Philoponus claims that the ὀπτικὸν πνεῦμα at the lens causes the κρίσις τῶν ὁρατῶν (350.25–26). Also note the denial of the extramission of πνεύματα at 339.4–5.

follows Aristotle in rejecting in favor of the view that light is the actualization of the transparent medium, and that vision occurs when the eye encounters such incorporeal actualizations.[37] The Galenic account is thus limited to the internal mechanism of vision, while the external situation is explained in Aristotelian terms. Apparently a similar compromise was reached by the later commentators, Averroes and Albertus Magnus, who shared Philoponus' knowledge of Galenic principles and used it in a similarly eclectic effort to maintain Aristotelian orthodoxy.[38]

Philoponus also spends considerable effort on refuting the view for which, as far as I know, there is no precedent, that when a "congealed fluid" (χυμὸς συνιστάμενος) on the surface of the eye is perceived as being outside it, then vision must be occurring by the extramission of πνεύματα that project this obstruction.[39] He argues *inter alia* that this effect is just analogous to vision through a colored mirror,[40] and reasons that such rheums are themselves visible because there is a medium within the eye between the lens and the cornea outside which the rheum is formed.[41] Now while there may be a parallel in Galen for the pathological case in-

volved here,[42] there is no indication that he used it to defend the extramission theory of vision. Again, while Galen's theory of vision in *De Placitis Hippocratis et Platonis* Book VII certainly includes criticism of the Aristotelian position defended by Philoponus, this commentator cannot be responding directly to that earlier discussion.[43]

Finally we must look at the internal senses, as they were known in medieval psychological theory. The division of these into the imaginative, the ratiocinative, and the commemorative, and their location in respectively the front ventricles, the middle ventricle, and the back ventricle of the brain, is a doctrine that Galen hints at rather than specifies.[44] Like the theory of three pneumata, it soon became part of an established Galenism and is codified in Nemesius of Emesa's *De natura hominis*.[45] In one passage Philoponus speaks of the sympathetic interaction between these ventricles, and the location of the memory in the back ventricle.[46] For the full system though, we have to turn to a passage in Sophonias' paraphrase of his commentary on *De an-*

---

[37] This is developed in a lengthy note on Aristotle, *De an.* II.7, 418b 9–10 at 324.25–342.16. The passage at 325.6–326.37 deals specifically with the emission of light rays. The whole subject of Philoponus' theory of light has recently been dealt with in detail by J. A. Christensen, "Aristotle and Philoponus on Light," (Diss., Harvard, 1979). The aspect of Philoponus' account noted here is, it should be stressed, one part of a larger picture developed in this thesis. I am grateful to Dr. Christensen for letting me see a copy of her thesis.

[38] See *Averroes: Epitome of Parva Naturalia*, trans. H. Blumberg (Cambridge, Mass., 1961), 18. For Albertus see the discussion in D. C. Lindberg, *Theories of Vision from Al-Kindi to Kepler* (Chicago/London, 1976), 105. On the rejection of Galen's theory of vision see also Temkin, *Galenism*, 122 with note 73.

[39] *De an.* 336.3–339.16. This χυμός is clearly a sore of some kind. Cf. 350.20–21 where ὑπόχυμα (a term that can mean "cataract") is used interchangeably with ὁ συνεστὼς χυμός. For συνίστασθαι meaning "to be compact" see LSJ, *s.v.* συνίστημι, B.V.

[40] See *De an.* 338.8–339.16, at 338.20–24. A series of other examples follows.

[41] *De an.* 350.24–351.7 apropos Aristotle, *De an.* II.7, 419a 11–13, where it is said that a colored object placed on the organ of vision eliminates sight because the intervening transparency is eliminated. On this same topic it is worth noting that at *De an.* 292.19–20 Philoponus says that we do not perceive our own sense organs because there is no intervening air: διὸ τῆς λήμης ἐν τῷ ὀφθαλμῷ οὔσης οὐκ ἀντιλαμβανόμεθα. The apparatus criticus shows λήμης to be written in an erasure by a second hand, while μήλης is found in another manscript. We can, I suggest, correct the latter case of iatism to μήλης, and accept it as the true reading partly in the light of the parallel at Olympiodorus, *Comm. on Phaedo* 4.7.7–8 Westerink. He refers to sense perception being defective because it recognizes only objects at a distance and adds: ἐπεὶ τὸν πυρῆνα τῆς μήλης τὸν ἐν τῷ ὀφθαλμῷ οὐχ ὁρᾷ, καὶ ἡ ἀφὴ δὲ διὰ μέσου ἀέρος ἀντιλαμβάνεται. This is essentially the Aristotelian context in which Philoponus' point

is made; cf. *De an.* 419a 20, and Philop. *De an.* 219.19. In another context I think that μήλη should probably be read at *De an.* 351.10, 15, 25, 27, 38. N.b. 351.25 where the reference to a ὑελίνη λήμη (a glass sore!) can hardly be plausible. Equally, doubt is now thrown on the reading λήμη in the discussion at 415.38–416.16.

[42] E.g., in the discussion of trachoma at *De compositione medicamentorum secundum locos*, IV.2, XII.709–711K, there is a reference to such a rheum. (I owe this reference to Emilie Savage-Smith.) But at *De Plac. Hippocr. et Plat.* VII.4, V.635–636K (Galen, *Doctrines* [ed. DeLacy], p. 468.2–6) cataracts are described as blocking optical pneuma; this presupposes extramission, and does not prove it.

[43] Thus Galen argues (1) that Aristotle cannot explain how we recognize the position, size, or distance of a perceived object (VII.7, V.637–639K [Galen, *Doctrines* (ed. DeLacy), pp. 470.17–472.2]), and (2) that he in fact invokes a theory of extramission in the explanation of rainbows (VII.7, V.639–641K [*Doctrines* (DeLacy), p. 472.3–24]). The latter must be a reference to Aristotle, *Meteorologica* III.3–4 (cf. especially 373b 33). Regarding (1) Philoponus deals only with the question of vision at a distance, and that only with reference to the general theory of vision by extramission and not to the case of πνεύματα; see *De an.* 334.30–336.3. As for (2), Aristotle is defended at 333.19–35 on the ground that he used this explanation as a hypothesis, but again the point is made in an entirely general context.

[44] *De sympt. diff.*, at VII.56K where the division into φανταστικόν, διανοητικόν, and μνημονευτικόν is found. Memory is associated with the back ventricle at *De loc. affect.*, III.9, VIII.173–175K.

[45] *De nat. hom.* chap. 13, pp. 204–6 Matthaei; cf. chap. 6, p. 173 Matth., and chap. 12, p. 201 Matth. On the codification of the three Galenic "spirits" see O. Temkin, "On Galen's Pneumatology," *Gesnerus*, 8 (1951), 180–89 (= *Double Face of Janus*, chap. 9). It would be perhaps profitable to compare and contrast Nemesius' and Philoponus' use of Galenic ideas in the search for the elusive Galenism available to non-medical authors in later antiquity.

[46] *De an.* 155.27–31.

imu III.3, a section that admittedly has no parallel
in the medieval Latin translation as an additional
control, but which can be fairly confidently attributed to Philoponus.[47]

In considering the senses and the sub-faculties
located in the brain we have moved to the limits of
a survey of purely anatomical and physiological
material, and are entering the wider field of the
general theory of the soul. For if the brain is the
central organ of the body, then its faculties must in
some way define the soul. We have so far said nothing about Philoponus' theory of the soul, nor about
its possible affect on his assimilation of medical material. That will be our concern next as we bring
his neoplatonism into the picture.

III. Philoponus, Neoplatonism, and Medical Ideas

We can best approach this issue through Galen's
own reflections about the status of pneuma in the
brain. He remarks in the *De Placitis Hippocratis et
Platonis* that if the soul is incorporeal "the pneuma
is, so to speak, its first home (πρῶτον οἰκτήριον),"
but if it is corporeal it is identical with the pneuma.[48]
And in a related passage he describes the relation
between the incorporeal soul and the pneuma as
one in which the latter was its "first vehicle (πρῶτον
ὄχημα)."[49] Galen himself may have vacillated about
the nature of the soul,[50] though in the *De Placitis*
he opts for the position that the pneuma was its
ὄργανον and that the soul itself was located not in
the ventricles but "in the actual body of the brain."[51]
We however need only emphasize that his account
of the status of the incorporeal soul in relation to
pneuma schematizes the theory found elaborated
in later neoplatonic psychology,[52] a theory that affects the way in which medical ideas are assimilated.

The account in question, as expounded in the
proem to Philoponus' commentary, envisages the
soul as preexisting and descending to a temporary
sojourn in the physical body. In this descent the
rational soul is complemented by the faculties of
the irrational soul—sensation, thumos, and desire;
these are said to inhere in a substrate, pneuma, that
serves as their vehicle (ὄχημα) in their descent into
a body that will have the vegetative functions that
will complete the hierarchy of souls in a living human being.[53] The sources of this theory and its
various elaborations need not concern us.[54] We need
only note that the three faculties of the irrational
soul are also involved, respectively, in the operation of the organs of brain, heart, and liver, that
we have been discussing. But they are said to have
a unity and identity independent of the body, and
this is expressed through a concept, pneuma, that
can also be used to explain the various psychical
functions of the body. What is the relation between
these two roles?

Our question is not formally raised. We do, however, encounter one passage in which both roles of
pneuma are acknowledged.[55] Here Philoponus argues that the removal of cataracts shows that the
faculty of perception is not itself a body that can
be affected by organic changes because "it has its
being not in our physical body but in the pneuma"
(the pneumatic substrate of the irrational soul, that
is).[56] But he goes on to illustrate this by referring
to the deterioration in the humors and tunics of
the eyes of old people; this, he says, blocks access
to the optical pneuma without the actual faculty of
perception being affected.[57] The faculty itself is then
an incorporeal (an unaffected) aspect of the pneumatic substrate, while the operations of the faculty
can involve sensory pneuma. The two accounts are

---

[47] Sophon., *De an.* 117.23–30. On the value of Sophonias in
reconstructing Philoponus see S. Van Riet, "Fragments de l'original grec du 'de Intellectu' de Philopon dans une compilation
de Sophonias," *Revue Philosophique de Louvain*, 63 (1965), 5–40.

[48] *De Plac. Hippocr. Plat.* VII.3, V.602K (= Galen, *Doctrines*
[ed. DeLacy], pp. 442.36–444.2).

[49] *De Plac. Hippocr. Plat.* VII.7, V.644K (= Galen, *Doctrines*
[ed. DeLacy], p. 474.26).

[50] For a recent discussion see P. Moraux, "Galien et Aristote,"
in *Images of Man in Ancient and Medieval Thought: Studia G. Verbeke . . . dicata* (Louvain, 1976), 127–46 at 136–42.

[51] *De Plac. Hippocr. Plat.*, VII.3, V.602K (= Galen, *Doctrines*
[ed. DeLacy], p. 444.4–6).

[52] This pasage is discussed in E. R. Dodds' discussion of the
development of this theory at *Proclus: The Elements of Theology*,
2nd ed. (Oxford, 1963), Appendix II, 316–17.

[53] Cf. *De an.* 5.29–33 for the acquisition of the irrational soul
in γένεσις. Also, note 18.15–16, and 52.4–7 for the acquisition
of πάθη in the descent of the soul into the physical body. For
pneuma as the substrate and vehicle of the irrational soul see
17.19–23. On the vegetative soul being inseparable from the
physical body see 16.26–17.19.

[54] In addition to Dodd's discussion cited in note 52 above see
A. Smith, *Porphyry's Place in the Neoplatonic Tradition* (The Hague,
1974), 152–58. This story is often presented as that of the three
"tunics," or vehicles of the soul, since in addition to the pneuma
and the physical body, the soul also has a "luminous vehicle"
that survives purification after death and is indestructible. The
latter aspect is touched on by Philoponus at *De an.* 18.22–33.

[55] *De an.* 161.3–27 à propos Aristotle, *De an.* 408b 20–22 where
in the context of a discussion of whether the intellect itself de-
cays, reference is made to the fact that an old man would have
the vision of a young man if he acquired a new eye.

[56] *De an.* 161.18–21.

[57] *De an.* 161.21–27.

set at different levels, and this presumably explains why metaphysics and medicine can be combined in this commentary.[58]

There are, however, passages in which the unity of the three faculties of the irrational soul in pneuma does place constraints on the implications of certain medical evidence. We mentioned above that the relation of the brain to the lower organs was in one place established with reference to certain clinical and pathological data (the application of the μηνιγγοφύλαξ, etc.).[59] In a subsequent passage this evidence is recapitulated,[60] but the commentator stresses that it does not prove that the three faculties are spatially separate. In neoplatonic terminology, the different organs in which they are located are differently suited for illumination by the faculties, but there is a continuity between them because those faculties are "related to the pneuma just as the vegetative faculties are to the tree, and they completely pervade pneuma."[61] In this way the wider psychological theory establishes a framework within which the medical evidence can be exploited in ways that we have already observed. This position does, however, create an ambivalence about certain passages. For example, Philoponus describes φαντασία as being "in the pneuma,"[62] and refers to pneuma as "the primary organ and vehicle of the senses."[63] In another place it is said to be "the common sense-organ of all the senses" because the common sense is located in it.[64] In such cases the unifying role of pneuma as a substrate overlaps with its functional role in the explanation of sensation and no real distinction can be drawn between the two.

It is worth adding that this particular combination of medicine and metaphysics may have evolved

in response to another neoplatonic version of the relation between the pneumatic vehicle and the body. Philoponus cites, and criticizes, an account (of which versions can be found in Proclus and Porphyry) to the effect that embodied pneuma risks pollution by a bad diet, and that the result of this would be a posthumous existence as a ghost around one's tomb.[65] This theory held no attraction for Philoponus. Among his criticisms is this dilemma.[66] Either those upholding this view must deny that the soul is distributed in the organs of the body (διωργανεῖσθαι), in which case the soul will not be the ἐντελέχεια of an organic body, as Aristotle had claimed, or they must grant that the soul is distributed in this way, and thus divided along with the parts of the body (i.e., the faculties are physically separate). Now we have seen that Philoponus rejects the latter option because of the basic unity of the faculties of the irrational soul in the pneuma. On the other hand he did think that there was a relation between those faculties and different organs, both on the evidence of medical data and in the light of the neoplatonic theory of illuminations from above. This position of compromise has to exclude the theory of pneuma as a substance in a condition often metaphorically described as one of threatened pollution by the body, "weighed down" or "nourished by material vapors" as Porphyry and Proclus put it. Part of the reason for Philoponus' position undoubtedly lies in the fact that he saw the relation between pneuma and the organic body in the neutral terms of medical theory, where an analysis of function excluded any moralizing notion of the pollution of the soul by the body.[67]

---

[58] At *De an.* 64.6–17 there is related support for this point. The discussion turns on the relation between θυμός and the body; θυμός is said to be in reason and τὸ πνεῦμα, but reason moves desire by means of pneuma, while pneuma moves the blood around the heart by means of desire. The basic physiology here may be Aristotelian rather than Galenic, but there is also a dual role assigned to the pneuma, as the substrate of a psychic faculty (cf. 64.14–15, where it is said to be separable from the physical body) and also as an agent in the operation of that faculty.

[59] Above, Part II, with note 28.

[60] *De an.* 201.1–15 apropos 411b 19–20, a query about the unity of the soul, given that plants and certain insects survive when divided.

[61] *De an.* 201.19–32. The translation is of 201.31–32.

[62] *De an.* 158.15–20; cf. Simplicius, *De an.* 214.4, 216.26–27. Cf. also Philop., 194.28–195.10 for a similar point about Plato's account of the organic distribution of the faculties in the *Timaeus*; there, however, there is no reference to the pneuma.

[63] *De an.* 162.14–15.

[64] *De an.* 433.34–35; cf. 438.34–35.

[65] *De an.* 19.18–20.9. There are, very briefly put, two aspects to this account: (1) the claim that the pneuma is polluted by being "thickened" by a bad diet in that it is "nourished by breaths" (δι' ἀτμῶν, 19.25–26); and (2) the theory that such pollution can cause visibility. On (1) cf. Proclus, *In Tim.* III, 331.6–9 Diehl, and *In rempub.* I, 119.11 Kroll; and Prophyry, *De ant. nymph.* 64.9–21 Nauck. On (2) cf. Plato, *Phaedo* 81c-d, Porphyry, *De ant. nymph.* 64.15–21 Nauck, *Sententiae* 29, 18.10–13 Lamberz, and Proclus, *In rempub.* II, 156.25–157.8, and 164.19–27 Kroll. These references are merely intended to suggest a background for the theory attacked by Philoponus; its details deserve closer attention.

[66] *De an.* 239.15–38, in response to a restatement of the view described in the previous note at 239.2–15. The Aristotelian text on which the debate is based is 413b 13–16, where Aristotle asks whether the faculties of the soul are themselves souls, or parts of the soul, and whether they are theoretically or physically separable.

[67] The view that θυμός and ἐπιθυμία are associated with the soul after death, and are involved in its purification, is developed at *De an.* 18.10–22 but in rather abstract terms.

Finally let us briefly note that neoplatonic psychology also conditions Philoponus' rejection of a Galenic doctrine that we mentioned earlier, the doctors' view "that the faculties of the soul follow the temperaments of the body."[68] I have considered elsewhere the exegetical context of this passage.[69] Here we shall see that the notion of the preexistent soul is a decisive consideration in his critique.[70] The commentator thus argues that the separable rational soul can oppose the dictates of the body; this means that mental conflict can occur, and that we can be said to act freely.[71] As for the πάθη of the soul, these are said to be an endowment of the soul "as it descends to creation;" they have, that is, pneuma as their substrate prior to embodiment, and although the κρᾶσις of the physical body may be a necessary condition for their embodiment they cannot be identified with it, or with any "product" (ἀποτέλεσμα) of it, as the medical theory envisages.[72] In neoplatonic language, the forms of the πάθη of the soul are engendered by "creative reasons" (δημιουργικοὶ λόγοι) in a "suitable blend of the elements."[73] This metaphysical superiority is emphasized finally by the claim that to deny the πάθη this status would be to make the worse (the κρᾶσις) the cause of the better, or something inanimate the cause of life, a line of criticism used elsewhere against the general theory, also attributed to "the doctors," that the soul is a κρᾶσις of the elements.[74]

A diametrical opposition emerges here between the medical explanation of the soul from matter "upwards," as a κρᾶσις of the elements, and the philosophical analysis of the soul's preexistence and metaphysical independence from the body. In this confrontation there is little sign that Philoponus has penetrated much beyond the title of the relevant Galenic treatise. He does claim that the doctors themselves admit that with the help of philosophy temperament may be resisted,[75] and this could be a reflection of Galen's own attempt in chapter 11 of the *Quod animi mores* to mitigate the deterministic implications of his general position. But otherwise Philoponus has invoked a Galenic principle as the occasion for the restatement of the first principles of his psychological theory. The contribution of medicine is relegated to defining the κρᾶσις of the elements; thereafter the philosopher takes over, and sets this factual data in its appropriate philosophical context. Here, as in all the examples that we have surveyed, medical material is firmly controlled by philosophical principles.

To conclude: the use of medical ideas represents only a minor aspect of Philoponus' exegetical output, yet its importance in his commentary on the *De anima* lies in the fact, noted at the outset, that it has no equal in the ancient and Byzantine Aristotelian tradition, not even when commentaries were written on medically more suggestive Aristotelian treatises. I have not, as I warned and explained earlier, been able to establish a clear historical context for my evidence. I hope though that something has been achieved by demonstrating that this early Byzantine commentary on Aristotle's *De anima*, whatever its precise antecedents, is a minor but noteworthy episode in the long history of the interaction between philosophy and medicine, as well as further evidence of the importance of the Philoponan corpus for the history of science in late antiquity.[76]

University of British Columbia

---

[68] See Part I, with note 18 above.

[69] See "Galenic Medical Ideas," 124–26.

[70] For an antecedent of Philoponus' critique see Proclus, *In Tim.* III, 349.21–350.8 Diehl.

[71] *De an.* 52.1–4.

[72] *De an.* 52.4–13. Cf. Philop., *De gen. et corr.* 164.4–19 for this argument against "the doctors'" theory of mixture. Cf. my paper "Some Concepts" (cited in note 2 above), 164.

[73] *De an.* 52.13–21. See "Some Concepts," 162–64 on this type of argument.

[74] *De an.* 52.22–25. Cf. *De an.* 35.27–30 for a similar argument against the general theory that the soul is a κρᾶσις. That theory is identified in an introductory doxography at *De an.* 9.21–35, and attributed to "the doctors" at 33.2. For an identification of the Galenic theory of the soul in these terms on the basis of the treatise *Quod animi mores corporis temperamenta sequantur* see Nemesius, *De nat. hom.* chap. 2, p. 86 Matth.

[75] *De an.* 51.29–34.

[76] Part of the research for this paper was conducted under grants from the Social Sciences and Humanities Research Council of Canada.

THE *HIPPIATRICA* AND BYZANTINE VETERINARY MEDICINE

ANNE-MARIE DOYEN-HIGUET

The history of veterinary medicine has not received the attention it deserves, although there is no lack of veterinary texts. I shall focus my discussion here on one branch of veterinary medicine, hippiatrics or horse medicine, which was particularly well developed as far back as in antiquity. With regard to Latin sources there are a number of important works: chapters 27–38 of Book VI of Columella's treatise *De re rustica*;[1] a large part of Pelagonius' treatise (recently re-edited by K. D. Fischer);[2] the *Mulomedicina Chironis*;[3] three of the four books of Vegetius;[4] paragraphs 22–28 of Book XIV of *De veterinaria medicina* of Palladius' agricultural treatise.[5] With regard to Greek sources we are less fortunate: the original writings of the Greek hippiatric authors, whose activity extended approximately from the third to the fifth century A.D.,[6] are not extant in their original form; there remains only a collection of excerpts.[7] The questions raised by the chronology, the structure, and the manuscript tradition of this compilation of texts are difficult and complex; the study of the individual texts requires considerable preliminary philological and editorial work. I propose now to provide a general survey of these Greek hippiatric texts[8] and to conclude with a few comments on the utilization of their contents and on their purpose.

THE SOURCES OF THE ORIGINAL *COLLECTION* AND THEIR CHRONOLOGY

In the original *Collection* of Greek hippiatric texts, seven authors were drawn on: Apsyrtos, Anatolios, Eumelos, Theomnestos, Hippocrates, Hierocles and Pelagonius. For every subject, the writer took the excerpts which he had found in his sources and arranged them in the alphabetical order of the names of the authors.[9] These sources were obviously not selected according to originality, and hippiatric authors repeat one another in many places in the *Collection*. They sometimes quote their predecessors, and this information is of great importance for the often difficult task of determining their chronology, which unfortunately has been, and still remains, uncertain.

Chronology hinges on the date of Apsyrtos. His work is cast in the form of letters. He writes at the

[The reader is referred to the list of abbreviations at the end of the volume.]

[1] Columella, *On Agriculture*, edited and translated by E. S. Forster and E. H. Heffner, II, Loeb Classical Library (London, 1954), 188–227.

[2] Fischer, ed., *Pelagonius*.

[3] Oder, ed., *Mulomedicina Chironis*.

[4] Lommatzsch, ed., *Vegetius*, 1–277. Book IV, taken straight from Columella, also survives, but deals with farm animals.

[5] Rodgers, ed., *Palladius*, 265, 6–272, 11. See also 135, 23–139, 18 (IV, 13–15); 283, 11–291, 10 (XIV, 39–65) *passim*.

[6] On the earlier works dealing with horses in Greek literature—Simon of Athen's treatise, Xenophon's *De re equestri*, Aristotle's *Historia animalium* (esp. V, 14; VI, 18 and 22–24; VIII, 8 and 24–25)—see K. D. Fischer, "Pelagonius on Horse Medicine," *Papers of the Liverpool Latin Seminar*, 3 (1981), 287.

[7] E. Oder and K. Hoppe, eds., *Corpus Hippiatricorum Graecorum*, I. *Hippiatrica Berolinensia* (Leipzig, 1924), II. *Hippiatrica Parisina Cantabrigiensia Londinensia Lugdunensia—Appendix* (Leipzig, 1927) (repr. Stuttgart, 1971); henceforth abbreviated as *CHG*. Book XVI of the *Geoponica* must be added to it (Beckh, ed., *Geoponica*, 451–68). The passages which are not contained in the *Collection* are published in the Appendix of Oder and Hoppe's edition (*CHG*, II, 325, 17–330, 15).

[8] I have already dealt with numerous problems raised by Greek hippiatric texts in an article entitled "Les textes d'hippiatrie grecque. Bilan et perspectives," *AntCl*, 50 (1981), 258–73. My present contribution complements this discussion and clears up some points. It also outlines the findings of my research, carried on during the last two years, which forms the subject matter of my Ph.D. thesis ("Un manuel grec de médecine vétérinaire. Histoire du texte, édition critique traduite et commentée. Contribution à l'étude du *Corpus Hippiatricorum Graecorum*," 5 vols. [in typescript, Louvain-La-Neuve, 1983]).

[9] The alphabetical order followed, of course, the Greek alphabet and took only the first letter of the word into account. This explains why, for instance, Anatolios follows Apsyrtos.

beginning of his letter on fever that he took part in a military campaign on the banks of the Danube (*CHG*, I, 1). This information recurs in the *Suda* (A 4739, *s.v.* Ἄψυρτος), which introduces Apsyrtos as a soldier and adds that the campaign took place in Scythia in the reign of the emperor Constantine:[10]

Ἄψυρτος, Προυσαεύς, Νικομηδεύς,[11] στρατιώτης, στρατευσάμενος ἐπὶ Κωνσταντίνου τοῦ βασιλέως ἐν Σκυθίᾳ παρὰ τὸν Ἴστρον. Ἱππιατρικὸν βιβλίον οὗτος ἔγραψεν καὶ φυσικὸν περὶ τῶν αὐτῶν ἀλόγων καὶ ἕτερα. . . .[12]

This information has been interpreted variously.

K. Sprengel first assigned Apsyrtos to the seventh century A.D., under the reign of Constantine IV Pogonates (668–685), who tried in vain to stop the Bulgarian expansion; he then dated Vegetius,[13] who quotes Apsyrtos, in the twelfth or thirteenth century A.D..[14] Later he admitted that he had

made a mistake, and assigned Apsyrtos to the fourth century A.D..[15] This dating was for a long time accepted, and it was generally agreed that the emperor in question was Constantine I (306–337), although opinions still diverged as to which campaigns were involved: some scholars believed that Apsyrtos took part in Constantine's campaign against the Sarmatians, from 320 to 323 A.D.;[16] others preferred the battles which Constantine fought successfully from 332 to 334 A.D. against the Goths, who were attacking the Sarmatians from Banat.[17]

G. Björck first took into account the difficulties arising from the date of Theomnestos.[18] Ch. Heusinger, who had only S. Grynaeus' edition[19] at his disposal, believed that Theomnestos was Theodoric the Great's (493–526) personal veterinary surgeon, and that he had been with him during his campaigns in Pannonia and Italy in 489 A.D.[20] Heusinger based his argument on information provided by Theomnestos at the beginning of his article on tetanus, where he states that he accompanied the emperor as a friend on his departure from Pannonia for Italy across the Alps (*CHG*, I, 183, 21–184, 6). The Parisinus Graecus 2322, however, has preserved a better text of this episode, which makes Heusinger's hypothesis hardly plausible. The additions of the Parisinus Graecus 2322 are shown between oblique brackets in the edition of E. Oder and K. Hoppe, whose text is reproduced here:

---

[10] Adler, ed., *Suda*, I, 444. According to the editor, this article is inspired by the Ὀνοματόλογος by Hesychius of Miletus.

[11] Apsyrtos' only homeland mentioned in the *Collection* is Clazomenae (Bithynia) (*CHG*, II, 96, 23). Probably he practised mainly in Prusa and Nicomedia, which would explain why these two cities were associated with his name.

[12] "Apsyrtos from Prusa, Nicomedia, a soldier, took part in a military campaign under the reign of Emperor Constantine in Scythia along the Danube. He wrote a book about hippiatrics, a book of magical nature about the same animals, and on other subjects. . . ." (The punctuation [·] placed in this edition between ἀλόγων and καὶ ἕτερα should, in my view, be omitted). φυσικὸν may be interpreted in two ways: either it is an adjective and refers to βιβλίον, in which case Apsyrtos' hippiatric treatise would also bear a "magical" aspect, or it is a neuter noun and Apsyrtos wrote, besides his treatise on hippiatrics, also a treatise of magical nature dealing with horses as well. The presence of αὐτῶν makes us prefer the second solution.

[13] It is generally agreed that the author of the *Mulomedicina* (Publius Vegetius Renatus) and the author of the *Epitome rei militaris* (Flavius Vegetius Renatus) are one and the same person. The dating for the writing of this second book has been discussed; it must have been written under one of Gratian's successors since he was given the epithet "divus" (*Epit. rei milit. I, 20*). A. R. Neumann, *s.v.* Publius (Flavius) Vegetius Renatus, *R-E*, suppl. X (Stuttgart, 1965), coll. 992–93, summarizes the various opinions and decides upon Theodosius I (A.D. 379–395). More recently W. Goffart, "The Date and Purpose of Vegetius' *De re militari*," *Traditio*, 33 (1977), 65–100, decided upon Valentinian III (A.D. 425–455). He was criticized by T. D. Barnes, "The Date of Vegetius," *Phoenix*, 33 (1979), 254–57, who believes this emperor is Theodosius I; G. Sabbah, "Pour la datation théodosienne du *De re militari* de Végèce," *Centre J. Palerne, Mémoires*, II (Saint-Etienne, 1980), 131–55, concurs. The *Mulomedicina*, in which Apsyrtos is mentioned in the preface and in other passages (see ed. Lommatzsch, XXVIII and XXXVI–XLII), does not contain any information that might enable us to date it with any precision.

[14] K. Sprengel, *Versuch einer pragmatischen Geschichte der Arzneykunde*, II (Halle, 1823³), 318 and 322.

[15] K. Sprengel, *Geschichte der Botanik*, I (Leipzig and Altenburg, 1917), 191, and "De Apsyrto Bithynio, hippiatro," *Opuscula Academica*, ed. J. Rosenbaum (Leipzig, 1844), 110–16.

[16] J. F. K. Hecker, *Geschichte der Heilkunde. Nach den Quellen bearbeitet*, II (Berlin, 1829), 245–46; Ch. Heusinger, *Recherches de pathologie comparée*, I (Cassel, 1847), 17–18; A. Postolka, *Geschichte der Periode der empirischen Tierheilkunde* (Vienna, 1885), 91–92; A. Baranski, *Geschichte der Thierzucht und Thiermedicin im Alterthum* (Vienna, 1886; reprint Hildesheim, 1971), 82; L. Moulé, "Histoire de la médecine vétérinaire dans l'Antiquité," *Bulletin de la Société Centrale de Médecine Vétérinaire*, 44 (1890), 580.

[17] E. Oder, "Apsyrtus. Lebensbild des bedeutendsten altgriechischen Veterinärs," *Veterinärhistorisches Jahrbuch*, 2 (1926), 121; E. Leclainche, *Histoire illustrée de la médecine vétérinaire*, I (Paris, 1955), 96.

[18] G. Björck, *Apsyrtus, Julius Africanus et l'hippiatrique grecque* (Uppsala, 1944) (Uppsala Universitets Årsskrift, 1944,4), 7–12.

[19] The *editio princeps* of the theologian and humanist Simon Grynaeus, Τῶν ἱππιατρικῶν βιβλία δύο. *Veterinariae medicinae libri duo a Joanne Ruellio olim quidem latinitate donati, nunc vero iidem sua, hoc est Graeca lingua, primum in lucem editi* (Basle, 1537), contains only the B recension. It has not been determined yet whether the manuscript(s) on which it is based is (are) among the known manuscripts of the B recension or not.

[20] Ch. Heusinger, *Theomnestus, Leibthierarzt Theodorichs des Grossen, Königs der Ostgothen* (Giessen, 1843), and *Recherches*, I (n. 16 above), 21–24.

Τοῦτο δὲ ἔγνων ἐγὼ γενόμενος ἐπὶ ⟨ . . .ἡμέρας κατὰ Κάρνον τῆς⟩ Παννονίας, βασιλεῖ παρεπόμενος καὶ ὡς φίλος σὺν αὐτῷ διάγων.[21] ⟨Ἀθρόως οὖν ἠπείχθη διὰ γάμον, καὶ ἀπὸ τῆς Κάρνου κατ' ἀρχὰς τοῦ φεβρουαρίου μηνὸς ὤδευσε τεταμένως εἰς τὴν Ἰταλίαν, ὡς δύο καὶ τρεῖς μονὰς μίαν ποιῆσαι. Διελθόντων δὲ ἡμῶν πᾶσαν τὴν Νωρικὸν καὶ λοιπὸν ἐπὶ τὰς Ἄλπεις ἐπιβάντων τὰς Ἰουλίας καλουμένας,⟩ χιὼν ἐξαίφνης κατερράγη πολλὴ περὶ πρώτην ὥραν, ⟨ἀναβαινόντων τὰς Ἄλπεις. Τότε⟩ καὶ οἱ στρατιῶται ἐπὶ τοῖς ἵπποις παγέντες ἀπώλλυντο, καὶ ἔμενον ἐπὶ τῶν ἵππων συντεταμένοι.

According to this passage, the emperor's trip took place in early February and hurriedly because of a wedding. As M. Haupt has shown,[22] the passage appears to refer to the emperor Licinius, who left Carinthia in the late winter of 313 A.D. for Milan to marry Constantine's sister.[23] This consequently makes Theomnestos much younger, since he quotes Apsyrtos.[24]

Now, if we stick to the facts found in the texts of Apsyrtos and in the *Suda*, it would seem likely that Apsyrtos would have written his work only after the military campaign, which would have enabled him to perfect his art through his contact with the Sarmatians. Oder and Hoppe assumed that Theomnestos then wrote at an advanced age what he had seen as a young man.[25] Björck considered this explanation not acceptable, for the following reason: the manner in which Theomnestos describes his relationship to the emperor implies that they were close in age, "and Licinius got married, it seems, when he was well over sixty."[26] This statement of Björck, however, contradicts the testimony of Aurelius Victor, according to whom Licinius was near sixty when he died in 325 A.D.[27] Björck further argues that Theomnestos prides himself on Licinius' friendship in his book, and that therefore the book can not have been published after the year

324 A.D., which marked Licinius' fall and condemnation. Björck concludes that Theomnestos published his work between 313 and 324 A.D., and that Apsyrtos should be placed before this period. He thinks that the note in the *Suda* comes straight from Apsyrtos' text; "consequently its dating is a conjecture without any historical value."[28] But it is not easy to define Apsyrtos' time. Björck notes that the city of Constantinople is not mentioned by the veterinary surgeon and that the names of his addressees are with one exception[29] classical, both of which led him to date Apsyrtos before 313 A.D. On the other hand, he thinks he has found in Apsyrtos' writings a quotation from Xenocrates of Aphrodisias (second half of the first century A.D.), which provides a *terminus post quem*;[30] this is confirmed by prosopography (some names seem to imply the series of emperors up to Nerva) and onomastics (the surname Fronto, found, among other places, in the Danubian provinces in the second century A.D. and in the early third century A.D., appears four times).[31] Thus, Björck proposes to assign Apsyrtos' activity between the years 150 and 250 A.D., although he cannot substantiate this hypothesis with any certainty.

In passing, it should be noted that Apsyrtos gives the names of the addressees in his letters;[32] he also mentions authors, peoples, cities and countries;[33] finally he himself is quoted by some of his col-

---

[21] After διάγων B has καὶ δήποτε ἐπὶ Ἰταλίαν διαβαινόντων ἡμῶν καὶ τὰς καλουμένας Ἄλπεις. . . .

[22] M. Haupt, "Varia, LIV," *Hermes*, 5 (1871), 23–25.

[23] This marriage is discussed by several authors: Lactantius, *De morte persecutorum* 43, 2 and 45, 1; Aurelius Victor, *De Caesaribus* 41, 2 and *Epitome* 41, 4; Eutropius, *Breviarium* X, 5; Orosius *Hist. adversum paganos* VII, 28, 19; Zosimus, *Hist.* II, 17, 2; Socrates, *Hist. eccl.* I, 2, 10; *Anonymus Valesii* 5, 13.

[24] *CHG*, I, 273, 15.

[25] *CHG*, II, IX.

[26] Björck, "Apsyrtus" (n. 18 above), 8.

[27] Aurelius Victor, *Epitome* 41, 8. One should probably not take the term ἐσχατογήρως literally. Eusebius of Caesarea (*Hist. eccl.* X, 8, 13) applies it to Licinius in a passage in which he is indignant at the emperor's lack of respect and reserve towards married women and young girls.

[28] Björck, "Apsyrtus" (n. 18 above), 9.

[29] Perhaps only the name Ἐπιφάνιος (*CHG*, I, 131, 2) is Christian.

[30] Björck, "Apsyrtus" (n. 18 above), 11. He compares this article (*CHG*, II, 49, 1–3) with a similar passage in Galen (ed. Kühn, XIII 846, 13–847, 1), where the name of Xenocrates also appears; he refers to M. Wellmann, "Xenocrates aus Aphrodisias," *Hermes*, 42 (1907), 614–29, especially, 620; some of his statements have been slightly altered by F. Kudlien, *s.v.* Xenocrates aus Aphrodisias, *R-E*, II, IX, 2 (Stuttgart, 1967), coll. 1529–31.

[31] Björck, "Apsyrtus" (n. 18 above), 12. He refers to L. R. Dean's thesis, *A Study of the Cognomina of Soldiers in the Roman Legions* (Princeton, 1916), 30, which I have not been able to consult, and goes so far as to identify one of Apsyrtos' addressees (*CHG*, I, 263, 48) with a certain Valerius Fronto, known in 155 (see *CIL* III, suppl. I, 7449).

[32] For an almost complete list of these, see *CHG*, I, pp. 451–52. There should be added: Γέλων ἱπποίατρος (Parisinus Graecus 2244, fol. 170ᵛ); Κιόστινος Μοσχίων, "Apsyrtos' doctor" (τῷ ἑαυτοῦ ἰατρῷ) (*CHG*, II, 96, 23–24); Οὖρσος στρατηλάτης (*CHG*, II, 216, 16–17); Παπίας Ἰοῦστος (Parisinus Graecus 2244, fol. 172ʳ); Πούπλιος Ἰούλιος Σπανός (Parisinus Graecus 2244, foll. 107ʳ and 171ᵛ); Ῥώμυλος ἑκατόνταρχος (*CHG*, II, 180, 22–23).

[33] Apsyrtos quotes Eumelos (*CHG*, I, 17, 10; 56, 17–18; 57, 23) and Mago (I, 168, 18–19 and II, 90, 20). Apart from the Danube, he mentions the Parthians (I, 77, 17 and 21), the Alexandrines (I, 96, 8), the Sarmatians (I, 97, 21; 102, 15; II, 70, 1) and their country (I, 102, 27–28) the Cappadocians (I, 425, 21) and the Syrians (I, 426, 2). As to the foreign names of the

leagues.[34] The study of this data, however, does not enable us to draw any literary or epigraphic parallel that would corroborate the hypothesis of Björck. Up to now, the traditionally accepted dating (first half of the fourth century A.D.) has been used as a *terminus post quem* for the *Mulomedicina Chironis*,[35] and it is in relation to Apsyrtos that other veterinary surgeons have been dated.

Eumelos from Thebes comes after Columella, whose sixth book he made much use of,[36] and before Apsyrtos, who quotes him;[37] he would come nearer to the latter. Traditional dating, which assigns him around 300 A.D. is challenged, of course, by Björck's hypothesis.

Rendering in more elegant Greek many articles of Apsyrtos, Hierocles literally pirated his predecessor's work.[38] There is no evidence which allows us to date with any precision this author, who appears to have been a learned lawyer.[39]

Anatolios is known from other sources: he is the author of a compilation on agriculture in twelve books, which Oder dates to the fourth or fifth century A.D.; and his work served as a basis, together with Didymus', for Cassianus Bassus' composition of the *Geoponica* in the sixth century A.D.[40]

As to Pelagonius, who also draws on Apsyrtos, it has for long been believed that his Latin text was but a translation of a Greek treatise, excerpts from which can be found in the *Collection*. However, the comparison of the two versions reveals the opposite, without it being possible to determine the date of the Greek translations.[41] As to the dating of Pelagonius' work,[42] written in the form of letters like those of Apsyrtos, the identification of two of his addressees with known people from the second half of the fourth century A.D. is not beyond doubt;[43] it seems also hard to draw any argument from the first words of the treatise, in which the circus and the sacred games are mentioned, and which were borrowed from Columella, another source of Pelagonius.[44] Nevertheless, Oder and Hoppe have deduced from them that the sacred games were not yet prohibited at the time when the treatise was written and that the writing had occurred therefore before 393 A.D.[45] Since the *terminus post quem* constituted by Apsyrtos has been challenged by Björck's hypothesis, the most reliable landmark now

marshmallow (ἀλθαία) he quotes the Romans, the Sarmatians, the Getae and the Thracians. He also mentions the areas where this plant grows: Asia (in particular, Smyrna, on the river Μέλης) and Sicilia (II, 45, 1–17). He says that he himself comes from Clazomenae (II, 96, 23). His addressees come from Alexandria (Alexandria Troas?), from Antioch (in Syria in Pisidia, or in Cappadocia?), from Callipolis (in Chersonese?), from Chalcedon (Bithynia), from Clazomenae (Bithynia), from Corinth, Ephesus, Laodicea (in Phrygia, in Lycia, or else in Syria?), from Nicaea (Bithynia?), from Nicomedia (Bithynia), from Tomi (Moesia) and from Spain. Most of these names were used for various cities, and it is difficult to locate those mentioned by Apsyrtos with any certainty.

[34] In the Greek *Collection*, Apsyrtos is quoted by Theomnestos (*CHG*, I, 273, 15) and by Hierocles (*CHG*, I, 55, 24; 58, 22; 59, 2; 63, 4; 98, 19; 121, 23, 128, 4–5; 129, 7; 171, 27, 181, 28; 182, 21; 205, 5; 207, 8; 221, 15 and 20; 224, 4; 231, 15; 232, 4; 241, 15; 264, 18; 300, 18; 302, 10; 314, 23; 342, 12; 348, 22; and II, 196, 22). On the Latin side, he is quoted by Pelagonius (ed. Fischer, 153), in the *Mulomedicina Chironis* (ed. Oder, 298), and by Vegetius (ed. Lommatzsch, 311).

[35] The *Mulomedicina Chironis* is a text contained in Monacensis Latinus 243, fifteenth century; which was discovered by W. Meyer in 1885 and edited by E. Oder in 1901; it is a compilation that includes texts by Apsyrtos among others; the *terminus ante quem* is Vegetius (ed. Lommatzsch, XXVIII and XXXVI-XLII).

[36] M. Ihm, ed., *Pelagonii artis veterinariae quae extant* (Leipzig, Teubner, 1892), 7–9.

[37] See n. 33 above.

[38] Possibly it was his correctness of speech that was responsible for the inclusion of his work in the *Collection* and for its translation into Latin and Sicilian in the Middle Ages (see Doyen, "Les textes" [n. 8 above], 267 and n. 51). E. Oder, "Beiträge zur Geschichte der Landwirthschaft bei den Griechen," *RhM*, 48 (1893), 34–35, suggests that Hierocles should not be placed after 500, because he avoids hiatus in his prologues, thus sticking to the rule applied by the sophists of the fourth and fifth centuries A.D. For want of something better, this weak argument was again used in the preface to the edition of the *Corpus* (*CHG*, II, XII).

[39] See the prologue to the first book, *CHG*, I, 3, 18–6, 21. He mentions in it Euripides, Pindar, Simon, Xenophon, the precis of *History of Animals* by Aristophanes from Byzantium, the brothers Quintilii and Tarentinus. In the prologue to the second book (*CHG*, I, 248, 13–250, 8), he mentions Hesiod and Aristotle.

[40] On the *Geoponica*, see E. Oder, "Beiträge zur Geschichte der Landwirthschaft bei den Griechen," *RhM*, 45 (1890), 58–98 and 212–22 and 48 (1893), 1–40, and more recently R. H. Rodgers, "Varro and Virgil in the *Geoponica*," *GRBS*, 19 (1978), 277–85 and M. Ullman, *Die Natur- und Geheimwissenschaften im Islam* (Leiden and Cologne, 1972) (Handbuch der Orientalistik, I, Ergb. VI, 2), 431 f.

[41] On the possible use of various versions of Pelagonius in the *Collection*, see K. D. Fischer, "Two notes on the *Hippiatrica*," *GRBS*, 20 (1979), 373–75.

[42] See Fischer, "Pelagonius" (n. 6 above), 286–88.

[43] *Ibid.*, 288–89. They are Arzygius, the dedicatee of the treatise, to whom letters III, VI, and XXIV are also addressed (ed. Fischer, 10, 6; 16, 24; 53, 9), and Astyrius, the addressee of letter IX (*ibid.*, 28, 7). The former could be Betitius Perpetuus Arzygius, consular to Etruria and Umbria after 366, in whose honor a statue was erected. The latter could be L. Turcius Apronianus Asterius, prefect of the city in 363, unless they are but relatives of these people (see *PLRE*, I, 88–89 and 688–89).

[44] *Equos circo sacrisque certaminibus quinquennes usque ad annum vigesimum plerumque idoneos adseverant, usibus autem domesticis a bimo usque in annum tricesimum necessarios esse apud diligentissimum dominum certissimum est* (ed. Fischer, 3, 2–5; cf. *Columella, Rust.*, VI, 27, 1 [ed. Forster and Heffner (n. 1 above), II, 188–91]).

[45] See *CHG*, II, XIII and K. Hoppe, "Die commenta artis medicinae veterinariae des Pelagonius," *Veterinärhistorisches Jahrbuch*, 3 (1927) (or *Abhandlungen aus der Geschichte der Veterinärmedizin*, 14 [Leipzig, 1927]), 193.

is Vegetius' treatise (between 383 and 455 A.D.), wherein he quotes and uses Pelagonius.[46]

Nothing is known about Hippocrates the veterinary surgeon, who is definitely not the medical doctor of Cos; there is no evidence for identifying him with Apsyrtos' correspondent.[47]

THE FOUR RECENSIONS OF THE *COLLECTION* AND THEIR EDITION

The chronology of the *Collection* also remains uncertain.[48] It has been maintained for a long time that the *Collection* was formed at the time of Constantine VII Porphyrogenitus, in the tenth century A.D. It is by no means impossible that the elaborately ornamented Berlin manuscript, the Berolinensis Graecus 134 (Phillippicus 1538) was intended for this sovereign.[49] The manuscript does not, however, contain the oldest stage of the *Collection*. Indeed, the *Collection* went through several successive redactions, characterized by the selection of authors used, the order in which these authors appear, their general organization, and their style. We know four of these recensions. They are referred to by the letters M, B, D (C and L) and RV.[50] The first three are characterized by a grouping according to the subject matter of the excerpts from various authors.

The M recension is known from a Paris manuscript of the eleventh century, the Parisinus Graecus 2322; it represents the oldest known stage of the *Collection*, nearest to the hypothetical archetype

of the *Collection* called A by Björck.[51] Like this, it still uses the seven authors mentioned above in the alphabetical order of their names.[52] From the discovery of this logical principle, still followed by the writer of M, there follows a major consequence for the study of the *Collection*: there is no reason why the attributions of M to such and such an author should be questioned; the M recension then forms a reliable basis for the identification of hippiatric texts that appear in the other three recensions, wherein authors' names do not occur with so much regularity; the general organization of M does not seem to correspond to any definite principle of classification.

The B recension, of which the oldest witness is the illustrated Berlin manuscript, appears in nine other manuscripts:

> Berolinensis Graecus 135 (Phillippicus 1539), sixteenth century;[53]
> Parisinus Graecus 2245, fifteenth century;
> Neapolitanus Borbonicus III d 26, fifteenth century;
> Oxoniensis Baroccianus 164, fifteenth century;
> Florentinus Laurentianus Graecus 75/6, fifteenth century;
> Londinensis Add. 5108, sixteenth century;
> Vaticanus Barberinianus Graecus 212, fifteenth century(?);
> Vaticanus Urbinas Graecus 80, fourteenth-fifteenth century;
> Romanus Bibliothecae Corsinianae 14.

Beside the seven authors whose excerpts do not appear any longer in the alphabetical order of their names, two new sources were used: a collection entitled Προγνώσεις καὶ ἰάσεις ("Prognoses and Treatments"), and Tiberius, an author about whom hardly anything is known, although it seems almost certain that he was inspired by Apsyrtos and Anatolios, and therefore would have to be dated after them. The information concerning the authors of excerpts in B never contradicts that in M. Unlike M, however, B contains many anonymous texts: if they appear in M as well, it is possible to identify their authors. The order of the subjects is more systematic in B than in M, and a stylistic

---

[46] See ed. Lommatzsch, XXVIII, XXXI–XXXV, and 311.

[47] *CHG*, I, 74, 15 and II, 143, 16.

[48] On the problems of chronology raised by the *Collection* and its various recensions, see Doyen, "Les textes" (n. 8 above), 269–72.

[49] On the discussions concerning the date of this manuscript, see *ibid.*, 270–71. On its illustrations, see especially: A. and W. Böckler, *Schöne Handschriften aus dem Besitz der Preussischen Staatsbibliothek* (Berlin, 1931), 7–8; R. Froehner, "Veterinärhistorische Abhandlungen über die griechischen Pferdeärzte des 4. Jahrhundert nebst Reproduktionen aus den *Hippiatrica* des Codex Graecus Berolinensis Phillippicus nr 1538 in farbigem Facsimiledruck, beigefügt der Festschrift von Hauptner, Rudolf," *80 Jahre H. Hauptner, 1857–1937* (1937), 24–44; J. Kirchner, *Beschreibende Verzeichnisse der Miniaturen-Handschriften der Preussischen Staatsbibliothek zu Berlin, I. Die Phillipps-Handschriften* (Leipzig, 1926), 16–17; K. Weitzmann; *Die byzantinische Buchmalerei des 9. und 10. Jahrhunderts* (Berlin, 1975), 1–18 and 71; and *Studies in Classical and Byzantine Manuscript Illumination* (Chicago and London, 1971), 194–95.

[50] M, B, and V, as well as C and L, are the initials used by Oder and Hoppe. It was Björck's suggestion to use D for the recension represented by the two English manuscripts (C and L) (G. Björck, *Zum Corpus Hippiatricorum Graecorum. Beiträge zur antiken Tierheilkunde* [Inaugural Dissertation, Uppsala, 1932], 20), and R for the Parisinus Graecus 2244 (G. Björck, "Le Parisinus grec 2244 et l'art vétérinaire grec," *REG*, 48 [1935], 508).

[51] Björck, *Zum Corpus* (n. 50 above), 20.

[52] See above p. 111 and n. 9.

[53] For most of the manuscripts of the B recension, the datings are those given in the catalogues. This information is not to be found by S. de Ricci, "Liste sommaire des manuscrits grecs de la Bibliothèque Barberina," *Revue des Bibliothèques*, 17 (1907), 97 (but see Björck, "Apsyrtos" [n. 18 above], 42), nor by G. Pierleoni, "Index codicum Graecorum qui Romae in Bybliotheca Corsiniana nunc Lynceorum adservantur," *Studi italiani di filologia classica*, 9 (1901), 475–76.

modification can be noticed, namely abridgment.[54]

The D recension, represented by two manuscripts kept in England, the Cantabrigiensis Collegii Emmanuelis III.3.19 (C), from the twelfth century, and the Londinensis Bibliothecae Sloanianae 745 (L), from the thirteenth century, is quite similar to B with regard to the sources used, the form, and the organization. In addition, the recension reflects other texts: especially excerpts from Julius Africanus;[55] texts about human medicine;[56] extracts from hippology, among which is the only passage known by Simon of Athens;[57] and a text of Timothaeus of Gaza on horse breeds.

There are many differences between the two manuscripts (C and L) in the internal organization of the chapters and the contents. Some texts of C are absent from L, but the reverse is more frequent. Among the excerpts contained in L only are: the letter on the vulture (*CHG*, II, 253, 13–255, 6)[58] and several passages of Tiberius. The attribu-

tions of C to such or such an author are generally confirmed by M or/and B or—for Tiberius' texts—by R, when the texts also appear in one of these recensions. But C sometimes gathers extracts from various authors, and the whole constituted in this way may bear the name of one of these authors. Many attributions of L are false, as comparison with M and B, or even C, when it is possible, demonstrates. C and L contain many anonymous texts, which one can sometimes identify by referring to M, B or R. But no means of verification is possible for the passages contained in L only.

The RV recension is known through two partly illustrated[59] manuscripts from the fourteenth century: the Parisinus Graecus 2244 (R) and the Leidensis Vossianus Graecus Q. 50 (V). It consists of several texts which do not follow the same principles as the other recensions.

The first part of R and V contains three books. The first two books are a reconstruction of Hierocles' two books. This reconstruction was in all likelihood carried out from recension B. The third book is a brief but thorough little treatise on hippiatrics attributed to Galen and Hippocrates, to which I shall return later (pp. 117–18 below). This "illuminated branch" of the hippiatric texts holds a special position in the manuscript tradition, because the texts of which it consists have been translated, together or separately, into Latin, Italian, and Sicilian, and sometimes illustrated.[60]

The second part of the RV recension presents without any illustrations several series of excerpts classified at times according to authors (Apsyrtos,

[54] See, for instance, the beginning of the first chapter on fever (*CHG*, I, 1) and Theomnestos' text on tetanus (*CHG*, I, 183, 14–186, 6). Cf. also *CHG*, I, 152, 19–24 (B, XXX, 8) and *CHG*, II, 95, 3–19 (M, 995) with the Latin source (Pelagonius 216 [ed. Fischer, 38, 12–23]).

[55] If Björck is to be believed, it seems likely that the writer referred to a compendium by Julius Africanus interpolated by extracts from Aelian (Björck, "Apsyrtus" [n. 18 above], 34; see 17–18 as well). This assumption is based on the analysis of a text in D attributed to Julius Africanus; the text is in fact that of Aelian (*CHG*, II, 161, 21–24 = Ael., *N.A.* 11–18 [Loeb, II (London, 1959), 384, 4–8]). This passage was also transmitted by Aristophanes of Byzantium II, 620 (S. Lambros ed., *Excerptorum Constantini De natura animalium libri duo Aristophanis historiae animalium epitome, subjunctis Aeliani Timothei aliorumque eclogis* [*Supplementum Aristotelicum*, I; Berlin, 1885], 152, 3–6). J. R. Vieillefond has republished and translated the thirty-nine paragraphs attributed to Julius Africanus by the Cantabrigiensis Collegii Emmanuelis, III.3.19 (*Les Cestes. Etude sur l'ensemble des fragments avec édition, traduction et commentaires*, Publications de l'Institut Français de Florence. 1ᵉʳᵉ série. Collection d'études d'histoire, de critique et de philologie, 20 [Florence and Paris, 1970], 215–55; see also 128–33, 138–39, 148–49).

[56] G. Björck has made up the list of these passages and put them side by side with passages from Oribasios, Aetios and Paulos Aegineta. He concludes that, following the example of other compilers in late antiquity, the writer of D seems to have used one or more collections and carefully remained silent about his direct sources, while at the same time mentioning the names of the authors in secondhand quotations. According to him this direct source is earlier than Oribasios since it contains excerpts from him (Björck, *Zum Corpus* [n. 50 above], 31–44).

[57] For the bibliography relating to these texts, see Doyen, "Les textes" (n. 8 above), 260–61, n. 19–25.

[58] Several Greek and Latin versions of this text are known. It shows interesting similarities with the sections on the eagle and the vulture in Book III of the *Cyranides* (D. Kaimakis, ed., *Die Kyraniden*, Beiträge zur klassischen Philologie, 76 [Meisenheim am Glan, 1976] 188–91 and 199–201). On the questions raised by the identification of the author (Bothros, Aretas, Alexander, or Teuthris), the sources (the same as the *Cyranides*?) and the way the contents have to be interpreted, see F. Cumont, "Le

sage Bothros ou le phylarque Arétas?," *RPh*, n.s., 50 (1926), 13–33; L. MacKinney, "An Unpublished Treatise on Medicine and Magic from the Age of Charlemagne," *Speculum*, 18:4 (1943), 494–96); A. A. Barb, "Birds and Medical Magic," *JWarb*, 13 (1950), 318–22.

[59] On the illustrations of the Parisinus Graecus 2244, see A. Grabar, "L'art profane à Byzance," *Actes du XIVᵉ congrès international des études byzantines, Bucarest, 6–12 septembre 1971*, I (Editura Academiei Republici Socialiste România, 1974), 328–29; Z. Kádár, "Le problème du style dans les illustrations du manuscrit hippiatrique de la Bibliothèque Nationale de Paris (Gr. 2244)," *ibid.*, II (1975), 459–61; K. Weitzmann, *Ancient Book Illumination* (Cambridge, 1959), 22–23 and *Studies* (n. 49 above), 42 and 194–95; K. Wessel, *s.v.* Buchillustration, *Reallexikon für byzantinische Kunst*, I (Stuttgart, 1966), 757–784 and *s.v.* Frontalität, *ibid.*, II (Stuttgart, 1971), 586–93. At the International Symposium on the History of Veterinary Medicine, held at Bärau bei Langnau in 1980, Dr. K. D. Fischer read a paper entitled "Griechische Pferdeheilkunde in spätmittelalterlichen Bilderhandschriften," which dealt with various Greek and Italian illustrated manuscripts, including the Vossianus Graecus Q. 50 and the Parisinus Graecus 2244. A summary of this paper was published in Society for Ancient Medicine *Newsletter*, No. 7 (October 1980), 5.

[60] For a list of the manuscripts containing these translations, see Doyen, "Les textes" (n. 8 above), 267, n. 51, and 273, n. 84.

Tiberius, Hieron), at other times according to subject matter. It is very hard to determine any principle of classification. In many respects, the second part is similar to the M recension.

The various interrelations of the recensions of the Greek hippiatric *Collection* are still far from being clear, but the fact remains that the *Collection* provides the historian of veterinary medicine with a considerable number of texts. Most of these texts were published by Oder and Hoppe in their Teubner edition of 1924 and 1927.[61] This edition does not enable the reader to form a clear opinion about the organization and the contents of the D and RV recensions. Therefore I have made a thorough inventory of the contents of these two recensions.[62] This endeavor does not suppress the drawbacks of an edition, which in other respects is of great value. At the same time it enables us for the time being to do without a complete edition of the four recensions of the *Collection*, which will definitely take several years to achieve.

Finally, some passages have not been edited in Oder and Hoppe's edition. They are the following texts:

1. Part of the *Hippiatrica* of the Parisinus Graecus 2244 (first part: foll. 1–195) and the Vossianus Graecus Q. 50:

> several chapters from the versions of the brief treatise on hippiatrics or *Epitome*[63] contained in these manuscripts;

> the text of a certain Lampudis on continuous fever;

> excerpts from Apsyrtos;

> various recipes, among which are included ophthalmic and cough remedies;

> a statement on *malis* by Hieron.

2. Two versions of the *Epitome*: one preserved in the Vaticanus Palatinus Graecus 365 (fifteenth century), the other in the Parisini Graeci 1995, 2091 and 2244 (second part: foll. 77–87) (fourteenth century).

3. Most of the texts on horses contained in the

Vaticanus Ottobonianus Graecus 338 (sixteenth century) and the Vaticani Graeci 114 (first and second part: foll. 118^r–141^v and foll. 142^r–145^v) (fifteenth century) and 1066 (fourteenth century):[64]

> a text concerning hippology, on the exterior of the horse, which opens the sections dealing with this animal in the Vaticanus Ottobonianus Graecus 338 and the Vaticani Graeci 114 (first part) and 1066;

> two series of excerpts from the *Epitome*, representing different versions of the three others mentioned above; they both appear in the Vaticanus Graecus 114 (first and second part). The beginning of the first part is also found in the Vaticanus Ottobonianus Graecus 338 and the Vaticanus Graecus 1066.

4. A treatise about how to determine the age of horses known through the Ambrosianus H 2 inf., fol. 225^{r-v} (sixteenth century). This last text has recently been edited with a commentary by K. D. Fischer and J. A. M. Sonderkamp.[65]

THE *EPITOME* OF THE *COLLECTION*

I have undertaken to prepare an edition of the *Epitome*, which has received little attention and has been completely neglected by previous editors. This Byzantine text is interesting for several reasons. First, its contents reveal that, to a very large extent, it is a summary of the *Collection* and that the manner of its compilation is contrary to that of the said *Collection*. Moreover, unlike the B recension, for instance, whose ten manuscripts offer the same text both in form and content, the *Epitome* is a living text which went through reshaping, undergoing sometimes very important alterations. I have therefore distinguished five stages of the text. Establishing any sort of affiliation between these different versions is, of course, out of the question, and it is impossible to clear up completely the problem of this living text's tradition, which eludes the classical laws of stemmatics: all the usual methods of combination fail one after the other. One particular circumstance, however, enabled me to carry further the study of the *Epitome*: several re-

---

[61] On previous edition, the turns taken by the project of editing the *Collection* in the nineteenth century, see *ibid.*, 259–62.

[62] This work is included in my Ph.D. thesis (n. 8 above), II, 8–79; it is accompanied by a detailed description of the recensions of the *Collection* (I, 8–41).

[63] This is the term used by Björck ("Le Parisinus" [n. 50 above], 511). Indeed, the title of a manuscript, Vaticanus Palatinus Graecus 365, containing the term, is: Ἰατρικὸν ἐν ἐπιτόμῳ ἄριστον περὶ ἵππων ἔχον κεφάλαια διάφορα (fol. 204^r).

[64] The chronological indications concern only the folios containing texts on hippiatrics or hippology. It is not always true for the entire manuscript.

[65] K. D. Fischer and J. A. M. Sonderkamp, "Ein byzantinischer Text zur Altersbestimmung von Pferden (Aus Ambrosianus. H 2 inf.)," *SA*, 64 (1980), 55–68.

censions of the *Collection* from which it comes are known, and it appears related to one of them, namely M. Therefore, I have tried to explore and use this relationship as much as possible. Before tackling the difficult problems of collating additions and omissions, I studied the arrangement, then I compared different passages from the text, not just within the versions of the *Epitome*, but with the various recensions of the *Collection* as well. Actually, only the study of the *Epitome*'s organization disclosed any new facts of value for the history of the text; subsequent research confirmed these facts.[66]

The history of the *Epitome*'s text shows that it does not stem from the M recension itself, but from a related recension. Does it then correspond to a later stage than M, or does it go back to an earlier stage, and why not to the original A *Collection*? If the second hypothesis were correct, the *Epitome* would be the oldest witness of the *Collection*. Unfortunately it is impossible to determine, and we know very little about the chronology of the *Epitome*. It is dependent on the chronology of the *Collection*, which constitutes the only *terminus post quem* of the treatise, whose oldest manuscripts date back from the fourteenth century, although an earlier *terminus ante quem* is provided by the Latin translation, which, in all likelihood, dates back to the second half of the thirteenth century.[67] Finally, it is important to point out that this technical text, without any literary claim, manifests some linguistic particularities which indicate real evolution in comparison with the entire *Collection*.[68]

PROSPECTS FOR THE STUDY OF THE GREEK HIPPIATRIC TEXTS

Such then are the Greek hippiatric texts which the historian of veterinary medicine has at his disposal. On one hand, there are the four known recensions of the *Corpus Hippiatricorum Graecorum*, to which must be added the sixteenth book of the *Geoponica* (see note 7 above); on the other hand, there are the five versions of the *Epitome*, which I have edited. There cannot be any really thorough

study of these texts until a complete edition, which considers all witnesses, is available. Nevertheless, it is possible to suggest the broad outlines of such a study by posing the main questions which will have to be answered.

The most urgent task—already undertaken at the beginning of this century by the veterinary surgeons L. Moulé, H. J. Sévilla, F. Simon[69] and W. Rieck,[70] and carried on in recent years in a masterly way by the distinguished historian of veterinary medicine, K. D. Fischer,[71] and with less satisfactory results by the veterinary medical students of Hanover and Munich[72]—falls within the prov-

---

[66] This study is found in my Ph.D. thesis (n. 8 above), I, 54–174 and II, 80–150.

[67] It is known through the Vaticanus Latinus 5366 (around 1300) and the Londinensis Add. 27 626 (fourteenth or fifteenth century?), which was edited by G. Sponer, *Die Pferdeheilkunde des Ipocras Indicus* (Vet. Diss., Hanover, 1966).

[68] I have made an inventory of all the grammatical matters in my Ph.D. thesis (n. 8 above), I, 175–212.

[69] On the bibliography of L. Moulé, H.J. Sévilla and F. Simon, see A. M. Doyen, "L'accouplement et la reproduction des équidés dans les textes hippiatriques grecs," *Annales de Médecine Vétérinaire*, 125 (1981), 552–53, n. 2–4.

[70] Dr. Wilhelm Rieck, professor emeritus from the Hanover School, is the author of many articles dealing with various periods in the history of veterinary medicine, including antiquity. He has studied primarily the history of ophthalmology ("Tieraugenheilkunde im Wandel der Zeiten," *Veterinärhistorisches Jahrbuch*, 8 [1936], 7–79) and the contents of the *Mulomedicina Chironis*. Among his recent articles, see "Die Blutentziehung in der anonymen Einleitung der *Mulomedicina Chironis*," *Et multum et multa* (Berlin, 1971), 307–12. He has also supervised several dissertations on such subjects. Thus, M. Skupas' dissertation: *Altgriechische Tierkrankheitsnamen und ihre Deutungen* (Vet. Diss., Hanover, 1962).

[71] K. D. Fischer and J. A. M. Sonderkamp's article, already mentioned (n. 65 above) is a model for this type of study. Edited with utmost philological rigor, the text from the Ambrosianus H 2 inf. is translated with great accuracy; there follows a detailed commentary. K. D. Fischer has also analyzed several terms from the vocabulary of Greek veterinary surgeons, in particular the names of diseases ("Two notes" [n. 41 above], 376–79, and "Wege zum Verständnis antiker Tierkrankeitsnamen," *Historia Medicinae Veterinariae*, 2 [1977], 106–11).

[72] In Munich the *Mulomedicina Chironis* has been completely translated and annotated by A. Baumgartner (Book I; 1976), R. Frik (Book II and Book IV, chapters 38–57; 1979), Th. Roeren (Book III; 1977), C. Guggenbichler (Book IV, chapters 1–37; 1978), H. Schwarzer (Book V; 1976), W. Wohlmuth (parts of Book VI and Book VII; 1978), W. Lamprecht (Book VIII, 1976); J. Krüger (Book IX; 1981) and C. Enderle (Book X; 1975). The *Corpus Hippiatricorum Graecorum* is now receiving the attention of several doctoral dissertations, supervised by Dr. J. Schäffer at the Institut für Paleoanatomie, Domestikationsforschung und Geschichte der Tiermedizin, headed by Prof. J. Boessneck. These include J. Schäffer, *Die Rezeptesammlung im Corpus Hippiatricorum Graecorum Band I (Kapitel 129, 130; Appendices 1–9)* (Munich, 1981); G. Reiter, *Die Kapitel über Erkrankungen an Kopf und Hals im Corpus Hippiatricorum Graecorum* (Munich, 1981); L. Zellwecker, *Die Kapitel über Erkrankungen an den Extremitäten im Corpus Hippiatricorum Graecorum* (Munich, 1981). These theses consist of a German translation (occasionally in need of correction) and a commentary which takes into account not only the pathological point of view, but the therapeutical questions as well. On the whole they are well researched. It is important that these hippiatric texts are also being examined by contemporary practitioners. It is, however, quite understandable that they do not attach much importance to philological study, which however constitutes the essential prerequisite to any subsequent analysis of the contents.

ince of the history of pathology.[73] The *Collection* deals with more than a hundred pathological cases. The descriptions of the "horse doctors" have to be examined closely and compared with not only the data of modern veterinary medicine, but also old texts of human medicine. Some diseases, of course, are only found in horses, such as μᾶλις, or κριθίασις (that is, founder or laminitis), but other diseases very frequently are discussed also in treatises on human medicine. Although it is occasionally possible to identify a disease described by the hippiatric authors simply by noting the described symptoms, it is most of the time necessary to consult the evidence provided by human medicine, so as to assess the data with regard to symptomatology, etiology, and pathology in general, and to interpret thus the veterinary writings. In several cases, such as in the case of epilepsy, it even appears that it is the influence of human medicine that justifies the presence of sometimes very long statements in the veterinary treatises. Otherwise one must suppose, to take the example of epilepsy again, that horses of long ago were more liable to that disease than their contemporary descendants, among which the disease is extremely rare.[74]

The influence of human medicine is therefore obvious, but it is very difficult to demonstrate which schools have exerted the most decisive influence. In the introduction to his medical work *De medicina*, Celsus puts the Methodists and the veterinary surgeons side by side;[75] indeed, the studies of some Latin texts, especially the *Mulomedicina Chironis*,[76] and the analyses made by Björck of a few passages of the Greek *Collection*[77] have shown the obvious contribution of the Methodists. The greater part of Greek hippiatrics, however, still has to be studied, and the task is all the more difficult since etiological information—as a rule the most interesting

information from this point of view—is generally very scarce and often only hinted at. Such a study, of course, will have to distinguish between the different authors' contributions to the *Collection*.

The influence of human medicine is visible not only in the pathological concepts and descriptions of diseases, but in therapeutical methods as well, and especially in the *materia medica*. Medicinal plants are essentially those used in human medicine, and some passages of the *Collection* were in fact written by medical doctors.[78] Thus, the issue of the specific character of the veterinary recipes is raised. A major problem is to prove that "horse doctors" did not content themselves with prescribing "kill-or-cure doses" of drugs borrowed from human medicine, but that they also had special medicines. Involved here are questions of quantification and the cost of the recipes. First it is essential to make a complete inventory of all the recipes, and there is a considerable number of them, even if we limit ourselves to Greek texts. Such a collation, it seems to me, makes the use of a computer almost unavoidable; and one must hope that the corpus of veterinary recipes will one day receive the same treatment as the recipes from human medicine studied in the THEOREMA project, now being carried out at the LASLA (Laboratoire d'Analyse Statistique des Langues Anciennes) at Liege University.[79] In this way it will be possible to survey all the veterinary recipes and to make the desired comparisons.

Finally, hippiatric texts raise a number of more general questions as regards the position of hippiatrics in ancient and medieval science, the status of "horse doctors" in society, their function, their education, their use of existing treatises, and the importance they gave to tradition. These last two aspects have to do with a recurrent problem in the history of the sciences, namely the relationship between theory and practice: what was the purpose of these texts, witnesses of the trend—so important and so little discussed in Byzantine scholarship—which resulted in the great collections of excerpts (on the military arts, alchemy, virtues and vices, etc.) and the summaries and abstracts of ancient science? At a time when knowledge was handed down orally, it is hard to believe that a book

---

[73] I have studied the contents of the *Epitome* from this point of view in my Ph.D. thesis (n. 8 above), V.

[74] At the International Symposion on the History of Veterinary Medicine held at Vienna in 1982, I read a paper entitled "Epilepsy in Greek Hippiatric Texts." A summary of it was published in *Historia Medicinae Veterinariae*, 7 (1982), 41. No one of the veterinary surgeons I have questioned, be he a practitioner, an inspector, or a professor, has even come across one case in his career.

[75] Celsus, *Prohoem.* 65 (ed. Marx, 27, 30–28, 1).

[76] See Rieck, "Die Blutentziehung" (n. 70 above). W. Rieck read a paper entitled "Krankheitsbegriffe der Methodischen Schule in der *Mulomedicina Chironis*" at the International Symposion on the History of Veterinary Medicine held at Vienna in 1982; a summary was published in *Historia Medicinae Veterinariae*, 7 (1982), 42.

[77] Björck, *Zum Corpus* (n. 50 above), 71 f.

[78] See K. Hoppe, "Über die Herkunft einiger Stellen im CHG II," *Veterinärhistorische Mitteilungen*, 7 (1927), 42–44 and 8 (1928), 1–2; Björck, *Zum Corpus* (n. 50 above), 32–44.

[79] See C. Opsomer-Halleux, "Prolégomènes à une étude des recettes médicales latines," *Centre Jean Palerne, Mémoires*, III, *Médecins et Médecine dans l'Antiquité* (Saint-Etienne, 1982), 85–104.

as bulky and wordy as the *Collection*, with its costly manuscripts, would have been found in the house of a "horse doctor" or a farrier. With regard to the subjects considered in the *Collection*, there are several statements, sometimes quite different, and a selection of various cures; with good reason any practitioner, who was little concerned with theories, would have been confused and disheartened.

The *Epitome* no doubt exerted a considerable influence, as is suggested by the various translations.[80] Moreover, several elements enable us to suppose that it was of much use to Byzantine veterinary surgeons. More concise than the *Collection*, the *Epitome* contains a short statement for each disease and a limited number of remedies. To these summaries, there is also a certain amount of practical information added (for instance, on the way of finding the vein to bleed), which must be due to someone in the profession. Finally there appear to have been several drafts, which would suggest that it was quite successful. Thus, I am inclined to think that the text of the *Epitome* did not go unheeded, but must have been used as a *vademecum* by the veterinary surgeons of the Byzantine period.[81]

Fonds National de la Recherche
Scientifique, Brussels

---

[80] See above, p. 116 and n. 60; p. 118 and n. 67.

[81] My warmest thanks to Dumbarton Oaks and to Prof. John Scarborough; I wish also to express my gratitude to Dr. Klaus-Dietrich Fischer; I am very grateful to Pierre Cossement and Dr. Joanne Phillips for their help in executing the English translation.

JOHN ACTUARIUS' *DE METHODO MEDENDI*—ON THE NEW EDITION

ARMIN HOHLWEG

Ἰωάννης Ζαχαρίας, which is the form of the name which has been transmitted to us by the majority of the manuscripts and letterheads of his contemporaries,[1] and who, on the basis of his position at the imperial court in Constantinople later held the title ἀκτουάριος, is generally considered to be one of the last great doctors in Byzantium.[2] Although this estimation is sometimes called into question, it is nevertheless advisable to stick to it for the moment as axiomatic. At the end of this essay we can return to the problem and pose the question anew.

The information concerning his life which one finds in the available textbooks is quite meager. To get beyond this information requires tedious effort, much like putting together a mosaic, and I cannot pursue it here *in extenso*. Precisely because this is the case, I would like to attempt a brief synopsis of the more certain data concerning his life.[3] Then I will treat of his medical education, and, fi-

nally, speak about his medical writings and the edition which has been begun.

Today it is the *communis opinio*, at least on the evidence of the pertinent compendia,[4] to place John's golden age in the years when the Emperor Andronikos III ruled. This view, however, must be complemented and corrected on the basis of John's correspondence, as well as on the basis of information which John himself gives in his writings. With the dedication of his major work, which I will designate with the brief Latin title *De methodo medendi*, to Alexios Apokaukos, we have a definite point of reference in time; for this Apokaukos is well known to us in the political history of the fourteenth century.[5] In the manucripts, we read that the work was written for the Parakoimomenos Apokaukos, who later received the title of a Megas Dux.[6] Apokaukos received the title Parakoi-

[The reader is referred to the list of abbreviations at the end of the volume.]

[1] Regarding the family name "Zacharias" in the Palaeologian period, cf. E. Trapp, *Prosopographisches Lexikon der Palaiologenzeit*, 3 Faszikel (Wien, 1978), 143–46.

[2] Several examples: H. Haeser, *Lehrbuch der Geschichte der Medicin*, 3rd ed., I (Jena, 1875), 481 ff.; H. Schelenz, *Geschichte der Pharmazie* (Berlin, 1904), 193; K. Sudhoff, *Kurzes Handbuch der Geschichte der Medizin* (Berlin, 1922), 134 f.; G. K. Pournaropoulos, Συμβολὴ εἰς τὴν ἱστορίαν τῆς βυζαντινῆς ἰατρικῆς (Athens, 1942), 170; P. Diepgen, *Geschichte der Medizin. Die historische Entwicklung der Heilkunde und des ärztlichen Lebens*, I (Berlin, 1949), 168 f.; H. Hunger, "Medizin," 312 f.; Sournia-Poulet-Martiny, *Illustrierte Geschichte der Medizin*, II. German edition under the direction of R. Toellner (Salzburg, 1980), 468.

[3] After completing the manuscript for this paper, I came upon the essay by S. I. Kuruses, Ὁ ἀκτουάριος Ἰωάννης Ζαχαρίας παραλήπτης τῆς ἐπιστολῆς ι΄ τοῦ Γεωργίου Λακαπηνοῦ. Τὰ βιογραφικά, Ἀθηνᾶ, 78 (1980–1982, published 1983), 237–76, referred to hereafter as "Kuruses II." Concerning John's biographical data, the pertinent results of Kuruses' study agree essentially with my own. For the epistolography of the time and the results which can be garnered from it concerning John Ac-

tuarius and his circle of friends, I refer to S. I. Kuruses, Τὸ ἐπιστολάριον Γεωργίου Λακαπηνοῦ καὶ Ἀνδρονίκου Ζαρίδου. Παρατηρήσεις χρονολογικαί, προσωπογραφικαὶ καὶ ἑρμηνευτικαί, Ἀθηνᾶ, 77 (1978–1979), 291–386; referred to hereafter as "Kuruses I."

[4] Krumbacher, 615; G. Sarton, *Introduction*, III:1, 889; H. Hunger, "Medizin," 313. Following Lambecius, Meyer, *Botanik*, III (1856), is somewhat more circumspect in his observations; he also rejects other data concerning John's life (cf. *ibid*. p. 383–90). Cf. K. Sudhoff, *op. cit.*, 134 and P. Diepgen, *op. cit.*, 168. This of course did not prevent some publications of the last decade from dating him in the twelfth or thirteenth centuries. Cf. M. Putscher, *Pneuma, Spiritus, Geist. Vorstellungen vom Lebensantrieb in ihren geschichtlichen Wandlungen* (Wiesbaden, 1973), 180, and L. J. T. Murphy, *The History of Urology* (Springfield, Ill., 1972), 126.

[5] Cf. R. Guilland, *Correspondance de Nicéphore Grégoras* (Paris, 1927), 299–301; *id.*, *Recherches sur les institutions byzantines*, I (Amsterdam, 1967), 210; G. Weiss, *Johannes Kantakuzenos—Aristokrat, Staatsmann, Kaiser und Mönch—in der Gesellschaftsentwicklung von Byzanz im 14. Jahrhundert* (Wiesbaden, 1969), 25–29 and *passim*; Johannes Kantakuzenos, *Geschichte*, ed. and trans. (German) by G. Fatouros and I. Krischer. Erster Teil. Bibliothek der Griechischen Literatur, 17 (Stuttgart, 1982), 221, note 47 with bibliography.

[6] ... τῷ παρακοιμωμένῳ τῷ Ἀποκαύκῳ τῷ καὶ ὕστερον χρηματίσαντι μεγάλῃ δουκί. Cf. G. A. Costomiris, "Etudes sur

momenos about 1321 from Emperor Andronikos II,[7] and he kept the title under his successor, Andronikos III, until he was named Megas Dux in 1341.[8] This means that the first book, in any case, of *De methodo medendi* must have been composed between 1321 and 1341. This time-span can, however, be narrowed down. This first book was given to Apokaukos on a diplomatic mission which he undertook in the fall; the second book was supposed to be finished upon his return in the following spring. In the meantime John wrote another composition for his teacher, Joseph the Philosopher.[9] If the latter died in 1330 or 1331, this means the first book must have been written in 1329 or 1330 at the latest.[10] Unfortunately, we are unable to date exactly the diplomatic mission of Apokaukos, and therefore cannot fix an exact date for the composition of these books.[11] Beyond scattered references in his own works, what we are otherwise able to ascertain regarding dates in John's life comes from the epistolography of the time and from the mention of his person in letters from his contemporaries, and there is a whole series of these. I wish to cite here the most important ones, in order to set some fixed points of reference in John's life, as far as this is possible.

From a letter of Georgios Lakapenos[12] in the fall of 1299,[13] we learn that John was staying at that time in Constantinople and was considering moving to Thessalonica. Lakapenos advises him against it. We learn also that John has his mother and other relatives in Constantinople and that he is engaged in the study of medicine, but that he has not yet completed his studies. Lakapenos speaks in this letter of the rather meager resources which John has at his disposal.[14] This is a rather general reference; but it could not have been made if Lakapenos did not know that John actually had no greater wealth at his disposal. Considering the circumstances, Lakapenos urges him to behave as a reasonable man and to prefer the quiet, ordered life in Constantinople to the difficulties which would be awaiting him in Thessalonica.

The tone of this letter permits us to conjecture that the author and the addressee are of approximately the same age. They are friends and have other friends in common. We can fix John's date of birth around 1275 or a bit later.[15] If we also consider the fact that Joseph the Philosopher (also known as Joseph Rhakendytes) was his teacher and friend, we can scarcely place the year of John's birth much earlier, since Joseph himself was born in 1260.[16]

Whether John followed the advice of Lakapenos and remained in Constantinople or whether he did go to Thessalonica, we do not know. From a later letter of Lakapenos, written before 1307,[17] and in all probability quite some time before 1307, we learn that John is well known by this time as ἰατρὸς ἀγαθός, as a good doctor, and that the author himself experienced this in a situation in which he himself was ill.

Here we can pinpoint one of John's character traits, namely, that he did not suffer from a lack of self-confidence. We should not ascribe that to some sort of Byzantinism, however; for this character trait is widespread in our own day, especially among doctors, not to mention scholars. Lakapenos was accustomed to reading to his friends the letters he was about to send. When John read the letter in which his friend's illness was mentioned, he protested quite loudly that he had been treated unfairly: Lakapenos neither related the case history nor did he report John's efforts and his contribution to healing the illness. This state of affairs is later set aright; Lakapenos admits the injustice and declares that he has only John to thank for the im-

---

les écrits inédits des anciens médecins. Cinquième série. XIIᵉ–XIVᵉ siècles," *REG*, 11 (1898), 414–45.

[7] Cf. especially Guilland, *Recherches*, I (Amsterdam, 1967), 210 with note 141.

[8] Joh. Kantakuz. III, 36 (Bonn ed., II, 218); cf. R. Guilland, *Recherches*, I *loc. cit.*

[9] *De diagnosi* I, 57 (ed. Ideler, II, 417; and II, prooem., 418).

[10] *Terminus ante quem* is the death of Joseph the Philosopher. He must have died before Theodoros Metochites (March 13, 1332), for the latter laments his death in a letter to a friend. John Zacharias does not mention Joseph's death. He also says nothing about the success of Apokaukos' diplomatic mission.

[11] Cf. note 75 below. The diplomatic mission was to the ὑπερβόρειοι Σκύθαι (Ideler, II, 353). The Mongols or Tartars are designated by historians of the time as ὑπερβόρειοι Σκύθαι (cf. G. Moravcsik, *Byzantinoturcica*, 2nd ed., II [Berlin, 1958], 228). Σκυθία is designated as their territory.

[12] *Georgii Lacapeni et Andronici Zaridae Epistulae XXXII cum epimerismis Lacapeni*, ed. S. Lindstam (Gothoburgi, 1924), *ep.* 10, p. 80–88.

[13] For dating this letter, cf. Kuruses I, 322–23, with information on pertinent bibliography; also in Kuruses II, 240.

[14] *Ep.* 10 (ed. Lindstam, p. 81, 32–82, 5 and 88, 10 f).

[15] One can conclude this form from the fact that G. Lakapenos was among the students of Maximos Planudes in 1293. Cf. Kuruses I, 370 with note 4.

[16] Joseph's date of birth can be inferred only approximately from information given by Metochites (M. Treu, "Der Philosoph Joseph," *BZ*, 8 [1899], 1–64, here 14, 2–3) that he was about 50 years old at the time of his death, perhaps somewhat younger, perhaps a bit older.

[17] *Ep.* 20 (ed. Lindstam, p. 128, 31–129, 21). In *ep.* 18 (p. 121, 16 Lindstam) John is designated as κορυφαῖος in his company of friends. For dating this corpus of letters within the years c. 1307–c. 1315, cf. Kuruses I, *passim* and also II, 250 f.

provement of his health.[18] One cannot overlook a certain irony on the part of Lakapenos.

John must have received the title of ἀκτουάριος[19] between 1310 and 1323. This can be verified in a letter of Michael Gabras, which was written in 1323. In the letter John is praised, but there is no mention made of the new honor. Therefore we can conclude that John did not receive the title just prior to the date of this letter.[20]

The date of John's death cannot be determined. We possess no news of him or about him which with certainty might be dated during the reign of Emperor Andronikos III. Gabras' last letter to John falls in the year 1327.[21] The work Περὶ ἐνεργειῶν καὶ παθῶν τοῦ ψυχικοῦ πνεύματος, which he wrote for his teacher Joseph, must have been completed before the latter's death in 1330 or 1331. At any rate, John does not mention Joseph's death. *De methodo medendi* was written after the work for Joseph, five books of it in any case. Whether John died in 1328, or shortly thereafter, must for the moment remain an open question. The silence of the sources concerning him could possibly be interpreted in another way.

After this brief synopsis of the most important external data concerning John, which on the basis of the sources must of necessity remain unclear in many points, I will attempt to say something about his education as a doctor and about his education in general.

With regard to questions concerning the professional education of doctors in Byzantium, we do not possess much certain testimony from the sources. Therefore, in this area, there are some unfounded suppositions and false hypotheses; so the information which we do possess on John in this regard can lead to a clarification on some points, at least for his own time. I have emphasized several times in other places that medical education in Byzantium must be seen in his connection with the ἐγκύκλιος παιδεία, and against the background of a correctly understood φιλοσοφία. Further, I think this is true not only for Byzantium and not only for the Middle Ages. On this point John is by no means the only witness, albeit a rather good one.

In his work *De urinis*, John speaks of the motives which led him to the pursuit of medicine, and the first one he names is a longstanding tendency toward the φυσικὸν μέρος τῆς φιλοσοφίας,[22] that is, to the natural sciences. He occupies himself with them as far as possible. His special love was for medical science, whose θεωρία he studied thoroughly. He took into consideration its φιλ-άνθρωπον as well as the θεραπευτικόν, but, on the other hand, he as also interested in its connection with φιλοσοφία.[23] He was always hesitant, as he says, to venture upon the treatment of sick people without first having thoroughly studied their illnesses. One must act with care and forethought (with λο-γικὴ ἐπιστασία).[24] In time he made progress, and in the belief that he could contribute to the τέχνη, he composed his work, in which theory and everyday experience are combined.[25]

So much for motives and consequences. In the report of sicknesses which he lists in *De urinis*, John gives a series of examples which testify to his attitude.[26] As for the course of studies itself, we must return to the letter of Lakapenos of fall 1299, which we used in our treatment of the particulars of John's life. From this letter we learn that John has not yet completed his medical studies, that he is not yet in possession of the τέχνη, and that he is improving his τέχνη through daily practice in a φροντι-στήριον.[27] If he were to go to Thessalonica, his friend explains to him, he would not have the appropriate opportunities for these pursuits. He has not yet arrived at the κολοφών, and therefore he has not yet received the κηρύγματα. I will explain below what is meant here. Lakapenos reproaches him: it is indeed poor, if someone entrusted to treat diseases which are not yet well known does not keep such clear and evident arguments in mind.

John practices daily in a φροντιστήριον. In Byzantine times this word designated a place of education, a school (διδασκαλεῖον), but also, and preferably, the monastery or the monk's cell, and finally the place for taking care of the poor, the weak and the sick.[28] This was, as we know, often connected

---

[18] *Ep.* 20 (ed. Lindstam, p. 129. 5–21).

[19] Cf. below p. 124–25, especially note 35.

[20] John is named three times as the addressee in the letters of Michael Gabras (G. Fatouros, *Die Briefe des Michael Gabras (ca. 1290–nach 1350)*, I.II, WByzSt, 10 [1973]): *ep.* 52, 310 and 439. In the last two instances he bears the title ἀκτουάριος. *Ep.* 310 should be dated in the 1323, *ep.* 52 in the year 130 (cf. Fatouros, I, 18).

[21] *Ep.* 439.

[22] Ideler, II, 190, 7.

[23] Ideler, II, 190, 11.

[24] Ideler, II, 190, 19 f.

[25] Ideler, II, 190, 20.

[26] Ideler, II, 50, 26–52, 1; 62, 29–63, 13; 92, 9–93, 3; 154, 31–156, 14; 162, 17–163, 27; 165, 9–166, 16; 166, 27–167, 8; 181, 12–183, 12; 186, 7–187, 4.

[27] *Ep.* 10 (ed. Lindstam, p. 82, 7–10).

[28] Cf. Lampe, *s.v.*; Anna Komnena, *Alexiad* III, 8, 2 (ed. Leib, I, 125, 31, in which the emperor's palace during the regency of Anna Dalassena is compared with ἱερὰ φροντιστήρια); VI, 3, 2

with a monastery. For this interpretation of the word we can cite numerous examples, from Gregory of Nazianzus and Emperor Julian to Anna Komnena and into the late Byzantine Era. A later scholium to our letter confirms the synonymity of the concepts φροντιστήριον and νοσοκομεῖον or ξενών.[29] We know that there was a series of hospitals in Constantinople and elsewhere in the empire.[30] We also know that into the late Byzantine period new ones were built and those that had fallen into disuse were restored to use. Just as well known is the fact that medicine was taught in such institutions. In the *Typikon* of the Pantokrator-Monastery,[31] mention is made of a διδάσκαλος τῆς ἰατρικῆς ἐπιστήμης, who instructed the παῖδες ἰατρῶν there.[32]

(Leib, II, 46, 19); XV, 7, 2 (Leib III, 214, 24 in connection with the Orphanotropheion); cf. also XV, 7, 7 (Leib III, 217); *Theophyl. Achrid. Opera*, ed. P. Gautier (CFHB, XVI, 1; 1980), 189, 17; *Nikeph. Bryenn.*, ed. P. Gautier (CFHB, IX; 1975), 103, 21 and 141, 1. Concerning the φροντιστήριον as a center of education which enjoyed a rank superior to that of the διδασκαλεῖον, cf. Agathias, *Hist.*, ed. R. Keydell (CFHB; 1967), V, 21 (p. 190, 32–191, 2); cf. also Zachar. Scholast., *De mundi opificio*, PG, 85, 1021 B and Manuel Moschopoulos in *Lexicon Philostr.*: φροντιστήρια· τὰ διδασκαλεῖα τῶν φιλοσόφων· λέγοντο δ' ἂν οὕτω καὶ τὰ παρ' ἡμῶν μοναστήρια. Cf. also *Hesychii Lexicon*, *s.v.*: φροντιστήριον· διατριβὴ καὶ τὸ οἴκημα Σωκράτους καὶ τὸ σχολεῖον καὶ μοναστήριον, and *Suda*, *s.v.*: φροντιστήριον· διατριβὴ ἢ μοναστήριον, ὅπερ 'Αττικοὶ σεμνεῖον καλοῦσιν.

[29] Cf. F. Fuchs, *Die höheren Schulen von Konstantinopel im Mittelalter* (Leipzig/Berlin, 1926), 61 with note 6.

[30] Cf. the compilation of D. J. Constantelos, *Byzantine Philanthropy and Social Welfare* (New Brunswick, 1968), 149–276, and more recently, K. Mentzou-Meimare, 'Επαρχιακὰ εὐαγῆ ἱδρύματα μέχρι τοῦ τέλους τῆς εἰκονομαχίας, Βυζαντινά 11 (1982), 243–308. Reference to specific bibliographical data can be overlooked in this context.

[31] Ed. P. Gautier, *REB*, 32 (1974), 1–145.

[32] Gautier, *REB*, 32 (1974), 107, 1313–16. On this point a brief excursus does indeed seem necessary, as certain wrong ideas crept in here, indeed in conjunction with a particular interpretation of the Hippocratic Oath—ideas, moreover, which are still lurking around as well in the most recent Byzantine professional literature. In the passage of the *Typikon* in question, this teacher was supposed to instruct the παῖδες ἰατρῶν, literally translated, "the children of the doctors." And because the genitive ξενῶνος (in the hospital) stands next to the expression, one always assumed that this man was charged with instructing the children of the doctors employed in the hospital. Such an interpretation makes no sense in the context of the whole regimentation. The doctors in the Pantokrator Hospital lived outside the hospital when they were not on night duty. Why would they bring their children along every day for instruction in the hospital? But apart from that, the concept παῖδες ἰατρῶν refers to the students of medicine and the young doctors. This can be verified at least since the time of Plato, and there is a great deal of evidence for it in the Byzantine literature, and indeed in the most differentiated genera of this literature. We have treatises for Byzantine hospitals, for example, with the title Προσταγαὶ καὶ τύποι τῶν μεγάλων ξενώνων ὅσα ἐκ πείρας ἰατρῶν παῖδες θεραπείας χάριν προσάγουσι . . . , and the παῖδες ἰατρῶν there are young doctors or assistants, who, however they may be trained, dispense medicine to the sick. A letter of Symeon Magistros (ed. J. Darrouzès, no. 68) clearly shows the application of

But let us get back to our letter of 1299. John has not yet completed his studies and has not yet received certification. He has not yet arrived at the endpoint, the κολοφών, and has therefore received as yet no κηρύγματα. These κηρύγματα represent the crowning point of the whole process. Whether or not this word is a *terminus technicus* we cannot say with certainty. In any case, it designated the public, legal character of the final examination. It is not necessary to cite legal texts, which treat of the examination of doctors and which regulate their teaching obligations according to the position they occupy, but clear, however, is the concern of the state for medical competence. In Byzantium this was much more distinctly regulated and defined than was the case in the West during the Middle Ages; and, of course, it can be verified at a much earlier date. We can observe this already in the time of the early Byzantine period, e.g., in the legal codices of Emperor Theodosios II and of Justinian. The already mentioned passage from the *Typikon* of the Pantokrator-Monastery in Constinople offers a good proof for the twelfth century, for which we also have other testimony at our disposal, e.g., a synodal decision of 1140.[33] Concerning the education of doctors, this decision stipulates that they are to have studied the λόγος ἰατρικῆς τέχνης, that they must have a lengthy education, and finally that they receive the σύμβολον ἐπικρίσεως. That is approximately the same thing which Lakapenos calls the κηρύγματα in his letter to John.

Whatever the case may be regarding John's residence in Thessalonica, in 1307, at the latest, he is considered an acknowledged doctor; and we know that from 1323 he uses the title ἀκτουάριος.[34] From the twelfth century for sure (and perhaps from the eleventh century as well),[35] we have testimony for

this concept to the doctors. John himself bears testimony to it also when he says that it is the business of the παῖδες ἰατρῶν to understand the salutary medicines and the anodynes and to dispense them. The question posed by Kuruses (II, p. 249) in connection with his reflections on this matter, namely, whether John's father was a ἰατρὸς ξενῶνος, appears to me therefore as irrelevant.

[33] V. Grumel, *Regestes des actes du patriarcat de Constantinople*, I, 3 (1947), no. 1007; *id.*, "La Profession médicale à Byzance (à l'époque des Comnènes)," *REB*, 7 (1949), 42–46; the text: Rhalles-Potles, Σύνταγμα τῶν θείων καὶ ἱερῶν κανόνων, V (1855), 76–82.

[34] Cf. above, p. 123.

[35] Whether the brother of the doctor whose death Psellos Laments (ed. K. N. Sathas, Μεσαιωνικὴ Βιβλιοθήκη, V (1876), 96–102), actually as a doctor bore the title ἀκτουάριος is uncertain. Concerning the development of this title, cf. the compilation in Kuruses II, p. 252–57; also regarding the ἀκτουάριοι of the Palaeologian period.

this title in Byzantium in connection with medicine, in the letters of Michael Italikos as well[36] as in the so-called *Ptochoprodromika*.[37] We are aware of ἀκτουάριοι during the whole late Byzantine period. It appears that this title signifies the highest echelon of the official medical hierarchy in the empire.

I would like to bring up two points in John's professional activity:

1. In the work *De urinis* there is a series of case histories[38] from which we can surmise that he made house calls, made diagnoses, and dispensed medicine. Frequently the patients in question are people who are personally known to John and who obviously wish to ask his advice, although they have already consulted other doctors. Again and again mention is made of the ἰατροὶ θαμίζοντες,[39] that is, of doctors who make frequent visits; and frequently these doctors prevail over John's opinion, indeed not always for the welfare of the patients. These cases are differentiated; they relate also to different specialized areas of medicine, and the patients frequently, though by no means always, belong to the highest levels of society. The question has, of course, been asked, whether John, perhaps even as ἀκτουάριος, had a practice, whether he made housecalls, and so on. He certainly made housecalls, but whether he did so as ἀκτουάριος seems questionable to me. It cannot, however, be ruled out considering his interest in the matter. It would scarcely have been the rule, however. Unfortunately, the reports do not offer more exact information which could be of help in setting down dates.

The reports show John's diagnostic as well as his prognostic abilities, they give information about the practice of medicine in Byzantium as well as about quackery, which obviously existed also. From the reports we clearly recognize that these Byzantine doctors, insofar as they took their profession seriously, always considered the entire person in making their diagnoses.

There is the case of a man suffering from a liver disorder who finally contracts jaundice;[40] this disease, apart from poor nutrition, is traced back to his psychic condition. He cannot overcome an injustice that has been done him.

In another case John diagnoses the malady of a wealthy woman[41] whose period does not take place. At first she thinks she is pregnant, but because she has a great deal of pain, she calls the doctors; in the fifth month of the illness John is called in for consultation. First he takes her pulse, which is very weak. The patient's skin color is sallow and looks like the color of someone suffering from jaundice. Around the face, hands and shoulders she is very thin; her body is very swollen. John does a uroscopy and finds blood in the urine. At this point in time John himself has only textbook knowledge of gynecology, and the other doctors who are present know nothing; they diagnosed dropsy. John studies the books of female diseases and compares what he has learned with the results of the uroscopy. And he arrives, as he says, at the correct diagnosis: ἐπίσχεσις ἐπιμηνίων, whereby he explains the blood in the urine on the basis of the proximity of uterus and bladder. Soon, severe hemorrhaging begins and the blood is mixed with pus. After a brief apparent improvement, the woman dies. On this occasion, one learns something of the psychic background of the case: the woman wanted to have another child and sought advice from other women as to how she might bring about a pregnancy. John indicates, albeit tactfully, that the advice was obviously not conducive to the woman's health. Here, as well as in another case in which an uneducated woman refuses the medicine proffered her by John, because in her folly she does not know what a φάρμακον is, we can take a look into the medical culture of that period, a glance at the cultural-historical source value of such professional literature, especially the case histories.

2. The second point concerns John's assertion that he frequently visited the ἰατρεῖον.[42] In all probability he had patients there and perhaps treated them. Whether he did so regularly, we do not know. By this ἰατρεῖον is obviously not meant a private practice. Otherwise John's manner of expression would not be intelligible when he says he often visited the place and learned of a particular case there. "*Iatreion*" is the term for the hospital. The word is thus used in the *Typikon* of the Pantokrator-Monastery as well.[43]

[36] Cf. P. Gautier, *Michael Italikos, Lettres et discours.* (Paris, 1972 [AOC 14]), 46–49, 111–15 (monody on the ἀκτουάριος Pantechnes); *ibid.* 209–10 (letter to an ἀκτουάριος [Pantechnes]).

[37] D. C. Hesseling-H. Pernot, *Poèmes prodromiques en Grec Vulgaire*, III, 415 (Amsterdam, 1910), 69.

[38] Cf. note 26 above.

[39] Ideler, II, 163, 19; 182, 18.

[40] Ideler, II, 154, 31–156, 14.

[41] Ideler, II, 181, 12–183, 12.

[42] Ideler, II, 95, 324–96, 6. Ἐγώγε μὴν καί τι τοιοῦτον μέμνημαι ἰδὼν περὶ τὸ ἰατρεῖον θαμίζων. . . .

[43] Ed. Gautier, p. 89, 1000 and 93, 1070. Nevertheless, the word is used in the same *Typikon* with a different meaning.

Now I would like to say something about the education of John in general, not only because it adds to a complete picture of the man, but also because it is fundamentally important for the attitude of the Byzantines toward education in general and, not least of all, toward the education of doctors.

In a letter of Georgios Lakapenos,[44] John is designated as the greatest credit to his circle of friends and as ἰατρός τ' ἀγαθὸς κρατερός τε φιλόσοφος, a good doctor and a great philosopher. In the manuscripts we meet him as σοφώτατος καὶ λογιώτατος βασιλικὸς ἰατρός,[45] the wisest and very learned doctor of the imperial court. In the letters of Gabras mention is made of the σὺν λόγῳ ζῶν, who loves everything which has to do with the τέχνη λόγων.[46] Gabras sends John a speech to the emperor for his evaluation. There is an interesting passage in the introduction to De urinis,[47] where John says he was considering returning to the λόγοι, whose charm lay in the reading of them; but he nevertheless recognized that, although educated in other fields, he would be wasting his time on this point. So he decided to occupy himself with that area of the λόγοι which would be of use to the others. Not the beauty of words about empty subjects should convince, but rather the content. Here is not the place to go into the contemporary historical-critical import of this passage; in any case it is telling for John. Even taking into account the character of captatio benevolentiae, the passage lets us see that John had made the usual ἐγκύκλιος παιδεία of the time his own and accordingly decided in favor of medicine. By no means did he deny the value of this ἐγκύκλιος παιδεία; we have sufficient evidence for this. For himself, however, with a view toward efficacy, he chose medicine.

The letters of this period offer a good insight into John's versatility. To arrange all of this in a systematic and perhaps even chronological way is a tedious piece of work that is hardly appropriate for a short paper. I will, therefore, summarize on this point and indicate the results.

John belongs to a circle of pupils under Maximos Planudes, who, in addition to grammar, rhetoric and prosody, occupied himself with mathematics, music and perhaps even with medicine.[48]

He is also a friend of John and of Andronikos Zaridas[49] and of Georgios Lakapenos, whose letters we have mentioned several times. They, too, are pupils of Planudes. Beyond that, they are men who concern themselves with a compehensive education, who collect books and copy them, just as did Joseph Rhakendytes,[50] who planned a comprehensive encyclopedia of all knowledge, and whose knowledge of medicine is not to be denied, although just how deep this knowledge went is another question.[51] We have already seen Michael Gabras among John's friends; other names could be mentioned, but I will stop here. The important thing is that John had good contacts with the ἄρχοντες in the imperial palace, and he belonged even to the circle of scholars in the company of Emperor Andronikos, so that he could use his influence for his friends there. We hear a number of times that he is asked to do so.[52] This circle around Andronikos II included the elite of the literary society of the time in the capital. Of course a significant role in this group was played by, as we would say today, the philologists. But to a certain extent, there is perhaps a problem of terminology or semantics. To be a philologos in the Constantinople of the fourteenth century meant much more than to be a philologist in the twentieth century, even if at a university. These people are not satisifed simply with Aischylos, Sophokles or Euripides. They are filled with a love and an enthusiasm for everything

---

[44]Ep. 20 (ed. Lindstam, p. 128, 32).

[45]For example, Paris. graec. 2256.

[46]Ep. 439 (ed. Fatouros, p. 677, 8).

[47]Ideler, II, 3.

[48]Cf. C. Wendel, "Planudes," RE XX, 2 (1950), 2202–53; id., "Planudes als Bücherfreund," Zentralblatt f. Bibliothekswesen, 58 (1941), 77–87.

[49]Ep. 18 (ed. Lindstam, p. 120–21); cf. Kuruses I, passim.

[50]Cf. M. Treu, BZ, 8 (1899), 1–64; R. Guilland, Nicéphore Grégoras, Correspondance (Paris, 1927), 338–42; B. N. Tatakes, Ἡ βυζαντινὴ φιλοσοφία, translated by E. K. Kalpourtzes. Ἐποπτεία καὶ βιβλιογραφικὴ ἐνημέρωση L. G. Benakis. Βιβλιοθήκη Γενικῆς Παιδείας, 5 (Athens, 1978), 228 f.; S. I. Kuruses, Μανουὴλ Γαβαλᾶς εἶτα Ματθαῖος μητροπολίτης Ἐφέσου (1271/2–1355/60), Α' Τὰ βιογραφικά (Athens, 1972), passim.

[51]G. E. Pentogalos, Οἱ ἰατρικὲς γνώσεις Ἰωσὴφ τοῦ Ῥακενδύτη καὶ ἡ σχετικὴ ἀνέκδοτη ἐπιστολὴ τοῦ Μιχαὴλ Γαβρᾶ (Athens, 1970). The letter in question is no. 293 (according to the edition of Fatouros). Apparently Joseph has sent him medicines, to which, along with Joseph's prayers, Gabras attributed the healing of his eye disease. Whether this means anything more than that Joseph had a certain pharmacological knowledge may be left undecided here. If he took care of the sick monk Merkurios over a period of years, he may have acquired such knowledge in the course of time. There remains the reference of John Actuarius (Ideler, I, 348, 32 ff.), that he himself had blood samples taken and discussed his own disease and its diagnosis with John. All this proves Joseph's interest in medicine, which perhaps can be traced back to a certain study of these things, which belong to the φυσικὸν μέρος τῆς φιλοσοφίας. This interest is apparent as well in the inclusion of medicine in the encyclopedia which was planned. It does not prove, of course, that Joseph was, or can be designated, ἰατρός in the technical sense.

[52]Mich. Gabras, ep. 22 (ed. Fatouros, II, 48 f.) to Georgios Lakapenos and John Zacharias Cf. Kuruses II, p. 251 f.; Georg. Lakapenos ep. 24 (ed. Lindstam, p. 150–54).

which was written in the past—and not only in the so-called Classical Age. Furthermore, they were eager to examine their own cultural heritage and, in a given case, to defend it against teaching and tendencies which had developed. To this cultural heritage belong, perhaps even preferentially, technical, geographical, mathematical, and astronomical texts. Thus the interest for the φυσικὸν μέρος τῆς φιλοσοφίας of which John speaks is quite suitable to this period. Already in the thirteenth century we notice a revival of those interests, and it continues into the fourteenth century. One is not satisfied with textbooks, but writes commentaries, e.g., on Euclid and Diophantos; one reads critically the *Geography* of Ptolemy of his *Tetrabiblos*, *Almagest*, or the commentaries of Theon, and so on.[53] Astronomy, although not totally separated from astrology, experienced a particular growth, and this is perhaps also a reason for the intense preoccupation with these topics in the circle of Emperor Andronikos II, who like no other Byzantine emperor was quite dependent on such things. That is indeed a different problem in conjunction with the decadent period of the empire. To this circle, which Nikephoros Gregoras designates as a *"gymnasion"* of rhetoricians and philosophers, and which stands far above the Platonic Academy, the Aristotelian "Lykeion" and the Attic Stoa,[54] belong—among others—Konstantinos Akropolites, Nikephoros Chumnos, Nikephoros Gregoras and also Theodoros Metochites, whose picture we recognize in a mosaic on the narthex of the Kariye Djami in Constantinople. Although he was truly a man of well-rounded education, he dedicated himself at the age of forty-three to the study of astronomy upon the advice of the emperor. Astronomy was the cardinal topic of the time, and it is not accidental that the proem to the Στοιχείωσις ἐπὶ τῇ ἀστρονομικῇ ἐπιστήμη of Theodoros Metochites includes a defense of astronomy and astrology. One can read more about the role of Metochites in this circle of men and in the context of these studies in the works of I. Ševčenko.[55]

I can now return to John Actuarius. Since he belongs to this group, then the question poses itself *eo ipso* (especially if one knows the rules according to which the learned discussions were conducted in this circle), whether John engaged in the study of astronomy. This question can be answered positively.

In the body of letters of Georgios Oinaiotes[56] there are four letters addressed to an unnamed ἀκτουάριος which fall within the years 1321 to 1327. There is no reason to assume that this ἀκτουάριος is not our John, even if we cannot explain exactly the relationship alluded to in the letters. We learn from these letters not only of John's interest in astronomy and that he wants to borrow one of Ptolemy's works from Oinaiotes, but also that his knowledge of astronomy is so great that Oinaiotes wants to be instructed by him. The instruction takes place, and Oinaiotes makes such good progress that he finally asks his teacher to get him into the circle of astronomers which has sprung up around Metochites. Gregorios Chioniades,[57] who turned to astronomy after first studying medicine, and who attained great prominence for the impetus given to astronomy in the late Byzantine period, is also counted among John's friends, as can be seen from one of his letters.

John testifies to his knowledge of, and interest in, astronomy in his own work. In the treatment of the κρίσιμοι ἡμέραι (critical days) in book II of his work on diagnosis, he includes his knowledge in a rather lengthy excursus.[58] That is, he determines not only the fourth, the seventh, the fourteenth,

---

[53] Cf. I. Ševčenko, "Theodore Metochites, the Chora, and the Intellectual Trends of His Time," in P. Underwood (ed.), *The Kariye Djami*, IV: *Studies in the Art of the Kariye Djami and Its Intellectual Background* (Princeton Univ. Press, 1975), 19–91, esp. 19–24.

[54] Nikeph. Gregoras, *Byz. Hist.*, ed. L. Schopen, X, 1 (ed. Bonn. I, 471, 11–12).

[55] Cf. esp. I. Ševčenko, *op. cit.*; *id., La Vie intellectuelle et politique à Byzance sous les premiers Paléologues. Etudes sur la polémique entre Théodore Métochite et Nicéphore Choumnos* (Bruxelles, 1962 [CBHByz Subsidia 3]); *id.,* "Théodore Métochites, Chora et les courants intellectuels de l'époque," in *Art et société à byzance sous*

les Paléologues. Bibliothèque de l'Institut Hellénique d'Etudes Byzantines et Post-Byzantines de Venise, 4 (Venice, 1971), 13–39; *id.,* "Society and Intellectual Life in the Fourteenth Century," *XIVᵉ Congrès Internat. des Etudes byzantines* (Bucarest, 6–12 septembre 1971) *Rapports* I, p. 7–30; cf. *id., Society and Intellectual Life in Late Byzantium* (London, 1981); also the discussion by A. Kazhdan, in *Greek Orthodox Theological Review,* 27 (1982) 83–97.

[56] G. Fatouros, S. I. Kuruses and D. Reinsch are preparing an edition of his letters. Here I am relying upon the references in Kuruses II, p. 260 ff., with pertinent bibliography (cf. Kuruses I, p. 380). Concerning John's knowledge of astronomy, cf. also I. Ševčenko, *Etudes sur la polémique, op. cit.,* 83, note 3 and 87, note 3, where this corpus of letters of Laur. marc. 356 is taken into account.

[57] Cf. D. Pingree, "Gregory Chioniades and Palaeologan Astronomy," 18 (1964), 134–60; L. G. Westerink, "La Profession de foi de Grégoire Chioniadès," *REB,* 38 (1980), 233–45. Letter no. 15 (ed. I. B. Papadopoulos [Thessalonike, 1929]) to a certain Ἰωάννης, a doctor, who is designated as γλυκύς, is not addressed to the later patriarch, as S. I. Kuruses in the Epimetron to his essay on John XIII Glykys (Ἐπ.Ἑτ.Βυζ.Σπ., 41 [1974], 372) has correctly demonstrated. It is rather a question of an allusion to the name "Zacharias" (cf. Kuruses II, p. 257 ff.).

[58] Ideler, II, 433–40; cf. also *De urinis* V, 10 (Ideler, II, 128–32) and *ibid.* VI, proem. (Ideler, II, 145).

the twentieth, the twenty-seventh day, which would actually be enough for a doctor; he also gives the reasons why this is so. He speaks of the influence of the sun on the seasons and especially of that of the moon on people. He is also conscious that he has gone rather far afield on this subject, for at the end of the chapter he calls himself back with the remark that he has said enough both for those who speak briefly of it and for those who wish to understand more about it. Therefore John studied astronomy, and we know also that he collected the pertinent literature in his library. One must keep in mind that, apart from the fact that this is suitable to John's time, in which astronomy was considered the κορυφαῖον μάθημα,[59] this science obviously—and even earlier—had a preferential place in the education of doctors. Michael Italikos in his monody praises the knowledge of astronomy of the ἀκτουάριος Pantechnes.[60] Finally we can go all the way back to Galen, who said of the doctors that they stood with the γεωμέτραι, ἀριθμητικοί, φιλόσοφοι, ἀστρονόμοι and γραμματικοὶ ἔγγιστα θεῷ, that is, in the closest proximity to God.[61]

Let me now come to John's works. In our present context we are interested in the medical writings.[62] Seen as a whole, they represent the last great compendium of Byzantine medicine. Here we have an accomplishment which for its penetration and thorough study of the material is not to be underestimated, even if the treatment is of uneven originality. Whatever John may have taken over from the past, and that is surely a great deal (that is in the nature of the thing), one must keep in mind that he arranged his material in a precise, systematic, and even stylistically pithy presentation, so that his work is not only handier and more synoptical but is also more useful than Galen's. A comment in the satire *Timarion* shows to what great extent the Byzantines, and particularly the Byzantine doctors, were put off by Galen's verbosity.[63]

The most important writings in his medical opus are three in number:

1. Περὶ οὔρων, in Latin *De urinis*, in seven books, is available in the edition of Ideler.[64] It was edited in Latin in 1519 in Venice, and then about another ten times in the sixteenth century. In 1531 an incomplete German translation appeared. Resting upon Galen's theory and evaluating the pertinent observations of Galen and Hippocrates, as well as of later Byzantine scholars—for example Theophilos—and frequently including his own experience, John offers in this work a compendium of the knowledge in this area which reaches up to his own time. Color, consistency and residue of the urine are extensively discussed, as well as the diagnostic/prognostic conclusions which one can draw. Even here diagnosis and prognosis are separated. I will make only two comments on this work, since it is not of primary importance to the topic of the new edition.

As the final chapter shows,[65] this piece of writing obviously represents John's maiden work in the field of medicine. He composed it in order to contribute to the understanding of medicine (τέχνη), as an expression of his knowledge. A doctor of his ability and with his ambitions had to give proof of his knowledge with one or more publications in order to develop a career. John also explains why, exactly, he chose this topic. There were many extensive writings in the other fields of medicine. In other authors he had found only scattered remarks concerning urine. He therefore consciously chose a topic which had not been treated to excess and with which he could help the τέχνη progress.

Another assertion is important in this context: in undertaking the work he observed the healthy people and the sick people with whom he had daily contact, and at the same time he compared the different λόγοι with one another.[66] Ten years ago a paper appeared under the title "Empirie und Theorie in der Harnlehre des Johannes Aktuarios."[67] In posing this question the author intended, as he says, to arrive at a "more concrete evaluation" of Byzantine medicine. This consists in his assertion that John attacks those doctors who

---

[59] Cf. Kuruses II, 262.

[60] Ed. P. Gautier, p. 110–15, esp. 112, 2.

[61] Galen (ed. Kühn), I, 7.

[62] In any case, we are acquainted with another letter to Theodoros Pediasimos (ed. M. Treu, *Theodori Pediasimi eiusque amicorum quae exstant*. Programm Victoria-Gymnasium Potsdam, Ostern 1899 [Potsdam, 1899], 39 f. and 59 f.). Cf. A. D. Komines, Τὸ βυζαντινὸν ἱερὸν ἐπίγραμμα καὶ οἱ ἐπιγραμματοποιοί (Athens, 1966), 183 f., with a reference to three more recent editions of one of the epigrams. The question about further writings of John, e.g., commentaries on Aristotle or Hippocrates, need not be dealt with here. Concerning translations from the Arabic, cf. below note 81.

[63] Ed. R. Romano, *Byzantina et Neo-Hellenica Neapolitana*, 2 (1974), 715 ff. (p. 75). Galen is not present at court. He had retreated in order to finish his treatment on fevers. The supple-

ments were to have a much greater range than what was already available.

[64] Regarding the older editions of John's works, which cannot all be listed here, cf. L. Choulant, *Handbuch der Bücherkunde für die ältere Medicin*, 2nd ed. (Leipzig, 1841; repr. 1956), 152–54; cf. also Sarton, *Introduction*, III, pt. 1, p. 889–92.

[65] VII, 18 (Ideler, II, 191–92).

[66] VII, 17 (Ideler, II, 190).

[67] F. Kudlien, *Clio Medica*, 8 (1973), 19–30.

refer only to the πεῖρα much more than Galen did; by λόγος John means simply physiological speculation; basically he assumes the mind-set of antiquity, and so forth. I am by no means certain whether the sequence in which the two concepts λόγος and πεῖρα appear in John's works (λόγος— πεῖρα or πεῖρα—λόγος) is really to be taken in the sense of a hierarchical ordering; and I cannot otherwise agree to each interpretation of the author. What is even more important, λόγος means the theoretical penetration of a subject which forms the presupposition for the results acquired from the πεῖρα. John distinctly emphasizes this at the conclusion of his work, when he points out that some details may be missing, but that they are contained implicitly. The work is written for the συνετοί, that is, for people with insight and understanding, for those who have daily practice with the λόγοι and who therefore could easily grasp the significance of something he may not have explicitly mentioned, and are thereby able to make the diagnosis or prognosis.[68] I cannot see any degrading of the πεῖρα when John says: "whoever possesses a sharp intellect and a natural talent for accuracy will easily arrive at the appropriate conclusions from what has been said as well as from what has not been said, even though he may have only the slightest practical experience."[69]

2. A second work by John bears the title Περὶ ἐνεργειῶν καὶ παθῶν τοῦ ψυχικοῦ πνεύματος καὶ τῆς κατ᾽ αὐτὸ διαίτης ("Concerning the activities and illnesses of the psychic pneuma and the corresponding mode of living"). It is the only work of John published also in the Greek language before the nineteenth century (in Paris 1557). It is also available today in the edition by Ideler,[70] and it is identical with John's two letters to Joseph Rhakendytes, contained in the cod. Riccardianus 31, and was supposed to be included in Rhakendytes' large encyclopedia.[71] It includes two books. The pneumatic theory is treated; and of the three types of pneumata—φυσικόν, ζωτικόν, ψυχικόν—the last receives preferential treatment. It deals with the influence of the pneuma on health and sickness and how physical diseases can also influence the soul. The following is discussed: the dependence of the material *pneuma psychikon* on the spiritual func-

tions—sense perception (αἴσθησις), imagination (φαντασία), power of judgment (μέρος δοξαστικόν), understanding (διάνοια), and reason (νοῦς)— as well as their relations to one another and the question of their localization in the particular parts of the brain. The second book contains dietetic and hygienic rules.

3. The third of John's comprehensive works on medicine is known in the current literary and medical history under an abbreviated title as the so-called Θεραπευτικὴ μέθοδος, in Latin *De methodo medendi*. In the introductory chapter John himself gives the title as βιβλίον περιέχον πᾶσαν τὴν τέχνην ἐν ἐπιτόμῳ and that is indeed correct; for *"De methodo medendi"* refers, strictly speaking, only to the second part of the work. In the introductory chapter, we read that it is a comprehensive medical handbook which John has written for his friend Alexios Apokaukos, when the latter had to undertake a diplomatic mission to the "hyperborean Scythians."[72] The work includes six books. The first two books deal with diagnostics in general, then with specific cases of disease. Both of these books appear to have circulated independently under the title Περὶ διαγνώσεως. They are edited in Ideler.[73] The Greek text of the rest of the work is not edited. Therapy is the theme of books III and IV. They are available only in the Latin translation of Mathisius (Venice, 1554). Finally, useful drugs for the treatment of internal and external diseases is the subject of the last two books (Latin translation by Ruelle, Paris, 1539). This work, a compendium of the entire field of medicine, is to be edited first. The manuscripts, which I will not go into further here, are numerous, regarding both the entire opus as well as the individual parts. Both the arrangement of the books as well as the subdivisions, particularly in the last two books about drugs, vary in the manuscripts. The enumeration of the books differs, according to whether the first two books under the title Περὶ διαγνώσεως are counted separately. The same is true, *mutatis mutandis*, also for the last two under the title Περὶ φαρμάκων συνθέσεως. To put it briefly, the history of the tradition puts up a series of problems which are not all clarified. We can pin down the following: that John himself had the idea of composing six books, two on diagnosis, two on therapy, and two on *pharmaka* or drugs. And he also followed through on this idea. In one manuscript we read: "Now that

---

[68] VII, 18, 10–11: Ideler, II, 192.
[69] II, 10, 16; Ideler, II, 42 f.
[70] Ideler, I, 312–86.
[71] Cf. M. Treu, *BZ*, 8 (1899), 45 f. and 63 f.; Pentogalos, (cf. note 51 above); cf. also R. Criscuolo, "Note sull' 'Enciclopedia' del filosofo Giuseppe," *Byzantion*, 44 (1974), 255–81.

[72] Cf. note 11 above.
[73] Ideler, II, 353–463.

diagnosis and the causes of diseases have been dealt with in the first two books, and therapy for individual maladies in the following two, the last two deal with *pharmaka* which are useful in treating internal and external diseases."[74]

The work is written for Alexios Apokaukos, and not on the command of the emperor as one so often reads. This opinion has crept into the pertinent literature because of an incorrect reference of a *genitivus absolutus*.[75] The question as to which diplomatic legation is meant shall not be discussed here,[76] any more than the question about the medical interests of Apokaukos, which must be seen in association with the well-known manuscript of Hippocrates (Cod. Paris. gr. 2144), and the question about the picture of Apokaukos there.[77]

In the preface of book I, John gives detailed information about the difficulties which resulted from the fact that the book is supposed to be a short one, a βραχυσύλλαβος δέλτος.[78] He is afraid of insulting the τέχνη by such a terse treatment. Besides, it is difficult to present the life of mankind and its lifestyles to someone who is unfamiliar with the material in just a few words. He is about to give up the undertaking, but the thought of friendship and the usefulness of the book for his friend prevent him from doing so; he wants to give it to him in remembrance of their friendship. When doubts once again assail him as to whether he can treat such a multi-layered topic in the brevity demanded, he recalls—and this is an important point regarding the problem just touched upon—that Apokaukos often made very sensitive remarks during their discussions of medical topics, such that John often challenged his friend to go deeper into the study of medicine.[79] Apokaukos was therefore in a position to understand correctly even a brief presentation. When one considers the extent of Galen's or Myrepsos' works, one cannot shrug off such remarks as a mere *captatio benevolentiae*. After

a brief recapitulation of those elements which a doctor must know *a priori*—such as the causes of illness, what is conducive to health, the natural resources of the living organism, which drugs are available—there is an outline of humoral physiology. Finally, and in some detail, the teaching concerning the pulse in its different aspects is treated, whereby psychic causes are also considered. Then the diagnosis of urine is briefly dealt with, and finally the diseases are listed according to the well-known principle *a capite ad calcem*.

From the introduction of the second book we learn that it was written in the following spring (after the first book had been written in the fall), when Apokaukos was expected to return from his diplomatic mission.[80] In the meantime, as already mentioned, Joseph Rhakendytes has asked John for a composition. The second book defines and treats the concept of fever and the κρίσεις, also the κρίσιμοι ἡμέραι, then the diseases of the skin and the individual parts of the body. At the end of the book, John says that he wants to write another dealing with the θεραπευτικαὶ μέθοδοι. In the introduction to the third book John refers to the two previous ones, in which he dealt with diagnosis per se and its relations to the individual parts of the body and with the causes of diseases; he also points out the methodical structure (ἐμμεθόδως) of his work.

Indeed, other authors of medical manuals in Byzantine times dealt with diagnosis and therapy, but not in this manner. For the most part, they dealt with diagnosis, therapy and drugs, one after the other. But John does not want to divide his compendium into small pieces; he sticks to the concept of a brief manual. If now and again he spends more time on a particular topic, then it is for the sake of clarity of presentation. If something appears to be missing, then he makes the required brevity the culprit. This is a convenient alibi; he must take more time with some illnesses in order to make the therapy clear. As an example of the versatility of the methods of treatment he cites phlebotomy. It constitutes the beginning of the third book, which deals also with purgation, suppositories, enemas, gargling, and so on, as well as the effects of baths, sleep, and gymnastic exercises. Therapy for the individual parts of the body is the subject of the fourth book. Of course in both these books drugs are named; but John says explicitly that he does not intend to treat the whole σύνθεσις, so as not to disturb the symmetry of the book. It seems preferable

---

[74] Cod. Monac. gr. 69, fol. 255ᵛ.

[75] Ideler, II, 353, 9–11. The "Illustrierte Geschichte der Medizin" (cf. note 2 above) speaks of a medical leader whom the emperor needed for his crusade against the Scythians (p. 468). Indeed, on the same page, in a legend to an illustration, mention is made that Apokaukos "went to the northern Scythians (Russians) in the capacity of ambassador" toward the end of the thirteenth(!) century. He took along the book on therapy, "which John Actuarius, his fellow-pupil, had composed at his request."

[76] This question will be dealt with elsewhere.

[77] Cf. H. Belting, *Das illuminierte Buch in der spätbyzantinischen Gesellschaft*. AbhHeidelberg, philos.-hist. Kl. 1970, 1 (Heidelberg, 1970), 59 f. and 83 f., with ill. 31 and 32.

[78] Ideler, II, 353, 14 f.

[79] Ideler, II, 354, 20 ff.

[80] Ideler, II, 418.

to him to write a separate treatise on the simple and compound drugs.

The recurring introductions clearly show, in my opinion, that the work was not written in a single sitting; perhaps it was given to Apokaukos piecemeal. Since John continually emphasizes and substantiates his principle of organization, we can conclude that it was not the usual one. And in fact, neither Aëtios, nor Alexander of Tralles, nor Paulos Aiginetes employed this principle. The symmetry of the individual books can scarcely have been the real reason for this manner of proceeding; rather it is an approximation to the system of medical instruction. Apart from that, there is a logical principle at work: from the general to the specific, from the cause to the therapy, including the help of the person's natural resources, up to the *ultima ratio*—the drugs. In the books dealing with therapy these drugs are generally simply named, the inducing effects are given but measures are not. At the end of the fourth book John explicitly states that another book is to follow, concerning the qualities and the quantitative composition of the drugs, which may not be used by everyone in the same way. Very important are the mixture, the person's habits and age, the season, and so forth. At the beginning of the fifth book, John explains that he does not intend to discuss the preparation of the drugs (cooking, grating, etc.) unless absolutely necessary. He specifies the composition, the indication, and the proportions as well as the specific peculiarities of those drugs which can be used for several diseases. For most of the drugs, the indications are recognizable from the headings; a specialist in diagnostics and therapeutics could put together other drugs according to the specified principles. This is one of John's basic ideas. In a general way he also lists his sources: he collected the drugs from different books (of other authors), but also from his own experience (πεῖρα), when they were nowhere written down. Finally he lists those which he himself has put together according to the ἰατρικὴ μέθοδος. Each individual drug has been experientially tested and is worthy of recommendation. He does not list the drugs in alphabetical order; the sequence corresponds to the one he used in his books on diagnosis and therapy. And there are always references to the pertinent literature in the other books. He goes from the more general to the more specific, and he also keeps the organizational principle of going from the internal to the external. After a brief discussion of the different forms in which the drugs can be administered

(τροχίσκοι, καταπότια, ἀντίδοτοι, ἀλοιφαί, etc.), the medicines for individual diseases follow. Obviously, among the multiplicity of drugs listed there is a high percentage of those for which only the name, the indications, the individual ingredients with ratios, and the dosage are given. There are, however, other medicines which include very exact data concerning their preparation, the manner in which they work during the course of the disease, the different methods of application, storage, and so on. What is offered is a *prima vista*, simply a long catalogue of formulae such as is found in Myrepsos' large collection, with which John must have been familiar. From the outset, John intends to list only the more effective prescriptions (χρησιμώτερα). He continually presupposes that the doctors know of the powers of *simplicia*, or ought to know of them. If that is the case, they can mix their own medicines, but they must always keep in mind the individual patient's constitution. This is emphasized over and over: one must carefully consider what is given to whom (ποῖα ποίοις); one must adapt the medicine to the sick person, just as the shoemaker adapts his shoemaker's last to the foot (καλαπόδιον). In these books about drugs there are evaluations of the formulae of different doctors, a series of personal assertions, that is, about medicines which John himself tested or put together. And several times he gives his sources, once again in a general way. They are Greek doctors of older and more recent times, but also foreigners (ἰατροὶ παλαιοί τε καὶ νέοι Ἑλλήνων καὶ βαρβάρων). If our information in the manuscripts is correct, then John translated Arabic medical writings or examined them for publication.[81]

I have already pointed out briefly the problems of textual transmission, and would like to say a few words about the new edition. In general I can say that the manuscripts offer no insurmountable problems, although some are in very poor condition and can no longer be photocopied. The transmission in the case of the two books about drugs is somewhat more problematic. It is a matter of technical literature, which demands suitable training. The preliminary work on other medical authors, which we do in Munich, is of great help here, especially the Oreibasios-Index. The publication will

---

[81] Concerning the tract on urine by ibn-Sīnā, the translation of which John improved, cf. Costomiris (note 5 above), 415; cf. also Ullmann, *Medizin*, 156. The text is edited in Ideler, II, 286–302. Cf. Costomiris, 416 concerning the translation of the writing Περὶ λοιμικῆς τοῦ Ῥαζῆ, which in Cod. Paris. gr. 2228 is attributed to John.

include an index of technical terms as well as an apparatus of testimonies. Here too, our preliminary work on other authors is useful. As far as the annotation is concerned, there are, corresponding to the nature of the matter, difficulties arising from the fact that not a few of the pertinent Greek texts are not available in appropriate editions; but that must remain a *cura posterior* which can finally be tackled only after appearance of the edition, as is usually the case with large publications in the field of natural science.

At the beginning I promised to return to the question of evaluating the accomplishments of John Actuarius, and I will do so very briefly. I will keep my remarks brief, with regard to the stage of the work, and I remind myself of the words of O. Temkin, who once said: "John Actuarius knows that he has something to say. Yet I hesitate to include him in my discussion. He lived at a time when the West had produced its great figures of scholastic medicine and when the influence of the West would have to be taken in account. As far as I know, not even the necessary philological preparation for such a task has as yet been made."[82] Some points in this statement will have to be completed and made more precise—a few perhaps even corrected—in the future, if the future blesses us with industrious scholars and the necessary leisure for science. What I can say today is the following:

1. John Actuarius systematically summarized the medical knowledge of his time, insofar as he condensed it into an ordered system. It is certain that some branches of medicine were quite strongly stressed, others less so.

2. John did not invent this system, but he did follow through on it. There are few passages in the work discussed in which he wears the topic out or gives himself over to his own fancies.

3. It is not a collection of popular medicine, but a work written for doctors by a doctor, and indeed by a doctor who possessed a great deal of practical experience. This is clear from his own opinions, prescriptions, evaluations of medicines of others, as well as from a whole series of personal assertions.

4. John rests upon the state which medicine has reached at his time, and in his cultural sphere in particular. That does not mean, however, that he simply took notes from the current medical literature, nor that he copied Galen or, as some assert,

Paulos Aiginetes. When one looks through the medico-historical literature, it is a favorite game to look for supposedly new discoveries by these Byzantine doctors, who are treated rather shabbily anyway. In John's case lead poisoning, for example, or trichocephalus dispar, would come into question. I do not wish to play this game at this moment. But I can give a brief example, which will clearly show the problematic involved in such matters. In an essay on John's ophthalmology[83] one can find the remark that in his valuation of the amblyopia he took the optic nerve into consideration. But one can confirm that Aëtios already spoke of the ὀπτικὸν νεῦρον. For another example, according to all appearances John praises, in a personal assertion, a prophylactic agent used in treating diseases of the eye which has been experientially tested, is quite excellent and also very well known. And then one ascertains that the same medication can be found among the *kollyria* of Aëtios, indeed that Galen had already described it. The manuscripts of our Actuarius do not allude to Galen. Here the question arises concerning the value of the personal statements, which in each case must be thoroughly scrutinized; and that is not always easy with the material at hand. Quite apart from the fact that John could scarcely afford to claim such a well-known medication for himself, it would be wrong, in my opinion, to shrug him off simply as a plagiarist. One must consider as well that the content of the concept "plagiarism" was entirely different in the Middle Ages than it is today, among other things.

On some points I have made comparisons, for example, with aural diseases. The result is that, in view of the multiplicity of descriptions, nuances and medicines, John describes exactly the more important symptoms and then cites the therapeutic methods. In the books on drugs, he offers the most important compounds, first the anodynes, and then the therapeutic drugs, whereby he does not forget the lifelong habits. Nothing is absolutely new. John says, to use his own words, what is necessary (τὰ δέοντα), and this is, apart from the systematical treatment, consistently and logically thought through. In the therapy it is the incentive for one who has studied the subject to arrive at new and better remedies.

It is similar with the affections of hair. Once again the systematic treatment is striking. John knows the

---

[82] "Byzantine Medicine: Tradition and Empiricism," *DOP*, 16 (1962), 97–115, esp. 114.

[83] J. Hirschberg, "Die Augenheilkunde bei den Griechen," *Archiv f. Ophthalmologie*, 33 (1887) 47–78.

available material well. He gives terse and exact definitions, in that he lists exactly the differences among the different forms of the disease. Again he differentiates between anodynes and therapy; and the drugs which he lists are well tested (διὰ πείρας βεβασανισμένα). In this connection there is a study of cosmetics, just as we saw with Galen and before him; but John emphasizes that medicine and cosmetics are two different things, and he mentions cosmetics in this case only because the remedies to be applied are in some instances the same. The reason why he speaks about it in connection with coloring agents for black hair is interesting: some consider white hair to be a sign of disgrace and old age. Actually one should not even talk about it. But he does so anyway, so as not to give the impression that he does not know anything about such matters. This criterion places him squarely in the tradition of Byzantine authors. One could further cite the description of sweats or that of fevers: everywhere the picture is similar.

John Actuarius was certainly a practitioner, but over and above that, he was a man of science who thoroughly studied his field and thought it through theoretically. Whether one can shrug all this off as physiological speculation, I am not so sure. He was not the revolutionary discoverer and research worker, but could he have been that? He was open to new knowledge, even if it came from foreigners. In my opinion, the historian of medicine, insofar as he is an historian, does not primarily have the task of evaluating the color of urine against its specific gravity.

I do not think that we will arrive at the day when we glorify Byzantine medicine as a whole, and I do not think that we should even attempt such a thing. I do believe, though, that we, as historians of Byzantine culture as well as of medicine, have the obligation to investigate matters thoroughly. When that happens, we can perhaps come to an evaluation against the entire backdrop of medical history; to raise or lower one's estimation of things beforehand merely blocks one's perception of things as they really were.

Institute for Byzantine Studies, University of Munich

INSANITY IN BYZANTINE AND ISLAMIC MEDICINE[1]

Michael Dols

The only detailed description of an early Islamic hospital is the account of the hospital founded by Aḥmad ibn Ṭūlūn in Egypt about A.D. 873. It was located near his famous mosque that still stands in the southern quarter of Cairo. By the early fifteenth century, however, no trace of the hospital had survived. Ibn Ṭūlūn apparently took a keen interest in his *māristān*, or hospital, generously endowing it and carefully stipulating its operation. The well-known Egyptian chronicler al-Maqrīzī tells us that the ruler came periodically to the hospital to inspect it and to see the patients, including the insane who were confined there. Al-Maqrīzī says:

Once he entered the hospital and stopped before one of the madmen who was shackled, and the madman shouted out to him: "Oh Amir, hear my words: I am not mad as you think, for I only acted that way as a ruse. I have a strong desire in my heart for a large pomegranate." So the governor ordered one for him immediately, and the man was delighted with it, tossing it in his hand and weighing it. Then, the madman, taking Ibn Ṭūlūn by surprise, threw the pomegranate at him. It splattered over his clothes, covering his entire chest. Thereupon, Ibn Ṭūlūn ordered them to guard the madman, and the governor did not return again after that incident to inspect the *māristān*.[2]

[The reader is referred to the list of abbreviations at the end of the volume.]

---

[1] For bibliographical references on this subject, I have relied on the following: H. Hunger, "Medizin," 287–320; and M. Ullmann, *Medizin.*

[2] Al-Maqrīzī, *al-Khiṭaṭ,* II (Būlāq, 1854), 405 f. Does the pomegranate symbolize the discontent of an overcrowded place? F. Rosenthal, *The Muslim Concept of Freedom* (Leiden, 1960), 76 f. quotes the verses of Ibn al-Muʿtazz:

Many a house did I visit where I felt
Crowded as if I were in a prison.
Only a pomegranate knows to jam seeds into its skin
As tightly as we (human beings) do.

Rosenthal adds that the pomegranate could be used as a metaphor for the greatest possible state of misery. Concerning the Islamic hospital, see below.

The vivid story of Ibn Ṭūlūn and the madman may be apocryphal, but there can be little doubt that hospitals were established in the Islamic empire from the early ninth century A.D., and that they provided care for the insane. These hospitals were a concrete expression of the Islamic indebtedness to Byzantine medical theory and therapeutics, for Islamic rulers clearly adopted the Byzantine institution of the hospital, and Islamic doctors clearly relied on Byzantine medical texts, especially for their interpretation of insanity. The fact that the insane received special attention in the Islamic hospitals, however, raises a number of questions about the understanding of insanity in both Byzantine and Islamic societies.[3]

---

[3] The literature on the history of the hospital is considerable. For the Byzantine hospital, see the following: D. J. Constantelos, *Byzantine Philanthropy and Social Welfare* (New Brunswick, N.J., 1968); A. Philipsborn, "Les premiere hôpitaux au moyen age (Orient et Occident)," *Nouvelle Clio,* 6 (1954), 137–63; *idem,* "Der Fortschritt in der Entwicklung des byzantinischen Krankenhauswesens," *BZ,* 54 (1961), 338–65; E. Jeanselme and L. Oeconomos, *Les oeuvres d'assistance et les hôpitaux byzantins au siècle des Comnènes* (Anvers, 1921); G. Rosen, "The Hospital: Historical Sociology of a Community Institution," in *The Hospital in Modern Society,* ed. E. Freidson (London, 1963), 1–36; G. Schreiber, "Byzantinisches und abendländisches Hospital zur Spitalordnung des Pantokrator und zur byzantinischen Medizin," *BZ,* 42 (1943–49), 37–76; G. E. Gask and J. Todd, "The Origin of Hospitals," in *Science, Medicine and History: Essays on the Evolution of Scientific Thought and Practice,* ed. E. A. Underwood, I (Oxford, 1953), 122–30; K. Sudhoff, "Aus der Geschichte des Krankenhauswesens im früheren Mittelalter im Morgenland und Abendland," *SA,* 21 (1929), 164–203; E. Wickersheimer, *Les édifices hospitaliers à travers les ages* (Paris, 1953). For the Islamic hospital, see the following: Aḥmad ʿĪsā, *Histoire des Bimaristans (hôpitaux) à l'époque islamique* (Cairo, 1928), and his revised and enlarged edition of this work, *Taʾrīkh al-bīmāristānāt fī l-islām* (Damascus, 1939); al-Bayān, *ad-Dustūr al-bīmāristān (Le formulaire des hôpitaux d'Ibn Abil Bayan, médecin du bimaristan an-Nacery au Caire au XIIIᵉ siècle),* ed. P. Sbath, in *BIE,* 15 (1932–33), 13–78; E. L. Bertherand, *De la création des hôpitaux arabes* (Algiers, 1849); D. Brandenburg, "Die alten islamischen Krankenhäuser in Kairo," *Forschung, Praxis, Fortbildung* (Berlin), 18 (1967), 524–30; J. Bravo, "Los hospitales en nuestra época musulmana," *Actas X. cong. intern. d'hist. méd.,* I (1935), 13 f., II (1935), 74–81; R. F. Bridgman, "Evolution compareé de l'organisation hospitalière en Europe et en pays d' Islam, influences mutuelles au

Before proceeding to the specific issues of medical theory and practice in the medieval Near East, I want to be as clear as possible about the subject. I have interpreted medicine and insanity in the widest sense. It would be very helpful to be able to define insanity concisely, but that is no easy matter, and the lack of precision seriously complicates the historical study of the topic.[4] First of all, we possess a very imperfect understanding of insanity today, so that we cannot confidently look into the past and clearly distinguish the various forms of insanity, as we can do for many physical illnesses. Mental illness is today a controversial subject, and some would argue that it is neither mental nor an illness. Perhaps the virtue of our ignorance is a greater empathy for those who had to grapple with the problem in the past. In any case, it seems best to define insanity as any behavior that is judged to be abnormal or extraordinary by a social group at a specific time and place. Within the wide spectrum of human behavior, members of any society set bound-

aries to what they believe to be acceptable or permissible behavior. This judgment depends generally on the degree to which an individual's behavior is disturbed and the attitudes of his or her social group toward those actions.[5]

To add to the complexity of the subject, culturally defined categories of abnormality shape the afflicted person's version of his inner experience and others' reports of his behavior. There is, then, a complex dialectical relationship between the reports of the experiences and symptoms of the mentally ill, the cultural categories of mental disturbances, and the theories of the practitioner and observer.[6] A good example in our period is the Saints' Lives, which may have gone a long way in creating such culturally shared categories.

The saints, especially the holy fools, in Byzantine and Islamic societies might be considered potential prophets—or dangerous lunatics.[7] Disturbed behavior usually poses a threat, so that some degree of fear has always influenced the social response to madness. George Rosen has shown how this fear was allayed by socially sanctioned forms of behavior in ancient Israel; abnormal behavior was channeled into religious rites. Prophecy, particularly, was a major and exceptional accommodation to individual deviancy. "The prophet was allowed to act as he wished even if some mocked

moyen-âge et à la renaissance," *Atti. Primo Congresso Europeo di Storia Ospitaliana* (Reggio Emilia, 1960), 229–339; idem, *L'Hôpital et la Cité* (Paris, 1963), 57–60; E. G. Browne, *Arabian Medicine* (Cambridge, 1962 rep.), 45 f., 56, 101 f.; J. C. Bürgel, "Secular and Religious Features of Medieval Arabic Medicine," in *Asian Medical Systems: A Comparative Study*, ed. C. Leslie (Berkeley, 1976), 44–62; M. Desruelles and H. Bersot, "L'Assistance aux aliénés chez les arabes du VIIIᵉ au XIIᵉ siècle," *Annales medico-psychologiques*, 96 (1938), 689–709; C. Elgood, *A Medical History of Persia* (Cambridge, 1951), s.v. "hospitals"; idem, *Safavid Medical Practice* (London, 1970 rep.), 27–29; *EI²*, s.v. "Bīmāristān" (Dunlop, Colin, and Şehsuvaroğlu), "Gondēshāpūr" (Huart and Sayili); S. K. Hamarneh, "Development of Hospitals in Islam," *JHM*, 17 (1962), 366–81; idem, "Medical Education and Practice in Medieval Islam," in *The History of Medical Education*, ed. C. D. O'Malley (Berkeley, 1970), 39–71; idem, "Some Aspects of Medical Practice and Institutions in Medieval Islam," *Episteme*, 7 (1973), 15–31; F. R. Hau "Die Bildung des Arztes im islamischen Mittelalter," *Clio Medica*, 13 (1978), 95–123, 175–200; 14 (1979), 7–25; D. Jetter, *Grundzüge der Hospitalgeschichte* (Darmstadt, 1973), 21–24; idem, "Hospitalgebäude in Spanien," *SA*, 44 (1960), 239–58; idem, "Zur Architektur islamischer Krankenhäusern," *SA*, 45 (1961), 261–73; idem, *Geschichte des Hospitals*, IV, *Spanien, von den Anfängen bis um 1500* (Wiesbaden, 1980); L. Leclerc, *Histoire de la médecine arabe*, I (Paris, 1876), 557–72; M. Levey, "Medieval Muslim Hospitals: Administration and Procedures," *Journal of the Albert Einstein Medical Center*, 10 (1962), 120–27; M. Meyerhof, "Von Alexandrien nach Baghdad," *SBBerl*, phil.- hist. kl., 23 (1930), 389–429; L. Torres Balbás, "El Māristān de Granada," *al-Andalus*, 9 (1944), 481–500; H. F. Wüstenfeld, "Macrizi's Beschreibung der Hospitäler in el-Câhira," *Janus*, 1 (1846), 28–39, Arabic text, i-viii; E. Bay, *Islamische Krankenhäuser im Mittelalter unter besonderer Berücksichtigung der Psychiatrie* (Diss., Medical Faculty, University of Düsseldorf, 1967); A. Terzioğlu, "Mittelalterliche islamische Krankenhäuser," *Annales Univ. Ankara*, 13 (1974), 47–76; idem, *Mittelalterliche islamische Krankenhäuser unter Berücksichtigung der Frage nach den ältesten psychiatrischen Anstalten* (Diss., Faculty of Architecture, Technical University, Berlin, 1968).

[4] See G. Mora and J. L. Brand, eds., *Psychiatry and Its History* (Springfield, Ill., 1976).

[5] G. Rosen, *Madness in Society, Chapters in the Historical Sociology of Mental Illness* (New York, 1969), 90. I have not considered in this paper the issue of group or collective hysteria; see, however, my remarks in *The Black Death in the Middle East* (Princeton, 1977), 24 *et passim*, and the tantalizing description of "madness" in Amida in 560 A.D. in Susan Ashbrook, "Asceticism in Adversity: An Early Byzantine Experience," *BMGS*, 6 (1980), 3f.

[6] See Ihsan Al-Issa, "Social and Cultural Aspects of Hallucination," *Psychological Bulletin*, 84 (1977), 570–87, which examines one aspect of mental illness with a sensitivity to its social context.

[7] On the phenomenon of the holy fool or holy wild man, see: W. S. Green, "Palestinian Holy Men: Charismatic Leadership and Rabbinic Tradition," *ANRW*, 19:2 (Berlin/New York, 1979), 619–47 for the historical background; P. Brown, "The Rise and Function of the Holy Man in Late Antiquity," in his *Society and the Holy in Late Antiquity* (Berkeley, 1982), 166–95; H. Petzold, "Zur Frömmigkeit der heiligen Narren," *Die Einheit der Kirche, Festgabe P. Meinhold* (Wiesbaden, 1977), 140–53; Penelope B. R. Doob, *Nebuchadnessar's Children: Conventions of Madness in Middle English Literature* (New Haven, 1974), chap. 4; L. Rydén, "The Holy Fool," in *The Byzantine Saint*, ed. S. Hackel, *Studies Supplementary to Sobornost*, 5 (London, 1981), 106–13; A. Y. Syrkin, "On the Behavior of the 'Fools for Christ's Sake,'" *History of Religions*, 22 (1982), 150–71; also, E. Benz, "Heilige Narrheit," *Kyrios*, 3 (1938), 1–55. The Islamic *majthūb* appears closer to the Hindu mystical tradition than does the Christian "holy fool" in Syrkin's study of the latter. The holy fool in Islamic society has not been adequately studied; see, however, A. Bausani, "Note sul 'Pazzo Sacro' nell'Islam," *StMSR*, 29 (1958), 93–107, and note 105 below.

him and others considered him mad, as long as what he said and did were not sufficiently threatening."[8] This view of Old Testament prophecy applies quite well to the life of Jesus. In the same Hebraic tradition, the abnormal inspirational states of Muḥammad are understood by Muslims as signs of unquestionable prophecy.[9] Medieval saints were seen, and saw themselves, in the light of this potent legacy.

Mental illness is, then, more intimately dependent on social attitudes and beliefs than is physical illness, and this social context largely determines the care and treatment of the mentally ill. Moreover, in most societies there is more than one view of mental disturbance and its treatment. As we shall see, there were in Byzantine and Islamic societies contending notions about insanity. It is a very untidy picture, in which there was no single socially chartered therapeutic system with final authority.[10]

The recent work of Peter Brown on Byzantine hagiography, however, suggests a useful conceptualization of medieval medicine. The bewildering diversity of medical beliefs and practices is evidence of the pluralism of pre-modern medicine and, particularly in the case of mental illness, the diversity is a direct reflection of its historical circumstances. It is interesting to note that insanity is one of the few areas in modern medicine that still retains strongly this pluralistic approach. In any case, I would like to push this view of medical pluralism much further. Briefly, I envision medieval pluralism as encompassing three ranges or spectra, which might be termed intellectual, sociological, and somatic or behavioral. The first is a continuum that runs from the strictly naturalistic explanation and treatment of health and illness to the strictly supernaturalistic. The second range represents roughly the continuum of an individual's social status based on wealth, education, religion, family, etc. And the third represents the range between an individual's health and illness; regarding insanity, it is a continuum between what was deemed normal and abnormal behavior.[11] The intersection of these

planes is the point where a decision about medical treatment is made. The model is not static due, particularly, to the variance between health and illness; nor is the medical decision exclusive, for successive judgments could be made that entailed concurrent but heterogeneous treatments. Despite some difficulties with this theoretical construct, it is a helpful framework for interpreting the historical evidence. There seem to me to be three distinct advantages in such a framework. First, it places medicine squarely in its social context as a malleable craft and emphasizes the role of the patient, rather than the doctor, in the determination of medical treatment(s).[12] Second, it avoids the mistaken notion that naturalistic medicine was the exclusive preserve of the upper class and, conversely, that the lower classes were devoted to magical and religious healing. And third, it emphasizes the continua in these three ranges, especially the intellectual, rather than the customary emphasis on conflict and tension. I do not mean to deny that conflicts and tensions, which imply clearly recognized polarities, did not exist in ancient and medieval medicine, but such a view does not account satisfactorily for the accommodation of eclectic and often contradictory beliefs and practices in the medical and historical texts and, presumably, in the lives of individuals.

In the often desperate search for methods of treating insanity, it appears from the medieval sources that the full range of possible judgments along the three continua were made. Although we have naturally tended to emphasize the medical texts, the professional medical approach was probably at a distinct disadvantage in relation to other forms of healing. The doctor's treatment was usually lengthy, expensive, sometimes painful, and frequently not very effective. Insanity is an elusive, complex and sensitive topic, yet sensitive to the values around which men and women have constructed and ordered their lives. It is a divining rod that may lead to a deeper understanding of medieval social relations.

Abnormal behavior posed in the medieval period, as it still does today, the question of its causation. Byzantine society could draw upon the naturalistic interpretation of the mind and its dysfunction that it had inherited from antiquity.[13]

---

[8] Rosen (note 5 above), 63.

[9] See O. Temkin, *The Falling Sickness*, 2nd ed. (Baltimore, 1971), 150–53, 370–73.

[10] V. Crapanzano, *The Ḥamadsha: A Study in Moroccan Ethnopsychiatry* (Berkeley, 1973), 133, cited in P. Brown, *The Cult of the Saints: Its Rise and Function in Latin Christianity* (Chicago, 1981), 114. See also L. M. Danforth, "The Role of Dance in the Ritual Therapy of the Anastenaria," *BMGS*, 5 (1979), 144–48.

[11] Although I am concerned here with illness, the model works reasonably well with regard to the regimen for the healthy, which was of considerable importance in pre-modern medicine.

[12] See Dols and Gamal, *Medieval Islamic Medicine: Ibn Riḍwān's Treatise "On the Prevention of Bodily Ills in Egypt"* (Berkeley, 1984), 39.

[13] For secondary works, see: B. Simon, *Mind and Madness in Ancient Greece: The Roots of Modern Psychiatry* (Ithaca, 1978); Ro-

Byzantine and, subsequently, Islamic medicine relied directly on the Hippocratic tradition as it had been elaborated by Galen in the second century A.D.[14] Insanity was generally explained according to the two fundamental theories of the humors and the spirits. Madness was produced by an imbalance of the humors, particularly an excess of black bile, which caused melancholy.[15] Medical treatment was intended to correct this imbalance by a manipulation of the humoral qualities; based on an allopathic principle of "contraries," successful treatment re-established a proper complexion or temperament. The second basic premise of Galenic medicine was the theory of the three *pneumata*—the vital, psychic, and natural spirits. A disturbance of the spirits was the second major cause of mental disorder. Generally, the theory of insanity crystallized in late antiquity around those concepts and was transmitted with astonishing literalness well into the nineteenth century, as can be seen in the works of Benjamin Rush and Philippe Pinel.[16]

It would be tedious to chronicle all the writings on insanity and its remedies that may be found in the Byzantine and Islamic medical texts, because they largely follow the lines of early Byzantine medicine.[17] I would, however, like to note some general characteristics of this literature.[18]

Unlike the classical writings, the medical texts of late antiquity contain more sustained discussions or descriptions of mental disturbances, particularly melancholy. The Islamic compendia of medicine (*kunnāshāt*), which followed the precedent set by Byzantine works of the late Alexandrian School, became popular systematic expositions of theory. The *Qānūn* of Ibn Sīnā was, perhaps, the most famous and influential on later works, but these authoritative encyclopedias were all quite similar.[19] They invariably dealt with psychic matters under various headings: the anatomy of the brain; the complexion of the brain; its faculties or powers (imagination, cognition, and memory); the psychic spirit that nurtured the brain; the preservation of mental well-being as one of the six "non-naturals"; psychic ailments as a part of the pathological description of the entire body; and the *materia medica* for the alleviation of mental disturbances. The description of psychic ailments, particularly, was non-clinical and was followed by a chapter on therapy. The maladies usually included epilepsy, mania, melancholy, phrenitis, lycanthropy (*quṭrūb*),[20] and passionate love (*ʿishq*), as in Ibn Sīnā's *Qānūn*.[21] The precedent for the presentation of the symptoms, causes, and therapies of psychic disorders in this manner may be traced back to Celsus; the immediate precedent for Islamic doctors was Alexander of Tralles.[22]

sen (note 5 above), chap. 3; Agnes C. Vaughan, *Madness in Greek Thought and Custom* (Baltimore, 1919); G. C. Moss, "Mental Disorders in Antiquity," in *Diseases in Antiquity*, ed. D. Brothwell and A. T. Sandison (Springfield, Ill., 1967), 709–22; J. L. Heiberg, *Geisteskrankheiten im klassischen Altertum* (Berlin/Leipzig, 1927); I. E. Drabkin, "Remarks on Ancient Psychopathology," *Isis*, 46 (1955), 223–34.

[14] Temkin, *Galenism, passim*; see especially S. W. Jackson, "Galen—On Mental Disorders," *JHBS*, 5 (1969), 365–84.

[15] For the central idea of *iʿtidāl* (humoral balance) in Islamic medicine, see J. Ch. Bürgel, "Adab und *iʿtidāl* in ar-Ruhāwīs Adab aṭ-ṭabīb: Studie zur Bedeutungsgeschichte zweier Begriffe," *ZDMG*, 117 (1967), 97–102.

[16] Simon (note 13 above), 43 f.

[17] The only surviving ancient text to contain a full and orderly discussion of mental illness is Caelius Aurelianus, *On the Acute and on Chronic Diseases*, trans. E. I. Drabkin (Chicago, 1950); the interpretation of the subject is, however, based on Methodist principles. Generally, the names given to mental disturbances in antiquity indicate a purely somatic approach, so that the disturbances were often not classified as mental illnesses, such as hysteria (the disturbance of the uterus) and hypochondria (disease below the diaphram); see note 21 below.

[18] In the present discussion, it is advantageous to bear in mind the contemporary European interpretation of insanity and the treatment of the insane, especially in view of the present-day revisionism of traditional historical treatments of the subject. See J. Kroll, "A Reappraisal of Psychiatry in the Middle Ages," *Archives of General Psychiatry*, 29 (1973), 276–83; Stanley W. Jackson, "Unusual Mental States in Medieval Europe, I. Medical Syndromes of Mental Disorder: 400–1100 A.D.," *JHM*, 27 (1972), 262–95; G. Mora, "Mind-Body Concepts in the Middle Ages: Part I. The Classical Background and Its Merging with the Ju-

deo-Christian Tradition in the Early Middle Ages," *JHBS*, 14 (1978), 344–61; *idem*, "Mind-Body Concepts in the Middle Ages: Part II. The Moslem Influence, the Great Theological Systems, and Cultural Attitudes Towards the Mentally Ill in the Late Middle Ages," *JHBS*, 16 (1980), 58–72; R. Neugebauer, "Treatment of the Mentally Ill in Medieval and Early Modern England: A Reappraisal," *JHBS*, 14 (1978), 158–69.

[19] For the analysis of major Islamic medical compendia, see the following: al-Majūsī, *al-Malakī*—M. Ullmann, *Islamic Medicine* (Edinburgh, 1978) and E. Ruth Harvey, *The Inward Wits: Psychological Theory in the Middle Ages and the Renaissance*, Warburg Institute Surveys, VI (London, 1975), 13–21; Kai-Kāʾūs, *Qābūs-Nāma*—F. Klein-Franke, *Vorlesungen über die Medizin im Islam*, in *SA*, Beihefte 23 (Wiesbaden, 1982), 77–81; G. Karmi, "A Medieval Compendium of Arabic Medicine: Abū Sahl al-Masīḥī's 'Book of the Hundred,'" *JHAS*, 2 (1978), 270–90.

[20] The syndrome of lycanthropy, which is lacking in Galen, was taken from Aetius of Amida, who reproduced it from Marcellus of Side (Ullmann [note 19 above], 22). See M. Ullmann, "Der Werwolf," *WZKM*, 68 (1976), 171–84; F. G. Welcker, "Lykanthropie, ein Aberglaube und eine Krankheit," *Kleine Schriften*, 3 (Bonn, 1850), 157 ff.

[21] Ibn Sīnā, *al-Qānūn fī ṭ-ṭibb*, II (Būlāq, 1877), 63 ff. Jackson suggests ("Galen—On Mental Disorders" [note 14 above], 371–76) that phrenitis, melancholia, and mania were "well-established as nosological categories" in antiquity, and he examines their description as well as related syndromes in Galen's works. The historical evolution of what comprised "mental illness" should be noted.

[22] Flashar, *Melancholie*, 74 f., 126–33; despite the title, the author masterfully surveys the topic through early Byzantine

Let me say something more about passionate love, which had been considered a sickness in antiquity.[23] In Persian and Urdu *sōdā* means both melancholy and passion. It comes from *al-mirra as-saudā'*, which is black bile, the source of melancholy and passion in the body. Dying of a broken heart is a well-known theme in oriental literature. Perhaps the best example is *Layla and Majnūn*, which tells the sad story of Majnūn, which means "madman," who is separated from his beloved; he wanders in the wilderness, is obsessed by his passionate love, and dies out of love for Layla.[24] In the medical literature, there are a number of anecdotes about famous doctors who detected, by feeling the pulse, an undisclosed love as the source of a patient's melancholy and were able to cure the patient.[25] These stories of pulse diagnosis are certainly not evidence of "psychiatry," but they are interesting instances of the physiological understanding of psychic illness.[26]

Aside from these compendia, a number of monographs were written on mental disturbances by Islamic doctors. Although non-clinical, they naturally contained a fuller discussion of theory and therapy, and they attest, through extensive quota-

tions, to their dependence on Greek medicine, particularly the work on melancholy by Rufus of Ephesus.[27] The most important such monograph was the early tenth-century *Maqāla fī Mālīkhūliyā* by Isḥāq ibn ʿImrān, which relied heavily on Rufus.[28] It is important because it was well known in the Islamic world and was translated into Latin by Constantinus Africanus in the eleventh century A.D., and the work appears to have significantly influenced Western views of mental illness. The notion of melancholy was used in these monographs as a catch-all expression, similar to our present-day "mental illness," for psychic disturbances of all kinds; that notion lasted until modern times.[29]

Generally, Rufus and his medieval followers recommended treatment with antidepressive drugs, psychotherapeutic remedies (particularly music),[30] and the psychic healing of manic delusions. One example of the third method may be helpful. A member of the Buyid dynasty suffered from the fixed idea of being a cow and refused all food; he even urged his attendants to have him slaughtered and roasted. The case was brought before the famous Ibn Sīnā, who proceeded as follows: First he

medicine. For a cursory review of Byzantine medical views of insanity, see G. Roccatagliata, *Storia della Psichiatria Antica* (Milan, 1973), chaps. 13–14. For Islamic medical views, see J. E. Staehelin, "Zur Geschichte der Psychiatrie des Islam," *Schweizerische Medizinische Wochenschrift*, no. 35/36 (Basel, 1957), 1151–53.

[23] According to Flashar, *Melancholie*, 79, the first connection of love-sickness with melancholy is in Aretaeus. See R. Walzer, "Fragmenta graeca in litteris arabicis: l. Palladios and Aristotle," *JRAS*, 1939, 407–22, and especially H. H. Biesterfeldt and D. Gutas, "The Malady of Love," *Journal of the American Oriental Society*, 104 (1984), 21–55. For the literary aspect, see Lois A. Giffin, *Theory of Profane Love Among the Arabs: The Development of the Genre* (New York, 1971). Ibn Sīnā's treatment of this "sickness" is instructive (*al-Qānūn*, II, 72 f.). He advises that the two lovers be united if it is permitted by Islamic law, but if not, the doctor should admonish the patient and even ridicule him. Ibn Sīnā mentions the usefulness of old women and effeminate men in discouraging such love by their slandering the lover's image of the beloved and transferring his affection to someone else. He also recommends entertainment and sports to divert the lovesick. The romantic aspect of ʿishq has clearly been lost in Ibn Sīnā's medical treatment of the subject.

[24] I. J. Kračkovskij, "Die Frühgeschichte der Erzählung von Macnūn und Lailā in der arabischen Literatur," trans. H. Ritter, *Oriens*, 8 (1955), 1–50; M. Gh. Hilal, *The Development of the Majnūn-Layla Theme in the Literature of the Orient* (Cairo, 1954), in Arabic. See the modern English translations of *Layla and Majnūn* of Nizāmī by R. Gelpke, et al. (London, 1966), and of Fuzūlī by S. Huri (London, 1970); and the play of Aḥmad Shawkī, *Majnun Layla*, trans. John Arberry (Cairo, 1933).

[25] J. Ch. Bürgel, "Psychosomatic Methods of Cures in the Islamic Middle Ages," *Humaniora Islamica*, 1 (1973), 157–72.

[26] Abū Saʿīd Ibn Bakhtīshūʿ, *Risālah fī ṭ-ṭibb*, ed. and trans. F. Klein-Franke, *Über die Heilung der Krankheiten der Seele und des Körpers*, in *Recherches*, nouvelle série: B. Orient chrétien, IV (Beirut, 1977), 29 f.

[27] See M. Ullmann, "Die arabische Überlieferung der Werke des Rufus von Ephesus," *The First International Symposium of Arab Science*, Aleppo, April 5–12, 1976, II (Aleppo, 1978), 348–57; Flashar, *Melancholie*, 84–104.

[28] Isḥāq ibn ʿImrān, "Maqāla fī l-Mālīḫūliyā" (Abhandlung über die Melancholie) und Constantini Africani "Libri Duo de Melancholia," ed. and trans. K. Garbers (Hamburg, 1977). See also R. Creutz and W. Creutz, "Die 'Melancholia' bei Konstantinus Africanus und seinen Quellen," *Archiv für Psychiatrie und Nervenkrankheiten*, 97 (1932), 244–69; G. Baader, "Zur Terminologie des Constantinus Africanus," *Medizinhistorisches Journal*, 2 (1967), 36–53; B. Ben Yahia, "Les origines arabes de De melancholia de Constantin l'Africain," *Revue d'histoire des sciences*, 7 (1954), 156 ff.

[29] The inclusive sense of "melancholy" may be found in the works of Aretaeus and Alexander of Tralles especially. There is an extensive literature on melancholy; see the following works: R. Klibansky, E. Panofsky, and F. Saxl, *Saturn and Melancholy* (New York, 1964); Flashar, *Melancholie, passim; idem*, ed., *Antike Medizin* (Darmstadt, 1971), especially W. Müri, "Melancholie und schwarze Galle," 165–91; A. Lewis, "Melancholia: A Historical Review," *The State of Psychiatry*, ed. A. Lewis (London, 1967), 71–110; J. Starobinski, *Histoire du traitement de la mélancolie des origines à 1900* (Diss., Faculty of Medicine, University of Lausanne, 1960); H. Schipperges, "Melancolia als ein mittelalterlicher Sammelbegriff für Wahnvorstellungen," *Studium Generale*, 20 (1967), 723–36; R. Burton, *The Anatomy of Melancholy*, ed. F. Dell and P. Jordan-Smith (New York, 1927).

[30] J. Ch. Bürgel, "Zur Musiktherapie im arabischen Mittelalter," in *Festschrift Arnold Geering*, ed. V. Ravissa (Bern/Stuttgart, 1972), 241–45; M. C. Yasargil, "Über die Musiktherapie im Orient und Okzident," *Schweizer Archiv für Neurologie, Neurochirurgie und Psychiatrie*, 90 (1962), 301–26; H. G. Farmer, *The Influence of Music: From Arabic Sources* (London, 1926); G. Bandmann, *Melancholie und Musik, ikonographische Studien* (Cologne, 1960); A. Süheyl Ünver, "Four Medical Vignettes from Turkey," *Int. Rec. Med.*, 171 (1958), 52.

transmitted a message to the sick man wherein he begged him to be in good spirits because the butcher was on his way to him, and the madman exulted. Soon afterwards, Ibn Sīnā entered the sickroom with a knife in his hand, saying, "Where is the cow, that I may slaughter her?" A lowing was the answer. Ibn Sīnā ordered him to be laid on the ground, his hands and feet bound, then he palpated his body and said, "She is too meagre to be slaughtered, she must be fattened!" The sick man thereupon began to eat, put on weight, lost his delusion, and recovered.[31]

It is obvious from the medical works that there was a common consensus that the brain, and not the heart, was the center of mental activity.[32] Furthermore, mental disturbance was an illness. As a natural phenomenon, no moral meaning was assigned to the disease—no guilt or shame was attached to the illness in the medical texts. Thus, the Dogmatic view of insanity was predominant, and it was both extended and refined by Islamic doctors like all other illnesses from a strongly somatic or physiological point of view. For example, Islamic doctors appear to have interpreted the ancient doctrine of temperament strictly in terms of a pathological humoralism.[33] Greco-Roman medicine, as in the works of Aretaeus and Caelius Aurelianus, differentiated between the divine or inspired madness and mental disorders arising from bodily disease.[34] I have not found, however, any survival of the Socratic categories of prophetic, telestic, or poetic madness in the Islamic medical texts.

Specifically with regard to the humors, we can see in Ibn Sīnā's discussion the culmination in the development of the notion that the various forms of mental illness were derived from the "scorching" or "burning" of each of the four humors, rather than just the black bile.[35] In this manner, the various forms of mental disturbance were given a "generic" cause. This theory also logically combined Galen's canonical theory of combustion with the doctrine of the four humors.

Concerning the bodily spirits, the Islamic doctors similarly extended and systematized Galenic theory. Where Galen "hardly incorporated the natural spirit in his system,"[36] the Islamic doctors rounded out the idea and gave all three spirits equal weight. Corresponding to the three spirits, Islamic writers adopted the triadic psychological system of Galen, who had taken it from Plato: the appetitive, irascible, and rational powers of the soul. The rational soul was located in the brain and was responsible for the psychic functions of voluntary movement, perception, and reason; the last comprised the three faculties of imagination, cognition, and memory. Unlike Plato's notion of the rational soul, however, Galen considered it to be corporeal; it was dependent on the harmonious relationship with the other two parts of the soul and on the physical well-being of the rest of the body.[37] Reason was the temperate complexion of the material psychic spirit, operating in the healthy cerebral ventricles. Consequently, the doctors were led to the treatment of disordered reason as though it were a purely physical function.[38] Medieval Islamic and European philosophers may have resented this presumption, but they relied on the information provided by the doctors; in the philosophers' psychological theory, human reason or the soul fell outside medicine. I do not know what the psychological theory of Byzantine philosophy was and its relation to medical thought. Nor can I deal here with the theological problem of the relationship of the psychic spirit with the soul in Christianity and Islam.[39] For the Islamic doctors, al-Majūsī summarizes the matter succinctly: "There can be no mind without the health of the rational soul, and the health of this is obtained only when the vital soul and the natural soul are healthy, nor can either of these be healthy without a healthy

---

[31] Bürgel (note 25 above), 164 f.; Browne (note 3 above), 88 f.

[32] On the Aristotelean view of the heart, see Simon (note 13 above), 223 f. To the ancient idea of melancholy arising from the disturbance of the stomach and affecting the brain, Flashar (*Melancholie*, 119 ff.) points out that Poseidonius is the only doctor who gives an exact anatomical foundation to this theory; opposed to the contemporary belief in demonic possession, Poseidonius localized psychic illness in the brain.

[33] On the post-Galenic development of the temperaments, see Flashar, *Melancholie*, 112 ff. For the temperaments in Islamic medicine, see Klibansky, et al., (note 29 above), 60 ff.; for example, Ibn Bakhtīshūʿ, *Risālah fī ṭ-ṭibb*, fol. 92ᵛ. Concerning the Dogmatic tradition in Islamic medicine generally, see Klein-Franke (note 19 above), chap. 6.

[34] Rosen (note 5 above), 102 f.

[35] Ibn Sīnā, *al-Qānūn*, II, 68. This humoral pathology was adopted by medieval Western medicine; see, for example, Ar-

noldus de Villanova, *De parte operative*, in *Opera Omnia*, ed. N. Taurelli (Basel, 1585), 271.

[36] R. E. Siegel, *Galen's System of Physiology and Medicine* (Basel, 1968), 186. See also O. Temkin, "On Galen's Pneumatology," *Gesnerus*, 8 (1951), 180–89, esp. 181; L. G. Wilson, "Erasistratus, Galen and the Pneuma," *BHM*, 33 (1959), 293–314.

[37] Jackson (note 14 above), 370 f.

[38] Harvey (note 19 above), 3, 7 ff.; see also Bürgel, (note 25 above), 160 ff.

[39] See Harvey (note 19 above), 31–61; F. Rahman, trans., *Avicenna's Psychology* (Oxford, 1952); Judith S. Neaman, *Suggestion of the Devil: The Origins of Madness* (Garden City, N.Y., 1975), chap. 2.

body, and this comes about from the balance of the humors."[40]

Another characteristic of the Islamic treatment of insanity was the general emphasis on the educative role of the doctor with regard to his patient's individual regimen. This aspect of medical practice can be traced back to antiquity, "but, overall, ancient medicine did not develop a concept of the healing power of words or dialogue, just as it did not develop a concept of disturbances of the mind apart from disturbances of the body."[41] Although rooted in traditional humoral theory, Aretaeus' discussion of melancholy marks the beginning of the psychogenic explanation, which was further developed in late antiquity.[42] Despite the dominance of the Dogmatic tradition in Islamic medicine, the psychic causation subsisted in the textbooks, and various forms of psychotherapy were evidently practiced. Although many of the therapies can be found in the works of late antique authors, the use of shock or shame therapy, particularly, by Islamic doctors seems to have been original.[43] Thus, it appears that some Islamic physicians drew upon their own experiences and often adopted a holistic approach to medicine.[44] The best representative of this minority view is the mid-eleventh-century doctor Saʿīd ibn Bakhtīshūʿ, who argued persuasively in one of his treatises for the psychic causation of illness, epitomized in his view by passionate love, alongside the somatic.[45] At the beginning of the fourth chapter of his work, Ibn Bakhtīshūʿ counters the neglect of the psychic element in illness by the ordinary doctor, "who has not entered the bīmāristāns and has not seen how the staff treats the sick—pacifying the nerves of some and busying the minds of others, diverting their anxieties and entertaining them with song and other things, exciting some of them by abuse and scorn and stirring their souls. . . ."[46]

This abrupt introduction to the māristān by Ibn Bakhtīshūʿ leads me to the actual treatment of the mentally ill. In Greco-Roman society, mental ill-

ness had been considered, generally, a private matter except where public safety or legal questions were involved. The handling of the insane varied according to circumstances, but the primary responsibility fell upon the family. The practice of allowing the disturbed who were not violent to roam the streets was followed only by the poorer classes and those who had no family. "Not infrequently they were followed by children or street loafers who mocked, ridiculed and abused them, and often threw stones at them. . . . Confinement at home was an accepted way of dealing with the mentally deranged who were disoriented and violent. When there was danger that a mentally ill person would injure himself or those associated with him, he was not only confined, but he was restrained as well. Such an individual might be bound or placed in the stocks. . . ."[47] The law did not define insanity, but concerned itself primarily with safeguarding private property. The insane were not held legally responsible for their actions, while a guardian or administrator might be appointed to protect their interests. The legal status of the insane remained roughly the same in Byzantine and Islamic societies, and this Greco-Roman legal view did not change appreciably until modern times.[48]

Within the Greco-Roman context, Christianity introduced a new and somewhat revolutionary idea. The infirm poor and other socially disadvantaged elements of society were no longer to be despised—they were to be honored. They became a communal responsibility. For the individual Christian, charity was a sure path to the atonement of his sins and to salvation. The bishop was to maintain a xenodochium, literally "a house for strangers," and supply needed social services.[49] With the recognition and eventual promotion of Christianity in the fourth century A.D., a widespread and highly developed welfare system was developed in Byzantine society. Subsequently, Muslims, similarly motivated by religious charity, imitated the Byzantine facilities in their newly created empire.[50] The

[40] Al-Majūsī quoted in Harvey (note 19 above), 14.

[41] Simon (note 13 above), 227.

[42] Flashar, Melancholie, 77 f.

[43] Bürgel (note 25 above), 171.

[44] See Klein-Franke (note 19 above), chap. 7.

[45] This seemingly paradoxical situation may be understood in the light of the history of psychiatry in the nineteenth century, when this science grew directly out of the somatic—that is, the neurological—approach to mental illness, especially in the work of Sigmund Freud. See the introductory survey by A. Scull in his Madhouses, Mad-Doctors, and Madmen (Philadelphia, 1981), 5–32.

[46] Ibn Bakhtīshūʿ, Risālah fī ṭ-ṭibb, fols. 74ʳ–74ᵛ.

[47] Rosen (note 5 above), 64 f.; see also 88 f.

[48] Ibid., 63–70, 121–29, 136; Neaman, Suggestion of the Devil (note 39 above), 68–110; Y. Linant de Bellefonds, Traité de droit musulman comparé (The Hague/Paris, 1965), 245 ff., 262; A. A. Fyzee, Outline of Muhammadan Law, 3rd ed. (Oxford, 1964), 88 et passim; G. H. Bousquet, Précis de droit musulman (Algiers, 1950), 120 et passim. Of considerable importance for Islamic society, beyond the legal sphere, is the Qurʾānic stipulation (4:4) to care for the incompetent (sufahāʾ); see below.

[49] G. Harig and J. Kollesch, "Arzt, Kranker und Krankenpflege in der griechisch-romanischen Antike und im byzantinischen Mittelalter," Helikon, 13–14 (1973–74), 274 f.

[50] See F. Rosenthal, "Sedaka, Charity," The Hebrew Union College Annual, 23 (1950–51), 411–30; N. A. Stillman, "Charity and

first major Islamic hospital was established in Baghdad by Hārūn ar-Rashīd in the early ninth century A.D. The inspiration for this foundation came, in a roundabout way, from the Nestorian physicians in Jūndishāpūr. Nestorian physicians organized and staffed the Baghdad hospital, and it served as a model for numerous hospitals in Islamic countries.[51]

The comparable development of Byzantine and Islamic hospitals highlights some essential features of the medieval institution. It is misleading, first of all, to call these institutions "hospitals," as I have done, because of the term's modern connotations. The medieval hospital was basically a civilian charitable institution, which more closely resembled a present-day convalescent or nursing home. The belief that the Byzantine hospitals were devoted only to acute illnesses is a very questionable assertion, especially if lepers were cared for in these hospitals. With the exception of a few major urban complexes, such as the Pantocrator Hospital, the Byzantine welfare facilities seem to have been small, undifferentiated, and very numerous. Islamic society, on the other hand, lacked such numerous small-scale facilities. The Islamic hospitals were usually grand structures, similar to the Pantocrator, and were confined to the important cities.[52] They were carefully planned, containing inpatient and outpatient departments with separate wards for male and female patients. Special wards or halls were devoted to surgery, eye diseases, bonesetting, and internal maladies, which roughly corresponded to the specializations of the medical profession. The most remarkable aspect of the Islamic hospitals was the inclusion of a section for the mentally ill.

It is remarkable because there is very little evi-

dence, to my knowledge, for the special care of the insane in the sophisticated and widespread Byzantine welfare system.[53] This lack of institutional specialization may be due to the equivocal status of insanity in Byzantine society, which will be discussed below.[54] It is, however, very likely that the Nestorian Christians in Jūndishāpūr did promote the special treatment of the insane in their famous hospital. Although we do not possess descriptions of the inner workings of the Jūndishāpūr hospital, we know that the city was the most important intellectual center in the pre-Islamic Near East. The Nestorian Christians were free from Byzantine constraints to pursue sedulously their scientific interests, so that their work provided eventually an important bridge between Hellenistic and Islamic learning.[55] Aside from the classical medical texts, a significant element of that learning was the Aristotelian tradition, which was decisive in the field of psychology.[56] At the same time, the eastern monasteries appear to have been refuges for the mentally disturbed. In one important instance, the Arabic sources mention an independent insane asylum at Dayr Hizqil (Ezechiel) in an-Nuʿmānija, which is located between Baghdad and Wāsiṭ in Lower Mesopotamia. It is probable that the asylum dated from before the Arab conquests; it clearly continued to function as a madhouse into the tenth century A.D.[57] In these circumstances, the Jūndishāpūr physicians, responding to their religious and professional obligations, may have promoted the

Social Service in Medieval Islam," *Societas*, 5 (1975), 105–15; S. D. Goitein, *A Mediterranean Society*, II (Berkeley, 1971), 3 *et passim*; Dols, "Islamic Hospitals and Poor Relief," *Dictionary of the Middle Ages*, in press.

[51] In his assertion of independence from Baghdad, Ibn Ṭūlūn may have sought to imitate the caliph by founding a comparable *māristān*. In any case, his hospital is a good example of the nature of medieval Muslim philanthropy. On the issue of the "first" Islamic hospital, see my "The Leper in Medieval Islamic Society," *Speculum*, 58 (1983), 891–916.

[52] Aside from mobile hospitals that accompanied armies in the field, rural medical facilities appear to have been quite rare. Elgood (note 3 above), 174 ff., gives the misleading impression that "moving hospitals" existed and were as common as "fixed hospitals"; his discussion is based on the exceptional instructions of the early fourth/tenth-century Baghdad vizier ʿAlī ibn ʿĪsā to the physician Thābit ibn Qurrah to provide medical care to the villagers in the Sawād. See H. Bowen, *The Life and Times of ʿAlī ibn ʿĪsā* (Cambridge, 1928), 184.

[53] The "sacred disease" in the Byzantine sources has often been misinterpreted to mean insanity; in the medieval period it almost invariably meant leprosy. See Mary E. Keenan, "St. Gregory of Nazianzus and Early Byzantine Medicine," *BHM*, 9 (1941), 18; PO, II, 85; and A. Philipsborn, "ΙΕΡΑ ΝΟΣΟΣ und die Spezial-Anstalt des Pantokrator-Krankenhauses," *Byzantion*, 33 (1963), 223–30.

[54] Secondary accounts of the history of the hospital often assert that there were mental asylums in early Byzantine civilization—a *morotrophium* in Jerusalem in A.D. 491 and another in Constantinople. This assertion is based on H. C. Burdett's greatly flawed *Hospitals and Asylums of the World*, I (London, 1891), 16, 38, 41, which is taken from U. Trélat, *Recherches historiques sur la folie* (Paris, 1839). Burdett contemptuously denies (p. 43) Desmaison's contention that the institutional treatment of the mentally ill originated in Islamic society; see J. G. Desmaison, *Des asiles d'aliénés en Espagne* (Paris, 1859), repr. in *Psychiatry in Russia and Spain* (New York, 1976). The latter initiated the modern controversy over the precedence of mental hospitals in Europe.

[55] Dols and Gamal (note 12 above), 4–6.

[56] See Heinz H. Schöffler, *Die Akademie von Gondischapur, Aristoteles auf dem Wege in den Orient* (Stuttgart, 1979).

[57] See Terzioğlu, *Mittelalterliche islamische Krankenhäusen* (note 3 above), 41 f.; Adam Mez, *The Renaissance of Islam*, trans. S. K. Bakhsk and D. S. Margoliouth, 1st ed. (Patna, 1937), 377; M. Streck, *Die alte Landschaft Babylonien nach dem arabischen Geographen* (Leiden, 1901), 2:301–303. My further study of this asylum and the oriental sources generally may clarify this issue.

institutional care of the insane in a manner that prefigured the well-documented Islamic hospital. But how was this possible? Why should insanity assume such a prominent place in the subsequent development of the Islamic hospital?

I would suggest that the answer lies in the different natures of the Byzantine and Islamic hospitals and, ultimately, in the different religious orientations of the two societies. The Islamic hospital was generally a secular institution; its legal status is markedly different from that of the Christian (Byzantine and European) hospitals.[58] The Islamic hospital was usually established by the local ruler as a personal monument—as a means of religious and political legitimation by the non-indigenous elites, which characterized most Islamic states from the ninth century A.D. The *māristān* was financed by the state and by private endowments, and it was administered by a highly-placed government official.[59] The chief physician or dean supervised the medical personnel; the institution was not staffed by clerics. The lay physicians placed an inordinate emphasis on the classical texts, primarily the works of Galen, as the sole criteria for professional status because of the lack of effective state regulation or self-regulation of medical practice.[60] Moreover, the preservation of Galenic medicine was reinforced by the close association of medical education with the hospital.[61] Consequently, it was possible for Christian and Jewish doctors to hold prestigious positions in the hospitals and to play a disproportionately large role in Islamic medicine during the medieval period.

On the other hand, there is no evidence of non-Christian practitioners in the Byzantine hospitals, which were closely tied to the Church. Invariably, they were administered by the Church, frequently being associated with monastic communities. Apart from strictly monastic medicine, there was also a strong tradition of priest-physicians, who combined religion with Galenic teaching.[62] Furthermore, monasteries and ecclesiastical schools seem to have been the main teaching centers of medicine.[63] Byzantine medicine appears, therefore, to have become deeply infused with Christian beliefs and practices.[64] I believe that this supernatural orientation may be seen most clearly and decisively in the case of insanity.[65]

The early Christian view of professional medicine was generally ambivalent, if not contradictory.[66] Mental illness, specifically, was believed to be demonic possession. The Apostles may have distinguished it from physical illnesses, but the subtlety of this distinction seems to have been lost from an

[58] See the concise comparison of Christian and Muslim law regarding hospitals in Bridgman, "Evolution comparée de l'organisation hospitalière (note 3 above)" 235–37, and *idem, L'Hôpital et la Cité* (note 3 above), 51 *et passim*.

[59] For example, hospitals in Mamlūk Egypt were major institutions; the budget of the Manṣūrī hospital, specifically, was the largest of any public institution in Egypt. See C. F. Petry, *The Civilian Elite of Cairo in the Later Middle Ages* (Princeton, 1981), 218; see also 140 f.

[60] See Dols and Gamal (note 12 above), 24–42; G. Leiser, "Medical Education in Islamic Lands from the Seventh to the Fourteenth Century," *JHM*, 38 (1983), 66–75; F. Rosenthal, "The Physician in Medieval Muslim Society," *BHM*, 52 (1978), 475–91.

[61] On Islamic medical education, see G. Makdisi, *The Rise of Colleges: Institutions of Learning in Islam and the West* (Edinburgh, 1981), 27 *et passim*; Leiser (note 60 above), 60 ff. In Europe, by comparison, such an association of medical education with hospitals was not made until the sixteenth century in Italy; see V. L. Bullough, *The Development of Medicine as a Profession* (Basel/London, 1966), 92. Concerning Byzantium, see V. Grumel, "La Profession medicale à Byzance a l'époque des Comnènes," *REB*, 7 (1949), 42–46, and the numerous works on the Pantocrator Hospital.

[62] For a general survey of this topic, see D. J. Constantelos, "Physician-Priests in the Medieval Greek Church," *The Greek Orthodox Theological Review*, 12 (1966–67), 141–53. In a recent paper, "Public Doctors in the Ancient and Medieval World," T. Miller states: "During Justinian's reign the *archiatroi* ceased to receive their pay from the city governments; they were now employees of the Church, working in the hospitals of Constantinople and in a few of the larger Byzantine towns" (Sixth Annual Byzantine Studies Conference, Abstracts of Papers [1980], p. 25). For specific examples of Egyptian physicians who became monks, see the Life of Severus, PO, II, 39, 43.

[63] O. Temkin, "Byzantine Medicine: Tradition and Empiricism," *DOP*, 16 (1962), 111 (= *Double Face of Janus*, 217–18).

[64] See P. Charanis, "Some Aspects of Daily Life in Byzantium," *The Greek Orthodox Theological Review*, 8 (1962–63), 53–70. Harig and Kollesch (note 49 above), 279–85, survey briefly the nature of the Byzantine hospitals, especially the financial support and personnel, and conclude that they became institutions with a "distinctly governmental-lay character" (285); furthermore, they assert (without any documentation) that the Islamic hospitals had a comparable character (287). The authors' argument for the character of the Byzantine hospitals is not persuasive; in fact, their data support the opposite conclusion. It is particularly hazardous to generalize about the vast Byzantine welfare system on the basis of the well-documented but exceptional Pantocrator Hospital, as the authors have done (289–92). Finally, they suggest that the Byzantine hospital was the model for hospitals in Russia, Georgia, Armenia, and Rumania (292). If this is so, it would be interesting to know how closely these institutions resemble the "Byzantine model" (?), particularly whether they cared for the insane.

[65] Concerning the closely related issue of epilepsy and its parallel development, see Temkin (note 9 above), 85–133.

[66] D. W. Amundsen, "Medicine and Faith in Early Christianity," *BHM*, 56 (1982), 326–50. Concerning the comparable tension between medicine and Islam, see F. Rosenthal, "The Defense of Medicine in the Medieval Muslim World," *BHM*, 43 (1969), 519–32; J. Ch. Bürgel, "Die wissenschaftliche Medizin im Kräftefeld der islamischen Kultur," *Bustan*, 8 (1967), 9–19; *idem*, "Secular and Religious Features of Medieval Arabic Medicine," 44–62; Klein-Franke (note 19 above), 87, 108–32.

early time.[67] In any case, demonology is conspicuous in early Byzantine writings, and there is good reason to believe that demonology was widespread throughout the Roman Empire at the time.[68]

> Christianity inherited the fateful legacy of an absolute division of the spiritual world between good and evil powers, between angels and demons. To men increasingly preoccupied with the problem of evil, the Christian attitude to the demon offered an answer designed to relieve nameless anxiety; they focused this anxiety on the demons and at the same time offered a remedy for it. . . . Hence, however many sound social and cultural reasons the historian may find for the expansion of the Christian Church, the fact remains that in all Christian literature from the New Testament onwards, the Christian missionaries advanced principally by revealing the bankruptcy of men's invisible enemies, the demons, through exorcisms and miracles of healing.[69]

[67] D. W. Amundsen and G. B. Ferngren, "Medicine and Religion: Early Christianity Through the Middle Ages," in *Health/Medicine and the Faith Traditions*, ed. M. E. Marty and K. L. Vaux (Philadelphia, 1982), 93–131; D. E. Aune, "Magic in Early Christianity," *ANRW*, 2:23:2, 1529 ff. The exorcisms of the Byzantine saints appear to differ from Jesus' in that the saints usually touched the demon-possessed individual.

[68] P. Brown, "Sorcery, Demons and the Rise of Christianity: from Late Antiquity into the Middle Ages," in his *Religion and Society in the Age of Saint Augustine* (London, 1972), 122. See also M. Smith, *Jesus the Magician* (New York, 1978), and Aune (note 67 above), 1507–57. The last is a masterful overview of the subject. Can we say, according to Aune (1515), that Christian healing practices were "religious" while Islamic healing practices were "magical," the latter being "means alternate to those normally sanctioned by the dominant religious institution"?

[69] P. Brown, *The World of Late Antiquity, A.D. 150–750* (London, 1971), 54 f. See also *idem, The Making of Late Antiquity* (Cambridge, Mass., 1978); *idem*, "Sorcery, Demons and the Rise of Christianity" (note 68 above) 132–38, emphasizes the Christian rejection of the sorcerer as the agent of misfortune and the concentration on the demons alone. R. MacMullen, "Two Types of Conversion to Early Christianity," *Vigiliae Christiane*, 37 (1983), 174–92. J. B. Russell, *The Devil: Perceptions of Evil from Antiquity to Primitive Christianity* (Ithaca, 1977), and his sequel, *Satan: The Early Christian Tradition* (Ithaca, 1981), is a more traditional survey of the subject. Temkin (note 9 above), 90 f., gives a good description of the probable pagan perception of Christian exorcism. Aline Rousselle, "From Sanctuary to Miracle-Worker: Healing in Fourth-Century Gaul," in *Selections from the Annales: Economies, Sociétés, Civilisations*, ed. R. Forster and O. Ranum, VII: *Ritual, Religion and the Sacred* (Baltimore, 1982), 95–127 (trans. E. Forster from *Annales* [1976], 1085–1107), especially 108 ff., for perceptive remarks about mental illness and the "miraculous" healing of psychosomatic illnesses. From a modern psychiatric point of view, Al-Issa (note 6 above), says (576): "By attributing [schizophrenic hallucinations] to the spirits, social expectations of their content and occurrence tend to be prescribed. What the spirits are expected to communicate to the individual may thus be socially stereotyped and could be predicted by the individual, his group, and the professionals. The general belief that external factors rather than individual ones are responsible for behavior during possession may very well facilitate social influence and cultural controls."

Concerning insanity as a theological issue, Origen's view of lunacy as intrusive possession appears to have been decisive.[70]

The claim of the Christian clergy as healers, especially as exorcists, was established and well known by the fourth century A.D.[71] At the same time, the instability of Late Roman society evoked an increase in both the number and quality of such miraculous healings.[72] There were three significant features of the reports of these healings: the successful management of supernatural powers was virtually always guaranteed; it was customarily free; and it was believed in by all classes of society. The last point needs to be stressed because of a common misunderstanding.[73] As Peter Brown has shown in a number of essays on the hagiographical literature, the belief in demonology and its association with religious healing were not confined to the common folk, but permeated at all levels of the social structure.[74]

Furthermore, it would appear from the Saints' Lives, for example the Life of Theodore of Sykeon, which is suffused with demons and their exorcism, that religious healing was sought primarily for chronic illnesses, while for acute illnesses a doctor might be recommended.[75] The recommenda-

[70] Temkin (note 9 above), 92. The groundwork had been prepared earlier by Christian apologists; see, for example, "The First Apology of Justin, the Martyr" and "A Plea Regarding Christians by Athenagoras, The Philosopher" in *Early Christian Fathers*, ed. C. C. Richardson (New York, 1970), 225–89 and 326–30 respectively.

[71] R. MacMullen, *Paganism in the Roman Empire* (New Haven, 1980), 50; MacMullen points out that "pagans lacked any corresponding deities, lacked temples known as places of resource for the possessed, on the model of Asclepieia, and had instead to trust to luck or to some not very respectable help bought in the shadows." It should be mentioned that the capacity to exorcise the possessed had its dangers for Christian healers. For example, St. Peter of Atroa became famous for his curing a consul's wife of madness; his unsuccessful rival healers claimed that his power came from the devil, so that the saint had to prove his orthodoxy; see Kathryn M. Ringrose, "Saints, Holy Men and Byzantine Society, 726 to 843" (Diss., Rutgers University, 1976), 89.

[72] Brown (note 68 above), 122 ff.; Amundsen and Ferngren (note 67 above), 103, give a number of reasons, but especially "an infusion of pagan modes of thinking into Christianity," which was stimulated by the mass conversions of the fourth century; A.-J. Festugière, ed. and trans., *Vie de Théodore de Sykéôn, SubsHag,* no. 48 (1970), I, xviii, and his *Les moines d'Orient* (Paris, 1961–65), particularly vol. I, chap. 1; Keenan (note 53 above), 16 f., a fine description of the interplay of Galenic medicine and Christianity in the fourth century A.D.

[73] E.g., Charanis (note 64 above), 96; MacMullen (note 69 above).

[74] Brown (note 10 above), 114 f.

[75] E. Dawes and N. H. Baynes, trans., *Three Byzantine Saints* (Crestwood, N.Y., 1977 rep.), 182 f. Similarly, *The Lausiac His-*

tion of doctors by Theodore may be exceptional.[76] The scholarly debate on this point indicates to me that there was no clear-cut division between religious and naturalistic healing in late antiquity. The *modus vivendi* for those entrusted with the care of the sick in a monastic infirmary or hospital is exceptionally well illustrated by the sixth-century A.D. correspondence of Saints Barsanuphius and John of Gaza. To summarize their view, they believed that medical science did not hinder one's piety; it should be regarded like the manual labor of other monks. While pride in medical expertise should be carefully guarded against, professional medicine was entirely compatible with a godly life.[77]

Nevertheless, the Saints' Lives reflect the omnipresence of demons in late antiquity. Dawes and Baynes have described this world-view well: "If we believe that the myriad bacilli about us were each and all inspired by a conscious will to injure man, we might then gain a realization of the constant menace that broods over human life in the biographies of Byzantine saints."[78] I have described this belief in demonology at length because I think that it greatly influenced the Byzantine attitude toward insanity. To paraphrase Nilsson, there was a "demonizing of medicine," despite the persistence of the Galenic tradition in the medical literature.[79]

Where were the mentally ill treated or, perhaps, incarcerated in Byzantine society? Consistent with the demonic nature of insanity, it would appear that most people eventually sought the aid of the Church, its saints and sacraments. Concerning the long-term care of the mentally ill, however, there were considerable discrepancies. The rich were able to pay for professional medical care and nursing in their homes. If we can judge from John of

Ephesus' account of Justin II's violent and prolonged madness, he was confined to the palace, where his chamberlains tried to calm the emperor by both restraints and entertainment.[80] The hostile allegation that the emperor's insanity was caused, in part, by calling in the Jewish physician, Timotheus, indicates that Justin was given professional medical attention.[81]

As for the lower classes, the harmless appear to have wandered at liberty, swallowed up among the mass of poor and homeless, which has been so well described by Patlagean for early Byzantine society.[82] Unlike the case in antiquity, however, the mentally ill appear to have resorted to the churches and saints. "The church building itself, in the practice of incubation becomes a hospital, and the sick lie about in the confines of the church awaiting a visitation from the physician-saints in the hope of being healed of their infirmities. 'Do you not know that our church has become the hospital ($\dot{\iota}\alpha\tau\varrho\epsilon\tilde{\iota}o\nu$) of the world?', ask the medical-saints, Cyrus and John."[83]

The Life of Andrew the Fool may reflect the common plight of the harmless madman in Byzantine society. Briefly, Andrew was a pious, well-educated, and trusted slave of a high court official in Constantinople. One night he received a vision that was interpreted to mean that he should devote himself to the spiritual life entirely, being "a fool for Christ's sake."[84] The following night he went into the garden of the house. Beside a well, situated close to his master's bedroom, he began to take off his clothes, tearing them with a sword, speaking unintelligible words, and making such an uproar that his master awoke suddenly and thought an evil spirit had emerged from the well. Then, frightened because he believed Andrew was possessed by a demon, the master sent him the next day to the Church of Saint Anastasius and commended

---

tory of Palladius, trans. Robert T. Meyer, in *Ancient Christian Writers*, no. 34 (Westminister/London, 1965) mentions a number of instances (83 f., 112 f., 136) of the treatment of ascetics by medical doctors, without any hint of hostility; moreover, *The Lausiac History* presents many of the themes related to insanity that are encountered in the later Saints' Lives: the cure of the possessed (57, 64, 79, 104, 121), the curse of insanity (120), the holy fool (96 ff.), and the restraint of the mad ascetic (85 ff.). On this work, see Rydén (note 7 above), 106 f.

[76] H. J. Magoulias, "The Lives of the Saints as Sources of Data for the History of Byzantine Medicine in the Sixth and Seventh Centuries," *BZ*, 57 (1964), 128 ff.

[77] *Barsanuphe et Jean de Gaza: Correspondance*, trans. L. Regnault, et al. (Sable-sur-Sarthe, 1972), 236–42; esp. 238.

[78] Dawes and Baynes (note 75 above), xii.

[79] M. P. Nilsson, *A History of Greek Religion*, 2nd ed. (Oxford, 1951), 72–78. See Temkin's remarks on this theme in his *The Falling Sickness* (note 9 above), 89 f.; he also points out a common compromise: the devil exerted his influence when the body's

humoral balance was upset (97 f.). See also *idem*, "Byzantine Medicine: Tradition and Empiricism" (note 63 above), 109 ff.

[80] John of Ephesus, *Ecclesiastical History* III.2, 89 ff.; see also P. Goubert, *Byzance avant l'Islam*, I (Paris, 1951), 53 f.

[81] Cited in Magoulias (note 76 above), 133. On the Jewish physicians in Byzantium, see A. Sharf, *The Universe of Shabbetai Donnolo* (Warminster, 1976), chaps. 6–7.

[82] E. Patlagean, *Pauvreté économique et pauvreté sociale à Byzance 4ᵉ–7ᵉ siècles* (Paris, 1977). The very pious but sane could easily be thought mad; see, for example, the incident in John of Ephesus, *Lives of the Eastern Saints*, ed. and trans. E. W. Brooks, PO, XVII (Paris, 1923), 169.

[83] Magoulias (note 76 above), 136.

[84] 1 Corinthians 4:10; see also 1:18–31.

him to a guard, to whom he gave a good tip.[85] Andrew stayed in the church with others, receiving numerous visions, speaking incoherently, and praying. When he had spent four months shackled in the Church of Saint Anastasius, the guards declared that, instead of being healed, his malady had worsened. His master was informed, and he ordered that they set Andrew free "as an incurable," ὡς ἤδη ἔξηχον καὶ δαιμονῶντα. From that time, Andrew spent his life roaming through the streets of Constantinople as a poor, ragged, and hungry beggar, preaching against avarice and luxury, speaking in tongues, and performing miracles.[86]

Related to the churches as refuges for the sick poor, the mentally disturbed probably sought assistance in the monasteries, particularly in the countryside. The following account from the Life of Theodore of Sykeon may be representative: "Another man, of the village of Salmania, was terribly abused by an unclean spirit. He went to the monastery [of St. Theodore]; because he was disorderly, St. Theodore ordered that he be tied to a post, and everyday the saint came to him and prayed for him. Consequently, the demon was so enflamed that he left the man and disappeared. At the end of two weeks the man was healed and returned to his home."[87]

This story of the man from Salmania in the monastery of St. Theodore finds a parallel in the Eastern Church. The biography of Rabban Bar-'Idtā (d. A.D. 612) tells the story of a Persian soldier who was brought to the monastery. "And through the violence of the devils in him he was bound carefully with cords. Now as they were bringing him into the martyrium to bind him with the chain which

was there, the coenobite Ṭēris-Ishōʿ happened to meet the soldier. And in the humility of the power of our Lord, he drew nigh, and took hold of the man's hands, and straightway his devil cried out and left him, and he came to his senses, and they brought the soldier to Rabban, and having learned about him he praised his Creator."[88]

Mental illness was, surely, not unknown among the monks themselves. According to the Life of St. Theodosius, the monks of the Syrian desert were overly zealous in their asceticism, so that their pride in spiritual athletics led to derangement. St. Theodosius set aside for these men a secluded section in his monastery, where he comforted them and urged them to be patient with the evils of this world.[89] The saint's special concern and plain counseling, amidst the numerous accounts of miraculous healings, strikes a responsive chord in the modern reader who is accustomed to "talk therapy."

The Life of Saint Maro also sheds some light on the plight of the insane. By feigning madness, the saint was unsuccessful in driving away the large numbers of sick and possessed who were attracted to him. The biographer of the saint says:

He would speak to the people with simple and ridiculous words and, like a fool, say, "Why do you come to a madman? Pray, have you seen anyone fouler than I am? For I am bound to this stone like a malefactor, or like a vicious dog that is bound by a chain, so that he may not escape and do harm. Do you not know that, if I were free to go, I should, like each of you, have both made a house for myself and had a wife and children? Or do you not understand that, in my case, also, it is on account of my sins and my spots and my crimes that God bound me to this stone, like a judge who puts a criminal in bounds?" But those who knew the blessed man's character and way of life used to say when they heard these things: "Yes, sir, we also are come as to a criminal, and as to one who is bound; for a man goes and sees even murderers when they are bound in prison."[90]

This brief account of the holy anti-hero, Saint Maro, is quite revealing about the cult of the saints; the allusion to the criminal, particularly, suggests the likelihood that violent or dangerous madmen

[85] According to the Life of Irene, the Church of the Blachernai also served as a refuge where the impoverished sick went to be cured; see G. da Costa-Louillet, "Saints de Constantinople aux VIIIᵉ, IXᵉ et Xᵉ siècles," *Byzantion*, 24 (1954), 187. Churches in fourth-century Gaul also appear to have harbored the possessed; see Rousselle (note 69 above), 171.

[86] PG, CXI, cols. 625–888. See Sara Murray, *A Study of the Life of Andreas the Fool* (Leipzig, 1910) for the older literature on this topic. Consult J. Wortley, "The Relationship between the *Vita* and the Cult of Saint Andrew Salos," *AnalBoll*, 90 (1972), 137–41 and C. Mango, "The Life of Saint Andrew the Fool Reconsidered," *Rivista di Studi bizantini e slavi*, 2 (1982), 297–313.

[87] Festugière, *Vie de Théodore de Sykéôn* (note 72 above) 83/85; see also II, 238 for other instances of restraint. In the medical literature, Paul of Aegina also recommended that patients suffering from mania "must be secured in bed, so that they may not be able to injure themselves, or those who approach them; or swung within a wicker-basket in a small couch suspended from on high" (trans. Adams, I, 385). The earliest recommendation of this latter therapy appears to be in Celsus (see Flashar, *Melancholie*, 75), and similar advice is given in Ibn Sīnā, *al-Qānūn*, II, 65.

[88] E. A. Wallis Budge, ed. and trans., *The Histories of Rabban Hōrmīzd the Persian and Rabban Bar-'Idtā*, II.1 (London, 1902), 220; see also 208, 261, 273, 278 f. for other instances of exorcisms. See the helpful survey by J. B. Segal, "Mesopotamian Communities from Julian to the Rise of Islam," *Proceedings of the British Academy*, 41 (1955), 109–39.

[89] *Der heilige Theodosios: Schriften des Theodoros und Kyrillos*, ed. H. R. Usener (Leipzig, 1890), 41–44; Festugière, *Les moines d'Orient* (note 72 above), III.3 (Paris, 1963), 125 f.

[90] John of Ephesus, *Lives of the Eastern Saints* (note 82 above), 68.

were put in prison, as in antiquity,[91] but I have found no evidence for this possibility.[92]

Some hospices also appear to have cared for the insane, although there is, again, no clear evidence that mental wards *per se* were created in Byzantine society. In the Life of Theodore of Sykeon we are told about the village of Germia in Galatia, where ancient tombs were disturbed when a cistern was being built. Evil spirits escaped and possessed the villagers, who sought shelter in their homes and hospices (ξενεῶνας).[93]

It may be concluded from these examples that the mentally ill often sought and received the care of the Church, which claimed the ability to exorcise the cause of the illness. Such beliefs and practices continued well into the Islamic era in the Middle East and formed the background to Muslim attitudes toward insanity. The continuity can be seen in an extraordinary incident in the Syriac Life of Rabban Hōrmīzd. The incident probably took place in the seventh century A.D. It is an unusually long account, not of an exorcism but of a resurrection. John, a twelve-year-old boy who was vexed by an evil spirit, was brought by his family to the monastery of Rabban Hōrmīzd, and the boy remained there for twenty-nine days. "And he was most grievously worked upon by that devil, for he was tortured by him in such wise that he broke his fetters and tore his garments in rags off his body, and bit off the flesh of his arms with his teeth and gnawed it, and those who were with him were in such sore tribulation that they were unable to leave him at any time, either by day or by night, lest quickly and speedily his life should be destroyed by the devil who was contending against the young man." While the whole monastic community prayed for him, the boy died. Rabban Hōrmīzd heard the cries of the family and joined them. Later, he returned disguised as a stranger, battled with Satan, and raised John from the dead.[94]

Concerning Islamic society, it would be quite reasonable to argue that the supernatural explanation and treatment of illness was just as prominent as in Byzantium. The evil jinn were the cause of sickness and disease for many, and madness (*junūn*) was literally possession by jinn.[95] The belief in jinn was inherited from pre-Islamic Arabia and is conspicuous in the Qurʾān.[96] Consequently, Christians and Muslims shared a common belief in demons as the agency of mental illness and a comparable reliance on religious and magical healing.[97] Yet, within the narrow confines of professional medicine, as encapsulated by the Islamic hospital, demonology did not encroach seriously on the Galenic tradition in the early Middle Ages, and some Islamic doctors were openly hostile to demonology.[98] As in the case of leprosy, the strength of the Galenic tradition in Islamic medicine appears to have allowed for a rational and noncondemnatory view of insanity.[99]

At the heart of the matter, Islam, in its high tradition (as distinct from ṣūfism), did not promote the doctrine of supernatural healing comparable to Christianity, nor did it possess a clergy empowered to perform exorcisms. From a different point of view, theodicy has played a very minor role in Islamic theology because of a quite different view from Christianity about the nature of human suffering—true pathology.[100] There was always a presumption of sin, however, in the chink of the Christian's baptismal armor, linking illness and sin. Madness, like other illnesses, was primarily a di-

[91] Rosen (note 5 above), 130.

[92] I have been unable to locate any study of prisons in Byzantine society, although prisons are frequently mentioned in the sources. For prisons in Islamic society, see Rosenthal (note 2 above), 35–77; ironically, he notes (60): "the evil custom of keeping people imprisoned in madhouses is attested from thirteenth-century Baghdad." See also M. M. Ziyādah, "As-Sujūn fī Miṣr," *ath-Thaqāfah*, nos. 260, 262, 279 (Cairo, 1943–44), 2123–25, 20–22, 424–26 respectively.

[93] Festugière, *Vie de Théodore de Sykéon* (note 72 above), 143 f., 147 f.; see also II, 265. Are not these malign spirits the *keres* of antiquity, who were originally the ghosts of the dead? See Rosen (note 5 above), 75 f.; "The First Apology of Justin, the Martyr" (note 70 above), 253.

[94] Budge (note 88 above), II.1.31–40; see the same incident in *The Metrical Life of Rabban Hōrmīzd*, II.2.346–355.

[95] See *EI*², *s.v.* "Djinn" (MacDonald, Masse, Boratav, Nizami, and Voorhaeve); E. Zbinden, *Die Djinn des Islam und der altorientalische Geisterglaube* (Berne, 1953); Klein-Franke (note 19 above), 8–27.

[96] On the pre-Islamic belief in gaddê or jinn, see H. Drijvers, "The Persistence of Pagan Cults and Practices in Christian Syria," in *East of Byzantium: Syria and Armenia in the Formative Period*, Dumbarton Oaks Symposium, 1980 (Washington, D.C., 1982), 38 and n. 26. See also K. Opitz, *Die Medizin im Koran* (Stuttgart, 1906), 22 ff.

[97] D. Brandenburg, *Medizin und Magie: Heilkunde und Geheimlehre des islamischen Zeitalters* (Berlin, 1975), *passim*. See, for example, the early account of the demoniac boy and St. Pisentius, who casts out the jinn in pre-Islamic Egypt, *The Arabic Life of S. Pisentius*, ed. and trans. D. O'Leary, in PO, XXII, 397 ff.

[98] See Klein-Franke (note 19 above), chap. 4.

[99] Dols, "The Leper in Medieval Islamic Society" (note 51 above).

[100] G. E. von Grunebaum, "Observations on the Muslim Concept of Evil," *Studia Islamica* (hereafter *SI*), 31 (1980), 117–34; Georges C. Anawati, "La notion de 'peche originel' existe-t-elle dans l'Islam?" *SI*, 31 (1980), 29–40; W. Montgomery Watt, "Suffering in Sunnite Islam," *SI*, 30 (1979), 5–19; L. E. Goodman, "Themes of Theodicy in the Exegesis of the Qurʾān and the Book of Job," presented at the Second Annual Conference of the Center for Islamic-Judaic Studies: "Scripture in Muslim and Jewish Traditions," April 17–18, 1983.

vine punishment for the sinful Christian; it might also be considered a purgation for the sinner or a test for the saint.[101] Yet, no such scenario existed for the faithful Muslim. According to the Qurʾān, the blind, the lame, and the sick bear no blame or guilt (*ḥaraj*) for their afflictions.[102] In addition, another Qurʾānic verse enjoins a benign attitude to the insane: "Do not give to the incompetent [*su-fahāʾ*] their property that God has assigned to you to manage; provide for them and clothe them out of it, and speak to them honorable words."[103]

In this study, I have devoted greater attention to the perceptions of insanity in Byzantine society and its care of the afflicted. Elsewhere I have described more fully the understanding of insanity and the status of the madman in Islamic society.[104] It may be sufficient to say that, like Byzantine society, there was a wide range of interpretations that allowed a broad diversity of treatments and a remarkable amount of personal freedom to the harmless madman. For example, as in Byzantine society, the *maj-dhūb*, or Muslim holy fool, was free to wander, testing other men's charity, if not their sanity.[105] The growth of ṣūfism in the later Middle Ages probably permitted an even wider latitude for abnormal behavior.

Yet, the development of ṣūfism throughout the Middle East from the eleventh century A.D. did not retard the establishment of *māristāns*. In fact, the advent of the Turks at this time marks the reinvigoration of Islamic learning. From the early thirteenth century A.D. the Turks created a number of hospitals in Asia Minor.[106] The Ottoman sultans

constructed insane asylums from the fifteenth century, and they survived until the early twentieth century.[107] In the later Middle Ages, Islamic hospitals were founded in non-Turkish territories as well. They were increasingly devoted to the care of the insane, so that in Arabic, Persian, and Turkish, *bīmāristān* or *māristān* became synonymous with an insane asylum.

To recall, finally, our madman with the pomegranate, one might be tempted to see the incarceration of the insane in Islamic hospitals as an expression of communal intolerance or concealment. Michel Foucault has suggested this "garbage can" view of hospitalization in early modern Europe,[108] but this interpretation appears inapplicable to the Islamic institutions because of the nature of the hospitals and of medieval Islamic society generally.[109] Islamic hospitals were not intended to be "cruel and unusual punishment" but were a pragmatic solution to a difficult social responsibility. They resulted from a combination of religious charity and medical science, in which Islamic doctors were able to interpret their Galenic heritage quite literally and to consider insanity as a mundane affliction like all other illnesses.

California State University, Hayward

---

[101] Doob (note 7 above), 3–10, 54–58 *et passim*; MacMullen (note 69 above), 180 ff.

[102] Qurʾān 24:60. See A. J. Arberry, *The Koran Interpreted*, II (New York, 1955), 54. Cf. S. D. Goitein, *A Mediterranean Society*, IV (Berkeley, 1983), 144.

[103] Qurʾān 4:4. See Arberry (note 102 above), I, 100.

[104] Dols, *Majnūn: The Madman in Medieval Islamic Society*, forthcoming. See H. Schipperges, "Der Narr und sein Humanum im islamischen Mittelalter," *Gesnerus*, 18 (1961), 1–12. Insanity appears to have played a considerable role in Islamic literature generally; see, for example, an-Nīsābūrī, ʿUqalāʾ al-majānīn, ed. W. F. al-Kaylānī (Cairo, 1924), and the brief study of this work by P. Loosen, "Die weisen Narren des Naisābūrī," *Zeitschrift für Assyriologie*, 27 (1912), 184–229. See also J. T. Monroe's treatment of the central story of the encounter in the asylum in "The Art of Badīʿ az-Zamān al-Hamadhānī as Picaresque Narrative," *Papers of the Center for Arab and Middle Eastern Studies (The American University of Beirut)*, 2 (1983), 1–176.

[105] *EI¹*, s.v. "Madjdhūb" (R. A. Nicholson); R. M. Eaton, *Sufis of Bijapur 1300–1700* (Princeton, 1978), 243–81, 288 f., and the healing of mental disorders at the saint's tomb, 295 f.; E. Lane, *The Manners and Customs of the Modern Egyptians* (London, 1966 rep.), 234 f.

[106] These structures do not appear to show a continuity with Byzantine institutions, but a reliance on Islamic precedents be-

cause of the destruction of the Byzantine cities by the Turks, the architectural form of the Turkish hospitals being distinctly Islamic (the *īwān* form), and the organization of their services, which included the care of the insane.

[107] A. Süheyl Ünver, "Sur l'histoire des hôpitaux en Turquie du moyen age jusqu'au XVIIᵉ siècle," *Comptes rendus du IXᵉ cong. intern. hist. méd.* (Bucharest, 1932), 263–78; *idem*, "About the History of Leproseries in Turkey," *Max Neuburger Festschrift* (Vienna, 1948), 447–50; E. M. Atabek, "Un Hôpital fondé en 1217 par les turcs seldjoukides et son influence sur l'enseignement de la médecine: l'hôpital de Sivas," *Atti del Primo Congresso Europeo di Storia Ospitaliera (6–12 Giugno, 1960)* (Reggio Emilia, 1960), 26–37; K. I. Gurkan, "Les Hôpitaux des Turcs Seldjoukides," *Société française d'histoire des hôpitaux*, 26 (1971), 33–54.

[108] M. Foucault, *Madness and Civilization: A History of Insanity in the Age of Reason*, trans. R. Howard (New York, 1973). See the trenchant criticism of this work by H. C. Erik Midelfort, "Madness and Civilization in Early Modern Europe: A Reappraisal of Michel Foucault," in *After the Reformation: Essays in Honor of J. H. Hexter*, ed. Barbara C. Malament (Philadelphia, 1980), 247–65.

[109] See M. G. S. Hodgson, *The Venture of Islam: Conscience and History in a World Civilization*, 3 vols. (Chicago, 1974); R. P. Mottahedeh, *Loyalty and Leadership in an Early Islamic Society* (Princeton, 1980); I. M. Lapidus, *Muslim Cities in the Later Middle Ages* (Cambridge, Mass., 1967); A. L. Udovitch, "Formalism and Informalism in the Social and Economic Institutions of the Medieval Islamic World," in *Individualism and Conformity in Classical Islam*, ed. A. Banani and S. Vryonis (Wiesbaden, 1977), 61–81; Dols, "The Leper in Medieval Islamic Society" (note 51 above), 914.

RABIES IN BYZANTINE MEDICINE

JEAN THÉODORIDÈS

Rabies, a terrible disease which has a uniformly fatal result if not prevented by vaccination, is a drama with three actors: the rabies virus, the biting mammal (dog, cat, wolf, fox, bat, etc.) and man. Known for at least 4,000 years in the Middle East, the disease spread into Asia and Europe.[1] Rabies was present in Greece in Homer's time (c. 800 B.C.),[2] and Xenophon's in the early fourth century B.C., and it is well described by Aristotle in the *Historia animalium*, as well as by various other Greek writers.

One of the few detailed French works on the history of rabies in ancient times is the medical thesis of M. de Tornéry,[3] of which the first fifty pages are devoted to classical antiquity and Byzantium. Although composed in the elaborate style typical of the end of the nineteenth century, de Tornéry set out some important conclusions:

1. Although absent from the Hippocratic corpus, rabies was known by the ancient Greek authors, medical and non-medical.

2. The most important source for the history of rabies in antiquity is Caelius Aurelianus (fifth century), who devotes eight chapters to this disease in his *Acute Diseases*.

3. The disease was well examined and studied by several physicians who lived in Ptolemaic Alexan-

[The reader is referred to the list of abbreviations at the end of the volume.]

dria, including Andreas of Carystos, Demetrios of Apamea, Artemidoros, and Gaios (a pupil of Herophilos).

4. Rabies is also considered by physicians of the Methodist sect, with early individuals listed as Artorios, Themison (who was probably afflicted with rabies), and his student, Eudemos; Soranos of Ephesos (second century A.D.) is the most prominent member of the sect in Roman times. Other authors also provide descriptions of rabies: Galen, Dioscorides, Rufus of Ephesos, and Poseidonios. Tornéry provides translations of the passages on rabies from Aristotle, Celsus, Galen, Oribasios, Dioscorides, Caelius Aurelianus, Aetios of Amida, and Paulos of Aegina; some further important Greek sources, however, are omitted by Tornéry. One such author, overlooked by Tornéry, is Philumenos.

PHILUMENOS ON RABIES

Philumenos (prob. *fl.* c. A.D. 180) is extant in Greek in a short tract on poisonous animals and remedies for their bites and stings. The sole surviving manuscript of this text was edited by Max Wellmann as a fascicle of the *Corpus Medicorum Graecorum*,[4] and a German translation later followed.[5] Philumenos considers rabies in the beginning of his *Poisonous Animals*, and this account apparently became very important for later Byzantine writers on the topic, as will be documented below.

Philumenos' first paragraphs deal with the description of the rabid dog: it contracts the disease when it is very hot or very cold; it does not eat or drink, has saliva flowing from its mouth, and appears irritable and aggressive. It does not bark,[6]

[1] The very ancient origin of this disease—sometimes challenged—is confirmed by P. B. Adamson, "The Spread of Rabies into Europe and the Probable Origin of This Disease in Antiquity," *Journal of the Royal Asiatic Society of Great Britain and Ireland*, 2 (1977), 140–44.

[2] B. Lincoln, "Homeric λύσσα: 'Wolfish Rage'," *Indogermanische Forschungen*, 80 (1975), 98–105.

[3] M. de Tornéry, *Essai sur l'histoire de la rage avant le XIXᵉ siècle* (Paris, 1893). On the ancient history of rabies, one may also consult: K. F. H. Marx, "Ueber das Vorkommen und die Beurtheilung der Hundswuth in alter Zeit," *Abhandlungen der Königlichen Gesellschaft Wissensch. Göttingen*, 17 (1872), 1–56; E. D. Baumann, "Über die Hundswut im Altertum," *Janus*, 32 (1928), 137–51 and 168–85; S. Winkle, "Die Tollwut im Altertum," *Die gelben Hefte*, 11 (1971), 34–44.

[4] M. Wellmann, ed., *Philumeni De venenatis animalibus eorumque remediis* (Leipzig, 1908 [*CMG* X 1, 1]).

[5] R. Froehner, "Philumenos über die Tollwut," *Archiv für Wissensch. u. prakt. Tierheilkunde*, 54 (1926), 512–18.

[6] This would suggest mute rabies (*rage mue*), a paralytic form of the disease in the dog.

and attacks both men and animals that chance to be in its path, whether they are familiar or not. Philumenos then describes the injuries caused to man by the bite of a dog that is rabid: the symptom called hydrophobia (characterized by spasms), and other disorders that affect the mind, followed by prostration, facial inflammation, and sweating. Sometimes there are also photophobia and anxiety. Some of the persons afflicted "bark like dogs" and attack other people, whom they bite, bringing to them the same illness. Except for one or two cases, Philumenos does not know of any cures for persons afflicted with rabies, and he quotes Eudemos,[7] a physician of the Methodist sect who lived in the first century A.D., and Themison,[8] a pupil of Asclepiades of Bithynia.[9] It may be possible that Eudemos and Themison suffered from rabies, but somehow they survived.

Philumenos next turns to the description of remedies for rabies. First mentioned is a mixture of powdered river crabs (probably crayfish, *Astacus fluviatilis*) calcinated over a fire made from vineyard branches combined with powdered gentian, all diluted in old wine. The patient was to drink this drug for forty days.[10] Philumenos says that the wounds which are deep and wide are less dangerous than simple scratches, since the major gashes allow the blood to flow out abundantly, carrying the "venom" of the disease; this is not characteristic of shallow wounds resulting from bites.[11] He therefore suggests that the wound be widened so that the "venom" (*ios*) could escape with the blood.

Philumenos also advises the physician to cauterize the wound, since fire has properties that would destroy the "venom" and could prevent its penetration into the body. Additionally, the wound has to be kept open for forty days, and this is promoted by the application to the wound of a plaster made of brine, crushed garlic, onion bulbs, and swollen grains of wheat (made moist by either soaking or chewing them). If the wound closes before the fortieth day, it should be reopened and recauterized.[12]

Chapter 4 of Philumenos' *Poisonous Animals* describes the diet which must be followed by patients afflicted by rabies.[13] The diet had to act against the "venom" and weaken its action. One should drink pure wine and sweet milk and eat garlic, onion, and leek. Suggested also are the multi-ingredient theriacs, the "Eupator" or "Mithridation."[14] The disease can be latent generally for forty days, but this stage can last much longer, from six months to as much as one year, or even seven years. If widening and cauterization of the bite have not been performed on the wound during the first days after it occurred, one then had to try to expel the poison by other means, including use of the "medicinal gourd" (*kolokynthē hiera*)[15] and sour milk. Inducing sweats before and after meals is also suggested, as well as the application of a depilatory ointment and strong plasters over the entire body. The most effective preventive remedy, however, is hellebore "to be used boldly, not only once or twice, but many times before and after the fortieth day."[16] Philumenos adds that "the remedy is so strong that it has cured rabid patients who had taken it at the very beginning of the course of the disease." Among the drug recipes that follow are pharmaceuticals mainly of animal origin, many of the so-called "Dreck-Apothek," including the curdled milk of a hare, dessicated dung of a dog, calves' fat, and the like. Philumenos writes that he is quoting these prescriptions from the writings of Theodoros the Physician,[17] who himself is quoting from Krates (otherwise unknown), who has written that the

---

[7] Eudemos is cited by Caelius Aurelianus, *Acute Diseases* III, 12.107; 15.125; and 16.134 (ed. Drabkin, pp. 368, 378, and 386) for his works and observations on hydrophobia and its treatment. Galen names a Eudemos among the Methodists in *Method of Medicine* I, 7 (ed. Kühn, X, 53), and he is probably the same person who appears prominently in accounts of the plot of Sejanus and Livilla to poison Drusus, son of Tiberius, in A.D. 23 (Pliny, *Natural History* XXIX, 20; Tacitus, *Annals* IV, 3 and 11).

[8] Themison traditionally is cited as the "founder" of the Methodist sect of physicians, and with the redating of the *floruit* of Asclepiades of Bithynia (n. 9 below), we can assume that Themison lived in the late second century B.C., since he was a student of Asclepiades (Pliny, *Natural History* XXIX, 6). Caelius Aurelianus, *Acute Diseases* III, 16.132 (ed. Drabkin, p. 384) and Philumenos, *Poisonous Animals* 1.4 (ed. Wellmann, p. 5) report that Themison contracted rabies but survived.

[9] Until recently, Asclepiades of Bithynia was dated as practicing medicine in Rome c. 90–70 B.C., but a close reading of the primary sources has shown that Asclepiades was dead by 90 B.C. Thus he must be redated at least fifty years earlier. See Elizabeth Rawson, "The Life and Death of Asclepiades of Bithynia," *CQ*, n.s. 32 (1982), 358–70. For references on Asclepiades, see Scarborough and Nutton, "Preface," 206–8.

[10] Philumenos 2.2–3 (ed. Wellmann, p. 5).

[11] Philumenos 2.6 (ed. Wellmann, p. 6).

[12] Philumenos 3 (ed. Wellmann, pp. 6–7).

[13] Philumenos 4 (ed. Wellmann, pp. 7–9).

[14] Philumenos 4.4 (ed. Wellmann, p. 7).

[15] Probably *Citrullus colocynthis* (L.) Schrader. Cf. Paul V, 3 (ed. Heiberg, II, p. 10), and C. E. Trease and W. C. Evans, *Pharmacognosy*, 11th ed. (London, 1978), 472.

[16] Philumenos, 4.10–11 (ed. Wellmann, p. 8).

[17] Theodoros was perhaps one of the first-century physicians of the Pneumatic sect. Pliny, *Natural History* XX, 40 and XXIV, 120. Diogenes Laertius II, 8.104. M. Wellmann, *Die Pneumatische Schule bis auf Archigenes* (Berlin, 1895), 13.

poison would be found in the urine of persons bitten by the animal.

The fifth chapter of Philumenos' *Poisonous Animals* considers the problems of persons bitten by rabid dogs or by rabid human beings.[18] Here are quoted recipes for drugs borrowed from Archigenes[19] and Straton (a pupil of Erasistratos):[20] one is to use ointments on the wound made from oil and the root of the fenugreek, ground in honey, or apply plasters that contain myrrh, terebinth-resin and copper sulfate mixed with honey, or calcined calves' bones mixed with soft pitch and honey. The most efficient plaster is made up of ground garlic or salt ground up in honey, and the "Dreck-Apothek" reappears with dried pig dung mixed with oil and leek. In addition to other recipes, two final prescriptions are given: fill up the wound with fire-dried dill, or lay on cabbage leaves, verdigris, rue, and salt.[21]

Quite probably derivative from Philumenos is the account of rabies found in the *Poisonous Animals* by a Pseudo-Dioscorides.[22] It is uncertain when this tract (along with another Pseudo-Dioscorides' *Poisons*) was added to the manuscript traditions of Dioscorides' *Materia Medica* and *Simples*,[23] but Photios knew these works as part of the collection of tracts written by Dioscorides.[24] Meyer speculated that Dioscorides' *Materia Medica* was combined with the *Poisons* and *Poisonous Animals* sometime in the seventh or eighth centuries,[25] an opinion shared by Berendes, who translated the two pseudo-Dioscoridean books into German.[26] It is, however,

our opinion that these two books are much earlier, even though Oribasios appears to know Dioscorides' *Simples* but not the Pseudo-Dioscorides *Poisonous Animals* and *Poisons*.[27] In chapters 1–3 of Pseudo-Dioscorides' *Poisonous Animals* occurs a description of rabies that is almost identical with that given by Philumenos.[28] Chapter 1 outlines the characteristic features of the rabid dog and the hydrophobic patient; chapters 2 and 3 list the remedies for persons bitten by a rabid dog and the various procedures employed to cure the wound (cauterization, scarification, application of plasters) and to expel the "venom." We make note, however, that the "Dreck-Apothek" present in Philumenos is absent in Pseudo-Dioscorides, and the anonymous author insists on the efficacy of the "medical gourd" and hellebore.[29]

ORIBASIOS ON RABIES

Oribasios, physician to Julian the Apostate (emperor 361–363), mentions rabies in several of his works.[30] In his *Synopsis*,[31] Oribasios gives a good description of the behavior of mad dogs, which lose both their voice and "understanding," not recognizing familiar persons. They do not want to eat and are thirsty; they pant and leave their ears hanging; much foamy saliva comes out of their mouths. When a person has been bitten by a rabid dog, the wound has to be cauterized and left open, then washed with an infusion of camomile or root of the wild patience-dock; the patient shuld also drink the juice of small buckthorn or *silphion*; *sil-*

[18] Philumenos 5 (ed. Wellmann, pp. 9–10).

[19] Archigenes was a physician of the Pneumatic sect (Pseudo-Galen, *Introduction* 9 [ed. Kühn, XIV, 699]), who probably *floruit* in the reigns of Nerva and Trajan, A.D. 96–117. Archigenes wrote tracts *On Fevers*, *On Pulses*, and some others (Wellmann, *Pneumatische Schule* [n. 17 above], 19–22, 84–85, and 170–71). Cf. Aetios XIII, 1 (ed. Zervos, pp. 264–65).

[20] Straton *floruit* in the third century B.C. as a younger contemporary of Erasistratos. See Galen, *On Bloodletting, against Erasistratos*, 2 (ed. Kühn, XI, 151 and 197). M. Michler, *Die alexandrinischen Chirurgen* (Wiesbaden, 1968), 95 with references.

[21] Philumenos 5.8 (ed. Wellmann, p. 10).

[22] J. Riddle, "Dioscorides" in *Catalogus*, IV, esp. 118–19.

[23] M. Wellmann accepted Dioscorides' *Simples* as "genuine," and prepared the edited Greek text which appears in Vol. III of his edition of Dioscorides (Berlin, 1914) as *Dioscuridis Liber de simplicibus* (pp. 149–326 [two books with a Greek *pinax*]). Arguments for Dioscorides as the author of *Simples* are given by M. Wellmann, *Die Schrift des Dioskurides* Περὶ ἁπλῶν φαρμάκων (Berlin, 1914).

[24] Photius, Cod. 178 (ed. Henry, Vol. II, p. 182).

[25] Meyer, *Botanik*, II, 110.

[26] J. Berendes, "I. Des Pedanios Dioskurides Schrift über die Gifte und Gegengifte. II. Des Pedanios Dioskurides Schrift über die giftigen Tiere und den tollen Hund," *Apotheker Zeitung*, 92–93 (1905), 908–10, 926–28, 933–35, and 945–54.

[27] Oribasios, *Medical Collection*, ed. Raeder, IV, p. 314 (index references to Dioscorides' *Simples*).

[28] C. Sprengel, ed., [Pedanii Dioscoridis] *De iis, quae virus eiaculantur, animalibus libellus, in quo et de rabioso cane* in *Pedanii Dioscoridis Anazarbei*, Vol. II (Leipzig, 1830 [C. G. Kühn, ed., *Medicorum Graecorum opera quae exstant*, Vol. XXVI]), pp. 42–91 (chs. 1–3: pp. 57–66).

[29] One may also mention the short paragraph on rabies by Theodorus Priscianus, physician to the emperor Gratian (A.D. 375–383). Priscianus composed the *Euporiston* as a guide to simples and diseases, and in Book, II, 8.26, one reads: "Some would declare that hydrophobias are caused by the bite of a rabid dog, others would say from the bite of a snake. But for us it is superfluous to seek out with an anxious care these causes. It is useless, in fact, for those afflicted by this disease to know its cause." A list of prominent symptoms follows, in turn followed by suggested pharmaceuticals, including powdered gentian root, which will be met in a number of Greek works on the topic. V. Rose, ed., *Theodori Prisciani Euporiston* (Leipzig, 1894), pp. 125–26.

[30] Generally we have used the edition of Oribasios edited and translated by Bussemaker and Daremberg (Paris, 1851–1876; 6 vols.).

[31] VIII, 13: Bussemaker and Daremberg, Vol. V, pp. 417–19 = Raeder, ed., *Synopsis*, pp. 250–51.

phion juice itself can be put into the wound, and the patient is advised that he can drink infusions of germander, gentian root, *polion*, and freshwater crabs (crayfish) with dill. Purgation is promoted by the use of a colocynth, and a piece of it (the size of a bean) is to be taken daily. One is supposed to take the bean-sized piece of the small gourd in a decoction of sage, or of the lodestone of Heracles, called *alyssos*, as an especially effective remedy against rabies. One can also take the drug made from the snake called the *echidna*, as well as various diuretics. One must also eat the liver of the dog that bit the victim, but this should not be done alone; one should take all the remedies together. Oribasios concludes his account on "Bites from Rabid Dogs" with the statement that Apollonios of Pergamon had reported that no hydrophobic patient had ever recovered when the disease resulted from the bite of a mad dog, but hydrophobia from other causes could be cured.

In his *Easily Procured Drugs Addressed to Eunapios*,[32] Oribasios gives a recipe for treatment of the bite of a rabid dog, in which he advises the roasting of freshwater crabs (crayfish), making them into a fine ash. Medical astrology adds its context here, since one is to prepare the crab-ash after the rising of Canis Major (the stellar constellation), when the sun is in the constellation of Leo and when the moon is in its eighteenth day. A compound drug is prepared which is made up of crab-ashes (ten parts), gentian root (five parts), and frankincense (one part). A large spoonful of this drug is to be put into water and drunk for forty days; if the treatment begins only a few days after the rabid dog bit the patient, two spoonfuls should be taken each day. A formula follows for making a salve which could be applied to the wound: Bruttian pitch (one Roman pound), strong vinegar (one *xestes* [c. one pint]), and opopanax (three Roman ounces).[33] Persons who use this drug are always safe after the bite of a mad dog. Oribasios concludes this terse consideration of treatment of the bites of rabid animals with additional suggestions of herbs used against the bites of poisonous animals (borrowed from Galen's *Mixtures and Properties of Simples*):[34] dried catmint (*kalaminthē*: *Napeta cataria* L.), betony (*kestros* = *bettonikē*: *Stachys officinalis* [L.] Trev.), the seeds of wild

rue, rennet from a young rabbit, and beet juice are all recommended. Another summary of treatments for the bites of rabid dogs occurs in Oribasios' *Medical Collection: Selection of Drugs*.[35] Here he repeats many of the drugs and herbs he has summarized in other texts (for example, pitch, vinegar, opopanax, freshwater crabs), but of special interest are several remedies made from animals, including the seahorse (*hippocampos*: 117.7 [Raeder, IV, p. 292 = Bussemaker and Daremberg, IV, p. 624]). In many instances, Oribasios' collection of descriptions and remedies for rabies becomes an important source for later Byzantine authors on the subject.

Rabies in Byzantine Veterinary Medicine

The main Byzantine veterinary materials are represented by the corpus of the *Hippiatrica*, which deals chiefly with horse medicine, but the date of the compilation is very uncertain.[36] Among the numerous extracts in the collection several authors are quoted by name, and rabies is mentioned frequently enough to suggest a knowledge and concern about the disease among domestic animals.

Apsyrtos was perhaps a veterinarian in the army of Constantine the Great (324–337), and he mentions rabies in horses. He believes that the main cause of the disease is the increase of heat, as well as the horses eating too much vetch. Apsyrtos suggests that cures can be effected with a number of remedies, including the root of the wild cucumber cooked in wine or black hellebore boiled in vinegar.[37]

Hierocles also mentions rabies in horses, but he has copied from Apsyrtos.[38] To Hierocles, the causes of the disease would be due to a large flow of blood into the meninges, the occurrence of bile in the blood, or the bad quality of the water. He says that the horse neighs without warning and will attack men. He advises the same remedies as Apsyrtos, adding crushed rue with mint, and bloodletting

---

[32] III, 72: Bussemaker and Daremberg, Vol. V, pp. 682–83 = Raeder, ed., *Libri ad Eunapium*, p. 432.

[33] The resin of *Opopanax chironium* (L.) Koch.

[34] *Simples* VII, 10.1 and 23 (ed. Kühn, XII, 4–5, and 23–24 and *passim*).

[35] 117 [118]: Bussemaker and Daremberg, Vol. IV, pp. 623–24 = Raeder, ed., Vol. IV, pp. 291–92.

[36] A.-M. Doyen, "Les Textes d'Hippiatrie grecque. Bilan et perspectives," *AntCl*, 50 (1981), 258–73. Cf. also by the same author, "The Hippiatrica and Byzantine Veterinary Medicine" in this collection. More particularly on rabies, cf. L. Moulé, "Histoire de la médecine vétérinaire," *Bulletin Société centr. Médecine vétérinaire*, 45 (1891), 285–86 [horses], 344 [bovines], 435–37 [dogs].

[37] *CHG*, I, 347.

[38] *CHG*, I, 347; II, 263.

performed on the throat. A drastic treatment included is the cutting of the horse's testicles.

Eumelos gives a good description of the rabid horse:[39] it breaks its rack, bites itself, and attacks men. It moves its ears, has staring and glowing eyes, and foam on the mouth. Eumelos advises that one should tie the horse up and draw blood from the leg or the cervical area, and then to rub its body with its own blood mixed with wine, as well as to cauterize its belly and temples. He also suggests castration. After the animal has become quiet, one should inject into the nostrils hemlock seeds crushed in water. Its belly should be released and its head rubbed with vinegar in which black hellebore has been boiled, then covered with sheepskins. Later on, crushed rue should be rubbed on its head, and the animal kept in a warm place.

Hippocrates[40] describes the symptoms that occur in a rabid horse:[41] its eyes protrude and are infused with blood, the veins on the body are prominent, and the animal has no appetite and is restless. Bloodletting in the veins of the neck is advised, and then the horse should be left in a dark and quiet place. In the evening, one may give it some water to drink, and this may be repeated the next day. During the first three days, its food and drink must be restricted, but afterwards the horse can be allowed to eat normally.

In the *Hippiatrica*[42] one also finds a recipe for the treatment of a bite from a rabid dog, which reads as follows: six Roman ounces of goat dung, six Roman ounces of old brine (or old salted fish), six Roman ounces of the berries of the dwarf elder (*Sambucus ebulus* L.), forty walnuts, all ground together. Another recipe for treatment of rabies in bovines combines animal, vegetable, and mineral substances: freshwater crab (crayfish), wild grapes (*agriostaphida*, or stavesacre [*Delphinium staphisagria* L. if *agriostaphida* = *staphis agria*] in Ranunculaceae), ground in vinegar; or Syrian sumac, man orchid (*satyrion: Aceras anthropophorum* [L.] Aiton fil.), and rock salt mixed with honey and cooked.[43]

As an appendix to the *Hippiatrica*, we may mention the tract *On Animals* by Timotheos of Gaza,

who lived in the fifth century.[44] Chapter 26 is devoted to the dog, and rabies is noted, along with two other diseases affecting this animal (dog-quinsy and podagra), paraphrased from Aristotle.[45] Timotheos then writes:

> They who are bitten by a rabid dog fear water [and] seldom live [that is, survive]. Drinking a pill with the right [side] of a hyena, they escape [death] [or] those who sacrifice a puppy and drink the curdled milk from its stomach with water.[46]

The commentators on Timotheos call attention to the venerated belief in the efficacy against rabies of hyena's meat, particularly from its right side, noted in the first century by Pliny the Elder in the *Natural History*: "[The Magi say] that to eat the flesh [of a hyena] renders harmless the bites of a mad dog, the liver being even more efficacious. . . ."[47] Timotheos continues: When one shows a mirror to people who have been bitten [by a rabid dog] and they see in it the image of a dog [then] they die, but when [they see the image] of a human being, they live. One recognizes the folkloristic elements in Timotheos' fragments, perhaps to be expected from a student of Horapollo,[48] author of the pseudo-learned *Hieroglyphica*, a prime example of the curious fusion of Egyptian with Greek learning in fourth- or fifth-century Byzantine Egypt. By contrast, the veterinary writers have inherited a lengthy tradition of meticulous knowledge of domestic animal lore, ultimately derived from many centuries of experience on Roman farms.[49]

CAELIUS AURELIANUS

Although not strictly within the Byzantine medical traditions, one must consider the important analysis and synopsis on rabies by Caelius Aurelianus in the fifth century.[50] Eight chapters of his *Acute Diseases*[51] are devoted to hydrophobia, and the account is rich in quotations from earlier authori-

---

[39] *CHG*, I, 349.
[40] On Hippocrates the veterinarian, see G. Björck, "Griechische Pferdeheilkunde in arabischer Überlieferung," *Monde Orient. Rev. Et. Orient (Uppsala)*, 30 (1936), 1–12. I thank Dr. A.-M. Doyen-Higuet for this reference.
[41] *CHG*, I, 350.
[42] *CHG*, I, 357.
[43] *CHG*, II, 50.

[44] F. S. Bodenheimer and A. Rabinowitz, *Timotheus of Gaza on Animals* (Leiden, 1949). See also M. Wellmann, "Timotheos von Gaza," *Hermes*, 62 (1927), 179–204.
[45] Aristotle, *Historia animalium* 604a22. The *podagra* here may perhaps be foot-and-mouth disease.
[46] *Timotheus* (n. 44 above), p. 33.
[47] Pliny, *Natural History* XVIII, 104.
[48] Wellmann, "Timotheos" (n. 44 above), 179 with n. 8.
[49] For a survey in English, see R. E. Walker, "Roman Veterinary Medicine," appendix in J. M. C. Toynbee, *Animals in Roman Life and Art* (London, 1973), 303–43 and 404–14.
[50] See the introductory essays in Drabkin, ed. and trans., pp. xi-xviii.
[51] Drabkin, ed. and trans., 361–89.

ties in Greek on the disease, so that Caelius Aurelianus is drawing on many of the same sources as would the later Byzantine medical writers, Aetios of Amida and Paulos of Aegina. Caelius Aurelianus begins with a definition of rabies, which he calls hydrophobia, from its most basic symptom, an excessive fear of water. Next comes a precise etiology:

> The antecedent cause of the disease is the bite of a mad dog or, as some say, of other animals that are subject to similar madness, such as the wolf, bear, leopard, horse, and ass, or the bite of a human being who has hydrophobia. . . . In some cases the patient is affected by rabies as a result of being injured by the claws of a rabid animal. And it is related that a woman became ill of hydrophobia when her face was slightly scratched by a small puppy. Again a case of rabies is said to have been caused by a slight scratch of a poultry-cock as it was struggling. And once when a seamstress was preparing to patch a cloak rent by the bites of a rabid animal, she adjusted the threads along the end, using her tongue, and then as she sewed she licked the edges that were being joined, in order to make the passage of the needle easier. It is reported that two days later she was stricken by rabies. Moreover, it is possible for the disease to originate in the body without any visible cause, when a state of stricture, such as that which comes from poison, is produced spontaneously. Now some incur the disease quickly after the bite. Others do so more slowly and are affected only after a year or even longer. But in most cases the disease comes after forty days.[52]

This etiology of rabies is one of the most important and significant for its time, because it broadens the modes of transmission of the disease in contrast to most other authorities, who limited rabies to the bites of wolves, dogs, and human beings. In addition, Caelius Aurelianus makes the distinction between hydrophobia contracted from the bite of a rabid animal and "spontaneous" hydrophobia.

In *Acute Diseases* III, 11–12 (Drabkin, 364–69), he details the symptoms of rabies in humans, and makes a careful distinction between them and those which arise from other, seemingly similar diseases: mania, phrenitis, and melancholia. Caelius Aurelianus is especially critical of Eudemos, a student of Themison, for his statement that melancholia is the same as hydrophobia.[53] *Acute Diseases* III, 15 (Drabkin, 371–75) is a careful discussion of various hypotheses proposed for the exact seat of the disease, and which parts of the body are affected by rabies. A number of authorities are cited, and the

suggested organs and parts are reviewed (nerves, meninges, diaphragm, esophagus, heart, etc.), but Caelius Aurelianus is wise enough not to give his own view. His therapeutics are, however, the weakest part of his contribution (*Acute Diseases* III, 16 [Drabkin, 380–89]), and he knows nothing of cauterization of the wound. Tornéry believes that Caelius Aurelianus' poor therapeutics result from the fact that he belonged to the Methodist sect, for whom therapeutics were only a contemplation of nature's efforts promoting recovery of the patients.[54]

ALEXANDER OF TRALLES, AETIOS OF AMIDA, PAULOS OF AEGINA

In the works of Alexander of Tralles (c. 525–605), one finds no mention of rabies.[55] Although he mentions in his first book various nervous diseases (epilepsy, paralysis, phrenitis, lethargia, etc.), there is nothing about rabies and its main symptom, hydrophobia. But in the works of Aetios of Amida and Paulos of Aegina, rabies is considered in some detail.

Although bites by human beings and dogs are considered in Book XIII of the *Tetrabiblos* by Aetios of Amida (c. 502–575), there is no mention of rabies.[56] But the disease is described in *Tetrabiblos* VI, which deals with various afflictions of the head and brain.[57] Chapter 24 begins with the disease in dogs, influenced by heat and hot weather, and cold and cold weather. Not allowed to drink water, they are seized by a great thirst which is why the "evil" (= damage) of the poison increases in intensity all the more. The symptomatology is as follows: rabid dogs are "speechless," that is, unable to bark and they do not recognize their masters; they are hungry and thirsty but unable to drink; they gasp for breath a great deal, exposing the tongue and leaving the mouth open; and they pour forth saliva that is both foamy and profuse. This is a classical description of what is called "dumb rabies" (*rage mue* or *muette*).

Aetios then describes the disease in humans:

---

[52] *Acute Diseases* III, 9.99–100 (trans. Drabkin, p. 363). Translation is Drabkin's.
[53] *Acute Diseases* III, 12.107–8 (Drabkin, p. 368).

[54] Tornéry, *Essai* (n. 3 above), 28.
[55] Employing the French translation of Alexander by F. Brunet (Paris, 1933–37).
[56] J. Théodoridès, "Sur le 13ᵉ Livre du Traité d'Aétios d'Amida, médecin byzantin du VIᵉ siècle," *Janus*, 47 (1958), 221–37.
[57] Aetios VI, ch. 24 in *Medicae Artis Principes post Hippocratum et Galenum, Graeci Latinitate donati* (Paris [Stephanus], 1567), Vol. II, cols. 260–63. I wish to thank Prof. J. Scarborough, who has kindly translated for me into English from the Greek of the Olivieri edition (*CMG*, VIII, 2) an important part of this chapter.

Everyone who is careless after having been bitten by a rabid dog . . . will either fear water or other liquids, some for forty days, but others for a longer time. The anxiety (*ekstasis*) is more painful for those who think [they see] water or some other translucent liquid in a mirror: they believe they see their own flushed faces with a keen look, full of rage. And this is the power over them, as some say, since the reflected image is that of the biting dog.

Then Aetios tells the story of a "philosopher" (Themison?) who had been bitten by a mad dog and who, while in his bath, saw its image. Reasoning to himself what was in common between the dog and the bath, he was cured. We have here a curious application of psychosomatics to "cure" an infectious disease! Aetios suggests various drugs and compounds, some of which are similar to those already listed by Galen and Oribasios (pitch, vinegar, opopanax, ashes of freshwater crabs, gentian, etc.). Another compound medicine which includes rock salt, chalk, squill, green rue, rosemary, and hoarhound seeds, will reappear in Paulos of Aegina. Still another compound recipe includes sagapenum gum from the stem of *Ferula persica* Willd., or possibly *F. scowitziana* D.C., still used in Arabic medicine, as well as opium, saffron, lycium (probably *Lycium intricatum* Boiss., which remains in the pharmacopoeia of Arabic North Africa), and fresh walnuts.

Kyphi, which is a compound incense,[58] is also advised, as well as eating the liver of the biting animal with salt and oil, an echo of the tradition recorded in Pliny. With this introduction into the *materia medica zoologica*, Aetios provides further similar examples: the fish, *hippocampos* (seahorse) has the same action as the biting dog's liver, which promotes the patient to drink, due to its blood, and it can be eaten or applied to the wound, ground up in vinegar (this had been mentioned by Oribasios); the rennet of a kitten; and hairs of bears, seals, and hyenas are burnt and given in a solution to drink to the patient. Aetios then speaks of the "test of the nuts," which is probably borrowed from Rufus of Ephesos.[59] Crushed walnuts were put on the wound suspected of being made by a rabid animal, and then the next day, the walnuts were given to a chicken; if the bird ate them and did not die, it meant that the biting animal was not rabid and thus the wound

was "safe." This curious means of diagnostics will be given again by Paulos of Aegina, John Actuarios, as well as by Rhazes, Avicenna, Albucasis, and Maimonides. Once the scar of the wound is formed, Aetios advises the use of white hellebore (*Veratrum album* L.) in order to prevent any further accident.[60] It appears that although Aetios has borrowed much from Rufus, Galen, Philumenos, and Oribasios, he provides a greater detail regarding rabies than his predecessors.

On rabies, Paulos of Aegina (*fl. c.* 640) differs little from Aetios, and the beginning sections of Paulos' medical encyclopedia account of rabies (Book V, 3) are paraphrases of Philumenos or the pseudo-Dioscoridean *Poisonous Animals*.[61] Paulos adds that among the people bitten, only those suffering from human bites have recovered. In Book V, 3, Paulos summarizes the accounts of Philumenos, Pseudo-Dioscorides, cites Rufus for a contrary opinion (rabies is a kind of melancholia), and quotes from Lycos, Oribasios, and—as apparent from the phraseology—Aetios. Paulos believes rabies is caused by a poison which has invaded the entire organism. He mentions the opinion of some physicians, according to whom the aversion to water would be due to a disordered dryness which brings a transmutation of all the body fluids. He further notes that Rufus thought that this aversion to water would be the result of the melancholy afflicting these patients, much as sufferers from melancholia generally fear one thing or another. Paulos also mentions the visual hallucinations of the patients and reports, as had his predecessors, that only one or two cases were known of persons escaping the disease after they had been bitten, and he insists that these people had been attacked by rabid men and not by animals. The "walnut test" follows, taken from Oribasios (so says Paulos), but which is almost identical with the similar passages in Aetios, who probably had also borrowed this diagnostic technique from Oribasios.[62] Paulos' pharmaceuticals for rabies are almost identical to those of his predecessors.[63] One prescription is, however, somewhat modified from the original: a mixture of gentian roots ground up in old wine given with two spoonfuls of partridge blood.

---

[58] For this compound incense, see the appendix to J. Scarborough, "Early Byzantine Pharmacology," pp. 229–32, below.

[59] Daremberg and Ruelle, eds., *Rufus*, pp. 371–75, consider the passage dealing with the "test of the nuts" as borrowed from Rufus, but in the apparatus criticus to the Greek text on p. 372, Ruelle expresses some doubt about this attribution.

[60] Aetios VI, 24 (ed. Olivieri [*CMG* VIII 2], pp. 166–67.

[61] Paul (ed. Heiberg), II, 7–8 = Paul (trans. Adams), II, 162–63.

[62] Paul (ed. Heiberg), II, 9 = Paul (trans. Adams), II, 163–64.

[63] Paul (ed. Heiberg), II, 9–10 = Paul (trans. Adams), II, 164–65.

Pseudo-Rabies in Agathias

Agathias (c. 537–c. 582) is the author of the important *Histories* which gives details of events in the sixth century.[64] In the *Histories* (II, 3.4–8), occurs a description of a strange disease which afflicted Leutharis, a leader of the "Barbarians" (Franks and Alamans) and his men, who were fighting the Romans, led by their general Narses. The peculiar events described in this passage took place in Venetia at the beginning of the year 553. The disease was an epidemic, characterized by the following symptoms: (1) agitation followed by falling, backward or forward; (2) foam coming out of the mouth; (3) staring eyes and rolling movement of the eyeballs; (4) the victims bit their own arms, tearing the flesh open and licking the blood; (5) fever and headaches; (6) paralysis and madness; and (7) death. Von Hagen presumed that this outbreak in Leutharis' army was rabies,[65] arguing for this diagnosis on the basis of the symptoms with the supposition that the disease would have been transmitted to Leutharis and his men by stray dogs.

In a recent paper considering this case,[66] I have concluded that the disease was an epidemic, since many persons became ill, and that it affected the nervous system. Although Agathias' description reminds one of ergotism, frequent in Europe in the Middle Ages, it lacks the digestive symptoms of ergotism, and ergotism lacks the fever which is present in the symptoms displayed by Leutharis and his army. I have, furthermore, discarded rabies, for the following reasons: (1) the occurrence of dogs is not mentioned by Agathias, who was writing at a time when rabies and its transmission to man by dogs was well known; (2) Agathias makes no allusion to hydrophobia, photophobia, and aerophobia, all characteristic of human rabies; and (3) in human rabies, no case history includes the patient biting his own upper limbs and tearing off the flesh. This last symptom is, however, typical of another disease of animals, which resembles rabies—Aujeszky's Disease, which was described in 1902 by a Hungarian veterinarian, and called also "Pseudo-Rabies." Aujeszky's Disease is caused by a virus of

the herpes group, and affects chiefly dogs, cats, cows and oxen, pigs, sheep, and horses. The main source of infection is the pig. Self-mutilations by dogs afflicted with this disease are frequent, and the animal dies after eighteen to thirty-six hours from bulbar paralysis. One is thus tempted to believe the disease described by Agathias is Pseudo-Rabies, or Aujeszky's Disease. The major difficulty with this diagnosis is that in the few cases of this illness known in humans, the symptoms were very mild and the patients recovered fully.

Two hypotheses seem reasonable: (1) there may have been, in the sixth century, a viral disease related to Pseudo-Rabies (Aujeszky's Disease), pathogenic for man as well as for animals, which has since disappeared; and (2) the strains of the virus of Aujeszky's Disease could have been, in Agathias' day, much more virulent than currently known, and it would affect humans as well as animals. With either hypothesis one may suppose that Leutharis and his men would have contracted the disease from eating pork, one of the usual parts of the diet of the Alamans. It may be that other Byzantine historical sources will reveal other descriptions of rabies in men and animals, but corollary materials have not emerged in the limited search made at this time.

The *Geoponica* and Rabies

It is of interest that only a few hints on rabies are to be found in the *Geoponica*, a Byzantine encyclopedia which is of uncertain date,[67] though the preface seems to indicate dedication to Constantine VII Porphyrogenitos.[68] Such passages as do occur in this agricultural compilation that are concerned with rabies consider very briefly remedies used against the bite of a mad dog, such as grapevine ashes, and the leaves of garlic and cabbage. One chapter, however, is extracted from Theomnestos, and suggests what should be done for female dogs that are rabid:

> One must lock up rabid bitches, and not allow them to eat during the day; then mix some hellebore into their drink. When they have been purged, one ought

[64] R. Keydell, ed., *Agathiae Myrinaei Historiarum* (Berlin, 1967 [CFHB, Vol. II]), and J. D. Frendo, trans., *Agathias: The Histories* (Berlin, 1975, [CFHB, Vol. II A]). *Histories* II, 3.4–8 = Keydell, pp. 43–44 = Frendo, pp. 34–35.
[65] B. von Hagen, *Lyssa, eine medizingeschichtliche Interpretation* (Jena, 1940).
[66] J. Théodoridès, "Quelle était la maladie décrite par l'historien Agathias (VIᵉ siècle A.D.)?," *Histoire des sciences médicales*, 15 (1981), 153–58.

[67] The only available edition of the Greek text of the *Geoponica* is that of H. Beckh (Leipzig, 1895). For the date of the collection, see E. Oder, "Beiträge zur Geschichte der Landwirthschaft bei den Griechen," *RhM* n.f. 45 (1890), 58–98, and 212–22, and *ibid.*, 48 (1893), 1–40, and M. Ullmann, in *HO*, VI (1972), 431 f.; see also H. Hunger, *Die hochsprachliche profane Literatur der Byzantiner*, 2 vols. (Munich, 1978), II, p. 273.
[68] *Geoponica*, Prooemium 11 (ed. Beckh, pp. 2–3).

to feed them bread made from barley. Persons bitten by rabid dogs should be treated in the same manner.[69]

Rabies in Later Byzantine Medicine

Rabies is mentioned by four physicians of the late centuries of Byzantium (tenth to the fourteenth centuries): Theophanes Nonnos, Nicholas Myrepsos, Demetrios Pepagomenos, and Joannes Actuarios. Theophanes Nonnos (tenth century) considers the disease in chapter 271 of his *Epitome de curatione morborum*,[70] devoted to the rabid dog and venomous animals. One finds here an abstract of what has already been said by Philumenos and his later commentators. The test of the nuts is also mentioned. Among the plasters recommended for application to the wound, we find the usual ones with vinegar, opopanax, balsam, garlic, onions, and salt. Another one, composed of grapevine ashes with oil and mint or honey or ashes of the fig tree, is proposed. The wound must be washed with an infusion of camomile or rumex (small sorrel) while some advise its cauterization. The absorption of a mixture of crayfish ash with gentian root in pure wine is also suggested, as well as the use of theriac, colocynth with a decoction of sage or heracleum, and also the liver of the biting dog. There are here very few original data, and in what concerns rabies Nonnos has to be considered a very poor compiler.[71]

Nicholas Myrepsos (thirteenth century) is the author of the *Dynameron*, an important treatise on pharmacology, which was used until the seventeenth century in western Europe as a work of reference. Among the numerous recipes and preparations given in the *Dynameron*, there is the following, prescribing a drink to be given to persons afflicted by rabies:

A wonderful potion against human rabies by the grace of God. Take about three ounces of the root of the soft esparto,[72] and take two ounces from it. After a careful cleaning and washing, have it boiled in six pounds of wine of good quality until a third of the wine is evaporated. Then have it filtered and take two ounces from it. To each of these portions add half an ounce of theriac and six ounces of Montbazillac wine.[73] To take it for twenty days while fasting proves to be a good remedy.[74]

Demetrios Pepagomenos (thirteenth century) is the author of, *inter alia*, a *kynosofion*, devoted to the diseases of dogs.[75] Rabies is mentioned and information given on its symptoms which is repetitive of earlier Greek and Byzantine texts on the subject. To detect the disease, one should give the dog a mixture of wild rose tree ground into a powder and then mixed with spring water. As a mode of prevention, Pepagomenos advises the removal of the "tongue worm," which looks like a white tendon. We have here a repetition of a belief recorded in the first century by Pliny in the *Natural History*. This operation was called everration, and remained recommended for dogs in Europe until the end of the nineteenth century as a method of preventing rabies. Pepagomenos also suggests some preventive remedies: (1) eating wild cucumber and old grease; (2) boiled ivy taken on the morning of a sunny day; and (3) birds' excrement and donkey's genitalia taken with good, strong, old wine. Pepagomenos also advises that rue leaves be applied to the wound of a dog that has been bitten.

The last Byzantine physician to mention rabies is Joannes Actuarios (fourteenth century) in his *De methodo medendi*. The disease is included in Book VI, chapter 10, along with the poisons,[76] and the section repeats and summarizes what had already been written on the subject by his predecessors. The only apparently original remark he makes is that the disease is a humoral one, induced by a warming of the bile. He advises the use of a plaster of white *iera* and a *catapotum* (= pill) of the size of an almond, the composition of which is not given.

In conclusion, one may say that the information given on rabies by Byzantine authors, whether physicians, veterinarians, or naturalists, is a repetition of what had been said on this disease in classical or post-classical Greek medicine. It appears that Philumenos' text is the major source for most later writers on rabies. In Greek and Byzantine medical theory, once the notion of a rabid dog passing venom had been proposed, this view would

---

[69] *Geoponica* XIX, 3.1 (ed. Beckh, p. 504). Translation by A.-M. Doyen-Higuet, whom I thank here.

[70] L. Felici, "L'opera medica di Teofane Nonno in manoscritti inediti," *Acta medicae historiae Patavinae*, 28 (1981–1982), 59–74.

[71] Rabies is also mentioned in a pharmacological tract, *De remediis*, ascribed to Nonnos; the first section is devoted to drugs and their use against biting and venomous animals. I thank here Mrs. Felici-Duimovich (Florence) and Dr. J. A. M. Sonderkamp (Berlin) for their useful and priceless assistance and references. On Nonnos, see also Dr. Sonderkamp's "Theophanes Nonnus: Medicine in the Circle of Constantine Porphyrogenitus," in this volume.

[72] A grass of the genus *Stipa*.

[73] A white, sweet wine, produced in the area of Montbazillac near Bergerac (Dordogne, France).

[74] *Medicae Artis Principes* (n. 57 above), II, col. 774. I thank Dr. T. Vetter (Strasbourg) for the translation.

[75] The text is included in R. Hercher, ed., *Varia Historica Epistolae Fragmenta* (Leipzig, 1866), 590–91, and 595.

[76] *Medicae Artis Principes* (n. 57 above), I, col. 330 and sqq.

be held for many centuries. Rabies was thought to be due to a "venom" or poison, and this is why the mad dog is always mentioned in chapters devoted to such venomous or poisonous animals as snakes or scorpions. Given this basic assumption, the chief aim of the Byzantine physicians was to try to prevent the penetration of this venom into the organism. Various procedures were used to do so, the major ones being the cauterization and scarification of the wound given to the patient by the biting animal. In treatment later on in the course of the disease, plasters composed of various substances of a chemical, vegetable, animal, or mineral nature were put on the wound to keep it open, and thereby prevent the penetration of the "venom." At the same time, or later on, the intake of purgative and diuretic remedies was advised, if the "venom" had already reached the organism due to an insufficient cauterization or scarification of the wound.

The main interest of the Byzantine texts on rabies lies on the compilation of the very rich and diversified polypharmacy, in which medicinal plants occupy the most important place.[77] Moreover, several of the Byzantine remedies against rabies are mentioned by Islamic authors.[78]

Two words borrowed from the title of an excellent paper on Byzantine medicine[79] rather well characterize what Byzantine medical authors have said about rabies as well as other subjects: "tradition" and "empiricism."

C.N.R.S. and
Université P. et M. Curie, Paris

[77] See Margaret H. Thomson, *Textes grecs inédits relatifs aux plantes* (Paris, 1955), for a number of these medicinal plants which were used against the bites of supposedly rabid dogs.

[78] J. Théodoridès, "Ibn Sinā et la rage," in *Actas XXVII Congr. intern. Historia Medicina (Barcelona 1980)*, Vol. II (1981), 756–60.

[79] O. Temkin, "Byzantine Medicine: Tradition and Empiricism," *DOP*, 16 (1962), 97–115 = Temkin, *Double Face of Janus*, 202–22.

MELETIUS' CHAPTER ON THE EYES: AN UNIDENTIFIED SOURCE

Robert Renehan

I

That the work of Meletius the Monk *On the Constitution of Man* is a profound treatise no one would maintain.[1] That it deserves more attention than it has hitherto received, and for more reasons than one, may appear from this paper. Such at least is its purpose.

Of Meletius we know only what he tells us himself, that he was a monk at the monastery of the Holy Trinity situated in the town of Tiberiopolis, belonging to the *bandon*[2] of Akrokos and the Opsikian Theme.[3] In another passage he states explicitly that he is a doctor, and that he practices cautery and blood-letting. He even gives us further, more personal, particulars: he is a Byzantine, the son of Gregory, short, blue-eyed, snub-nosed, afflicted with gout, and with a scar on his forehead.[4] What we would most like to know he does not tell us—his dates. I have seen him placed as early as the fifth century A.D., which is clearly impossible. The latest author identified as a source for Meletius is Maximus Confessor (see below), who

died in 662 A.D., so that Meletius cannot have lived before the seventh century. It is customary to place him, for no very compelling reason, in the ninth century. Most recently, M. Morani has argued that Meletius, in his borrowings from Nemesius, used a Dresden codex, or a copy of it, which would require a dating in the late twelfth or early thirteenth century.[5] If Meletius is that recent, it is all the more interesting that he still had access to some of the works, now lost, which he used. Meletius' own manuscripts provide an absolute terminus: one at least is of the thirteenth century.[6]

Meletius' prefatory remarks make it perfectly clear that he himself believed that he had produced a new type of treatise, namely a concise, but complete, account of the nature of man. He claims no originality of thought for himself, but does insist, somewhat naively, that his treatise is the first synthesis to cover all aspects of the subject. Human anatomy and physiology, the relationship of body and soul, the names and etymologies of the parts of the body—a very important question for Meletius, as for the Greeks in general since the time of Plato's *Cratylus* and before—these and similar topics, occasionally seasoned with pious ejaculations of admiration for the Deity, constitute Meletius' chosen theme. That his work enjoyed a certain success in late Byzantium is suggested by the number of

---

[The reader is referred to the list of abbreviations at the end of the volume.]

[1] The work is printed by J. A. Cramer in his *Anecdota Graeca e codicibus manuscriptis bibliothecarum Oxoniensium*, vol. III (Oxford, 1836; repr. Amsterdam, 1963), 1–157, and is usually cited by Cramer's page and line numeration. There is also a text of it in Migne, *Patrologia Graeca* vol. 64, coll. 1075–1310. The PG edition uses one additional manuscript (cod. Parisiensis 2299 = P) and adds the Latin version of Nicolaus Petreius (Venice, 1552). Neither edition is satisfactory.

[2] For βάνδον, originally a military term, see Du Cange's *Glossarium ad Scriptores Mediae et Infimae Graecitatis* and Lampe, *s.v.*

[3] p. 1.6–8 C.

[4] p. 155.1–3, 11 C. Meletius does not furnish these particulars about himself from mere whimsy; he is illustrating the meaning of "individual" (ἄτομον) and "person" (πρόσωπον) and chooses himself as an example.

[5] M. Morani, *La tradizione manoscritta del De natura hominis di Nemesio* (Milan, 1981), 147–55. A caveat: I have not yet seen this work and know of it from R. Browning's review in *CR*, n.s. 32 (1982), 149–51. Browning (p. 151, n.1) accepts Morani's argument. If this dating is correct, the treatise entitled Σύνοψις εἰς τὴν φύσιν τῶν ἀνθρώπων by a certain Leo the Physician, whoever he was, will also have to be given a correspondingly more recent date, inasmuch as it consists almost entirely of excerpts from Meletius. See R. Renehan, ed. and trans., *Leo the Physician: Epitome on the Nature of Man* (Berlin, 1969 [*CMG* X, 4]).

[6] See Diels, *Handschriften*, II, 62–64 and *Nachtrag*, 58–59.

manuscripts still extant. Even more significant, not to say astonishing, is the existence of manuscripts in which the name of Meletius is explicitly linked with the august names of Hippocrates and Galen, as a kind of medical trinity. Historically this is of some importance. In late Byzantium Meletius seems to have acquired the status of a standard medical author. Neither original nor profound, he owed such success as he attained to the convenient format of his treatise. A medical and anthropological catechism, accessible and not unduly difficult, would find a ready audience in that period.

Thus Meletius' composition is of some interest as an historical document illustrating the tastes of the literate Byzantine public. Quite apart from this, the work is of considerable importance precisely because it is so unoriginal and derivative, paradoxical though that may sound. For Meletius has put together a pastiche consisting almost entirely of quotations and adaptations of earlier writers, medical and patristic. Scholars, especially Georg Helmreich,[7] have succeeded in identifying a number of Meletius' sources.

One use to which this information can be put is as a supplementary corrective to the direct manuscript tradition of those authors whom Meletius transcribes. Occasionally he can be a valuable witness. Far more interesting is the fact that Meletius had access to earlier sources now lost. To give a surprising example, Meletius alone preserves a small fragment from a classical Greek tragedy;[8] perhaps even more surprising, his source, direct or indirect, for this piece of verse was none other than Soranus of Ephesus, one of the greatest of Greek doctors, on whom more below.

Let us consider briefly what Meletius himself says of his sources, and then what the realities are. He mentions Hippocrates, Galen, "Socrates," and the church fathers Basil the Great, Gregory of Nyssa, John Chrysostom, Cyril. Of these Hippocrates is clearly window dressing cited to lend a spurious authority to the work.[9] Meletius does quote several

works from the Galenic corpus, especially the *Definitiones medicae*, which is generally recognized as spurious. The mention of Socrates is more problematic; Meletius writes Σωκράτης δὲ ἐτυμολογίας μᾶλλον μορίων καὶ ὀνομάτων ἐν τῷ περὶ φύσεως ἀνθρώπου συντάγματι αὐτοῦ ὡς γραμματικὸς ἢ φιλόσοφος συνετάξατο.[10] Meletius in fact pays particular attention to anatomical nomenclature and the corresponding etymologies (often, needless to say, fanciful). It happens that the source for his information in this area is not in doubt—the great Greek physician Soranus who wrote a treatise on this topic.[11] The proof for this assertion is simple and certain, even though the name Soranus appears nowhere in the manuscripts of Meletius: (1) Many anatomical etymologies given by Meletius have strikingly parallel entries in the Byzantine lexica, such as the so-called *Etymologicum Magnum*,[12] and these lexica on occasion specifically name Soranus' etymological work as their source. (2) Meletius both preserves a number of etymologies not to be found in the other Byzantine sources and also, in some cases where there are parallel entries, Meletius' account is fuller. Therefore Meletius does not take his material from these lexica. He is in fact the most important source for recovering what we can of Soranus' lost work; this alone would make his treatise most valuable for us. There may be other grounds for considering it a precious document. Before looking into this we must first attempt to solve a puzzle.

Meletius, as we have seen, makes no mention of Soranus; he mentions rather Socrates. What are we to make of this? There are at least three possibilities. Voigt assumed the existence of an otherwise unknown Socrates (the name is not uncommon) who excerpted Soranus' treatise and who was Meletius' immediate and acknowledged source. This is improbable. In the paragraph in question Meletius is clearly indulging in some innocent name-dropping; an obscure grammarian named Socrates is no fit

---

[7] *Handschriftliche Studien zu Meletius* (Berlin, 1918).

[8] p. 83.7–8 C.= *Trag. Frag. Adesp.* 305a Kannicht-Snell; see *RhM* 109 (1966), 185–86.

[9] p. 1.15–16 C.: Ἱπποκράτης περὶ φύσεως παιδίου καὶ ἀνδρὸς γράψας. If the reference is to the Hippocratic treatises Περὶ φύσιος παιδίου and Περὶ φύσιος ἀνθρώπου, neither of which Meletius quotes, the replacement of ἀνθρώπου by ἀνδρός in the title may be significant; Meletius is perhaps alluding to a work of which he had only heard and not read, hence the confusion. There are five brief Hippocratic quotations, three from the *Aphorisms* and two from *Nutriment*. Of these at least two are taken from Soranus (*Aph.* 2.21 = p. 89.28 C.; *Aph.* 1.15 = p. 101.4–

5 C.) and three, or rather all, are familiar sentences which Meletius could easily have known at second hand only (*Nutr.* 55 = p. 18.25 C.; *Nutr.* 8 = p. 101.13 C.; *Aph.* 5.48 = p. 115.21–22 C.). For example, knowledge of the epigrammatic ὑγρασίη τροφῆς σχῆμα (= *Nutr.* 55) hardly proves direct acquaintance with the Hippocratic work whence it comes.

[10] p. 1.21–23 C. L. Cohn wished to delete the καὶ after μορίων.

[11] See especially P. Voigt, *Sorani Ephesii Liber de etymologiis corporis humani quatenus restitui possit* (Griefswald, 1882), and L. Scheele, *De Sorano Ephesio medico etymologico* (Argentoratum, 1884).

[12] The parallelism extends even to the mutual inclusion of illustrative poetic quotations from works now lost.

company for Hippocrates and Galen, Basil and Gregory. Scheele therefore conjectured that Σωκράτης in the manuscripts was a corruption of Σωρανός and that Meletius had in fact mentioned Soranus here. Much as we would welcome such an explicit testimony, the context argues against Scheele's conjecture.

"In his treatise *On the Nature of Man* Socrates compiled his etymologies," writes Meletius, "more like a grammarian *than a philosopher*." Had Meletius been referring to the physician Soranus, he would have written "more like a grammarian *than a doctor*." The word φιλόσοφος points unmistakably to the famous Socrates, who certainly is fit company for Hippocrates and Galen.[13] Meletius obviously thought that he was using a work by *the* Socrates. What he must have had to hand was a treatise under the name Socrates in his manuscript copy. Whether this was Soranus' original treatise, perhaps in an abridged form, the name Soranus having been corrupted to Socrates at some earlier stage of the transmission *before reaching Meletius*, or whether after all there really was a grammarian named Socrates who excerpted Soranus' work and who was Meletius' immediate source cannot be determined. In either event Meletius believed that he was in possession of a genuine work by the philosopher Socrates, and that tells us something about the level of his erudition.[14]

Meletius thus, at the very beginning of his work, cites famous names, some of whom he has actually used.[15] He goes on to state explicitly what his practice will be, namely, to collect scattered excerpts into a single volume: οὐδεὶς μέντοι γε τῶν προειρημένων ἀνδρῶν ἢ τῶν ἁγίων τούτων συναγαγὼν φαίνεται τὴν ὅλην ὑπόθεσιν τοῦ μίαν πραγματείαν

ἀποτελέσαι. τὰ οὖν διεσπαρμένως ἐν ταῖς τούτων βίβλοις ἐγκείμενα αὐτὸς ἐκλαβὼν τὸ παρόν, ὡς ἐνόν, συνεστησάμην δὴ σύγγραμμα.[16] What Meletius neglects to mention is a complete list of all his sources. To give a telling example, he probably quotes Nemesius' treatise *On the Nature of Man* more often than any other work, yet he never acknowledges the fact. The reason is clear: the name of Nemesius was not grand enough; it would not have lent sufficient authority to Meletius' work.[17] The practice is not unknown among the Byzantines, who loved to display a sham learning by appealing to the great names of antiquity. But Meletius' practice approaches the bizarre. Almost immediately after the words just quoted he indulges in a typical *captatio benevolentiae*. "You must read this," he writes, "in an unofficious manner, with love and fear of God; do this for edification and do not hunt for inelegant expressions with which to criticize the author. For in my opinion the things compiled here are not so readily comprehensible by all, but many of them, in the case of most people, require considerable examination."[18] Such an appeal to the reader's goodwill of course follows a long tradition and there would appear to be nothing unusual about it. It was a shock to discover that the passage had been lifted almost word for word from the prologue to one of Maximus Confessor's works.[19]

The foregoing analysis was necessary in order to establish Meletius' principles of composition. I regard the following as certain. First, Meletius' treatise is almost entirely derivative not only in content but in the actual wording, even when it is a question not of the formal subject matter itself but merely of incidental literary embellishment. Meletius' own main contribution consists in the patching together of excerpts from various writers into

[13] For the collocation of philosopher and physician compare, for example, Galen's *De Placitis Hippocratis et Platonis*, ed. and trans. P. DeLacy (*CMG* V 4, 1, 2 [Berlin, 1978–1980; 2 vols.]).

[14] By "Socrates" he would have understood the Socrates of the Platonic dialogues. Failure to distinguish between (*a*) Plato and (*b*) Socrates as represented in the dialogues of Plato has been common since antiquity—and not merely in casual allusions. The PG edition of Meletius actually prints here Σωκράτης . . . ἐν τῷ Περὶ φύσεως ἀνθρώπου συντάγματι αὐτοῦ [*sc.* in Timaeo] . . . ! (Περὶ φύσεως—without ἀνθρώπου—was the "Thrasyllan" subtitle of the *Timaeus*; whether this is behind the comment "*sc.* in Timaeo" I cannot say. Compare also perhaps the garbled reference to "Timaeus" at p. 60.17 C.)

[15] Galen, as we have seen, Meletius does quote; for Hippocrates compare above, n. 9. Of the church fathers, he often quotes Basil, Gregory of Nyssa, and also Gregory of Nazianzus (not mentioned here). As for Chrysostom and Cyril, hitherto one passage from the former, none from the latter, has been detected.

[16] p. 2.3–7 C. Let the reader be advised that the text of Meletius which I print will on occasion (as here) differ from that of Cramer or Migne or both. I have access to collations of manuscripts, some made by Helmreich and others by myself, not known to the editors. This is not the place to indicate every minor departure from the printed texts.

[17] In some manuscripts Nemesius' work is attributed to Gregory of Nyssa, so that some may wish to assume that Meletius believed that he really was quoting Gregory. I consider this most unlikely. Meletius also used Gregory's similar work Περὶ κατασκευῆς ἀνθρώπου (presumably the original cause of the confusion of ascription in the manuscripts of Nemesius), so that he knew the difference between the two. Moreover, in the Dresden codex of Nemesius which Meletius is believed to have used, directly or indirectly (see above, n. 5), the work is ascribed to Nemesius, not Gregory.

[18] p. 2.10–14 C.

[19] PG 90.960 B, 961 A.

a unified whole, and he tells us as much himself (p. 2.3–7 C.; see above). Secondly, Meletius often fails to name his sources; to judge from the cases of Nemesius and Maximus, the less eminent, and perhaps also the more recent, the authority, the more likely that Meletius will be silent.

In short, that practically everything in Meletius is borrowed goods is more than a working hypothesis; rather it is as certain as such things can be. Many passages in Meletius have been tracked down to their sources; there remain many, primarily of medical content, for which no known source exists. Given the extent of the patristic and later Greek medical corpora—and some works are preserved only in manuscript even today—it is possible that such sources are lurking somewhere, undetected still. But it is far more likely that they have not survived. Herein lies Meletius' chief significance for us. He is the repository of some lost Greek medical work(s) waiting to be recovered from his pages.

I propose to illustrate this by an analysis of his longest chapter, that on the eyes (pp. 61.7–72.20 C.).

II

The contents of the chapter are briefly as follows. A short introductory paragraph (p. 61.10–21 C.) announces the topics to be treated. Next comes a paragraph (p. 61.22–62.13 C.) dealing with the general "blend" (κρᾶσις), shape, and size of the eye. No one has discovered a source for this section, although I may note that the subject matter and, to some extent, the wording, is similar to a passage in Galen's *Ars medica*, which, however, is probably not the immediate source.[20] The next brief paragraph announces further topics: the causes of the various colors found in eyes, the several Greek names for "eye," its constituent parts, humors and tunics in particular, the functions and activities of the eye (p. 62.14–21 C.). Then comes a potentially significant passage, a discussion of the optic nerves and thalami and of four tunics of the eye (pp. 62.21–65.3 C.). Etymologies are given for θάλαμος and for the names of several of the tunics; some at least of this section must go back to Soranus, and we shall return to it.[21] The two following sections take

up respectively the functions of the optic "pneuma" and the causes of the several colors of the eye (pp. 65.27–67.12 C.); there are no known sources.[22] Next comes a transitional paragraph summing up what Meletius has thus far discussed (pp. 67.13–68.2 C.). Herein occurs a significant statement: ἐπεὶ οὖν τὰ περὶ τῶν ὀφθαλμῶν ἐρευνῶντες ἐξεθέμεθα . . . πῶς ὁ μὲν ἀμφιβληστροειδὴς καὶ ὁ ἐπιπεφυκὼς καὶ ὁ ῥαγοειδὴς ἔχουσι φλέβας, ὁ δὲ κερατοειδὴς ἄφλεβός ἐστι. . . . (p. 67.13–18 C.). Meletius has in fact mentioned no such detail. This is a clear indication not only that he has been excerpting a fuller account but also that, in all probability, this summation itself is copied from his source. He carelessly fails to notice that, in making his abridgment, he omitted the particular piece of information which he now claims to have given above.[23]

Meletius proceeds to announce his next topics, the definition of "eye," the various words for it in Greek, and the etymologies of these words; eyelids, eyelashes, eyebrows are also discussed (pp. 68.3–70.3 C.). First he gives a definition: ὀφθαλμοί, φησιν, εἰσὶν οἱ συνεστῶτες ἐκ τεσσάρων χιτώνων, καὶ ὑγρῶν διαφερόντων τριῶν· νευρώδεις· αἰσθητικοὶ τῶν ὑποκειμένων χρωμάτων καὶ μεγεθῶν καὶ σχημάτων. The wording is almost identical to that of a definition in the Pseudo-Galenic *Definitiones medicae*.[24] The rest of the section is chiefly concerned with the etymological derivations of "eye" words and certainly goes back almost entirely to Soranus. However, several phrases concerned with the eyelids and eyebrows have close verbal parallels in a homily of John Chrysostom, and either Meletius has here borrowed from Chrysostom or both

---

[20] I.329–30 K. Compare below, n. 49.

[21] The etymology of θάλαμος (p. 62.29–63.6 C.) has a parallel entry in the so-called *Etymologicum Magnum*; this and the fact that Meletius quotes the poet Hesiod in illustration are clear signs that Soranus is the source of this much at least. (Whether Meletius used θαλάμη or θάλαμος as the technical optical term is unclear; the MSS have at p. 62.29 C. the variants τὰς λεγομένας

θαλάμας, τὰς λεγομένας θαλάμους, τοὺς λεγομένους θαλάμους, and at p. 63.7 C. τὰς θαλάμους and τοὺς θαλάμους.) The usual term for bodily cavities, in the earlier period at least, is θαλάμη, which Galen used for the optic thalami. See further J. Hyrtl, *Onomatologia Anatomica* (Vienna, 1880), 539–41.

[22] Similar language and content for some of this material (pp. 66.29–67.7 C.) may be seen in Galen's *Ars medica*, I.330–31 K., but again this passage does not appear to be Meletius' immediate source. See however below, n. 49.

[23] I have cited some examples of this sort of careless abridgment from the work of Leo Medicus in *RhM*, 113, (1970), 79–81.

[24] p. 68.4–7 C. = Galen XIX.358–59 K. φησιν in Meletius (p. 68.4 C.) probably is an explicit indication on his part that he is quoting a specific source. I say probably, and not certainly, because the singular φησί can be used idiomatically much like the plural φασί = "they say," "people say," and Meletius himself so uses it (p. 6.23 C., where there is a variant φασί). For examples of this usage see Epictetus 2.9.2, 3.20.12; Hippolytus, *Refut. omn. haeres.* V.17, p. 134 ff. Duncker-Schneidewin = V.7.2, p. 79 Wendland; *RhM*, 113 (1970), 84.

draw from a common source.[25] The next paragraph deals concisely with the question of relative eye sizes and concludes with a mention of λιϱόφθαλμος, an adjective meaning "having large eyes," for which an etymology is given, a probable sign that some of this paragraph as well derives from Soranus.

We are approaching the end of the chapter. The next paragraph discusses the muscles of the eye in language very close to a passage in Galen,[26] though there may be an intermediary source, then defines ὅϱασις in agreement with the definition in Pseudo-Galen,[27] and concludes with some echoes of Gregory of Nazianzus, who is explicitly acknowledged (κατὰ τὴν τοῦ Θεολόγου φωνήν).[28] Finally, several pages are devoted to the nature of vision and the views of various thinkers on this subject. The entire passage is copied from Nemesius.[29]

I summarize the results of this survey. In Cramer's edition of Meletius the chapter on the eyes occupies almost eleven and a half pages, or 341 lines. If we tally up all the passages therein for which a definite source has been identified (including the etymological passages which may be safely assigned to Soranus, even though he is not named), the total is approximately 122 lines. Another thirty lines or so, very similar in content to passages in Galen, although not quite close enough in language to guarantee direct borrowing, may be added for good measure. This gives us some 150 lines, or approximately five pages, for which we can account. That leaves more than half the chapter, some six pages, still unassigned. Inasmuch as Meletius, by his own admission, is but a derivative compiler of other writers' works and no original author himself, this is a veritable treasure trove. Let us see what we can discover there.

III

"The number and character of the ocular tunics furnished abundant discussion and controversy in ancient and medieval times. *Quot homines quot sententiae* was the rule of ocular anatomy in those early days."[30] Meletius devotes two pages to the ocular tunics;[31] his source is unknown. The fact that there was such diversity of doctrine in regard to the ocular tunics provides us with an excellent clue, if not for discovering the actual name of Meletius' source, at least for narrowing the field by process of elimination.

Modern anatomy teaches that there are three tunics of the eye: the first (from without inward) consists of the sclerotic and cornea; the second is the uvea, composed of the choroid, ciliary body, and iris; third and last is the retina (see figure 1). Various causes were responsible for the confused state of affairs in antiquity and the middle ages. First of course was the imperfect knowledge of ocular anatomy at the time, although so far as the tunics were concerned, the Greeks did make some progress. Herophilus, the great Alexandrian anatomist, bears an honorable name in this connection.[32] A second, more specific cause of confusion lay in the fact that several of the ocular tunics are composed of more than one part, continuous in each instance. Thus, for example, some Greek physicians recognized the division of the first tunic into the sclerotic and cornea; others did not, as a consequence often using a name strictly appropriate to part of the composite tunic for the whole tunic. Finally, the Greeks, even when they agreed in doctrine, had no uniform terminology for the ocular tunics, especially in the earlier period. A given tunic, or component thereof, could be called by several names. This chaotic situation can be put to advantage in the case of Meletius. We need only compare his "system" and nomenclature with those found in earlier treatises which have survived; any work fundamentally inconsistent with Meletius' exposition can be immediately eliminated as a source, direct or indirect.

Meletius states that there are four ocular tunics

---

[25] p. 69.21–23 C.: . . . κόνιν καὶ κάρφη [κάρφος C.] καὶ πάντα τὰ προσπίπτοντα τοῖς ὀφθαλμοῖς ἔξωθεν ἀποκρούονται, καὶ οὐκ ἐῶσι παρενοχλεῖσθαι αὐτοὺς ὑπ' οὐδενός ~ Chrys., PG 49.123: . . . κόνιν καὶ κάρφη καὶ πάντα τὰ διενοχλοῦντα ἔξωθεν ἀποκρουόμεναι τῶν ὀφθαλμῶν, καὶ οὐκ ἐῶσαι ἐνοχλεῖσθαι τὰ βλέφαρα. p. 69.28–70.2 C.: αἱ μὲν τῆς κεφαλῆς τρίχες αὔξουσί τε καὶ ἀποκείρονται· αὗται δὲ αἱ βλεφαρίδες . . . ἐκωλύθησαν αὐξάνεσθαι ~ Chrys., PG 49.123: αἱ μὲν τῆς κεφαλῆς αὔξονται τρίχες καὶ ἀποκείρονται, αἱ δὲ τῶν ὀφρύων οὐκέτι. (Both also mention, with different wording, the problems the very aged experience in this regard.) Note how Meletius has confused eyelashes (βλεφαρίδες) with eyebrows (ὀφρύες), one more indication of careless abridgment (whether of Chrysostom or of a common source).

[26] p. 70.20–27 C. ~ Περὶ μυῶν ἀνατομῆς, XVIII B.932–33 K.

[27] p. 70.27–30 C. ~ *Definitiones medicae*, XIX.379 K.

[28] p. 71.2–5 C. ~ PG 36.609 B.

[29] pp. 71.7–72.20 C. ~ Nemesius, pp. 179–89 Matthaei (excerpts).

[30] C. A. Wood, *Benevenutus Grassus of Jerusalem De Oculis Eorumque Egritudinibus et Curis. Translated with Notes and Illustrations from the first printed edition, Ferrara, 1474 A.D.* (Stanford, 1929), 28 n. 2.

[31] p. 63.7–65.3 C.

[32] See the interesting paper of H. Oppermann, "Herophilos bei Kallimachos" in *Hermes*, 60 (1925), 14–32. See also G. W. Most, "Callimachus and Herophilus," *Hermes*, 109 (1981), 188–96.

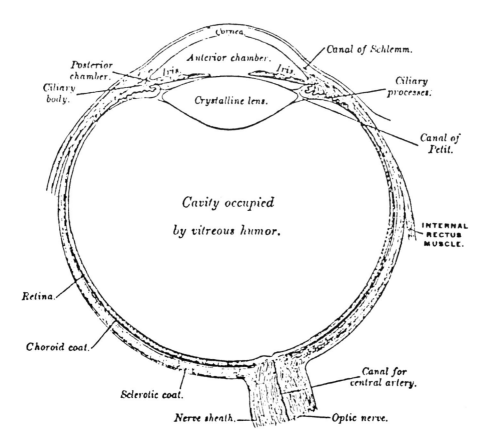

1. After Gray's Anatomy

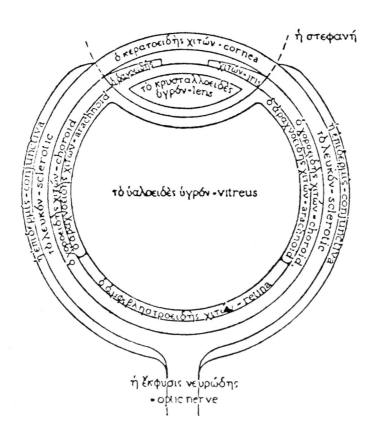

2. Diagram of Eye Reconstructed from Descriptions of Rufus
   of Ephesus (from Charles Singer, *A Short History of Anatomy
   and Physiology from the Greeks to Harvey*

(χιτῶνες), namely, starting from within outwards, ὁ ἀμφιβληστροειδής, or retina; ὁ ῥαγοειδής, corresponding to our uvea (= choroid, ciliary body, and iris);[33] ὁ κερατοειδής, corresponding to the sclerotic and cornea; and, finally, ὁ ἐπιπεφυκώς, or conjunctiva. This last, a mucous membrane lining the eyelids and reflected over the fore part of the sclerotic and cornea, is not classified as a tunic proper of the eye by modern anatomists.[34]

Let us survey briefly the competing anatomical doctrines of the Greeks as they relate to the tunics of the eye. The Pseudo-Galenic treatise entitled *Introductio sive medicus* puts it succinctly: ὁ . . . ὀφθαλμὸς συνέστηκεν μὲν καθ' Ἱπποκράτην ἐκ χιτώνων δύο, οὓς μήνιγγας ὁ Ἱπποκράτης καλεῖ, ἐπειδὴ ἐκ τῶν μηνίγγων ἐκπεφύκασιν. κατὰ δὲ τοὺς νεωτέρους ἐκ τριῶν, κατ' ἐνίους δὲ ἐκ τεσσάρων.[35] Here is explicit testimony for a four-tunic system. The author proceeds to name the four: ὁ κερατοειδής, ὁ ῥαγοειδής, ὁ ἀμφιβληστροειδής, and, lastly, "a fourth tunic, introduced by some, which they also call ἄδηλος." What is this fourth "unclear" tunic? It certainly cannot be the conjunctiva, for that is excluded by the description of it which Pseudo-Galen gives.[36] The term ἄδηλος apparently occurs only here; LSJ state that it refers to the hyaloid membrane of the eye. This seems to be an error. The adjective ὑαλοειδής is used primarily of the vitreous humor, τὸ ὑαλοειδὲς ὑγρόν (see figure 2), but also as another term for the retina: ὁ ὑαλοειδὴς χιτών = ὁ ἀμφιβληστροειδὴς χιτών,[37] so that the

"hyaloid membrane" should be the retina, which has just been mentioned in explicit contrast to the fourth tunic, ὁ ἄδηλος. This latter is probably to be identified rather with the capsule of the lens, which Herophilus discovered and added as a fourth tunic, as can be deduced from the accounts given by Rufus of Ephesus and the Pseudo-Rufus, both of whom explicitly set out a four-tunic scheme which includes the capsule of the lens as the fourth tunic.[38] There is other evidence for such a scheme, but we need not pursue it further, for it clearly differs from Meletius' account, in which the conjunctiva constitutes the fourth tunic.

Galen approaches the problem of ocular nomenclature with a good deal of common sense. Although his own detailed account of the anatomy of the eye is flawed in certain particulars—how could it be otherwise at the time?—he recognizes the differences of opinons as to the names and number of the tunics, explains why such a state of affairs has come about, and avoids excessive dogmatism. On occasion he recommends as the best procedure simply to follow the common usage of anatomists. As examples of his lack of dogmatism I may mention that he acknowledges both that some physicians regard the capsule of the lens as a tunic (this, it will be recalled, was Herophilus' view), and that the first and second tunic from without inwards may be regarded as two or four tunics, as one likes.[39] Despite this rather flexible attitude, Galen nowhere mentions the particular set of four tunics which Meletius adopts.

When we turn to the Byzantine period, there is a dramatic change. Not only does Meletius' list (ἀμφιβληστροειδής, ῥαγοειδής, κερατοειδής, ἐπιπεφυκώς) appear, it seems to have won the field and acquired the status of an orthodox canon. What is most characteristic of this list, as we have seen, is the inclusion of the conjunctiva (ἐπιπεφυκώς) as one

---

[33] For these terms see J. Hyrtl (n. 21 above), 588–91.

[34] Compare also Rufus, *Onom.* 28 (Daremberg-Ruelle, p. 137): ἐπίκειται δὲ αὐτῷ [sc. τῷ κερατοειδεῖ καὶ λευκῷ χιτῶνι] ἄνωθεν ἡ καλουμένη ἐπιδερμίς κτλ. Rufus does not here include the conjunctiva (= ἐπιδερμίς, a meaning not recognized in LSJ) among the tunics. See figure 2. Aetius VII, 1 (Olivieri, II, p. 254, 11–12, 26–27) who does list the ἐπιπεφυκώς as a tunic (compare below), then proceeds to call it a membrane: τὰ δὲ βλέφαρα συνίστησιν ὁ ἐπιπεφυκὼς ὑμήν.

[35] XIV.711 K. The Hippocratic corpus has little to say; see, however, *Loc. hom.* 2 (VI.280 Littré) = Joly, ed., *Hippocrate* XIII, p. 40: μήνιγγες δὲ τρεῖς εἰσιν αἱ τοὺς ὀφθαλμοὺς φυλάσσουσαι, ἡ μὲν ἐπάνω παχυτέρη, ἡ δὲ διὰ μέσου λεπτοτέρη, ἡ δὲ τρίτη λεπτὴ ἡ τὸ ὑγρὸν φυλάσσουσα.

[36] τρίτος δὲ ὁ ἀμφιβληστροειδής, ἐγκολπούμενος ὥσπερ καὶ δεχόμενος ἐπ' ἄκρῳ τὸν . . . τέταρτον χιτῶνα, ὃν καὶ ἄδηλον προσαγορεύουσιν. ἔστι μὲν γὰρ ὑμὴν σμικρότατός τε καὶ ἰσχνότατος (XIV.712 K.).

[37] For ὑαλοειδής as a synonym of ἀμφιβληστροειδής see Rufus *Onom.* 153, p. 154.10 Daremberg-Ruelle, and Pseudo-Rufus, *Anat.* 15, p. 171.11–12 Daremberg-Ruelle. (When LSJ s.v. ὑαλοειδής, state ". . . ὁ ὑ. χιτὼν ὀφθαλμοῦ the *crystalline* lens of the eye, Medici ap. Poll. 2.71," they are perpetuating Pollux's error: he has confused the names for two tunics, as is clear from a comparison with Rufus. Cf. Pollux II, 70–71 (ed. Bethe, vol. I, pp. 104–05). Eduard Zarncke (*Symbolae ad Iulii Pollucis tractatum De partibus corporis humani* [Leipzig, 1884]), showed that

Pollux derived much of his anatomy from Rufus. For the tunics, see esp. pp. 26–27.

[38] Rufus, *Onom.* 153, p. 154; Pseudo-Rufus 10–17, pp. 170–72. For further details see H. Opperman's article (n. 22 above), with references.

[39] For Galen's views, see esp. *Anatomical Procedures* X, 2–4 (ed. Simon [Arabic], pp. 40–63; trans. Duckworth, Lyons, Towers, pp. 33–50), and *De usu partium* X, 1–7 (ed. Helmreich, II, 54–81; trans. May, *Parts*, II, 463–82). For the capsule of the lens as tunic: Duckworth, p. 40, and for the first and second tunics as two or four, *ibid*, p. 42. For the *De usu partium* both Daremberg, I, pp. 607 ff., and May, trans., *Parts*, II, pp. 463 ff., have very useful notes. See also Galen, *De medendi methodo* 1.6, X.47 K., for yet another list of four tunics, namely, κερατοειδής, ῥαγοειδής, ἀραχνοειδής, ἀμφιβληστροειδής. The ἀραχνοειδής, elsewhere identified with the ἀμφιβληστροειδής or retina, here seems to be a section of it. (Compare fig. 2.)

of the tunics. Such is not the practice now, nor does it appear to have been a common view in the pre-Byzantine period. In Byzantium not only Meletius' list, but even his order, starting from within outwards, seems to be standard dogma. Thus Aetius of Amida in the sixth century has the same four tunics in the same order.[40] In the seventh century (?) Theophilus Protospatharius also names these four.[41] So too does Leo the Philosopher, whoever he may have been, in his *Synopsis of Medicine*;[42] the work perhaps dates from the tenth century. None of these works is directly dependent on any of the others, so far as we can tell; so this gives us a fair representation of the distribution of the doctrine. One might thus be tempted to conclude that Meletius is simply reproducing a typical and specifically Byzantine medical teaching and let it go at that, were it not for several complicating factors.

First, there is at least one medical treatise from the pre-Byzantine period in which this list of tunics, same names and same order, can be found, to wit the Pseudo-Galenic *Definitiones medicae*.[43] Second, Meletius quotes this very work a number of times. Third, most of the anatomical details in Meletius' chapter on the eye cannot derive from the *Definitiones medicae* for the very good reason that these details do not occur in this latter work. Jutta Kollesch, the leading authority on the *Definitiones medicae*, dates that treatise to the last quarter of the first century A.D.[44] If this dating is even approxi-

mately correct, a fact of some historical importance emerges. There must have existed in the Roman period a general anatomical treatise[45] which taught a doctrine different from that of Herophilus (as preserved in Rufus and Pseudo-Rufus, Pollux, Celsus etc.), Galen, and the few other medical writers known from this earlier period. This treatise was used by the author of the *Definitiones medicae*, probably in the first century A.D., and then seems to vanish for centuries. It is as if it disappeared into the sea and, to paraphrase the poet, sailed along some underwater stream to the holy city of Byzantium.

If I may continue this image for a moment, the waters of source criticism, or *Quellenforschung*, can become very muddy indeed, and I shall exercise a certain restraint here, with fear and trembling that A. E. Housman's shade may appear of a sudden and contemptuously hiss that *Quellenforschung* is but a longer and nobler word for fudge. Still Meletius undoubtedly did have access, one way or other, to at least one lost first/second century source, Soranus, and that alone, to repeat, makes his work very precious. Kollesch rightly stresses that we cannot identify, for want of evidence, the specific author from whom Pseudo-Galen took his anatomical definitions.[46] The same, alas, is true of Meletius. We do not know the name of his source. We cannot even say whether he still had direct access to this lost work or used it only indirectly. Nevertheless, in the midst of this uncertainty, we would do well to remind ourselves that the existence of some lost source, hitherto unrecognized, has been detected. That is a real gain. Perhaps we can go a bit further.

IV

Some at least of the Byzantine medical epitomizers are capable of expressing their borrowed doctrines in their own words. *Rem tene, verba sequentur.* Theophilus may be cited as an example. Contrast, for instance, his description of the tyrant Dionysius' brightly illuminated room, constructed directly over the darkened prison chamber for the

[40] Aetius VII, 1 (ed. Olivieri, II, p. 254.5–14 = J. Hirschberg, ed. and trans., *Die Augenheilkunde des Aëtius aus Amida* [Leipzig, 1899], p. 2.10–21).

[41] *De corporis humani fabrica* 4.20, p. 161.15–19 Greenhill. Theophilus has gotten the order confused: ἔστι δὲ ἡ τάξις τῶν χιτώνων αὕτη· πρῶτος ὁ κερατοειδής, δεύτερος ὁ ῥαγοειδής, τρίτος ὁ ἀμφιβληστροειδής, καὶ τέταρτος ὁ ἐπιπεφυκώς, ὁ λευκός. As (1) the first tunic (from without) was sometimes divided into two parts, called respectively ὁ λευκός and ὁ κερατοειδής (whereas more often ὁ κερατοειδής came to be used for the whole tunic), and (2) the ἐπιπεφυκώς was also described as λευκός (see Meletius, p. 64.30 C.), a certain confusion was inevitable. Thus Greenhill in his note to Theophilus p. 159.13 (on p. 309) writes: "... hoc nomine [sc. τῷ λευκῷ] Noster videtur designare non solum *Tunicam Albugineam*, verum etiam *Membranam Scleroticam*, quod ἐπιπεφυκώς etiam appellatur.... (p. 161.l.18) Adeo tamen temere talia vocabula antiqui (atque etiam nonnumquam recentiores,) usurpant, ut saepe difficillime percipias quid quisque eodem nomine significare voluerit." See Hyrtl (n. 21 above), 15–17, 146–47.

[42] Printed by Ermerins, see p. 129. The manuscript which Ermerins used was missing a folium at the critical point. J. F. Boissonade supplied the deficiency from another manuscript in his *Anecdota Nova* (Paris, 1844, repr. Hildesheim, 1962), 367.

[43] XIX.358 K.: ὀφθαλμοί εἰσιν οἱ συνεστῶτες ἐκ τεσσάρων χιτώνων, ἀμφιβληστροειδοῦς, ῥαγοειδοῦς, κερατοειδοῦς, καὶ ἐπιπεφυκότος κτλ.

[44] *Untersuchungen zu den pseudogalenischen Definitiones Medicae* (Berlin, 1973), 66.

[45] I say general, rather than specifically ocular, treatise because, as will be seen, the work which Meletius used was not confined to the anatomy of the eye, since he used it also in those chapters which deal with certain other anatomical subjects. For this reason it is unlikely that Meletius' proximate source was a specialist treatise on the eyes, such as the famous Περὶ ὀφθαλμῶν of Demosthenes. See M. Wellmann in *Hermes*, 38 (1903), 546–66, and J. Hirschberg, "Die Bruchstücke der Augenheilkunde des Demosthenes," *SA*, 11 (1918), 183–88.

[46] Kollesch (n. 44 above), 93.

express purpose of damaging the eyes of the prisoners as they were suddenly exposed to the bright light after a long stay in utter darkness, with the similar account in Galen's *De usu partium*, his source.[47] Theophilus' language is obviously indebted to Galen's, but he has introduced numerous variations. He is his own man. Meletius cannot, or will not, exercise even this much independence; he is little better than a copyist. It bears repeating that for us this is his chief merit.

Now if we study Meletius' language more carefully, there appear slight, but unmistakable, signs of an original writer. Certain stylistic features stand out which set his treatise apart from other Byzantine medical catechisms. Of course what we are seeing is the hand not of Meletius, but of his source. It is the odd detail of style that turns up here and there, rather than the content, which leads me to believe that Meletius had access not merely to a routine Byzantine handbook but, directly or indirectly, to a medical work of more importance. That he actually possessed a copy of a first-century work I consider unlikely, but possible; more probably he used a later abridgment which preserved reasonably faithfully the contents and, to some extent, the language of a lost work which we should be very glad to have. In the absence of it Meletius assumes an importance of his own.

I give some typical examples of the style. On p. 63.7–11 C. Meletius writes: διασχίζεται δὲ τὰ νεῦρα εἰς τὰς θαλάμους, ὥσπερ εἴ τις λαβὼν πάπυρον, ταύτην εἰς λεπτὰ κατατεμών, διασχίζει ἀναπλέκει τε πάλιν, καὶ ποιεῖ χιτῶνα τὸν λεγόμενον ἀμφιβληστροειδῆ, ὅμοιον ἀμφιβλήστρῳ· ὄργανον δὲ τοῦτο θηρευτικὸν ἰχθύων. Rufus of Ephesus attests that Herophilus coined the name ἀμφιβληστροειδής; it is not uncommon for medical writers to make the obvious etymology explicit, that the tunic was so called because of its similarity to a net. Thus far Meletius' account contains nothing out of the ordinary, unless it be the identification of ἀμφίβληστρον specifically with a *fishing* net. I do not recall that detail in other accounts, but, since that is what the word most often means, we prob-

ably ought not to press that too much. However, the comparison with papyrus, to the best of my knowledge, does not occur elsewhere, and that has the ring of authenticity. A practicing anatomist, which Meletius hardly was, first introduced that illustration. He continues, p. 63.11–14 C.: μετὰ τοῦτον δὲ τὸν χιτῶνα ἔστι δεύτερος χιτὼν λεγόμενος ῥαγοειδής, ὅτι ῥαγὶ σταφυλῆς ἔοικε κατὰ τὸ σχῆμα· καὶ καθάπερ ἐπὶ τῆς σταφυλῆς ὁρῶμεν τὰ μὲν ἔσω δασύτερα, τὰ δὲ ἔξω λεῖα, οὕτως καὶ ἐπὶ τοῦ ῥαγοειδοῦς ἔστιν ἰδεῖν. The technical term ῥαγοειδής and the explanation that it is so called because it is similar in shape to a ῥάξ, "grape," had long been traditional. The expansion of this by means of an explicit comparison ("just as ... so also") is not usually found; the device is similar to what we saw above (ὥσπερ εἴ τις κτλ.) and may be a stylistic mannerism of a specific author. As one reads on, this impression is confirmed, p. 64.17–20 C.: διὰ τοῦτο μάλιστα ἐδεήθη ἐκ διαφανεστάτης οὐσίας τὸν κερατοειδῆ γενέσθαι· καὶ ὥσπερ ὁρῶμεν ὅτι τῶν κερατίνων ἔνδοθεν φανῶν περιεχόμενος ὁ λύχνος τὸ φῶς τὸ οἰκεῖον ἔξω πέμπει, μηδὲν ἐμποδίζοντος τῷ λύχνῳ τοῦ σώματος, οὕτω κἀνταῦθα ὁ κερατοειδὴς διαφανὴς ὢν οὐκ ἐμποδίζει τὸ ὀπτικὸν πνεῦμα διεξιέναι κτλ. Once again an explicit comparison is used by way of illustration. The following passage employs the same device, p. 66.19–27 C.: εἰ μὲν οὖν πολύ ἐστι τὸ ᾠῶδες ὑγρόν, ποιεῖ τὸν γλαυκὸν ὀφθαλμόν, καὶ ὀλίγη γίνεται ἡ παρ' αὐτοῦ ἔκλαμψις διότι βαθύνεται τὸ κρυσταλλοειδὲς ὑγρὸν καὶ ἡ κόρη. τοῦτο δὲ καὶ ἐπὶ λίμνης ὑδάτων ἴδοις γινόμενον· τὰ γὰρ ἐν βάθει αὐτῆς ὁρᾶν οὐ δυνάμεθα· οὐ μὴν οὐδ' εἰ τεθολωμένον εἴη, ἐπιτήδειόν ἐστι δέξασθαι χρῶμα τὸ οἷονοῦν. τοῦτο γὰρ καὶ τὰ θολερὰ τῶν ὑδάτων ποιοῦσι καὶ ἰλυώδη, μὴ συγχωροῦντα τὰς ἀκτῖνας τοῦ φωτὸς δι' αὐτῶν διέρχεσθαι καθαρῶς κτλ. One more example must suffice. Meletius states that it is not always easy to determine the constitution of the eye in specific cases: a "hard and dry" eye is difficult to identify by direct examination: οὐκοῦν ἐκ τῆς ἔξωθεν βασάνου διαγινώσκεται· πολλοὺς γὰρ ὁρῶμεν ἐν καπνῷ στῆναι μὴ δυναμένους, ἀλλὰ δακρύοντας πολλά, ἄλλους δὲ σφόδρα πρὸς τὸν καπνὸν ἀντιτείνοντας· καί εἰσιν οἱ μὲν πρῶτοι ὑγροί τε καὶ εὐπαθεῖς, οἱ δὲ δεύτεροι σκληροί τε καὶ δυσπαθεῖς (pp. 61.29–62.3 C.).[48]

---

[47] Theophilus IV.20.7, p. 162.9–163.3 Greenhill ~ Galen, *De usu partium* 10.3, II.66.23–67.6 Helmreich. Galen is said to be the only source for this anecdote; considering Plato's well-known relationship with the tyrant Dionysius, I have often wondered whether the famous parable of the cave in the *Republic*, where it describes prisoners forced to look suddenly up at the light with the attendant pain (see 515 C), may not have been intended in part as an oblique criticism of the tyrant. This is indeed speculative, perhaps too much so, especially since we do not know whether Galen's anecdote is historical, but still . . .

[48] Compare J. Locke, "Gypsy Life in Shropshire—As It Was and As It Is," in *Journal of the Gypsy Lore Society*, Fourth Series, 1:1 (1974), 19: "You may have noticed that you seldom see a Romany wearing glasses—even at 60 or 70. I don't know why this is, unless our camp fires have something to do with it. If a

It is time to summarize the results of this enquiry. Meletius had access to a treatise on human anatomy and physiology which has not survived. Comparison with other chapters of Meletius, where this same treatise was also clearly used, proves that it was a general study and not a special treatise on the eyes alone.[49] Its four-tunic theory probably goes

back at least to the first century A.D., although this doctrine does not appear to have become common before the Byzantine period. It is true that we know neither the author nor the date of this lost treatise;[50] we do not even know whether Meletius used it directly or in a later abridgment.[51] But such a treatise there was. It is safe to assume that Meletius, such being his practice, has copied his source fairly closely, if selectively. Moreover, the characteristic mannerisms of style illustrated above do suggest that the *ipsissima verba* of the author have been preserved to some extent, even if there was an intermediate source involved.

The present paper is thus of a preliminary nature; its purpose has been merely to call attention to the existence of this anonymous treatise embedded in the pages of Meletius. Perhaps even this veil of anonymity can in time be stripped away. Much remains to be done; much can be done. If we scholars are prepared to gird up our loins and dig long and deep, who is to say that one fine day we will not at last discover the crock of gold?

University of California, Santa Barbara

---

gorgio [= non-gypsy] comes to our fire, the wood smoke makes his eyes water. It does not seem to affect our eyes, and perhaps over the years the smoke has made our eyes stronger."

[49] I give one example: What Meletius says in his chapter on the head concerning the relative merits of small and large heads, and their signification (pp. 56.23–57.13 C.), and what he says about small and large eyes in the chapter under consideration (pp. 62.4–13 C.), are obviously derived from the same work, as a comparison of the two passages will immediately show. Meletius himself—or his source—makes a cross-reference, p. 62.8–9: καθὰ καὶ περὶ τῆς κεφαλῆς εἴρηται. (R. Foerster in his *Scriptores Physiognomonici Graeci et Latini* [Leipzig, 1893], II.315–16, includes Meletius, pp. 56.23–57.13 C. Presumably he knew no immediate source for the passage.) As an illustration of the complexity of *Quellenforschung*, note that the statement ἡ μὲν οὖν μικρὰ κεφαλὴ μοχθηρᾶς ἐγκεφάλου κατασκευῆς ἴδιον σημεῖον (p. 56.23–24 C.) occurs verbatim in Galen, *Ars medica* I.320.4–6 K., in a passage of very similar content, though its relationship to Meletius is problematic. (Benedict Einarson also called my attention to Galen's *Commentary on Hippocr. Epid.* VI.XVII A.818–19 K., another, but less close parallel, for the statement.) Compare also Galen I.320.6–10 ~ Meletius p. 57.8–11 C., though here too the verbal correspondences should be closer if Galen is the immediate source. In this same section Galen discusses, among other topics, the question of the head which is εὔρυθμος σχήματι; Meletius does not. However, in the chapter on the eyes Meletius does introduce the corresponding topic: ὁ τοίνυν ὀφθαλμὸς ἢ μέγας ἐστὶν ἢ μικρὸς καὶ ἢ εὔρυθμος ἢ ἄρυθμος κτλ. (p. 62. 4 ff. C.). The same topic occurs in Galen's *Ars medica*, which, as in the case of the head, so also with the eyes, shows close correspondences with Meletius; compare *Ars medica* I.329–331 K. with Meletius, pp. 61.22–62.13 and pp. 66.28–67.7 C. Presumably Meletius' immediate source, whatever its relation to Galen, dealt with the εὐρυθμία and ἀρυθμία of both head and eyes; Meletius omitted the relevant sentences in the case of the head. (This assumes, to repeat, that Meletius did not in these cases borrow directly from Galen. We cannot be absolutely certain of that and the presence in both authors of an identical sentence such as ἡ μὲν οὖν μικρὰ κεφαλὴ μοχθηρᾶς ἐγκεφάλου κατασκευῆς ἴδιον σημεῖον [see above] may strike some as decisive. The situation is not so simple. For example, in Paul of Aegina VI.61 = 2.101.13–16 Heiberg, the following sentence occurs: οἱ δὲ παραστάται καὶ κρεμαστῆρες ὀνομαζόμενοι ἐκφύσεις εἰσὶν τῆς τοῦ νωτιαίου μυελοῦ μήνιγγος σὺν φλεψὶν ἀρτηριωδέσιν ἐν τοῖς διδύμοις καθήκουσαι, δι' ὧν ἡ τοῦ σπέρματος εἰς τὸ αἰδοῖον γίνεται πρόεσις. The same sentence occurs in Meletius, p. 113.17–20 C. with only the slightest of

variants [οἱ καὶ κρεμαστῆρες λεγόμενοι for καὶ κρεμαστῆρες ὀνομαζόμενοι and τοῦ νωτιαίου μυέλου τῆς μήνιγγος for τῆς τοῦ νωτιαίου μυελοῦ μήνιγγος. In Meletius read ἐκφύσεις εἰσὶν for ἔκφυσίς ἐστι of the printed editions; there is MS authority for εἰσὶν.] This is not an isolated case of Meletius' borrowing from Paul; rather both go back to a common source—and that source, in the last analysis, may well be Soranus, to judge from the surrounding context in Meletius.)

[50] Soranus, whom Meletius certainly used, cannot be excluded as a candidate. Unfortunately, too little is known about the format and extent of his work on the names and etymologies of the parts of the body. It may have been fairly detailed. What his teaching on the ocular tunics was is also unknown. I call attention only to the fact that he seems to have had a fondness for the mannerism, found in Meletius, of explaining his point by "just as . . . so also" clauses. See, for example, his *Gynaeceia* 1.26, p. 16.26 ff. Ilberg; 1.35, p. 25.4 ff.; 1.36, p. 25.11 ff.

[51] There are occasional unclassical usages in the passages cited: p. 64.20 C. μηδὲν ἐμποδίζοντος, rather than οὐδὲν ἐμπιδίζοντος; p. 66.25–26 μὴ συγχωροῦντα for οὐ συγχωροῦντα; p. 66.22 ἴδοις, potential optative without ἄν. But such lapses from "pure" Attic style occur long before the Byzantine period and can tell us little. Manuscript spellings such as γίνεται tell us nothing.

HELLENISTIC AND BYZANTINE OPHTHALMOLOGY: TRACHOMA AND SEQUELAE

EMILIE SAVAGE-SMITH

As a case study in the transmission and elaboration of a medical idea through Hellenistic, Byzantine, and Islamic cultures, I have chosen to trace the diagnosis and treatment of three ocular conditions. These three are trachoma, trachomatous pannus, and pterygium. The latter two were viewed by medieval physicians as sequelae of trachoma.[1] These three conditions were selected because trachoma was, and still is, a major cause of blindness in the Near East, and indeed in the early centuries of our era it must have been much more common in southern Europe than one would suppose from its incidence there today. The treatment of these diseases involved both drug and surgical therapy—thus allowing a variety of techniques and terminology to be developed and expanded by subsequent medical writers. In addition, the affliction called today trachomatous pannus and the surgical treatment of it were well described very early in the Islamic literature, yet whether or not it was recognized in the Byzantine literature and earlier Greco-Roman writings is problematic. More, however, will be said on that shortly.

The present paper is concerned with the Byzantine medical literature, and the Hellenistic writings on which it was primarily based, with the purpose of surveying the identification and description of these conditions along with the surgical therapies. A separate study will examine and compare in detail the compound drug remedies for these conditions, again with a view to tracing the transmission of such recipes and the maintenance of the integrity of the more frequently cited compound drugs. Future studies will be concerned with the reception of the Greek descriptions and practices in the Islamic world and the elaboration of the ideas and techniques by subsequent writers.[2]

A brief word is necessary here concerning the conditions themselves. Trachoma (from τράχωμα 'roughness') was considered by early Byzantine and later Islamic physicians to consist of four stages and to be a disease of the eyelid.[3] Today it is viewed as a disease of the conjunctiva in which dense, hard-packed papillae form on the inner surface of the eyelid, resulting when untreated in several complications and sequelae. The condition known today as pterygium (from πτερύγιον 'wing') is a triangular-shaped ingrowth of the conjunctiva onto either side of the cornea, most frequently on the nasal side. It was early classified as a disease of the conjunctiva and removed surgically. Pannus is an invasion of the cornea by vessels from the limbus; occasionally the entire cornea becomes vascularized and the overlying corneal epithelium becomes irregular and shows small punctate ulcers.[4] It was

[The reader is referred to the list of abbreviations at the end of the volume.]

---

[1] At least by the tenth century A.D. pannus was recognized as being a characteristic companion of trachoma. Later Islamic physicians considered pterygium to be related to, and a form of, pannus and hence also a sequela of trachoma. Byzantine physicians did not ever spell out a direct relationship between trachoma and pterygium, although they used much the same drug therapy for both conditions. Today no direct relation between trachomatous pannus and pterygium is recognized. Islamic physicians also recognized trichiasis and entropion (ingrown eyelashes and rolled-in eyelids) as sequelae of trachoma, but for this survey only trachoma, trachomatous pannus, and pterygium are to be dealt with.

[2] For a thirteenth-century Islamic analysis and treatment of these three conditions see Emilie Savage-Smith, "Ibn al-Nafīs's *Perfected Book on Ophthalmology* and His Treatment of Trachoma and Its Sequelae," *JHAS*, 4 (1980), 147–206; and *id.*, "Drug Therapy in Trachoma and its Sequelae as Presented by Ibn al-Nafīs," *PH*, 14 (1972), 95–110.

[3] See M. Meyerhof, "The History of Trachoma Treatment in Antiquity and During the Arabic Middle Ages," *Bulletin de la Société d'Ophtalmologie d'Égypte*, 29 (1936), 25–87; and Hirschberg, *Geschichte*, 130–39.

[4] For all three conditions see P. D. Trevor-Roper, *The Eye and Its Disorders* (Oxford/London, 1974), 404–10 and 461.

classified by medieval Islamic physicians as a disease of the conjunctiva. It is, however, a puzzle for historians to what extent, if at all, this condition was recognized by Hellenistic or Byzantine physicians.

The first definite description we have of pannus is by the ninth-century Islamic physician Yūḥanna ibn Māsawayh.[5] By the tenth century, Islamic physicians knew it to be always associated with trachoma and advocated removing it surgically by a procedure known later in the West as peritomy. Certainly no such surgical procedure is mentioned in the extant Hellenistic and Byzantine sources surveyed here. The usual Arabic name for it is *sabal*, meaning rain, although Ibn Māsawayh also used the Arabic *rīḥ al-sabal* and the Persian *bārandagī*, both of which mean "the pouring of rain." However, the ninth-century oculist and translator Ḥunayn ibn Isḥāq stated that there was a Greek name for this condition.[6] Ḥunayn wrote the word as *qīr-sūfthālmīya* which suggests a Greek word from κιρσός, meaning an enlargement of a bloodvessel, and ὀφθαλμία, a disease of the eye. The ninth- and early tenth-century physician Abū Bakr Muḥammad ibn Zakarīyā' al-Rāzī (Rhazes), citing Ḥunayn as a source, stated that the Greek name is derived from the word *al-dawālī*, apparently trying to define the transliterated Greek word given by Ḥunayn:[7]

> Ḥunayn said: *al-sabal* is vessels filled with blood and thickened and swollen, and there is with it in most cases watering of the eyes and lacrimation, itching, and redness, and its name in Greek is derived from the name *al-dawālī*.

The Arabic word *al-dawālī* is an early technical medical term for varicosity.[8]

While the term κιρσοφθαλμία would fit well the vascularization of the cornea which is the hallmark

of pannus, it is unfortunately not known to occur in any extant Greek medical writing. Nor could I locate a passage in any known Hellenistic or Byzantine tract which describes a condition which could be interpreted as pannus.

Nonetheless, al-Rāzī[9] in his extensive book on eye diseases, which formed part of his *Kitāb al-Ḥāwī fī al-ṭibb*, appears to have felt that some Greek writers did in fact describe a condition which he termed *al-sabal*, or pannus, for he cites three such passages. In all three cases only the title of the work is given (in Arabic), and the author's name omitted; the titles, however, of the Hippocratic and Galenic writings are quite uniform in the Arabic literature. One passage given by al-Rāzī is from Galen's *De usu partium*:[10]

> In the tenth [book] of *On the Uses of the Parts* (*Manāfiʿ al-aʿḍāʾ*) he said that *sabal* (pannus) is a wasting (*nuqṣān*) occurring in the pupil, and because of that the body of the eye is weakened and becomes small, and in most cases it occurs in one eye [only]. The recognition of it is easy because the healthy eye reveals the diseased one.

When we turn to the corresponding portion of *De usu partium* we find a discussion of the wrinkling and atrophy of the eye in a context not of eye afflictions but a discourse on the nature of the aqueous humor. The Greek text reads as follows:[11]

> Thus the wrinkled condition of the hornlike tunic itself in old persons is proper to old age because of weakness and the lack of pneuma coming down from above. The affection called *phthisis* is a shrinking of the pupil itself without any separate involvement of the hornlike tunic. Hence in most cases it occurs in [only] one of the eyes so that it is readily recognized and does not escape the notice of any physician; for the healthy eye beside it indicates the failure of the one affected.

Since contraction and atrophy of the cornea or pupil are not among the hallmarks of pannus, we are at first puzzled by al-Rāzī's misinterpretation of the atrophy of the eye for pannus—until, that is, we look at the Arabic translation that Ḥunayn ibn Isḥāq prepared of *De usu partium*. There we find the following rendering of the same passage:[12]

---

[5] M. Meyerhof, "Neues zur Geschichte des Begriffes Pannus," *SA*, 19 (1927), 240–52. For Ibn Māsawayh, see Ullmann, *Medizin*, 112 and 205; and Sezgin, *Geschichte*, III, 231–36.

[6] Ḥunayn ibn Isḥāq, *The Book of the Ten Treatises on the Eye Ascribed to Ḥunain ibn Isḥāq (809–877 A.D.). The Earliest Existing Systematic Textbook of Ophthalmology*, ed. and trans. M. Meyerhof (Cairo, 1928), 57.

[7] Al-Rāzī, Abū Bakr Muḥammad ibn Zakarīyā', *Kitāb al-Ḥāwī fī al-ṭibb. Rhazes' Liber Continens. An Encyclopedia of Medicine. Part II. On the Diseases of the Eye. Edited by the Bureau, based on a unique Escurial MS.* (Hyderabad, 1374/1955), 145. See also M. Meyerhof, "Nachträge zur Geschichte des Begriffes Pannus," *SA*, 20 (1928), 391.

[8] For examples of its use see P. de Koning, *Trois traités d'anatomie arabes par Muḥammad ibn Zakariyya al-Rāzī, ʿAlī ibn al-ʿAbbās et ʿAlī ibn Sīnā* (Leiden, 1903), 817.

[9] For the writings of al-Rāzī see Ullmann, *Medizin*, 128–36.

[10] Al-Rāzī, *Kitāb al-Ḥāwī* (n. 7 above), 119 (juz 2, bāb 3).

[11] Galen, *De usu partium* (ed. Helmreich), II, 73; Galen, *Parts* (trans. May), II, 477. The translation is that of May.

[12] The tenth chapter of the Arabic version has not been edited. The passage here translated is to be found in the following two MSS: Escorial, Bibliotheca del Monasterio de San Lorenzo el Real de El Escorial, Arabic MS 850, fol. 118a; and Paris, Bib-

And the wrinkling (shanaj) of the cornea occurs in old men because of the weakness of the tunic itself which occurs in old age[13] from their age and because of the smaller amount of pneuma which comes to the eye. As for the disease which occurs in the eye and is called *al-sill* (wasting away), it is a wasting (nuqṣān) of the eye itself in that it exists when the pupil alone diminishes in size without there being any of the symptoms in the cornea itself. For this reason it occurs in most cases in one eye only, and the recognition of it is easy and is not hidden from even one of the physicians, for the healthy eye discloses the diseased eye and reveals it.

As can be seen, Ḥunayn translated the Greek term φθίσις, meaning wasting away or atrophy, with the Arabic word *sill*, which means basically the same thing and is a standard rendering of *phthisis*.[14] Al-Rāzī, however, did not apparently recognize the word, and hence interpreted *al-sill* as *al-sabal*, which in Arabic involves only a slight change in the formation of the word. Thus al-Rāzī incorrectly extracted and summarized this passage as an example of Galen's knowledge of pannus.

A similar mistake in interpreting the Arabic may well have accounted for al-Rāzī's extracting another statement concerning the atrophy of the eye and asserting that it was about pannus. Al-Rāzī refers to Galen's tract *Methodus medendi* when saying:[15]

The third [book] of *Ḥilāt al-bur³*: he said *al-sabal* (pannus) happens to the eye when its nourishment and its humor are diminished, so it [the eye] is diminished and lessened.

Although I have been unable to locate the equivalent passage in *Methodus medendi* and have not seen the Arabic version, it is likely that a mistake similar to that just illustrated resulted in this inclusion of a statement which in fact applies not at all to trachomatous pannus. Consequently neither of these citations supports the notion that pannus was described by Galen.

The third passage is more puzzling. In citing a treatise entitled *Kitāb taqdimat al-maʿrifa*, which is

the usual Arabic title of the Hippocratic treatise *Prognostic* (Προγνωστικόν),[16] al-Rāzī says:[17]

Concerning *al-sabal*: He said in *Kitāb taqdimat al-maʿrifa* in the first section (maqāla) that indeed it is possible for the vessels in the eye to become red so that the eye appears red, indicating repletion (imtilāʾ) in the brain and its "mater"; and as for the acrid swelling there, when it is in that state it is fitting for the pannus (al-sabal) that the brain be purged and strengthened with strong substances and abstention from whatever irrevocably fills it.

And after this he said that it connected with the conjunctiva by the vessels in it, and on account of these there is no [effective] care inside or outside, for anointing is without good effect.

In the Hippocratic text *Prognostic*[18] there is no such passage, but only a brief reference, in part two and not part one, to some ocular ailments to be noted by physicians:[19]

For if they shun the light, or weep involuntarily, or are distorted, or if one becomes less than the other, if the whites be red or livid or have black veins in them . . . all these symptoms must be considered bad.

This passage certainly does not merit the rendering of it presented by al-Rāzī, if indeed this is the passage he had in mind. It is possible that al-Rāzī was actually using the commentary by Galen on the Hippocratic text *Prognostic*, for Galen in the first book of his commentary says, regarding the passage just cited:[20]

The whites of the eyes becoming red, such as in ophthalmias and in some people who are intoxicated, is an indication of repletion (πλῆθος) in the brain and membranes (μήνιγγας, dura and pia mater), and indeed sometimes inflammation has occurred in them. Either way, the blood is forced to the veins of the eyes, for which reason the white part in them appears red—that is, the area all around what is called the "ring" (the limbus, στεφάνη) which we have learnt through dissections to be a point of union of all the membranes and tunics of the eye.

---

liothèque Nationale, arabe MS 2853, fol. 175b. For a general discussion of the nature of Ḥunayn's translation and an edition of the sixteenth book, see E. Savage-Smith, "Galen on Nerves, Veins, and Arteries: A Critical Edition and Translation from the Arabic, with Notes, Glossary and an Introductory Essay" (Dissertation, University of Wisconsin, 1969).

[13] *shaykhūkha* in Escorial, Arabic MS 850, fol. 118a; and *shuyūkh* "old men" in Paris, arabe MS 2853, fol. 175b. Cf. Galen, *Parts* (trans. May), II, 477, note 29.

[14] See, for example, E. W. Lane, *An Arabic-English Lexicon*, part 4, (London, 1872; rpr. Beirut, 1968), 1396.

[15] Al-Rāzī, *Kitāb al-Ḥāwī* (n. 7 above), 117 (jūz 2, bāb 3).

[16] Ullmann, *Medizin*, 29. The citation occurs in the midst of citations from Galenic works, which supports the interpretation given below that al-Rāzī was actually using the commentary by Galen on the Hippocratic treatise *Prognostic*.

[17] Al-Rāzī, *Kitāb al-Ḥāwī* (n. 7 above), 118–19 (jūz 3, bāb 3).

[18] Littré, II, 140–90; *Hippocrates* (ed. and trans. Jones and Withington), II, 1–55.

[19] *Hippocrates* (ed. and trans. Jones and Withington), II, 10–11.

[20] Galen, *In Hippocratis prognosticum commentaria tria* I, 10, ed. J. Heeg (CMG V, 9, 2) (Berlin, 1915), 222. I wish to thank Professor John Duffy for bringing to my attention the tendency of medieval Islamic authors to confuse the Galenic commentaries with the Hippocratic treatises themselves.

If this was the passage which al-Rāzī had before him when preparing his collection of abstracts, then he took the first sentence of Galen's commentary, inserted an idea of his own in which he mentions pannus, and then in rendering Galen's second sentence misinterpreted it. In any case, neither Galen nor al-Rāzī refer to the cornea being red and engorged, which is the characteristic of pannus. If it is assumed that the text which al-Rāzī was referring to is now lost or unidentified, this third passage from al-Rāzī still cannot be used as conclusive evidence for early knowledge of pannus, since, as we observed above, al-Rāzī had earlier used the term when the original did not warrant it.

For these reasons we cannot rely upon the citations given by al-Rāzī as proof that trachomatous pannus was recognized in the Hellenistic literature. It has been brought to my attention that Galen, in his treatise *On Examining Physicians*, may refer to pannus. This treatise is lost in the original Greek; the Arabic translation is currently being edited, but until it is published no definite conclusions can be drawn regarding Galen's knowledge of the condition.[21]

We are then left with the statement by Ḥunayn ibn Isḥāq that there did exist a Greek word for the condition. But since neither the word, nor a similar word, nor a description in general terms of this ailment, can be found in the Hellenistic and Byzantine writings themselves, it is still an unsettled question. What can be said with certainty, however, is that it was not widely recognized in Byzantine practice, for it occurs in none of the treatises to be discussed shortly. For this reason little reference will be made to pannus in what follows. It is to be understood that it is not found in any Greco-Roman or Byzantine writing which has been examined.[22]

In the collection of Hippocratic writings there are no references to what might be considered trachoma,[23] although there is a brief reference to a sequela of trachoma, trichiasis, in a late appendix to the important Hippocratic treatise *Regimen in Acute Diseases*.[24] It is only in another late Hippocratic tract, *On Vision*,[25] that we encounter what must be a treatment for trachoma, although no name or detailed description is given for the condition:

> When you scrape the eyelids you must scrape with pure and thick Milesian wool rolled around a wooden rod. Be mindful of the limbus [and cornea] and do not cauterize through to the cartilage (χόνδρος). The indication of when you are to stop scraping is when there is no longer pure blood, but a blood-colored or watery liquid. After this it is necessary to rub on one of the liquid drugs, such as that from ἄνθος χαλκοῦ ("flower of copper," fine granulated copper). Afterwards, following the scraping and cauterizing,[26] when the scabs (ἐσχάραι) have fallen off and the ulcers are cleansed and producing flesh, it is necessary to incise the parietal bones. When the blood streams forth, one must treat with a drug for staunching blood. After that, cleanse the head.

---

[21] I wish to thank Dr. Vivian Nutton for drawing this to my attention. The editor of the Arabic text, A. Z. Iskandar, published a few paragraphs of this Galenic tract in English translation (giving no Arabic text), in one of which, according to Iskandar, Galen states "you should also praise those who treat with drugs ailments of the eyes which others treat by excision. Such ailments are e.g. pterygium, trachoma, pannus, chalazion. . . ." A passage from al-Rāzī's treatise *On Examining Physicians*, which Iskandar compares with this Galenic statement, is nearly identical except for omitting the reference to pannus. See A. Z. Iskandar, "Galen and Rhazes on Examining Physicians," *BHM*, 36 (1962), 363. Several Arabic paragraphs from Galen's treatise *On Examining Physicians* were published by A. Dietrich; in these published sections there is no mention of pannus, although there is a list of diseases treated by surgery which includes cataract, pterygium, and trichiasis (but omits pannus). See A. Dietrich, *Medicinalia Arabica. Studien über arabische medizinische Handschriften in türkischen und syrischen Bibliotheken* (Göttingen, 1966), 190–95. When the complete Arabic text is available more can be said regarding Galen's knowledge of pannus.

[22] The fact that there is no conclusive evidence at this point that Galen recognized pannus is one reason for supposing that the treatise extant in Arabic under the title *Jawāmiʿ Kitāb Jālīnūs fī al-amrāḍ al-ḥāditha al-ʿain* ("Summary of Galen's Book on the Diseases of the Eye") is in fact based upon spurious Galenic writings, for this treatise discusses *al-sabal*. I am in the process of editing and translating this treatise and shall include a discussion of it in a future study on the Islamic knowledge of Greek sources. For manuscript copies of this tract see Ullmann, *Medizin*, 56, and Sezgin, *Geschichte*, III, 101–102.

[23] In the Hippocratic tract *Epidemics III* there is a reference to "growths on the eyelids, internal and external, in many cases harming the sight, which are called σῶκα (figs)." See Hippocrates, (ed. Littré), III, 84–85. This passage is not specific enough to warrant the interpretation of it as a description of trachoma; it is likely only a reference to styes or possibly warts on the eyelids, even though the author does speak of "figs" and the papillary stage of trachoma was later called σύκωσις. See J. T. Pearlmann, "Hippocrates and Ophthalmology," *American Journal of Ophthalmology*, 68:6 (1969), 1072, who considers it a description of trachoma.

[24] Hippocrates, *Du régime des maladies aiguës, Appendice*, ed. and trans. R. Joly (Hippocrate, VI, 2) (Paris, 1972), 95–96; Hippocrates (ed. Littré), II, 516–18; cf. III, xliv and X, xv–xvii.

[25] Pseudo-Hippocrates, *De visu* 4, 5; Hippocrates, (ed. Littré), IX 156–9 = Joly, ed., *Hippocrate*, XIII, 169–71. See also Hirschberg, *Geschichte*, 130–31; Meyerhof (n. 3 above), 27; and A. Haras, *Die hippokratische Augenheilkunde* (Inaug. Diss. Erlangen, 1896), 14.

[26] ξῦσις and καῦσις. Cautery here seems to refer to the use of a caustic solution rather than cauterizing with heat. It may be that the author intended for the wool on the wooden rod to be soaked in a caustic, since he warns of cauterizing into the "cartilage" before he mentions using the liquid remedy. See J. Sichel, "De la vision," in Hippocrates (ed. Littré), IX, 122–61.

If the lids are more thick than normal, try to cut as much of the flesh as is easily possible on the underside. After that cauterize the lids with [a cautery] which is not red-hot, being mindful of the nature of the hairs [lashes], or shrink it with burnt and pulverized "flower of copper." When the scab falls off, treat the rest.

The condition known today as pterygium is mentioned briefly by name (πτερύγιον) in the Hippocratic treatise *Prorrhetikon II*.[27] There is, however, no reference to a surgical operation to remove it nor a detailed description of it. There appear to be no further references in the Hippocratic corpus to trachoma or pterygium, nor to pannus or other sequelae.

Hellenistic physicians were clearly aware of trachoma and the scraping of the eyelids to relieve it.[28] Medical practice current in the first century A.D. is reflected in the encyclopedia of Celsus written between A.D. 18 and 39. In the medical portion of the Latin encyclopedia (*De medicina* VI.6.26–28) it is said that trachoma (*aspritudo*) follows inflammation (*inflammatio*) of the eyes, and that, as a result of trachoma, running eye (*lippitudo*) occurs which aggravates the trachoma. Some physicians, Celsus noted, scrape the thickened and hard (inner surface) of the eyelids with a fig leaf, or a corrugated probe (*asperato specillo*) or a scalpel, and rub medicaments daily under the eyelid. Celsus warned, however, that such scraping should only be done when there is marked and inveterate roughness, and then not very frequently. It is better to treat by diet and by proper medicaments, for which Celsus recommends exercise, frequent baths, washing the eyelids with hot water, eating food which is acrid and attenuating, the use of the compound remedy called *Caesarianum*, a collyrium named after a certain Hierax,[29] and those collyria called *Canopita* (from the town Canopus in Egypt), *zmilion* (from σμιλίον 'the little scalpel' because it stings), *pyxinum* (kept in a box-wood case), and *sphaerion*, the last two recipes having been invented by Euelpides.[30] Celsus gives the recipes for the col-

lyria at various places in the writing on medicine.[31] When none of these remedies are at hand, Celsus states (VI.6.28) that goat's bile or the best grade of honey are suitable for treating trachoma.

In the chapter on surgical procedures (VII.7.4) Celsus discusses pterygium. Throughout the descriptions of pterygium in Hellenistic, Byzantine, and Islamic literature, there is no distinction made between the two conditions which we today call true pterygium and pseudo-pterygium. Pseudo-pterygium is a fold of conjunctiva resembling a pterygium which has become secondarily adherent to marginal ulcers on the cornea, caused by burning or other injury. Pseudo-pterygium can be distinguished from true pterygium in that a probe can be easily passed under it, for a bridge forms over the limbus in the case of pseudo-pterygium. Such a distinction, however, between those pterygia which can easily have a probe passed under them and those which cannot is not remarked upon in the ancient or medieval literature.

According to Celsus (VII.7.4) *unguis*, which he notes was called in Greek *pterygion*, was "a little sinewy membrane" (*membranula nervosa*) arising from the angle of the eye [canthus], most often from the nasal side, and sometimes spreading until blocking the pupil. It was to be treated by drugs if of recent origin, but if it was thick and of long standing then it had to be excised. For this operation, the patient was to be either seated in a chair facing the physician, or turned with his back to the physician so that his head rested upon the physician's lap. Some physicians preferred the former position if the left eye was affected and the latter if the right eye was afflicted. One eyelid was opened by the physician and the other by an assistant, and a hook inserted to lift the growth while a threaded needle was passed through it. After laying aside the needle, the physician then took both ends of the thread and raised up the pterygium by means of the thread and separated it from the eyeball by using the handle of a scalpel. By then pulling and slackening the thread he determined its point of origin. Celsus then warns the surgeon:[32]

> There is a double danger, that either some of the pterygium is left behind and, if this ulcerates, it is hardly ever amenable to treatment; or that with it part of the

[27] Hippocrates, *Prorrhetics II*, 20, in Hippocrates (ed. Littré), IX, 48–49.

[28] See Meyerhof, "Trachoma" (n. 3 above); and Hirschberg, *Geschichte*, 132–35.

[29] Nothing is known of where or when Hierax lived. See H. Gosson, "Hierax (12)," *RE*, VIII (Stuttgart, 1913), col. 1411. The statement of Celsus, "*id quod Hieracis nominatur*," is better interpreted as a proper name than from the Greek ἱέραξ 'falcon' as Hirschberg preferred; see Hirschberg, *Geschichte*, 263.

[30] The last two collyria, *pyxinum* and *sphaerion*, also appear as names of collyria engraved on extant Roman collyria seals. See H. Nielsen, *Ancient Ophthalmological Agents* (Acta Historica Scientiarum Naturalium et Medicinalium, 31) (Odense, 1974), 22–23.

[31] Celsus (ed. and trans. Spencer), II, 214–7, 211 and 213.

[32] Celsus, *De medicina* VII, 7.4 (ed. and trans. Spencer, III, 331). Translation is that of W. G. Spencer.

flesh is cut away from the angle; and if the pterygium is pulled too strongly, the flesh follows unnoticed, and when it is cut away a hole is left through which there is afterwards a persistent flow of rheum; the Greeks call it *rhyas* (ῥυάς).

Once the true point of origin at the canthus is observed, then the pterygium was cut with a knife so that no part of the canthus was hurt; Celsus does not mention procedures for excision near the cornea. Afterwards, flax (*linamentum*) soaked in honey was put on the eye with a linen cloth (*linteolum*) over it and either a sponge (*spongia*) or unscoured wool (*lana sucida*) on top of that. The eyes were to be opened daily to prevent adhesion and then anointed with a collyrium which would cicatrize the ulcers. The procedure should ideally be carried out in the spring and certainly before winter. Celsus adds that lesions (*vitia*) can arise when treating pterygium as well as from other causes, and sometimes when not all the pterygium has been cut away, a small tumor arises in the corner of the eye.[33]

The encyclopedia of Celsus is important for our knowledge of early Roman practices, although his treatise had little direct influence on later Hellenistic and Byzantine physicians and was unknown in the Islamic world. Nonetheless, many items which occur in later works first appear in the account of Celsus, and must reflect practices current in his day which were transmitted to later writers by sources now unknown.

The Roman physician Scribonius Largus, a younger contemporary of Celsus, included in his *Compositiones*, also written in Latin, six compound remedies for trachoma, including one called *hygra* because it is a liquid (ὑγρά) to be used against "very long-standing roughness of the lids and granular flesh which is called σύκωσις."[34] The latter term, which Scribonius gives in the Greek, means "fig-like," and is a reference to the papillary stage of trachoma, resembling the inner surface of a ripe fig.[35]

After giving directions on how to compound this collyrium, Scribonius goes on to say that the eyelid should be everted and the remedy carefully rubbed in until lacrimation ceases (*delacrimatio*). When the stinging stops, the lid is again everted and the membranes (*membranae*, eschar caused by the caustic substances) are removed with the thumb from the inner surface of the lid, which, he adds, is easily done. After this the lids are to be anointed with a thick ash-colored collyrium diluted in water. The procedure, Scribonius continues, "removes in a few days the chronic roughness (*callos*) and trachoma (*aspritudines palpebrarum*) even in cases which were given up by oculists (*oculariorum*)." Scribonius gives five other recipes for trachoma, in addition to the ash-colored ones;[36] there is no mention of pterygium, however.

Yet another near contemporary of Celsus, who wrote, however, in Greek rather than Latin, was the army physician Dioscorides, born in Anazarbus, near Tarsus in Cilicia, on the southern coast of Asia Minor. His extensive treatise on *materia medica*, Περὶ ὕλης ἰατρικῆς, was a major source for Galen and subsequent writers when compiling compound remedies. While discussing various substances, Dioscorides recommends eight for use in trachoma (τραχέα βλέφαρα, τραχώματα ἐν ὀφθαλμοῖς, τραχύτης βλεφάρων), including items such as fig leaves and hematite.[37] For pterygia, three are specified, including rock salt and licorice, while for both conditions three items are advocated—aloe, iron oxide, and "bone" of cuttlefish (*sepia*) made into collyria.[38] The simples recommended by Dioscorides and their subsequent use will be treated in greater detail in a separate study of drug remedies. Suffice it to say at this point that he served as

---

[33] Celsus, *De medicina* VII, 7.4 (ed. and trans. Spencer, III, 328–33); cf. Hirschberg, *Geschichte*, 271–73.

[34] Scribonius Largus 37 (ed. Helmreich, p. 18; ed. Sconocchia, p. 27). Helmreich retains the Greek (inserted by Jean Ruelle in his edition of Largus [Paris, 1529]), but Sconocchia has restored the Latin on the basis of fresh MS readings. See F. Rinne, "Das Receptbuch des Scribonius Largus," *Koberts historische Studien aus dem pharmakologischen Institut der kaiserlichen Universität Dorpat*, 5 (1896), 1–99 [p. 14]; and W. Schonack, *Die Rezepte des Scribonius Largus* (Jena, 1913), 22–23, no. 37. See also Meyerhof, "Trachoma" (n. 3 above), 29; Hirschberg, 297, no. 37; and Nielsen, *Ancient Ophthalmological Agents* (n. 30 above), 26.

[35] For a modern discussion of the four stages of trachoma, see Trevor-Roper, *The Eye* (n. 4 above), 404–10.

[36] Nos. 24, 28, 32, 33, 35, and 36 of his collection of recipes (ed. Sconocchia, pp. 23, 25, 26, and 27). Schonack, *Die Rezepte* (n. 34 above), 20–23; and Hirschberg, *Geschichte*, 296–97. These included one collyrium called ἅρμα (chariot) "because it has four parts, as a chariot has four horses and has quick results," and one called *stratioticum* "soldier-like," a name which also occurs on extant Roman collyria seals; see Nielsen, *Ancient Ophthalmological Agents* (n. 30 above), 22–23.

[37] *De materia medica* I, 64.4 (myrrh) and 128.6 (figs); II, 5 (Pontic mussel) and 74.4 (lanolin), V, 5.2 (unripe grape juice), 78.2 (oxidized copper = "verdigris"), 99.2 (copper ore), and 126.1 (hematite); (ed. Wellmann, Vol. I, pp. 59, 119, 123, and 150; Vol. III, pp. 5, 47–48, 69–70, and 94).

[38] *De materia medica* I, 101.2 (acacia); III, 5.2 (licorice); V, 109.2 (salt); and II, 21 (sepia); III, 22.4 (aloe); V, 80.1 (iron oxide); (ed. Wellmann, Vol. I, p. 93; Vol. II, pp. 9–10; Vol. III, pp. 52–53. For aloe, see J. Scarborough, "Roman Pharmacy and the Eastern Drug Trade," *PH*, 24 (1982), 135–43. For sepia, see D. W. Thompson, *A Glossary of Greek Fishes* (London, 1947), 231–32.

a major figure in the development of treatment for these conditions, even though he provided no general discussion of the afflictions or their general therapy.[39]

The second-century A.D. physician Antyllus[40] wrote a treatise on surgery, Χειρουργούμενα, which is lost to us today except through quotations from later writers. In the case of his surgical treatment of pterygium we have a quotation by al-Rāzī in Kitāb al-Ḥāwī fī al-ṭibb:[41]

> Concerning the excision of pterygium, Anṭīlus said that what is left of it remains always. If you extirpate it in ignorance, there will also be cutting into the flesh which is in the canthus; and there will occur from that lacrimation and separation between the flesh and the pterygium. If the pterygium is white and the flesh black, and [or?] the flesh loose and the pterygium hard, then excise it. Then drop into the eye salt and cumin and dress it with egg white and oil of rose. Then after some days anoint with the Red [Collyrium].

The admonitions to physicians to avoid leaving any behind after extirpation and cutting into the flesh in the canthus were made in the first century A.D. as well, according to Celsus. On the other hand, the use of oil of rose and the Red Collyrium is typical of Arabic literature on the subject, and not encountered in the Greek. It is quite possible, in light of the liberties which al-Rāzī took in his summary of Galen quoted earlier, that these latter items were added by al-Rāzī onto his summary of Antyllus's description. However, it might be that Antyllus first prescribed such things, but they were not noted in the later Byzantine writings. Antyllus's statements concerning when to excise the pterygium are obscure as transmitted by al-Rāzī.

Galen, also writing in the second century A.D. discussed both trachoma and pterygium at various places in the large corpus of his extant writings. Of trachoma he had the following to say in De compositione medicamentorum secundum locos IV, 2 (Kühn XII, 709–11):

> ... roughnesses (αἱ τραχώτητες) of the eyelids, because of which, as in ophthalmia, the tunics of the eyes, being constantly hit, suffer pain. We venture to mix with the drugs appropriate to inflammation a small amount of the cleansing (ῥυπτικά) drugs, like the trachomatikon collyrium[42] from wine, so as to stop whatever is growing upon the eyelids, and once the inflammation of the eyelids has subsided to scrape the roughness. In the case of those having ulcers along with stinging discharges, it is not possible to use these medicaments, for the "hornlike" [cornea] is then even more erroded and the prolapsis of the "grapelike" [uvea] is great, and very much pain seizes the patient, and the malignant discharge (κακόηθες ῥεῦμα) is brought on.

In severe cases the physicians have invented, in their perplexity, a singular cure, which is to cleanse the everted eyelids and scrape them without the use of drugs. Some scrape superficially with the spoon of the scalpel (τῷ κυαθίσκῳ τῆς σμίλης) and then with a soft sponge wipe off the discharge, using caustics on the eyelids for the remainder of the roughness, while others employ the superficially rough skin of certain marine animals (θαλαττίων ζώων) for the same purpose. One of my teachers made a collyrium from pumice (κίσσηρις) and scraped the roughness with it after everting the eyelids. Obviously it is necessary to pulverize the pumice first and then mold it with tragacanth or gum.[43] After the discharge has ceased through the action of the collyria, then we may venture to apply to the lids cleansing drugs, at first in a weak mixture and then gradually increasing the strength when it appears the patient can bear it. After the discharge has dried up and the eyelids are moderated, it is necessary to fill the empty ulcers (ἕλκη) with a collyrium of frankincense, mixing at first a very little bit of it with wine, and then increasing the strength of the mixture, so that the eyelids will no longer harm the tunics of the eye and the ulcers will be clean and precisely filled and cicatrized.

In another treatise, De simplicium medicamentorum XI, 27 (Kühn XII, 347–48) Galen described another scraper for trachoma, made from cuttlefish "bone":[44]

---

[39] In Dioscorides's treatise entitled Εὐπόριστα or Περὶ ἁπλῶν φαρμάκων I, 44.2, there occurs the statement that "callused lids" (τετυλωμένα βλέφαρα) must be everted and scraped with the rough leaves of a fig tree, or with a scalpel, or with the "bone" of cuttlefish formed into a collyrium, and also verdigris, which with gum is formed into a collyrium (ed. Wellmann, Vol. III, p. 167). Other references collected in Thompson, Fishes (n. 38 above), 232. For the "genuineness" of Dioscorides's Simples, see M. Wellmann, Die Schrift des Dioscurides Περὶ ἁπλῶν φαρμάκων (Berlin, 1914). For this and other writings, see J. M. Riddle, "Dioscorides," in Catalogus IV, 3–143; and Scarborough and Nutton, "Preface," 187–94. For the problem of Dioscorides as an "army doctor," see ibid., 213–17.

[40] See M. Wellmann in RE, I, part 2 (Stuttgart, 1894), cols. 2644–45; Ullmann, Medizin, 78; Sezgin, Geschichte, III, 63–64; and R. L. Grant, "Antyllus and His Medical System," BHM, 34 (1960), 154–74.

[41] Al-Rāzī, Kitāb al-Ḥāwī (n. 7 above), 150, cf. 138 (jūz 2, bāb 4).

[42] A trachomatikon collyrium was any of a class of collyria designed specifically for combating roughness, cicatrices, and trachoma.

[43] A similar statement concerning items for scraping the "fig-like" (σύκωσις, the papillary stage of trachoma) is found in Galen's commentary on the Hippocratic treatise Epidemics VI (Kühn XVIIA, 901–2); Galen, In Hippocratis epidemiarum librum VI commentaria I-VIII, ed. E. Wenkebach and F. Pfaff (CMG V, 10, 2, 2) (Berlin, 1956), 62–63.

[44] For further discussion of the use of the bony shell embedded in the mantle of cuttlefish (genus: sepia), a genus of cephalopod mollusks, and related items used for scrapers in trachoma, see the separate study, forthcoming, of drug remedies employed in Hellenistic and Byzantine practice. In using cuttlefish "bone" Galen may well have been following Dioscorides.

The hard shell of cuttlefish (τὸ σηπίας ὄστραχον) is sufficiently porous so that it is not [like] the stony shells of oysters. . . . Being suitable for roughness, we are also accustomed to use it against the severe roughnesses in the eyes which are called "fig-like" (σύχωσις, the papillary stage of trachoma), carving from it something resembling a [molded] collyrium in form and rubbing the roughnesses until they bleed. Having done this, the caustic (καθαιρετικά) collyria function better on them.

In *De compositione medicamentorum secundum locos* IV, 8, Galen specified fifteen compound remedies for trachoma,[45] all drawn from the immediate source of Asclepiades Pharmacion, who wrote about the third quarter of the first century A.D.[46] A few of the recipes bear the names of persons who possibly were their supposed inventors. There is the σκυλάκιον ("young puppy," but possibly from Scylacium in southern Italy) collyrium of Apollonius the Physician which is said to be the same as the "hawkweed" (ἱεράκιον) *trachomatikon* collyrium which is labeled Phoenix (Φοίνιξ). Galen gives a variant recipe for the Phoenix collyrium as he found it in the collection of remedies by Areius of Tarsus,[47] and also a collyrium for trachoma by Paccius, as excerpted by Asclepiades.[48]

Concerning the nature of pterygium, there is the following statement in the probably spurious Galenic tract *De remediis parabilibus* II, 4 (Kühn XIV, 410–11):

Pterygium is a sinewy (νευρώδης) projection of the conjunctival membrane beginning from the corner and proceeding to the limbus (στεφάνη) until it increases and even covers the pupil (κόρη).[49] When large and long-lasting, surgery is indicated. Recent and moderate-sized pterygium is removed by abrasives (σμηκτικά) such as burnt copper or χάλκανθος (an impure sulfate of copper), with gall of swine. Another very efficacious [medicament] is one part χάλκανθος and one part gum arabic. Another is lycium and henna with water.

Here, as earlier in Celsus, the wing-shaped ingrowth of the conjunctiva forming pterygium is described as "sinewy." It is probable that Hellenistic physicians intended this adjective to mean "fibrous" in this context. This particular definition, given in what is likely a spurious Galenic tract, was to have a long history in the Byzantine literature, as well as in the Islamic medical literature.

In *De compositione medicamentorum secundum locos* IV, 4 (Kühn XII, 717) Galen states:

In the case of pterygia and the "fig-like" [papillary stage of trachoma] the cleansing (ῥυπτικά) drugs are helpful, both those molded in the form of a collyrium and those dried without being molded, with which there is mixed a small amount of the caustic (σηπτικά) drugs. Related to these are those [drugs appropriate] for dry and itchy scaling (ψωρώδεις διαθέσεις) in the eyelids [blepharitis], and because of this they are called ψωρικά drugs. Of all those things, the strongest, which destroy old calluses and cure that called pterygia, are combinations of cleansing and caustic drugs.

In *Methodus medendi* XIV, 19 (Kühn X, 1018) Galen again[50] says that the small and soft varieties of pterygium can be healed by means of cleansing drugs, such as those called *trachomatika*, while the large and hard require surgery (χειρουργία), adding the following notion:

Inasmuch as pterygium is unnatural (ἀλλότριον) in the healthy constitution, I consider it to be generally evident that it is nonetheless not unnatural in relation to its own substance (κατὰ τὴν οὐσίαν), as are ἀθέρωμα (a tumor full of gruel-like matter) or μελικηρίς (a kind of cyst with a honeycomb interior).

In his discussion of the use of cuttlefish "bone" in which he mentions its use as a scraper for trachoma, Galen also described its use as an agent to dissolve pterygia (*De simplicium medicamentorum* XI, 27; Kühn XIV, 410–11):

---

[45] Several are called simply *trachomatikon*, that is, belonging to the class of collyria especially for use against trachoma. Some have special names associated with them. There is the saffron (κροκῶδες) collyrium of Antigonus, which Galen states is labeled "the small lion" (λευντάριον) since it is stamped with the image of a small lion (Kühn XII, 773). Galen mentions (K. XII, 775–76) a *trachomatikon* collyrium τοῦ ἱέραχος, literally "of the hawk," but here probably intended as the proper name Hierax, a man whom Celsus had earlier mentioned as having a collyrium for trachoma (see n. 27 above). One collyrium (K. XII, 779) is called "the small chariot" (ἁρμάτιον) for the rather cryptic reason that Ptolemy the King used it. Another (K. XII, 780) was termed ἀρτεμώνιον (? "the small foresail") because it was used by Bassos the Comrade-in-Arms (Βάσσος ὁ ἑταῖρος). The ingredient hematite determined the name of three collyria (K. XII, 732, 775, 779). One collyrium (K. XII, 783–84) is labeled simply "the orange one for general use" (κιῤῥὸν πάγχρασον), while another (K. XII, 785–86) has the more prestigious title of "worth its weight in gold" (ἰσοχρύσον).

[46] Fabricius, 192–98.

[47] Kühn XII, 776. For Areius of Tarsus see Scarborough and Nutton, "Preface," 198–99; and for Apollonius, see Fabricius, 180–83.

[48] For Paccius (Πάκκιος), a Roman physician of the first century A.D., see H. Diller, "Paccius (4)," *RE* XVIII(2)2 (Stuttgart, 1942), col. 2063; and Fabricius, 226.

[49] For similar statements elsewhere in the Galenic corpus see *De tumoribus praeter naturam* (Kühn VII, 732) and the pseudo-Galenic *Definitiones medicae* 366 (Kühn XIX, 439).

[50] The word πτερύγιον is also employed in the Galenic corpus for other skin conditions. See, e.g., Galen, *In Hippocratis prognosticum commentaria tria*, ed. I. Heeg (*CMG* V, 9, 2) (Leipzig, 1915), 212 and *In Hippocratis epidemiarum librum VI commentaria I-VIII*, ed. E. Wenkebach and F. Pfaff (n. 43 above), 19.

Being composed of very small parts, it [cuttlefish "bone"] is selected as appropriate for other things, for which reason we use it burnt against a dull-white leprosy (ἀλφός),[51] rough spots or freckles on the face (ἔφηλις), moles (φακά) and dry itch (ψώρα). But when mixed with quarried salt it dissolves the pterygia formed on the eyes. But before it is burned, when baked and smooth, it polishes teeth and dries ulcers.

The compound remedies offered for pterygium are given in a different treatise from the one presenting remedies for trachoma—that is, in *De compositione medicamentorum per genera* V,[52] where ten recipes are given for *trochiskoi*, or small tablets which are to be prepared specifically for use in pterygium, as well as in other conditions, such as different types of ulcers and skin disorders. These tablets at the time of application are to be mixed with water or honey. As developers of these troches Galen cites Heracleides of Tarentum, a well-known first-century B.C. physician of the Empiric school, Aristarchus of Tarsus, Areius of Tarsus, Aelius Gallus, one Magnus Philadelpheus, and a certain Diodorus.[53] Curiously, none of these remedies seem to have passed into subsequent literature. There is only one mention of pterygium among the conditions for which the remedies are prescribed in *De compositione medicamentorum secundum locos*—a short recipe given among ocular remedies ascribed to Archigenes, a physician originally from Syria who lived at the time of Trajan.[54] The latter remedy is advocated by later physicians.

Although pterygium is defined and described, there is no account of the surgical excision of pterygium in the extant Galenic corpus. Galen is of course known to have written a separate work on

the diagnosis of eye diseases and possibly another on the therapy as well.[55] These are lost to us today.

An important physician of the fourth century A.D. and model for later Byzantine physicians was Oribasius, who was friend, advisor, and physician-in-ordinary to the emperor Julian the Apostate.[56] Unfortunately his major encyclopedia, Ἰατρικαὶ συναγωγαί, or *Collectiones medicae*, is not extant today in its entirety. This enormous medical compendium relied heavily on extracts borrowed, frequently verbatim, from Galen and other Greek physicians. Neither trachoma, pterygium, or pannus are mentioned in the extant sections. Oribasius does make a very brief reference to pterygium and its treatment by surgery in his collection of easily obtained remedies compiled for the use of laymen entitled Περὶ εὐπορίστων.[57]

Another treatise on easily obtainable, common medicines also written in the fourth century was that by Theodorus Priscianus, who served the emperor Gratian (A.D. 367–383) as physician-in-ordinary (ἀρχίατρος). In this compilation, written first in Greek and then in Latin, entitled *Euporista*, Theodorus Priscianus mentions what appears to be a somewhat novel treatment of trachoma, by taking a garlic and inserting the head of a probe in the center of it and, squeezing the juice, anointing the eye with it.[58] His work combined elements of traditional medicines along with more learned medical practices.

Another compiler of popular and traditional medicines alongside excerpts from scholarly writings was Marcellus, later surnamed Empiricus, of Bordeaux. He was *magister officiorum* under Theodosius I (A.D. 379–395) and in the first decade of the fifth century composed *De medicamentis liber*, containing medicaments and recipes for treating

---

[51] For the significance of these terms for skin eruptions, see Paul (trans. Adams), II, 17–20. For a general discussion of leprosy and certain skin disorders, see M. W. Dols, "Leprosy in Medieval Arabic Medicine," *JHM*, 34 (1979), 314–33.

[52] *Comp. med. per gen.* V, 11 (Kühn XIII, 824–25, 829); V, 12 (Kühn XIII, 836–37); V, 13 (Kühn XIII, 838); and V, 15 (Kühn XIII, 856–57).

[53] For Heracleides of Tarentum, see H. Gossen, "Herakleides (54)," *RE* VIII(1) (Stuttgart, 1913), cols. 493–96, and Scarborough and Nutton, "Preface," 203. For Areius of Tarsus and Aristarchus of Tarsus, see Fabricius, 92–93, 97, and 225; and Scarborough and Nutton, "Preface," 198–99, 215, and 217. For Aelius Gallus, see M. Wellmann, "Aelius (59)" *RE* I(1) (Stuttgart, 1894), col. 493. Galen also gives one troche called Bithynian which he says was made in Cilicia.

[54] Galen, *Comp. med. sec. loc.* IV, 8 (Kühn XII, 802). For Archigenes, see M. Wellmann, "Archigenes," *RE* II(1) (Stuttgart, 1896), cols. 484–86; Sezgin, *Geschichte*, III, 61–63; and Fabricius, 198–99. In *De simpl. med.* VI, 9 (Kühn XI, 858), Dioscorides is cited as recommending the use of the dried root of licorice, pulverized in a mortar, as a powdered drug for treating pterygia.

[55] See, for example, J. Hirschberg, "Die griechischen Sonderschriften und Abhandlungen über Augenheilkunde," *Archiv für Augenheilkunde*, 85 (1919), 153–57; G. Bergsträsser, *Ḥunain ibn Isḥāq über die syrischen und arabischen Galen-Übersetzungen* (Abhandlungen für die Kunde des Morgenlandes XVII, 2) (Leipzig, 1925), item 54; and see above, note 22.

[56] See H. O. Schröder, "Oreibasios," *RE* suppl. VII (Stuttgart, 1940), cols. 797–812; and F. Kudlien, "Oribasius," *DSB*, X, 230–31.

[57] *Euporistes (Libri ad Eunapium)* IV, 24 (ed. Bussemaker and Daremberg, V, 714, cf. VI, 545–46); *Libri ad Eunapium* (ed. Raeder, 448). Eye diseases are also discussed in *Synopsis ad Eustathium*, (ed. Raeder), 262–69 although there appears to be no reference to the diseases under consideration here.

[58] *Euporiston* I, 12.37 (V. Rose, ed., *Theodori Prisciani Euporiston* [Leipzig, 1894], p. 37); see the German trans. in T. Meyer, *Theodorus Priscianus und die römische Medizin* (Jena, 1909), 109–10.

the diseases from head to foot. In his discussion of eye remedies Marcellus effectively plundered Scribonius Largus, with entire sections agreeing nearly word for word. To these excerpts Marcellus added a few recipes, most of which have an ample portion of a narcotic medicament.[59] Neither Theodorus Priscianus or Marcellus added significantly to the diagnosis or treatment of these three eye diseases in their accounts.

In the middle of the fifth century one Cassius Felix compiled for his son a medical encyclopedia in Latin[60] based, according to the author's own statement, upon Greek sources, but showing perhaps a few signs of personal experience as well. In his discussion of the treatment of trachoma he presents quite a detailed description of the scraping procedure, followed by the expression "*miraberis hoc factum,*" which might indicate actual experience with it. Cassius Felix heads his discussion of trachoma[61] with "*ad trachomata id est asperitates palpebrarum et ad sycosin, quam nos ficitatem dicimus,*" which seems to indicate that he considered σύκωσις, or the papillary stage of trachoma to be a disease distinct and separate from trachoma. He continues by saying that the latter is called *sycosis* or *ficitas,*

> since the roughnesses on the eyelids appear similar to the seeds of a fig. For the cure you painstakingly rub the *asperitates,* with the eyelid everted, with either pumice or soft "bone" of cuttlefish—that is, with the cortex removed (*osso sepiae molli hoc est detracto cortice*) until it is bloody. Then you carefully clean and astringe them with a sponge (*penicillo*) squeezed with cold vinegar-water. After that you use the *trachomaticum* collyrium which they call *paedicon,* that is, for a child, since it is appropriate for small children. For *reumata* and *trachomata* it is beneficial if you loosen them with water and anoint under the eyelid (*sub palpebro*) or under the lids (*sub ciliis*) which the Greeks call *ex hypoboles.*[62] *Miraberis hoc factum.*

After this there follows a recipe.

The next source chronologically was written some four hundred years after the time of Galen. Aëtius of Amida was born in Amida on the upper Tigris river, now Diyarbakir in Turkey, and resided in By-

zantium. He carried the title *comes obsequii,* which was not introduced until the reign of Justinian I (A.D. 537–567). The title implies a high rank at court, possibly military, and it has been suggested that he might have been court physician to Justinian.[63] Aëtius's medical encyclopedia, Βιβλία ἰατρικὰ ἑκκαίδεκα, consisted, as the title implies, of sixteen books. The seventh book of this compendium is devoted to ophthalmology and is a rich source of information on the practices of oculists prior to Aëtius whose works would otherwise be unknown to us today.

In Book VII, chapter 45, Aëtius presents[64] a discussion of trachoma taken from Severus, a physician and oculist at the time of Augustus.[65] Severus, according to Aëtius, said that roughnesses (τραχώματα), which many call rawnesses (δασύματα), occur often as a result of unskilled treatment. The condition also, he says, arises following a chronic, very non-pungent discharge (ἐκ ῥεύματος πολυχρονίου ἀδηκτοτέρου), "for if it were acrid (δριμύς) it would destroy the eye before establishing disease on the eyelid." Severus says (according to Aëtius) that occasionally the condition arises without a preceding discharge and with no apparent cause. In the latter circumstances, however, there is something like small grains of millet or small peas protruding on the inner surface of the eyelid. When there is a preceding discharge, the everted lids appear somewhat raw, rough and blood-red. He then states that the following distinctions should be drawn in the development of trachoma:

> [1] The rawness (ἡ δασύτης) is superficial and accompanied by redness; [2] the rough state (ἡ τραχύτης) has greater irregularity and protrusion, accompanied by pain and heaviness. Both [of the first two stages] are accompanied by watering of the eyes. [3] The so-called fig-like (ἡ σύκωσις) shows higher protrusions which seem to be notched and resemble nothing as much as a fig ripe to bursting. [4] The forming of calluses (ἡ τύλωσις) is [a feature] of inveterate roughness and shows the altered parts to be hardened and calloused.

Severus says that some physicians try to shave off the roughness using a knife or fig leaves, but he

[59] Esp. Marcellus Empiricus, *De medicamentis liber* VIII (ed. Liechtenhan, I, pp. 110–69). For general comments regarding Marcellus, see H. J. Rose, *A Handbook of Latin Literature* (New York, 1960), 428.

[60] V. Rose, ed., *Cassii Felicis De medicina ex graecis logicae sectae auctoribus liber translatus sub Artabure et Calipio consulibus (anno 447)* (Leipzig, 1879). Little is known of this particular figure.

[61] Cassius Felix XXIX (ed. Rose, p. 55).

[62] ἐξ ὑποβολῆς, an expression used by Antyllus according to Oribasius (X, 23.24) and by Severus according to Aëtius (VII, 32), and later in the ninth century by Leo to mean "by interposition" or beneath the eyelid. For Aëtius and Leo see below.

[63] See F. Kudlien, "Aëtius of Amida," *DSB*, I, 68–69.

[64] Aëtius (ed. Olivieri [*CMG* VIII, 2]), pp. 297–300; *Die Augenheilkunde des Aëtius aus Amida,* ed. and trans. J. Hirschberg (Leipzig, 1899) 107–15. For an English translation see T. H. Shastid, "History of Ophthalmology," *The American Encyclopaedia and Dictionary of Ophthalmology,* ed. C. A. Wood, XI (Chicago, 1918) 8662–64.

[65] See F. E. Kind, "Severus (48)," *RE,* II(2) (Stuttgart, 1923), cols. 2010–11. Aëtius's seventh book is our major source of information on Severus.

warns that this is harmful, for usually the formations are only increased and hard scars produced. He does recommend as treatment for trachoma (τὰ τραχώματα), when there is no ulcer (ἕλκος) in the eye nor inflammation, everting the lids and anointing with remedies prescribed for children, and massaging them for a long time with the head of a probe (μήλη); if rubbing is stopped too soon, greater roughness and discharges to the eye are produced. If the trachoma continues, stronger remedies are recommended. Aëtius notes that he has found the dry collyrium of Severus to be extremely useful, after which he gives recipes for six compound remedies.[66]

Aëtius states[67] that when inflammation of the eyes accompanies the trachoma, it is necessary to add some of the cleansing (ῥυπτικά) drugs to the remedies specifically for inflammation (φλεγμονή). He repeats the warning of Galen that if there is an ulcer with acrid discharge the usual drug remedies are not to be used, for the cornea will be corroded, prolapse of the iris will increase, and the pain for the patient and the corrosive discharge will be made worse. For these patients he recommends, as did Galen, the collyrium of finely powdered pumice combined with tragacanth or gum. He then presents the rest of the therapy as described by Galen in *De compositione medicamentorum secundum locos* IV, 2, given above.

In chapter 60 of the same book Aëtius discusses pterygium in general, with drug remedies given in chapter 61 and the surgical procedure in chapter 62. In this account Aëtius cites no particular authority as a source. He begins with the statement:[68]

> It is said to be pterygium (πτερύγιον) when upon much growth (αὐξηθέντος) or excess flesh (ὑπερσαρκώσαντος) of the white of the eye, as a result of blepharitis (ψωροφθαλμία) or oppresive discharge, an outgrowth spreads contrary to nature (παρὰ φύσιν).

He adds that it usually begins at the larger, nasal canthus, but may occur at the other canthus or even closer to the upper or lower lid, and in all cases extends to the dark of the eye and may even reach the pupil, in which case it interferes with vision. Aëtius distinguishes different colors of pterygia: white with a small base which he says is easy to cure; the contrary (ἐναντία) are difficult, for those which are somewhat reddish tend after surgery to cause necrosis (σφάκελος) and hemicranial headaches, although after these symptoms are removed the eye is well. He does warn, however, that pterygia which are accompanied by the onset of cataract (ὑπόχυσις) cannot be treated, for if pterygium is removed the cataract will develop more quickly. Nor should one treat pterygia which are thickened, rolled outward, protruding, hard, and accompanied by sympathetic headaches, for these are malignant (κακοήθη) and cancerous (καρκινώδη). In the case of pterygia which have covered the pupil, Aëtius notes that their removal will free the eye of discharge, but the operation will result in a scar (οὐλή) near the pupil which will nonetheless impair vision. The pterygia which are large and cover the dark of the eye (cornea) must be removed surgically, while those restricted to the white of the eye can be shrunk with drug therapy. There then follow in the next chapter twenty recipes, including the one from Archigenes which Galen had earlier given.[69]

Aëtius's description of the surgical procedure omits any statement as to the position of the patient, although he does say that if the patient refuses to open his eyes, a blunt hook should be gradually slipped between the upper lid and the eyeball and then drawn up, after which one can operate. The technique for the surgery is basically the same as that described by Celsus: a tiny hook inserted into the middle lifts the growth away from the eye, so the epidermis (ἐπίδερμα) of the cornea will not be detached, for he warns that if the latter occurs, a severe inflammation will result. A horse-

---

[66] This includes one recipe drawn from Apollonius and one attributed to a certain Theophilus. Brief mention is also made of a collyrium called the Phoenix and one called Dionysius. For Apollonius, a name also associated with a trachoma remedy by Galen, but one of different composition see above, note 47. Galen also advocated a Phoenix collyrium.

[67] Aëtius of Amida (ed. Olivieri), 313–16; ed. J. Hirschberg, 145–51. See also Shastid, "History" (n. 64 above), 8672–74.

[68] Following the reading of Olivieri, who reads αὐξηθέντος "growth" instead of ἑλκωθέντος "ulcers," and ὑπεροχή τις παρὰ φύσιν ὑποστῇ "an outgrowth spreads unnaturally" instead of ὑμὴν λεπτὸς καὶ νευρώδης ἐπιδράμη τὸν ὀφθαλμόν "a delicate, tendon-like membrane spreads over the eye;" Aëtius (ed. Olivieri, 313). This corrects the conjectural reading of Hirschberg. See also A. Olivieri, "L'Oftalmologia di Aetios nel cod. Laurenziano 75,5," *Studi italiani di filologia classica*, 12 (1904), 274.

[69] Following the text edited by A. Olivieri, which has twenty recipes instead of thirteen as in the Hirschberg edition (see above, note 64). Among the compound remedies advocated by Aëtius is the Theodotian (θεοδότιον) collyrium of Severus, that is, the collyrium attributed by Severus to Theodotus. The collyrium of Theodotus is also given by Celsus (VI, 6.6), though no specific mention is made of using it for trachoma or pterygium. This reference by Severus (as related by Aëtius) to a compound drug by Theodotus gives scholars the *terminus post quem* for Severus himself; see Kind, "Severus (48)" (n. 65 above). Aëtius also recommended all the cleansing collyria used for trachoma, as well as those used for "flyhead" (μυιοκέφαλον), a condition in which the uvea protrudes like a fly's head, and staphyloma (σταφύλωμα), the best of which he says contain wine.

hair and a linen thread are inserted into a needle and passed under the raised pterygium. The physician then holds the horsehair and linen thread in both hands and moves them about under the pterygium to separate the growth from what is under it, beginning at the cornea and moving to the canthus. Aëtius says the pterygium is removed from the cornea by means of the horsehair and thread, while the attachment to the canthus is removed with the "pterygium knife" (πτερυγοτόμος), taking care not to injure the lids or the canthus itself, for that will cause adhesions or, if the canthus is completely removed, a running of tears. Aëtius states that if it is not entirely excised it will recur.[70] After the operation salt water should be dropped into the eye, and then wool soaked in egg white should be applied and the eye bandaged. On the next day it should be anointed with the White, Mild Collyrium of Severus and on the fourth day with one of the "collyria for eye diseases" which he says consist of the one from nard and the one of Theodotus;[71] for the rest of the treatment one should avoid the gentle (ἀπαλά) and flesh-forming (σαρκωτικά) collyria.

The account by Aëtius of the treatment of pterygium and trachoma is the most complete to come down to us from Byzantine literature.

Born in the first half of the sixth century A.D. in Lydia, a province of Asia Minor, Alexander of Tralles composed a Θεραπευτικά in eleven books, the second of which was concerned with the therapy of the eyes. He was the son of a physician Stephanus, and had four learned brothers, one of whom was also a physician. It seems that for a while he practiced in Rome, and he mentions having traveled to Spain and Gaul. His writings were widely read and used in the Islamic world.[72]

Alexander employed the writings of Oribasius, Galen, and Aëtius as sources, although he did more than simply compile excerpts from previous writers, as had been the practice of Aëtius and Oribasius before him. While not usually naming sources, he appears either to have employed some writings now unknown to us or to have incorporated material originating from his own experience. This is particularly evident in some of his writings on other topics.[73] Compound remedies dominate his chapter on eye diseases in the Θεραπευτικά.[74] Four recipes are given for use against trachoma (τραχέα βλέφαρα, σύκωσις), only one of which bears a special name, the Great Theodotian. This is similar in composition to that associated with the name of Theodotus by Aëtius as drawn from Severus. For pterygia he specifically recommends the Hecatomb (ἡ ἑκατόμβη) collyrium consisting of fifteen ingredients, while four additional recipes can be employed in both conditions.

There is no general definition or description of either pterygium or trachoma, nor anything which might be interpreted as pannus, nor are there instructions for the surgical removal of pterygium or even basic steps in the scraping of trachoma. There is only a short paragraph[75] following one of the *trachomatika* collyria reminding the reader that when ulcers occur along with the trachoma, the lids should be everted and wiped with the curve of a probe or leaves of a fig tree. (Note that this is precisely the opposite of what Aëtius advocated.) Some, Alexander says, use the "bone" of the cuttlefish or a very rough skin, while others rub in one of the collyria made with pumice. When the eyelids are quieted and attenuated, the ulcers are to be treated with either the Libian (λιβιανόν) or Celestial (οὐράνιον) collyrium. If the case is not very severe the Theodotian collyrium can be employed directly.

The Libian collyrium is one of a class of collyria known also to Galen, while the Celestial collyrium, as well as the Hecatomb and some of the unlabeled compounds, appear to be new introductions into the extant literature. In regard to the nature, diagnosis and general therapy of these particular conditions, however, this treatise is far from as informative as its predecessors.

In his Θεραπευτικά Alexander of Tralles mentions having written an earlier treatise on the diagnosis, causes, and therapeutics of eye diseases, as well as on collyria.[76] This treatise is now lost to us. An anonymous treatise on eye diseases was found bound with a manuscript copy of the Θεραπευτικά of Alexander of Tralles. The editor of this anonymous tract[77] suggested that it in fact was written by Alexander of Tralles in his youth while

---

[70] The earliest reference to what must have been the observation that the recurrence of pterygium is quite usual. This recurrence defies all medical techniques known today; see Trevor-Roper, *The Eye* (n. 4 above), 461.

[71] See above, note 69.

[72] See F. Kudlien, "Alexander of Tralles," *DSB*, I, 121; Ullmann, *Medizin* 85–86; and Sezgin, *Geschichte*, III, 162–64.

[73] See F. Kudlien, "Alexander of Tralles," *DSB* I, 121.

[74] Alexander (ed. Puschmann), II, 2–60, esp. 46–53 and 64–65.

[75] *Ibid.*, 48–49.

[76] *Ibid.*, 2.

[77] T. Puschmann, *Nachträge zu Alexander Trallianus. Fragmente aus Philumenus und Philagrius nebst einer bisher noch ungedruckten Abhandlung über Augenkrankheiten. Nach den Handscriften heraus-*

in Asia Minor. More evidence is needed to confirm this assertion, however.

The tract has no recipes, for the third book, devoted to compound remedies, is now missing. Pterygium is defined with a slight reworking of Galen's definition in *De remediis parabilibus* quoted above:[78]

> What is pterygium? Pterygia are sinewy outgrowths (αἱ νευρώδεις ἐπιφύσεις). The origin of them is from the large canthus. Gradually around the limbus it grows upon the black. Sometimes, when it has grown beyond the normal amount (πέρα τοῦ δέοντος) it also impedes the pupil.

Nothing else is said of pterygium, although when discussing adhesions of the eyelids the author says that such adhesions are frequently treated with "the surgery of pterygia" (χειρουργία πτερυγίων).[79]

The first two stages of trachoma are treated together, while the third and fourth are treated quite separately, with discussions of other conditions intervening, as if the author did not realize that all four were really stages of the same disease. No general term for trachoma occurs.

Of the first two stages (δασύτης and τραχύτης) it is said that they:[80]

> ... develop on the inside of the eyelids. They differ from one another in that the first consists for the most part of redness while the second has more unevenness, with pain as well as discomfort. Both cause the eye to water.

Further on,[81] the anonymous author says of the fourth or cicatricial stage of trachoma: "τύλωσις is a chronic roughness (τραχύτης χρονία) having irregularities which are hardened and coarse." Four paragraphs later the third stage is characterized:[82] "σύκωσις has large and separated papillae (ὑψηλότεραι) and resembles an opened fig." Nothing further is said of these conditions.

Little is known of the life of the seventh-century Byzantine physician Paul, who was born on the island of Aegina in the Saronic Gulf and was trained at Alexandria. He also practiced in Alexandria, but it is uncertain how much of his tenure there overlapped with the Islamic invasion and occupation after A.D. 640. Paul of Aegina covers trachoma and pterygium in his discussion of diseases of the eye

which comprises the twenty-second chapter of the third book of his ὑπόμνημα (*Memorandum*), with the surgical removal of pterygium described in the eighteenth chapter of the sixth book, which is devoted to surgery.[83] Trachoma (τὰ τράχωμα), he says, is a roughness (τραχύτης) on the inside of the eyelids. An advanced form appears like clefts, for which reason it is called fig-like (σύκωσις), while it is called callosity (τύλωσις) when it is long-lasting and callous. In this, Paul follows Aëtius in his terminology, although without the explicit four stages. Paul mentions briefly that if the callosity is hard, then one must rub the lid with pumice, or with cuttlefish "bone," or fig leaves, or with the instrument called βλεφαρόξυστον "the eyelid scraper."

When describing pterygium (Book III, 22, sec. 25) Paul repeats Galen's basic definition that it is a "sinewy" (νευρώδης) projection of the conjunctival membrane. Paul's discussion consists of a nearly literal quotation (without citing Galen) of Galen's description of pterygium in *De remediis parabilibus* quoted above, without adding anything new except for a compound remedy and the note that some mix the gall of a goat with honey and anoint with it, the latter being a practice mentioned by Celsus.

In drug therapy Paul cites Oribasius as one source and appears to have relied as much upon Alexander of Tralles, or a common source, as upon Galen. For trachoma he recommends eight compound remedies.[84] One unnamed dry collyrium is identical to that given by Alexander of Tralles, though he is not cited as a source. Another is attributed in the text to Galen though it differs from any extant recipe of Galen.[85] The ἁρμάτιον collyrium given by Paul is identical to that given by Galen (Kühn XII, 779), which he drew in turn from Asclepiades Pharmacion. A Cygnus collyrium (κυκνάριον) mentioned by Paul is quite similar to that known to Celsus (VI.6.7) as *cycnon*. The saffron collyrium, however, as prescribed by Paul differs markedly in composition from those of the same designation advocated by Aëtius, Galen, and Celsus. Both saffron and cygnus, however, are names given to entire classes of collyria.

---

gegeben und ins Deutsche übersetzt (Berliner Studien für classische Philologie und Archaeologie, V, 2) (Berlin, 1886), 130–33.

[78] *Ibid.*, 142–43.
[79] *Ibid.*, 146–47.
[80] *Ibid.*, 144–45.
[81] *Ibid.*, 146–47.
[82] *Ibid.*

[83] Paul (ed. Heiberg), I, 176 and 181–82; and II, 58–59; Paul (trans. Adams), I, 414 (cf. 428), 418–19 (cf. 432–33), and III, 275–77.

[84] The collyria are given in Book VII, chapter 16. Some recipes state that they are to be used for trachoma or pterygium. Others are cited by name in Book II, 22 and Book VI, 18 of the treatise.

[85] I have been unable to find the recipe given by Paul among those listed by Galen, although it does bear some resemblance to that called βασιλίδιον (Kühn XII, 786–87).

For pterygium Paul advocates one remedy from Oribasius plus all those employed for trachoma and a condition called leucoma. These include a Hecatomb collyrium identical to that of Alexander of Tralles and one called ῥινάριον "small file" which differs substantially from remedies with similar names in earlier writings.[86]

In the treatment of pterygium presented among the surgical procedures, Paul again defines pterygium and says it can obstruct the movement of the eyeball,[87] as well as cover the pupil and thus obstruct vision. Paul states that the thin and white type is easiest to cure and should be excised, omitting a discussion of other types and complications of pterygia which had concerned Aëtius. His account of the surgical procedure and care following excision is a shortened version of Aëtius's description, with no new additions.

Paul made no claim to originality in his writing.[88] And indeed, as can be seen in the preceding summary, he drew heavily, and at times word for word, from Aëtius and from Galen, as well as other sources such as Oribasius and perhaps Alexander of Tralles. The precise debt to Oribasius in this context is of course difficult to assess, since the section of Oribasius's treatise which was concerned with these conditions is lost. Even the surgical treatment displays no new techniques or personal experience on the part of the author. His medical encyclopedia was, however, of enormous influence in subsequent medical thought, especially in Islamic lands, where it circulated widely.[89]

When we turn to the ninth-century medical epitome written by Leo, we find a succinct but well-written summary of the nature and treatment of pterygium along with some new compound remedies. Leo was a physician and philosopher living at the time of the emperor Theophilus (A.D. 829–842). He wrote his Σύνοψις ἰατρική for a younger physician, Georgius.[90] Concerning pterygium Leo says:[91]

> Pterygium is an excess of flesh (ὑπερσάρκημα) of the conjunctiva beginning from the large canthus and extending up to the pupil, at which point, when it has grown large, it obscures it. Therefore we use pterygotomy, inserting with a needle (βελόνη) a horsehair and thus cutting; and then we use collyria suited for staunching (κατασταλτικά) and attenuating (λεπτά), such as the one of Constantine, the one made of hartshorn, and the one made of mussel. Pterygium rarely occurs from the small canthus.

When defining pterygium as an excrescence, Leo has dropped the adjective "sinewy" (νευρώδης) used by most of his predecessors. The term πτερυγοτομία for excision of pterygium appears here for the first time in the literature surveyed. The three collyria are also new to the accounts.

It is evident from Leo's discussion of trachoma that a complete appreciation of the four stages of trachoma as stated by Aëtius was lacking in the literature available to Leo in the ninth century. In chapter eight of the third book Leo has the following to say:[92]

> It is called trachoma (τραχώματα) when you turn the eyelids inside out and you see on them something of a seed (κεγχραμίς) having some roughness like those in figs. For these we use the collyria called trachomatika, such as that made with wine, the one made of two stones, and similar ones. When the trachoma becomes very old and stone-like it is called τύλωσις (callosity).

Yet in chapter ten of the same book he says:[93]

> Fig-like (σύκωσις) is when you evert the eyelids and you find excess flesh of some redness, like figs. And these are treated with trachomatika collyria, which we anoint from beneath (ἐξ ὑποβολῆς, that is, under the eyelid).

From this it appears that Leo considered σύκωσις, the fig-like papillary stage which Aëtius and Paul viewed as the third stage, to be a separate ailment which was, however, to be treated in the same manner as τραχώματα. Under the latter term he grouped the first two stages and the fourth, consisting of τύλωσις, or the formation of calluses. This evident separation of the papillary stage of trachoma from the other stages, to be seen also in the writings of Cassius Felix in the fifth century, may simply have been an outgrowth of a custom evident in writings prior to Aëtius in which the papillary stage is sometimes discussed separately from general roughness of the eyelids, with no mention of well-defined stages of trachoma. This tendency can be seen, for example, in Galen's discussion of trachoma in *De compositione medicamentorum secundum locos* and *De simplicium medicamentorum* quoted

---

[86] Galen has one collyrium called ῥίνημα "small filings" (Kühn XII, 778–79) and Celsus (VI, 6.30) one called *rinion*. Both are very different.

[87] It can indeed mechanically interfere with the movement of the eye when very extensive.

[88] See P. D. Thomas, "Paul of Aegina," *DSB*, X, 417–19, and E. F. Rice, Jr., "Paulus Aegineta," *Catalogus*, IV, 145–91.

[89] See Ullmann, *Medizin*, 86–87; and Sezgin, *Geschichte*, III, 168–70.

[90] See Hunger, "Medizin," 305; and Hirschberg, *Geschichte*, 365–66.

[91] *Conspectus medicinae* III, 20 (in Ermerins, 136–37).

[92] *Conspectus medicinae* III, 8 (in Ermerins, 130–31).

[93] *Conspectus medicinae* III, 10 (in Ermerins, 130–31).

above. If such is the case, it would indicate that for the diagnosis of the condition, the early writings were of greater influence than those of Aëtius and Paul. It is notable that Leo makes no mention of the quite common practice of scraping trachoma. Perhaps the practice was becoming less common. Could he in this regard have been following the advice of Aëtius to avoid scraping rather than that of Paul and others who completely overlooked Aëtius's warning? Leo's synopsis, of course, may well have been based upon sources unknown to us today, with some personal experiences as well determining his selection of comments.

In the tenth century, Theophanes Nonnus compiled an epitome of therapeutic practices which for our purposes is very limited. This abstract from older medical writings was prepared at the request of Constantine VII Porphyrogenitus.[94] The synopsis was based to a large extent, and often very literally, upon Oribasius—so much so in fact that one copyist indicated in the margin of his copy that he supposed the entire writing to be by Oribasius.[95] Unfortunately we are missing the equivalent sections of Oribasius's tract and so cannot compare them. It appears that in the case of eye diseases, however, Theophanes was highly selective, for only pterygium is mentioned by him. There is no discussion whatsoever of trachoma. Of pterygium, Theophanes says simply:[96] "Pterygium is an excess of flesh of the conjunctiva beginning at the large canthus and spreading out to the pupil." Following this nearly word-for-word repetition of the definition given by Leo, Theophanes gives two untitled compound remedies. No mention is made of surgical treatment.

Moving ahead two centuries,[97] the next text, chronologically, to contain pertinent material was written between 1270 and 1280 by Nicolaus Myrepsus, court physician (ἀκτουάριος) at Nicaea

under the emperor John Vatatzes.[98] Myrepsus composed a treatise on compound remedies (Δυναμερόν) which was to have great influence through Latin translations as late as the seventeenth century. The work may well reflect his own experience in the field of drug making, since the name by which he became known, Myrepsus (μυρεψός) is equivalent to the Latin unguentarius, one who prepared unguents, although it is possible that the title was given him after his death on the basis of his having compiled the treatise rather than for his expertise during his lifetime.

The twenty-fourth chapter of his treatise concerns collyria.[99] Collyria given numbers 1, 20, and 21 are all recommended for pterygia and bear special names. They do not appear in previous literature. Their names are κολούριον σωτρία μανιθῶνος (sic) "the salutary collyrium [called] Manithonos (?)"; the collyrium called ἱερὰ ἄγγυρα (sic) ἐκ τοῦ ποντικοῦ "the sacred anchor of the one from Pontus"; and κολούριον θεοδώρητον ἀσκληπιάδου "the God-given collyrium of Asclepiades."

Collyrium number 42 is one "called that made with Scylacian stones" (τὸ διὰ λίθων σκυλακίων λεγόμενον), to be used for trachoma (τραχώματα) and the fig-formation (σύκωσις). The recipe is nearly identical in composition to that given by Paul of Aegina (VII, 16) as a collyrium "from two stones" which was also cited by Leo as a treatment for trachoma.[100] Myrepsus has a collyrium (no. 36) titled κολούριον μονοήμερον τὸ περιβόητον "the much-

[94] See Hunger, "Medizin," 305–6; and Hirschberg, Geschichte, 366–67.

[95] Hirschberg, Geschichte, 366 note 5.

[96] Epitome de curatione III, 63 (ed. I. O. S. Bernard, I [Gotha, 1794] 240–41).

[97] It had been my intention to compare the tenth- or eleventh-century Greek translation made of the treatise entitled Kitāb zād al-musāfir wa qūt al-ḥāḍir ("Provisions for the Traveler and Food for the Settled") with the Arabic original written by Abū Jaʿfar Aḥmad ibn Ibrāhīm ibn Abī Khālid al-Jazzār, who died about A.D. 1004 (see Ullmann, Medizin, 147–49, and Sezgin, Geschichte, III, 304–7). The Greek translation under the title Ἐφόδια mentions pterygia as well as some other conditions. Neither the Greek text nor the Arabic have been published. I examined the Greek copy in Oxford, Bodleian Library, MS Laud. Gr. 59 (the ophthalmological section occupies fols. 89ʳ–99ᵛ); however, the tract did not in any way line up with the one com-

plete Arabic copy, of the same title, available (Bethesda, Md., National Library of Medicine, MS A92, item 2, fols. 1–33a, with ophthalmological material fols. 2a–6b). Consequently, further evaluation of the Greek rendering of the text and its faithfulness to the original, as well as its relationship with subsequent Greek texts, will be postponed until another complete copy of the Arabic can be studied.

[98] See Hunger, "Medizin," 312; and K. Vogel, "Byzantine Science," CMH, IV, pt. 2, ed. J. M. Hussey (Cambridge, 1967), 291.

[99] Unfortunately the Greek text of this important treatise still remains unedited. I have for this study employed Oxford, Bodleian Library, MS Barocci 171, which is a fifteenth-century copy of the treatise. The chapter on collyria occupies fols. 115ʳ–121ʳ. Each recipe is numbered within each chapter. The numbers in the manuscript do not always correspond with those given in the Latin translation by L. Fuchs, Nicolai Myrepsi Alexandrini Medicamentorum Opus, in sectiones quadragintaocto digestum, hactenus in Germania non uisum, omnibus tum Medicis, tum Seplasiarijs mirum in modum utile (Basel, 1549), of which Chapter 24 occupies cols. 373–90. For the confusion of Latin texts associated with the name Nikolaus, see F. K. Held, Nicolaus Salernitanus und Nikolaos Myrepsos (Inaugural Dissertation, Leipzig, 1916).

[100] Myrepsus differs from Paul in having saffron instead of cassia and adding myrrh in his list of ten ingredients. The word σκυλάκιον calls to mind the σκυλάκιον collyrium of Apollonius given by Galen (Kühn XII, 776) and also Aëtius (VII, 112), but the recipe of Myrepsus is entirely different. Myrepsus also shows

talked-about curing-in-one-day collyrium," whose only specified use is in treating pterygia. The name μονοήμερον is a very common one for a collyrium; many different recipes are found under this title, and indeed Myrepsus himself has four different compounds under that name. The name, which occurs on Roman collyria seals as Monohemerum,[101] is also used by Paul, Aëtius and Marcellus Empiricus, though their recipes bear no resemblance to the one cited by Myrepsus for pterygia. From the name of the collyrium Phoenix (no. 31), also to be used in pterygia, one would expect the composition to be similar to that given by Galen and Aëtius for the same purpose. But such is not the case, for the eleven ingredients are totally different from the six in the earlier versions. What is more interesting, Myrepsus has interpreted the name Phoenix literally—that is, as date-palm (φοίνιξ) and so has included in his recipe "stones from the fruit of date-palm trees, burnt and ground." In the early recipes the Phoenix collyrium had nothing to do with date-palms.

In this limited sampling we see that Myrepsus displays some dependence upon the recipes transmitted by Paul, but virtually none upon those of Aëtius and Galen, and that he, or some unknown intermediate source, introduced new collyria with new names and apparently reinterpreted some of the older names. It is of interest that five of the six recipes are for pterygia. The one mentioning trachoma also names the "fig-like formation" (σύκωσις), suggesting that once again the two were viewed as separate conditions.

The last figure to be included in this survey is Johannes Actuarius, court physician (ἀκτουάριος) in Constantinople to the emperor Andronicus III (A.D. 1328–1341). Johannes Actuarius has rightly been praised as a physician, though firmly within the Galenic tradition, demonstrating personal experience and observation in his writing.[102] These qualities are displayed in his treatise on urine, a tract on pneuma concerned in part with the powers and disorders of the mind, and in parts of a

large book on *Methods of Treatment* (Θεραπευτικὴ μέθοδος). Of the latter treatise only the first two books, on diagnosis (Περὶ διαγνώσεως), have been edited.[103]

The discussion of trachoma and pterygium by Actuarius is at first encounter disappointing because of the nearly literal extraction of passages from earlier writings. The short entry on pterygium is nothing but an almost word-for-word transcription of Galen's first sentence in *De remediis parabilibus*, quoted above, with an additional phrase or two. Actuarius says:[104]

Among the diseases of the eye belong pterygium, which is a "sinewy" (νευρώδης) projection of the conjunctival membrane beginning at the canthus and going forward to the limbus; if by chance the pterygium can grow no larger (ἄν γε μὴ ὑπεραυξηθὲν τὸ πτερύγιον τύχῃ) it also covers the pupil itself and hinders the vision (τοῦ ὁρᾶ κωλύει).

Nothing else is said of this condition.

When writing the entry on trachoma, however, Actuarius seems to have been more concerned than previous writers with the differential diagnosis of trachoma from other conditions of the eyelid. To achieve this end Actuarius took the first sentence of Paul of Aegina's paragraph on trachoma, the first sentence of his statement on chalazion and the first sentence of his description of the stye.[105] To these Actuarius then added a sentence of his own:[106]

Trachoma (τράχωμα) is a roughness of the inner surface of the eyelid. When intense, having the appearance of incisions, it is called σύκωσις "fig-like." When chronic and thus made callous, it is called τύλος "callus." From these chalazion (χαλάζιον) differs, being a concretion of water on the eyelid. But that called stye (κριθή), as all know, is an elongated abscess (ἀπόστημα) on the inside of the eyelid. When the eyelids have lice, and the disease from them is clearly visible, it is called phthiriasis (φθειρίασις, pediculosis palpebrarum); and to those observing sharply they appear living animals and to be moving.

These abstracts were arranged by Actuarius in such a way as to give them more significance for comparative diagnosis than they had had in the original work of Paul. The last sentence is not in the

---

dependence upon Paul in the twenty-seventh collyrium, called πρωτεύς, recommended for cicatrices and calluses. It is very similar to that given by Paul (VII, 16) for the same purpose. Since Proteus is a common name on Roman collyria seals, it is likely a name of a group of recipes (see Nielsen, *Ancient Ophthalmological Agents* [n. 30 above] 23).

[101] See Nielsen, *Ancient Ophthalmological Agents* (n. 30 above), 22–23 and 87.

[102] See Hunger, "Medizin," 312–13; Vogel, "Byzantine Science," *CMH*, IV, pt. 2 (1967), 291; and Kudlien, "Alexander of Tralles," *DSB*, I, 121.

[103] Ideler, II, 354–464. The ophthalmological portion (pp. 444–49) was reprinted and translated into German by J. Hirschberg, "Die Augenheilkunde bei den Griechen," *Archiv für Ophthalmologie*, 33:1 (1887), 48–78.

[104] Hirschberg, *ibid.*, 56–57.

[105] Paul of Aegina III, 22 (ed. Heiberg, I, 176–77).

[106] Hirschberg, "Die Augenheilkunde bei den Griechen" (n. 103 above), 54–55.

treatise of Paul, although he does mention a compound remedy for treating lice. Actuarius's productive arrangement of the abstracts from an earlier writer, alongside a note possibly from his own observations, resulted in a concise but useful, even though derivative, guide to the diagnosis of trachoma and its differentiation from other conditions which Actuarius thought might be confused with it.[107]

Even though we possess now only a few pertinent texts from a span of time extending over a thousand years, we may still venture some conclusions regarding the general development of Byzantine ophthalmological knowledge and care. In the early Byzantine literature, written from the fourth through the seventh centuries, when Alexandria was still the center of activity, we see the great reference works being compiled. It was indeed a formative, although perhaps not highly original, period when the great encyclopedists Oribasius, Alexander, Aëtius, and Paul composed their summaries of previous theory and practice. From our perspective, the importance of Oribasius and Alexander is difficult to evaluate, since most of their writings on our topic are now lost. Certainly Aëtius supplied the fullest account of trachoma and pterygium and their treatment in the Greek literature, based according to his own account to a large extent upon the first-century B.C. physician Severus. Aëtius's masterful account presented definitions, causes, complications, concomitant afflictions and their effect upon the treatment, as well as therapy for the ailments, which included drug treatment and intricate surgical procedures, with admonitions to physicians on things to avoid.

As early as the seventh century, however, in the encyclopedia of Paul there are indications of a beginning lack of interest in the theoretical aspects of the causes and interrelationships of diseases. While Paul does have the observation that pterygium can obstruct the movement of the eyeball, there is not as much in his presentation that betrays actual experience as is evident in that given by Aëtius (or by Aëtius's immediate source). Even the surgical section of Paul, for which he was to become so

renowned, is in this case an inferior restatement of that given earlier by Aëtius.

When we turn to the middle and late Byzantine periods centered in Constantinople, it is true that our sources grow less numerous. But it is also true that what ones we do have show less and less interest in theoretical matters and in surgery—in fact in any therapy except drug therapy—and even very little interest in regimen or accurate diagnosis. Confusion increases, for example, about the stages of trachoma, with some writers apparently considering them to be distinct diseases. On the other hand, it should be noted that the Byzantine writers did not err in regarding pterygium as one of the sequelae of trachoma, as did the Islamic physicians. In general the descriptions of these diseases become more succinct, pedantic, repetitive, and less useful, and thereby, one might conclude, reflecting little personal experience.

What appears to be happening is an increasing lack of interest in diagnosis, general therapy, surgical therapy and even in regimen. The only subject that really holds the attention of late Byzantine physicians with regard to these conditions is drug therapy, and to that they added new compound remedies, but not (at least for these diseases) new simples. The other aspects—accurate diagnosis (with the exception of Johannes Actuarius, who does at least display a concern over this matter), the interrelationship of diseases, regimen, and surgical therapy—which were of considerable concern to the early Byzantine writers, were not maintained, much less built upon. Did the rôle of the learned physician change so much in a thousand years that he had no need for accurate diagnosis or productive therapy? Could the physician have been as successful with only his drug therapy as others had earlier been with their surgical techniques and scraping? Were the surgical techniques perhaps not as widespread or as effective (sepsis being a major but unrecognized problem) in Roman and Hellenistic medical practice as one might be led to think on the basis of the medical texts? Was the warning given by Aëtius against what he considered to be the harmful procedure of scraping trachomatous eyelids singled out and followed by the late Byzantine physicians even though Paul and others completely ignored the advice? Was the incidence of trachoma and pterygium much less in Constantinople than it had been earlier in Alexandria or even southern Europe?

With regard to the problem of whether or not Hellenistic and Byzantine physicians knew of tra-

[107] Actuarius does not discuss the surgical treatment of these conditions, although he does give pertinent compound remedies in the last section of his therapeutic manual. The latter has not yet been printed in the original Greek, but is at the moment available only in the sixteenth-century Latin translation made by Corneille Henri Mathys, published first in 1554 under the title *Methodi medendi libri sex* and reprinted many times, including as a part of *Medicae artis principes post Hippocratem et Galenum* (n.p., 1567).

chomatous pannus, we are again reminded of the fact that we are working with a very limited sampling of all that must have been written on the topic. We cannot rule out, particularly given the assurance of Ḥunayn ibn Isḥāq that there was a Greek term for pannus, that some Greek physician did identify the disease and possibly even tried to remove it surgically. While we cannot argue from the silence of the extant texts that the condition was unknown to Hellenistic and Byzantine physicians, we can nonetheless confidently assert that it was not at all widely known. The treatises we do possess were written by highly placed physicians, many of them court physicians or physicians-in-ordinary to emperors. One would assume that they were in a position to acquire the best texts available in their day, and to meet the most experienced practitioners. Yet they are silent on the subject. Although the topic has not been exhausted, the Byzantine texts, in regard to these three conditions, reflect no influence from Islamic physicians, whose knowledge, speculation, and treatment of them, from the tenth through the fifteenth centuries, show much evolving and development over that found in the earlier writings of Galen, Aëtius, Alexander and Paul.

It is often said that late Byzantine medicine is highly derivative, but what is apparent from this sampling is that it is not derivative enough—for if writers were simply repeating, reorganizing, and preserving earlier writings, then there would still be accounts of the causes and relationships of diseases, regimen, and surgical therapy, for all of these aspects were well covered in the early Byzantine compilations. Three of the four early Byzantine encyclopedists whose works form the basis of the later knowledge included surgical practices in their reference works. Only Alexander of Tralles omitted surgery. Yet the tradition was broken, for reasons now unknown or little understood. Surgery was not of much concern to the later authors of medical tracts and appears to be left to another segment of society. There are no suggestions of new materials with which to scrape trachomatous eyelids, which one would expect if the practice were being continued, and which indeed one does find in the contemporaneous Islamic writings. When there is any reference to surgery, there are no apparent refinements in techniques—no preferences as to the number and position of hooks or the use of probes or couching needles, as one finds in the Islamic writings of the same period.

While later Byzantine writers may have been uncritical of earlier medical writers, they were not sufficiently in awe of them to make a really concerted effort to transmit accurately and fully all they said. In fact their own lack of interest in topics dictated their selection and, even more to the point, their omission of material from earlier writers.

Gustave E. von Grunebaum Center
for Near Eastern Studies
University of California, Los Angeles

TWO LISTS OF GREEK SURGICAL INSTRUMENTS AND THE STATE OF SURGERY IN BYZANTINE TIMES

Lawrence J. Bliquez

The object of this study is to inquire into the state of the surgical art in Byzantine times, with particular emphasis on the Middle Byzantine Period. As will soon be apparent, I have concluded that a very fruitful approach is through references to the actual surgical tools employed; therefore I shall often be obliged to deal in specifics. However, the larger question must always remain in view: How advanced was surgery from the time of Constantine the Great to Constantine XI Dragases?

To be sure, the period opens very auspiciously. True, there is almost nothing of interest on surgery in the surviving work of Alexander of Tralles (525–605); but we are amply compensated for his deficiencies by the contributions of Julian's doctor, Oribasius, of Aetius of Amida, physician to the court of Justinian I, and of the great scholar/physician of the seventh century, Paul of Aegina. Paul in particular is a mine of information, providing in the sixth book of his *Epitome* extraordinarily detailed descriptions of over 120 operations and the instruments employed in them.[1] While Paul's surgery is venturesome enough to attempt mastectomy and operations for hernia, tumors and bladder stone, still, like all surgeons prior to modern times, the better part of his efforts were confined to the sur-

face of the body or to those areas where natural openings like the nasal and genital passages allowed surgical instruments to be utilized internally. Even so, Paul, Aetius, and Oribasius represent the culmination of all surgery up to their time, demonstrating clearly how much had been achieved since the days of the great Hippocrates.

If, however, we look beyond Aetius and Paul to the accomplishments of surgeons from the time of the Isaurian dynasty to the Palaeologi and the fatal year 1453, this auspicious beginning does not at once seem to be followed by activity of comparable interest. I have found nothing to match Paul's sixth book in subsequent Byzantine medical literature. And if one looks away from the literature and concentrates on the material evidence, that is, the actual surviving surgical instruments of the Byzantine period, the results here too are hardly spectacular. I have assembled as much information as I could on surviving tools, based on my own knowledge and that which came to me through approximately fifty-five letters of inquiry to individuals and museums in fifteen countries. It is appropriate to provide here a catalogue of every object known to me which *could* have been employed for surgical purposes in Byzantine times.

I

A. A series of fifteen objects from Byzantine Corinth are of interest. These were published by G. R. Davidson in *Corinth*, Volume XII, *The Minor Objects* (Princeton, 1952), nos. 1377–1391. All the pieces are of bronze; most of them were discovered in assuredly Byzantine contexts (at Corinth = ninth to twelfth centuries). I must emphasize that, so far as

[The reader is referred to the list of abbreviations at the end of the volume.]

I wish to express my gratitude to Professors Henri Amin Awad, Gerhard Baader, Imre Boba, Alexander Kazhdan, Ernst Künzl, Pierre MacKay, John Scarborough, and especially Timothy Miller for their help in the preparation of this paper. I also wish to acknowledge the assistance provided by the American School of Classical Studies in Athens. For the views expressed herein I alone bear responsibility.

[1] For Paul I have used the Greek text edited by Heiberg.

I know, none were found in any medical context. Even so, the shape, size, and aesthetic detail of some of the pieces suggested to Professor Davidson that they may have been the property of Byzantine physicians. These pieces include:

1. Seven bifurcated instruments (nos. 1377–1383; fig. 1) the remnants of which range in length from 0.073 m. to 0.145 m. Decor consists of incised linear or circular patterns, in many cases on nicely turned shafts. Some of the pieces were probably inserted in wooden handles. These "forks" could very well have served to stretch wide wound openings in the removal of arrowheads, etc. (cf. Celsus VII, 5). They closely resemble items in the British Museum believed to have been used for this purpose.[2]

2. A simple probe (no. 1384; l. 0.073 m.; fig. 2). The shape of the piece somewhat resembles a probe in the British Museum (cf. L. J. Bliquez, "Greek and Roman Medicine," *Archaeology*, 34 [1981], 17), and one in Mainz (cf. J. Hassel, Ernst Künzl, "Ein römisches Arztgrab des 3. Jahrhunderts n. Chr. aus Kleinasien," *Medizinhistorisches Journal*, Band 15 (1980), 408, Taf. III, no. 10). Both date to the Roman Empire.

3. A spatula (no. 1385; l. 0.141 m.; fig. 3). Very likely there was an olivary enlargement on the broken end. The type is exceedingly common throughout antiquity (cf., e.g., Milne, 58–61 and Pls. XII–XIII).

4. Knife (no. 1386; l. 0.102 m.; fig. 4). A piece of great interest. It probably served as a lancet or phlebotome. While its particular triangular shape does not resemble that of any surviving Roman phlebotome, such angular designs are familiar from the manuscripts of Albucasis.[3] For this reason the piece most likely is Byzantine, although Professor Davidson could not exclude the possibility that it is Roman.

5. Bronze instruments of unknown purpose (nos. 1387–1390; l. 0.107–0.09 m.; fig. 5). These are peculiar pieces in that the blades or spatulas are split at the ends. Decor consists of incised lines and circles and elaborately turned handles.

6. Bronze handle (no. 1391; l. 0.077 m.; fig. 6). On such a sturdy, well turned handle a medicament spoon or large spatula might have been mounted (cf. Milne, Pl. XIX, nos. 1–3).

B.   A second group of objects to consider was once a part of the collection of the Russian Baron Ustinov and is believed to have come from Palestine and/or Syria. S. Holth, believing that most of these objects were surgical instruments, purchased them in Oslo in 1918/19, and, after studying them, published his findings in *Skrifter utgit av Videnscapsselskapet i Kristiania*, 1919 (I Matematisk-Naturvidenskabelig Klasse), 3–20 + Pls., I–IV. Altogether, Holth acquired thirty-five objects plus a balance or steelyard. Of these pieces some, he concluded, were Greco-Roman or even modern; these need not occupy us. There were also, however, a number of pieces which differed in shape and decor from Greco-Roman tools. These are:

1. Four bronze spoon spatulas (nos. 11–14; l. 15.8–7.5 cm.) decorated with twined patterns of an oriental character. One (no. 11) actually carries an inscription in Arabic, Atiʿakāb, a Palmyrene proper name—apparently that of the owner or maker.

2. Six bronze double sounds with handles, square in section, centered at midshaft (nos. 16–21; l. 15.8–7.3 cm.).

3. A bronze remnant believed by Holth to be the handle for a cataract needle (no. 23; l. 7.5 cm.).

4. A silver knife handle (no. 35; l. 9.7 cm.; fig. 7). This piece features what look to be hunting scenes on both sides, and on both sides an inscription: Θές με, κλέπτα ("Put me down, thief!") and κῦριν ἔχω ("I have a master already!")[4]

Holth argued that the hunting scenes are not good evidence that the piece was a hunting knife. At 9.7 cm. it is too small for that purpose but is of the proper size for a scalpel handle; and like so many surviving Greco-Roman scalpel handles it has lost its blade which, being of steel, has now rusted away.

---

[2] Cf. L. J. Bliquez, "Greek and Roman Medicine," *Archaeology*, 34 (1981), 17; J. S. Milne, *Surgical Instruments in Greek and Roman Times* (repr. New York, 1970) (hereafter Milne), 83 and Pl. XXII.

[3] Cf. M. S. Spink and G. L. Lewis, *Albucasis on Surgery and Instruments* (Berkeley, 1973), chap. 46, figs. 88–90.

[4] Holth would restore κῦρι[ο]ν and suggests (p.12) that the absence of ο shows that the engraver may not have been a Greek. The form κῦρις is, however, attested: cf., e.g., Theophanes, *Chronographia*, ed. C. de Boor, (Leipzig, 1883), I, 673, 3, ὁ κῦρις Βουλγαρίας.

The letters of the inscription could be as early as the third century but they could also be later.

In short, we seem to have here a number of pieces which postdate the Roman Empire. In my experience some instruments of the classical period from the outer reaches of the Empire have a provincial air,[5] but Holth's pieces are rather more exotic. If, then, they are later, they must be Byzantine (especially the knife) or early Islamic. If the former, they will not be later than the seventh century, when Syria and Palestine were lost to the Arabs.

C. Finally, a number of objects in Cairo may be relevant. These consist of fifty-six pieces in the Coptic Museum, forty-three of them having been donated by Dr. Henri Amin Awad, who kindly called my attention to them and sent on photographs. Dr. Awad believes that these pieces qualify as Byzantine surgical instruments, and will soon set forth his views in a study which he is currently preparing on surgical instruments found on Egyptian soil. The collection in the Coptic Museum contains a rich variety of tools, including what appear to be probes (?), scoops and spoons, a chisel, scrapers, forceps, spatulas, a pair of shears, a retractor (?), and a container, perhaps for medicaments. Types vary considerably: some objects closely resemble pieces produced in the Roman Empire (for example, no. 3 below), some resemble pieces from Byzantine Corinth (for example, no. 4), some are similar to pieces published by Holth (no. 5), and still others are sui generis. A number of pieces are attractively turned and decorated with stamped or incised lines, concentric circles (already familiar from Corinth), and finials in the form of birds and the cross. I can supply no measurements, nor am I certain that all the pieces are of bronze. Some of the more interesting of these pieces are:

1. A probe (?) (no. 5219; fig. 8) decorated with stamped or incised circles on its shaft and surmounted by a cross.

2. A small chisel (no. 5009; fig. 9).

3. A "cyathiscomele" (no. 7278) which resembles many such pieces produced by the Romans.

4. A knife (no. 5759; fig. 10) rather like the triangular piece from Corinth (no. A, 4 above). It ap-

pears to have a three-pronged retractor at its other end. For a double retractor cf. R. Caton, "Notes on a Group of Medical and Surgical Instruments Found near Kolophon," *JHS*, 34 (1914), 115, IV and Pl. X, no. 16.

5. Eight double probes? (one bears the number 5240, the rest belong to the Awad collection) resembling six similar pieces published by Holth (cf. B, 2 above).

6. A gouge? (no. 1212; fig. 11) with a nicely turned shaft and a finial in the shape of a bird or cock.

7. A medicament container in the shape of a fish decorated with what appear to be floral motifs (Awad Collection).

8. Two probes (?) surmounted by finials in the shape of birds, one bird decorated with circles (fig. 12; Awad Collection).

Dr. Awad also calls my attention to what appears to be a probe with a finial in the shape of a cross in the Museum of Islamic Art, Cairo. I have no other information on this piece.

This is the material evidence for Byzantine surgery of which I am aware. It will be seen at once that without further discoveries, the material evidence surviving from the Byzantine period is not abundant. And, since it is so far impossible to demonstrate that many of these pieces are in fact surgical tools, or in some cases that they are even Byzantine, the evidence may even be called meager. This is disappointing in view of the rich survival of instruments of the Roman Empire. We must remember, however, that where the Roman Empire is concerned, we owe our good fortune to the practice which prevailed then of burying deceased physicians with their instrumentaria. Were it not for this practice (and for the chance eruption of Vesuvius in 79 A.D. which preserved the instruments in Pompeii), we would probably have very few instruments from the Roman Empire as well, and their function as surgical tools might also be disputed. It is worthwhile noting that among the Greeks of the Classical Period it was not the custom to bury instruments with the dead physician, as it apparently was not among the Byzantines. Thus, as there are few remaining instruments from Byzantine times, so also there are none known to me (with the exception of a few bleeding cups) from the age of Hippocrates, and few if any survivals from the fourth century B.C. and the ensuing Hellenistic Pe-

[5] See, e.g., L. J. Bliquez, "Roman Surgical Instruments in the Johns Hopkins University Institute of the History of Medicine," *BHM*, 56 (1982), 197–202.

riod.[6] Perhaps, then, we should be grateful for such Byzantine remains as there are.

In any case, if it be conceded that a number of the objects presented here were employed by Byzantines as surgical tools (and I for one believe this), then we at least have a few samples from various times and locations.[7] Based on these pieces it appears that in some cases Roman types and shapes were closely adhered to, even into the twelfth century, whereas in still other cases local preferences in shape and decor prevailed to a much greater degree than in Roman times. Perhaps factors like the looser composition of the Byzantine empire and its short life in some areas account for the variations.

II

If the material remains do not amount to much, neither, as I have stated, is one particularly impressed with the literary treatment of surgery by Paul's successors. For neither in the texts of the great handbook names nor in the pages of lesser authors is there anything to equal Paul's sixth book. For example, although Theophanes Nonnus deals with countless conditions in the medical encyclopedia which he composed in the tenth century, he has little to say about surgery, aside from references to cupping and bloodletting. Of the most significant authors of the eleventh century, Michael Psellus supplies only a few items of interest in his dictionary of diseases, in his medical poem in 1,373 trimeters, or in his other works; and Symeon Seth confines himself to investigating the properties of foods and herbs in his most important contribution. Finally, while John Actuarius in the fourteenth century wrote voluminously, he will be remembered far longer for his acute knowledge of the properties of human waste products than for anything he had to tell us about the surgical art.

Of all Byzantine medical authorities, the only one who supplies any extensive information about sur-

gery is the ninth-century figure Leon, the Learned Physician (ἰατροσοφιστής). In his *Epitome of Medicine*[8] there can be found references to over forty operations, and approximately fifteen surgical instruments and parasurgical items.

However, Leon almost never enters into any detail as to the actual mechanics of a particular operation; often enough he is content merely to mention in passing that conditions like hydrocele, cirsocele and various eye complaints are dealt with διὰ χειρουργίας.[9] The same lack of attention to detail usually prevails when Leon refers to the actual instruments used in operations. For example, when the name of a specific tool within a class is desired, he often supplies only the generic term, for instance, καυτήρ as opposed to τριαινοειδὲς καυτήριον (Paul 6.48), μαχαιρωτὸς καυτήρ (Paul 6.42), πυρηνοειδὲς καυτήριον (Paul 6.25), γαμμοειδὲς καυτήριον (Paul 6.62), μηνοειδὲς καυτήριον (Paul 6.57), etc.[10] Furthermore, Leon's surgery seems limited. Although he is willing to operate for tonsils, gangrenous uvula, the usual eye conditions, tumors, cysts, hemorrhoids, and fistula, and quite ready to cup and bleed for headache and female complaints, it is noteworthy that he does not mention surgery as a remedy for the treatment of empyema or bladder stone; and he is remarkably silent in other areas. He says nothing of the more adventuresome operations which appear in the Roman Empire and the Early Byzantine Period—mastectomy for example. He does not treat of weapons or tooth extraction or bone surgery or trephination or amputation of any type. Moreover, to read Leon one would think that all Byzantine women gave birth with ease, as he has no comment at all on problems which might confront the physician in this sphere. It cannot be argued that Leon does not discuss these topics because he disapproved of surgery as a remedy for them. In section III, xxi, for example, he asserts that prophysis or symphysis of the eyelids is incurable, although some dare to operate for it. Clearly Leon sees no point to surgery for these conditions; the point is, he mentions it as an option exercised by some, nevertheless.

In short, although there is much to interest the student of surgery in Leon's *Epitome*, the fact remains that Leon simply pales in the presence of

---

[6] See E. Künzl, J. Hassel and S. Künzl, "Medizinische Instrumente aus Sepulkralfunden der römischen Kaiserzeit, *BJb*, 182 (1982), 125–26. V. Lambrinoudakis may have recovered some pieces of the classical period in the shrine of Apollo Maleatas; see his Ἱερὸν Μαλεάτου Ἀπόλλωνος εἰς Ἐπίδαυρον, Πρακτ.Ἀρχ.Ἐτ., 1975:1, p. 175 with pl. 149; and Ἀνασκαφὴ στὸ ἱερὸ τοῦ Ἀπόλλωνος Μαλεάτα, Πρακτ.Ἀρχ.Ἐτ., 1976:1, p. 209 with pl. 148.

[7] I favor especially the probe and lancet from Corinth (A, 2 and 4 above) and the scalpel (B, 4 above) published by Holth. It is premature to pronounce on the pieces in Cairo.

[8] I have used the text in Ermerins.

[9] III, xl, xli; VI, xii, xiv.

[10] An exception: συριγγιακὸς καυτήρ (III, xxi).

Paul, his predecessor of two centuries before; and, as I have said, there is no other commanding literary presence in the field of surgery after Leon. Since, then, there seem to be few survivals of the surgical instruments used by Byzantine χειρουργοί, and since later Byzantine medical literature dealing with surgery is not nearly as impressive as earlier Byzantine work on the subject, one might be tempted to conclude that the state of surgery actually declined in the Byzantine world as time passed.[11] Fortunately, two documents which have previously received only limited attention now acquire considerable importance. As it turns out they are the best, if not the sole evidence, that this was not the case.

III

By chance, the documents to which I refer each contain a list of surgical instruments and paraphernalia. The oldest of the two lists, Codex Parisinus Latinus 11219, dates to the ninth century. Following the heading "Incipiunt ferramentorum nomina. Necesse est universorum ferramentorum nomina dicere ita," it supplies in some remarkably barbaric Latin spellings the names of sixty-six instruments, all of them Greek save two.[12] The more recent list occurs on Laurentianus gr. LXXIV 2, a manuscript of the eleventh century. After the title ὀνόματα τῶν ἰατρικῶν ἐργαλείων κατὰ στοιχεῖον ἃ ἐν ταῖς χειρουργίαις χρώμεθα it provides (in more or less alphabetical order) eighty-nine entries, all in Greek. Both of these lists were published together for informational and comparative purposes by Hermann Schöne in 1903.[13] At that time Schöne did not inquire into the origins of either list. He merely stated his opinion that they derived from independent sources because, although both often name the same instruments, in many cases one list gives the diminutive while the other does not; and of course there are numerous instances in which one list supplies a name omitted by the other. For our purposes, however, it is necessary to speculate on the circumstances under which these lists might have been created and perpetuated, and the time when this occurred.

Lists of surgical instruments and attendant par-

aphernalia in Greek can be found at least as early as Pollux (second century A.D.),[14] and lists or glosses in Latin at least as early as Isidor of Seville (ca. 560–636).[15] These lists, however, are nowhere near as comprehensive (Pollux, twenty-two names;[16] Isidore, 12[17]) as those being considered; furthermore, they do not exist independently, but are included in works on a variety of subjects circulated under the name of an author. Schöne's lists, on the other hand, have about them the air of simple inventories or checklists detailing the surgical apparatus respectable medical establishments might be expected to have on hand. For example, they seem perfectly at home in the carefully detailed atmosphere of establishments like the famous hospital of the Pantocrator monastery, the *Typikon* of which enumerates the interesting responsibilities of the ἀκονητής or "sharpener":

> He must keep clean all of the surgical instruments which are stored in the ξενών and used for operations on the sick. For there will always be stored in the ξενών itself lancets, cauterizing irons, a catheter, a tooth forceps, instruments for the stomach and head, and in short those (instruments) necessary for all operations. Furthermore, there shall always be on hand bronze wash basins of every type in which the physicians can wash themselves after treating the patients in a manner suitable to the care of each.[18]

In view of the affinity between Schöne's lists and this passage from the *Typikon*, I suggest that these documents may have originated as checklists on the basis of which functionaries like the ἀκονητής secured and maintained the surgical equipment of Byzantine hospitals and clinics.

As it now stands, the list in Latin letters is probably no more than the bookish compilation of someone in the West who tried to assemble the names and (less successfully) proper transliterations ("necesse est . . . dicere ita") of as many ("universorum") instruments as he could.[19] His list,

[11] This may be the view of Mario Tabanelli, who in his *Studi sulla Chirurgia Bizantina* (Florence, 1964) confines himself to Paul.
[12] *Acus, auriscalpium.*
[13] "Zwei Listen Chirurgischer Instrumente," *Hermes*, 38 (1903), 280–84.

[14] See *Onomasticon* 10, 149 (Bekker edition); see also St. John Climacus, *Liber ad pastorem*, PG, 88, cols, 1168–1169.
[15] *Etymologiarum*, IV, XI, 1–7.
[16] σμίλη, ὑπογραφίς, ὠτογλυφίς, ψαλίς, μηλωτρίς, μήλη, ὀδοντοξέστης, ὀδοντάγρα, ἐξάλειπτρον, λουτήριον, σικύα, ὑπόθετον, λεκανίς, σπογγία, ἐπίδεσμα, σπληνίον, λαμπάδιον, ποδοστράβη, κλυστήρ, βάλανος, ῥάκια, κηρωτή.
[17] *Phlebotomum, smiliaria, angistrum, spatomele, guva, cucurbita, ventosa, clistere, pila, pilum, mortarium, coticula.*
[18] P. Gautier, "Le Typikon du Christ Sauveur Pantocrator," 1270–1280, in *REB*, 32 (1974), 1–145 (see 105).
[19] I had entertained the notion that the Latin list had in some way to do with the foundation or improvement and maintenance of the surgical instrumentarium for a hospital or clinic in

however, obviously depends on a Greek original which, like the eleventh-century list and its antecedents, very probably had a practical (ἃ ἐν ταῖς χειρουργίαις χρώμεθα) end in view. Thus my suggestion that both lists originated as checklists in Byzantine times.

To support this position we must ask when Schöne's lists were first compiled, assuming that both are copies of earlier documents. In view of their extensive detail it is clear that they must be later than Pollux and Isidore. A more significant point is that, between them, the two lists attest to approximately thirty-two names which, to the best of my knowledge, are not found in Paul or before.[20] Of these thirty-two names, nine occur in both lists, nineteen only in the Greek list, and four only in the Latin list. Now a few new terms might not amount to much, but the occurrence of thirteen new names in the Latin list seems to me to constitute reasonably strong grounds for contending that its original was created well after Paul's time; and this is even more obvious in the case of the Greek list, which features twenty-eight new names. It is quite probable then that these lists date to well into the Byzantine period and are not copied from classical originals. So, in terms of their chronology at least, nothing prevents the lists from being associated with Byzantine hospitals.

The most important consideration, however, is this. Whether the lists have anything to do with hospitals or not, unless—contrary to received opinion—the Byzantine medical profession was given over to antiquarian pursuits, the very fact that lists of surgical gear were being copied out by Byzantines in the ninth to eleventh centuries should mean that their contents were then important in a practical sense, that is, that the items detailed in the lists were actually in use (ἃ . . . χρώμεθα) at the time each was composed. If this is true, then it must also be the case that if there existed in the ninth to eleventh centuries instruments which were employed for operations centuries earlier, the same operations must also have been performed for the

most part in this period. To be sure, this is less certain in cases where a generic instrument is attested, for example, μαχαίριον or scalpel, since this type of instrument was used in any number of surgical procedures. In the case of specific types, however, such as ἀντιοτόμον (tonsil knife), ἐμβρυοτόμον (embryo knife), λιθοτόμον (bladder stone knife), πτερυγοτόμον (pterygium knife), σταφυλοτόμον (uvula knife), συριγγοτόμον (fistula knife), βλεφαροτόμον (eyelid knife), and κατιάς (a type of phlebotome), we are on a firmer ground; and a significant number of the instruments on the lists are of this type. Thus, as I have stated, Schöne's lists are a tremendously important factor in determining the state of surgery in the ninth to eleventh centuries; for they show, as Leon, Theophanes Nonnus, Michael Psellus, and Symeon Seth do not, just how enterprising the surgeons of the Middle Byzantine Period were, at least in some places at some times.

And indeed the lists offer a full repertoire of surgical tools. As previously noted, there are knives of all types: special models for excision of polyp, tonsil, uvula, pterygium, and fistula, in addition to colorless generic names like μαχαίριον or σμίλη. And there are listed the λιθοτόμον or knife for excision of bladder stone, and surgical scissors. Probes abound on the lists, which feature, in addition to the generic term μήλη, specific types such as those with double olivary enlargement, the ear probe and the spatula probe. There are retractors and various needles; the tongue depressor is mentioned. There are forceps of all types, those for eye work, those for gripping various types of tissue, and heavy-duty models for bone and teeth. There are all sorts of other bone and tooth instruments listed: drills, trephines, saws, chisels, guards, levers, files, scalers, and impellents for weapons extraction. One could be as easily purged to distraction in the ninth to eleventh centuries as in the time of Oribasius, since clysters occur on the lists in profusion; and all the specialized tubes needed for drainage and extraction are attested—for instance, the cannula and the pus extractor. Byzantine mothers in difficult labor who were ignored by Leon could hope for some assistance at the appearance of an ἰατρός equipped, as the lists direct, with uterine dilators, various specula, embryo hooks, the cranioclast, and special bodkins and knives for the destruction and excision of an impacted fetus. In addition to various accoutrements and aids to surgery, the lists also provide approximately twenty-five names of objects whose identity is doubtful. In some cases names appear to be hopelessly corrupted. In the cases

---

the West. Owing to the skillful arguments of Prof. Baader, I have abandoned this view.

[20] ἀντιβολάδιον / *antiboladium*, ἀντόπτρα, ἀ⟨πο⟩ξυστήρ, βλεφαροτόμον, βούγλωσσον, γραμμιστήρ / *grammister*, ἐθειρόλογος, ἐντε⟨ρο⟩φύλαξ, ἐπικρούστιον, κέστρος / *cestros*, καυλοκλυστήρ, κυνορράφιον, λεπτάριον, λεπτομήλη, μασχαλολαβεύς / *mascalolabeos*, μητρανύκτης, ὀστεγχύτης, ὀσταναλαβεύς, ὀφθαλμοστατήρ / *ostalmostater*, παραστολεύς / *parastoleus*, περιλαβεύς / *peribabeos*, πλευροπριστήρ / *pliroprister*, πρασία / *prasia*, ῥινοσπάθιον, σκυθομήλη, σκηνορράφιον, σταφυλολαβίς, ὑπερβιβαστήρ, *epibastes*, *cefaloclases*, *deltarium*, *ostanaboleos*.

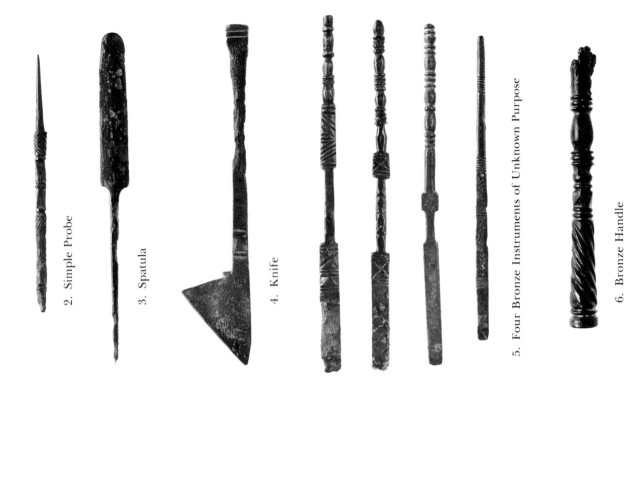

2. Simple Probe

3. Spatula

4. Knife

5. Four Bronze Instruments of Unknown Purpose

6. Bronze Handle

Surgical Instruments from Corinth

1. Seven Bifurcated Instruments

Corinth Museum (American School of Classical Studies)

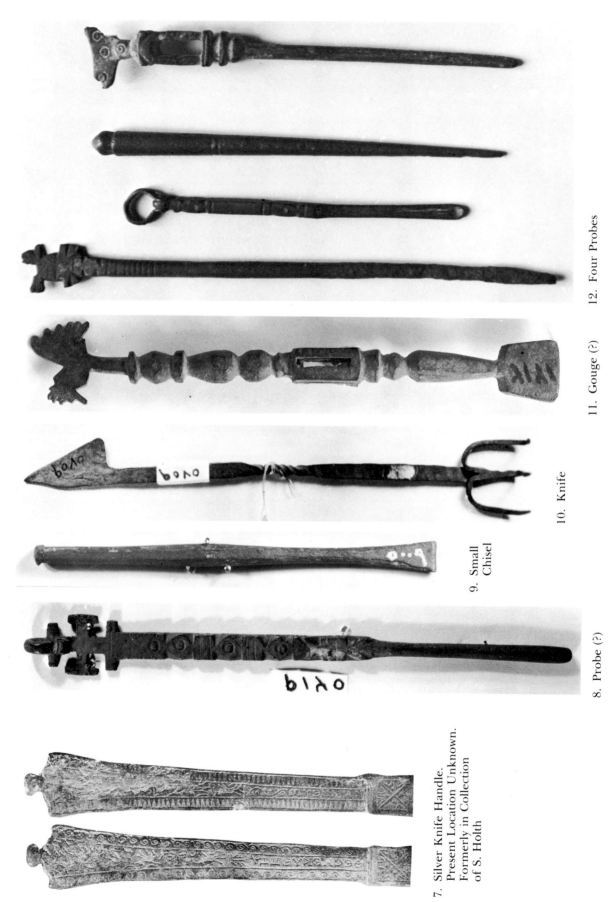

7. Silver Knife Handle. Present Location Unknown. Formerly in Collection of S. Holth

8. Probe (?)

9. Small Chisel

10. Knife

11. Gouge (?)

12. Four Probes

Cairo, Coptic Museum. Surgical Instruments from Egypt

where they are not corrupted, we can sometimes make a good guess as to the identity of an instrument (see Appendix I below). In sum, the lists detail almost every instrument known to Paul and his predecessors—with two remarkable exceptions. Nowhere is there any reference to the bleeding cup, and it is likely that the cautery too is omitted. Certainly the generic καυτήρ or καυτήριον does not occur in the case of the latter. Possibly dubious terms like βούγλωσσον (instrument shaped like an ox tongue), *deltarium* (delta-shaped instrument?) or *fenicus* (if = a wedge-shaped cautery attested by Hippocrates) refer to cauterizing instruments; but we cannot know. If no cauteries are attested, as certainly seems to be the case with bleeding cups, that is indeed cause for surprise. Perhaps the lists do not contain such instruments because they were too common to deserve mention. In any case, their existence in this period cannot be doubted because they are abundantly attested in other sources.[21]

To repeat, the two lists we have discussed are the firmest evidence at hand that most of the major surgical tools employed by Paul and his predecessors (and therefore most of the operations for which they were employed) were in use from at least the Macedonian dynasty through the Comneni. It appears, therefore, that the state of surgery did not decline significantly in the Middle Byzantine Period. It may be that in some respects it even advanced a bit. Certainly the surgeons of the capital did not seem reluctant to undertake operations previously unattested. One such spectacular operation took place in the tenth century when, in the reign of Constantine VII Porphyrogenitus, Siamese (actually Armenian) twins connected at the upper abdomen were separated after one of them had died. The operation was not a success, however, as the remaining twin died three days later.[22]

But it is probably unwise to conclude that there was any significant change in the state of surgery. My feeling is that things probably stayed about the same as in Paul's time; so, there was no subsequent author among later Byzantines to eclipse him.[23] For this reason the critical acumen of one Nicetas, who sometime between the ninth and early twelfth centuries extracted from the surgical chapters of

Paul and a few of his predecessors, is to be commended.[24] Only the lists, however, show to what extent all the operations detailed in Paul were still practiced.

It is commonly said that in the sciences the Byzantines originated little but passed on a great deal. If so, my own investigation into Byzantine surgery seems to bear out this conclusion.

IV

A few final observations on the conditions under which surgery was practiced in Byzantine times are in order.

It appears that dissection of the human body was practiced continuously, so that surgeons were directly acquainted with the anatomy. [St. Eustathius of Antioch] attests to the practice in the fourth century, noting that the bodies of condemned criminals were used for the purpose.[25] There is one grim account of actual vivisection in the reign of Constantine V Copronymus. Under the year 765 Theophanes chronicles the arrest of one Christianus, prince of the Scamari, who (apparently for religious deviations) was given over to physicians who dissected him alive on the mole of St. Thomas in the capital.[26] Finally, autopsies performed by physicians on corpses are mentioned by St. Symeon the New Theologian around the turn of the eleventh century, and George Tornices describes them in the twelfth.[27] It is doubtful that these exercises resulted in new knowledge about the human anatomy; at least so one gathers from the anatomical treatises that survive from the Byzantine Period. On the other hand, if, as I argue, Byzantine surgery did not slide backwards, I think it very likely that autopsy was a key factor in preventing decline. Contrast the situation in the Latin West, where autopsy was abandoned and where the decline of surgery through the Middle Ages is well known.[28]

---

[21] See Appendix II below, *s.vv.* καυτήρ, σικύα.

[22] See G. E. Pentagalos and J. G. Lascaratos, "A Surgical Operation Performed on Siamese Twins during the Tenth Century in Byzantium," *BHM*, 58 (1984), 99–102.

[23] And of course the Persians and Arabs, who were influenced by the Greeks, owed much to Paul but not later Byzantine surgeons.

[24] F. Kudlien may have had the last word. He argues for the tenth century; *Die handschriftliche Überlieferung des Galenkommentars zu Hippokrates, De articulis* (Berlin, 1960), 11 ff.

[25] [Eustathius], Spuria, *Comment. in Hexaemeron*, PG, 18, cols. 788–789.

[26] Theophanes, *Chronographia* (ed. C. de Boor [Leipzig, 1883], I:436, 16–21.

[27] Syméon le Noveau Théologien, *Traités théologiques et éthiques*, ed. J. Darrouzès (Paris, 1967), vol. 2, 138–40; Georges et Demetrios Tornikès, *Lettres et discours*, ed. J. Darrouzès (Paris, 1970), 225. I am indebted to Prof. Alexander Kazhdan for these references.

[28] A. Kazhdan and I will disucss these passages and the conclusions drawn from them more fully in a future issue of the *Bulletin of the History of Medicine*.

For those who had lost limbs it is clear that artificial substitutes were available, as was the case in the Classical Period.[29] Whether these limbs amounted to more than peg legs and hooks for hands is not certain; but, as the Byzantines were clever workmen, it seems quite possible that some of their artificial productions would have been not only functional, but fashioned to resemble the lost part.[30]

Although modern antiseptics were of course unavailable, Byzantine surgeons seem to have attempted to observe elementary rules of sanitation, donning aprons and towels for operations and employing sponges and tepid water in the course of them. Care was also taken to see that operations were conducted in favorable temperatures.[31]

There are frequent testimonia to operations performed in public, the physicians creating a kind of operating theater out of the attending crowd. Various motives are adduced for this practice. St. John Damascene thought that the physicians were anxious to demonstrate how science overcomes disease;[32] John the Faster speculated that the onlookers might be moved to contrition by observing the sufferings of others;[33] and St. John Chrysostom asserted that by witnessing the misfortunes of others we might become inclined to protect our own health, in particular our spiritual health.[34] St. John Chrysostom appears himself to have been particularly inspired by such spectacles, as he leaves behind the most detailed description of them; and he gives good reason for supposing that general anesthesia was no more widely used in his time than it had been earlier.[35] "At these operations," he says, "you can see the flesh being cut, the blood flowing, gangrene being removed; and one has to endure a good deal of unpleasantness arising from the spectacle and a good deal of pain and grief, not only from the sight of the wounds but also from the suffering of those being cauterized and cut. For no one is so made of stone that, as he stands by those undergoing these operations and hears their cries (ὀλολυζόντων), he does not break down, feel troubled, and become despondent in his soul."[36]

As the surgical gear of the Classical Period is remarkable for the aesthetic care lavished on it, so too such surviving Byzantine tools as appear to have been used for surgical purposes are, in many instances, carefully turned, decorated with various motifs, and are sometimes made of precious metals. In the second century the satirist Lucian of Samosata complained that quacks enticed the naive with such fancy equipment;[37] but for competent physicians, there must be another explanation. In a period when there were few antiseptics and little if any anesthesia, all surgery—no matter how accomplished the surgeon—must have been extremely painful and downright dangerous. Attractive instruments must have helped surgeons as they attempted to inspire confidence in their patients, just as nowadays we relax a little when the dentist has one of those new "painless" drills. We can therefore be thankful that, however advanced surgery had become in the time of Paul of Aegina and his successors, we ourselves have the good fortune to live in modern times.

University of Washington

[29] See R. Guillard, *Correspondance de Nicéphore Grégoras* (Paris 1927), 193.

[30] At least one such limb survived classical antiquity, the famous Capua leg of ca. 300 B.C. Unfortunately, it was destroyed in 1941 when the Museum of the Royal College of Surgeons in London was bombed. See W. R. Brunn, "Der Stelzfuss von Capua und die antiken Prothesen," *SA*, 18 (1926), 351–60 and L. J. Bliquez, "Classical Prosthetics," *Archaeology* (1983) 25–29.

[31] St. John Climacus, *Liber ad pastorem*, PG, 88, col. 1169; Διήγησις τῶν θαυμάτων τοῦ ἁγίου ᾿Αρτεμίου (*apud* A. Papadopoulos-Kerameus, *Varia Graeca Sacra* (St. Petersburg, 1909), 41, 20; *idem* (ed.), ᾿Εξήγησις ἤτοι μαρτύριον τῶν ἁγίων πατέρων . . . , *Pravoslavnij Palestinskij Sbornik*, 19, 3 (1907), 31–32.

[32] *Sacra parallela*, PG, 96, col. 121.

[33] *Sermo de poenitentia*, PG, 88, col. 1973.

[34] *Ecloga de adversa valetudine at medicis*, Homil. XIII, PG, 63, col. 656.

[35] See Celsus VII, Prooemium, 4, and Hippocrates, *Haem.* 2, both of whom mention the cries of the patients.

[36] *In paralyticum demissum per tectum*, PG, 51, col. 55.

[37] *Ind.* 29; cf. also St. John Damascene (*Sacra parallela*, PG, 96, col. 61), who may have Lucian in mind.

APPENDICES[38]

APPENDIX I

NOTES ON SCHÖNE'S LISTS

When Schöne published the two lists together in 1903 he wished merely to present the names which they contained and to correct spellings, sometimes using one list against the other for this purpose. He did not attempt to identify the names on the list with putatively surgical instruments which had been recovered from excavations and chance finds, but specifically left this work to others. In 1907, there appeared the standard work on Greco-Roman surgical gear, J. S. Milne's *Surgical Instruments in Greek and Roman Times*. In his book Milne attempted to match surviving objects with names and descriptions in Greek and Roman medical texts from Hippocrates to Paul. However, not every name for the instruments of the Classical and Early Byzantine Periods can be found in Milne; and of course Milne made no attempt to collect the terms used in later Byzantine times. It seems worthwhile, therefore, to provide here information about those items on the lists which are not included in Milne, or about which some comment is warranted for one reason or another. I do this following the order of the names in Schöne's publication.

While no name ever occurs twice on either of the lists, it does appear that in a few cases two different names for the same instrument can be found.[39] These instances, however, are few in number. Therefore, in attempting to identify a name, I have generally assumed (unless I had good reason to believe otherwise) that it does not duplicate other items on its list.

ἄγκιστρα / angistrum
Milne certainly includes the term, identifying it as a sharp hook or retractor, many examples of which survive (see App. II below, *s.v.*). Noteworthy here is the fact that the eleventh-century list uses the plural, probably because these tools were so often used in quantity that they were frequently referred to in the plural (cf., e.g., Paul 6.35, 37, 39). Cf. also ῥαφίδες below.

ἀκμάδιον
The name was dubious to Schöne, who seems to have entertained ἀκονάδιον or "little whetstone," the emendation of Dietz, a previous editor. But Ps.-Moses (M.

Bertholt, *Collection des anciens alchimistes grecs* [Paris, 1888], p. 39 B) attests to ἀκμάδιον as a conical crucible; and, as there are a number of parasurgical items on the lists (e.g., πύαλος, *incliridium*), this interpretation is preferable to an emendation which is, as far as I can see, completely unattested in the literature.

ἀντιβολάδιον / antiboladium
Otherwise unattested. That the term is a diminutive of ἀντίβολον (= copy, transcript), from ἀντιβολέω, is impossible. Very likely it derives from ἀντιβάλλω, which occurs in Palladius, *in Hip. Fract.* 12.285c (in R. Charterius, *Hippocratis et Galeni Opera*, Vol. XII [Paris, 1679]) in the sense of "put back protruding bone." Thus the instrument would be a type of bone lever; cf. ἀναβολεύς, μοχλίσκος, App. II below, *s.vv.*

ἀντιοτόμον / antiothomum
A tonsil knife, see Galen (ed. Kühn), 14.785.

ἀντόπτρα
Otherwise unattested. All similar terms have to do with instruments used to dilate the rectum and the female genitals, e.g., διόπτρα, κατοπτήρ. I have not encountered the latter in a Byzantine text, so perhaps it was replaced by ἀντόπτρα; cf. διαστολεύς below.

ἀ⟨πο⟩ξυστήρ
Otherwise unattested. A type of raspatory, cf. περιξυστήρ below.

βλεφαροτόμον
Otherwise unattested. Obviously a small scalpel for work on the eyelid. Very likely therefore the ἀναρραφικὸν σμιλίον, which is attested for work on a variety of eye conditions, but does not occur in the lists (see App. II below, *s.v.*)

βούγλωσσον
Otherwise unattested. LSJ would make it a tongue depressor, but the name is equally suggestive of other instruments (e.g., a cautery) and the γλωσσοκάτοχος or tongue depressor is already included on the eleventh-century list.

γραμμιστήρ / grammister
Otherwise unattested. Galen (ed. Kühn), 2.673 uses the word γραμμή in the sense of the edge of a knife, so a kind of scalpel could be meant. But, more likely than not, we have here an instrument for making a line, a γράφιον therefore or stylus. These were used for various surgical procedures (see Milne, 72–73).

διαστολεύς
For Milne (81–82, 150) this term meant only uterine dilator or vaginal speculum. Paul, however, clearly intends by διαστολεύς a rectal speculum (6.78); and, since this is the only other occurrence of the word which I have encountered in a Byzantine text, I believe that is what we should understand here.

ἐθειρόλογος
Otherwise unattested. A tweezer for plucking hairs

---

[38] In the appendices the following abbreviations and editions have been used: Galen = ed. Kühn, cited by volume and page; Orib. = ed. Raeder, *Oribasii Collectionum Medicarum*; Aetius = ed. A. Olivieri, *Libri Medicinales* V–VIII; Psellus, Ποίημα ἰατρικόν, in Ideler, I, 203 ff.; Michael Italicus, *loc. cit.* = Michel Italikos, *Lettres et discours*, ed. P. Gautier (Paris, 1972), p. 114, ll. 20–25; M–S = T. Meyer-Steineg. *Chirurgische Instrumente des Altertums* (Jena, 1912); S (9th and 11th) = The ninth and eleventh century lists edited by H. Schöne (see note 13 above); *Varia Graeca Sacra* (see note 31 above); *Typikon* (see note 18 above). For the editions of Paul and Leon, see notes 1 and 8 above.

[39] ἐθειρόλογος—τριχολάβον (epilation tweezer), ὀστanalaβεύς—ὀστάγρα (bone forceps).

(ἔθειρα), probably in treatment of granular ophthalmia. If so, the instrument is the same as the τριχολάβον which is also included in the eleventh-century list.

ἐνετήρ
Widely attested as a type of clyster: see Cassius Felix 48; Alexander Trall. 8.2; Severus, περὶ ἐνετήρων (title); Stephanus, *In Galenum, in Hippocratem* 1.331 D.

ἐντε⟨ρο⟩φύλαξ
Otherwise unattested. An analogy is provided by the μηνιγγοφύλαξ, an instrument generally used to protect membranes during surgical operations on bone (see Milne, 126 and Pl. XL, 3) Thus, the present piece should be some sort of plate which, to judge by its name, was especially designed to protect the inner parts of the abdomen while, e.g., a rib was being sawed through. It is worthwhile noting that Paul mentions sawing operations on ribs (6.77, 96), though he only mentions the μηνιγγοφύλαξ in connection with them. It should also be noted that a special rib saw seems to have been developed by the Middle Byzantine Period (see πλευροπριστήρ below).

ἐπικρούστιον
Otherwise unattested. Perhaps a hammer (cf. ἐπικρουστήριον *s.v.* in the *Corpus Glossariorum Latinorum*) and indeed the hammer is not elsewhere attested on the lists. Very likely, however, we are dealing here with a type of phlebotome; cf. φλεβοτόμον ἐπικρουστικόν (Aetius 6.8) which may be the type of phlebotome figured in Milne, 35 and Pl. VIII, 3.

κέστωρ / cestros / κέστρος
Otherwise unattested as a surgical instrument. Entries in LSJ include a serrated tool for encaustic painting (Pliny, *N.H.* 25.84), a bolt shot from a catapult (Polyb. 27.11.1; Dion. Hal. 20.1.1) and roughness of the tongue (Hsch., *s.v.*). This seems therefore to be a shaftlike instrument with a roughened surface. Perhaps, then, it is a kind of file (although the file, ῥινοτορίνιον, is included on the lists) or even something like a screw probe, at least one sample of which survives and the name for which is unknown (see Milne, 68 and Pl. XXI, 5).

καυλοκλυστήρ
Otherwise unattested. Obviously a type of clyster. The noun καυλός may be descriptive of the instrument ("stem," "stalk"), or more probably of its function. Under the meanings of καυλός LSJ also lists the urethra, the penis itself, and the cervix. This instrument is therefore likely to be a clyster for irrigation of the genital passages.

κυνορράφιον
Otherwise unattested. Obviously a type of needle, cf. σκηνορράφιον, ῥαφίδες below. LSJ takes κυν- as = *frenum praeputii*. If so, a special needle for stitching the prepuce. Operations on the prepuce are described by Oribasius (50.3) and Paul (6.54), but no needle is mentioned.

λαβίς
Attested as a forceps in Hippocrates (*Steril.* 244) and Galen (ed. Kühn, 12.659). The former describes it as λεπτοτάτη and the latter uses it to extract objects which have fallen into the ear canal. So a small slender type of tweezers is meant.

λεπτάριον
Otherwise unattested. A small and slender instrument, to judge by its name. Some cauteries are called λεπτόν (see App. II below, *s.v.* καυτήρ) as is the λαβίς (above) and the λεπτομήλη (below). Unfortunately, the possibilities are too numerous for an intelligent guess.

λεπτομήλη
Otherwise unattested. The name indicates that it is a "fine probe," very likely of the type designated as ἀπυρηνομήλη, i.e., a simple shaft without the usual olivary enlargement.

μασχαλολαβεύς / mascalolabeos
Otherwise unattested. A type of forceps (λαβίς, -λάβον) for gripping the arm pit (μασχάλη) seems pointless. Some instruments of reduction were designed to support the arm pit (cf. App. II below, *s.vv.* ὕπερον, ἄμβη), and this may be what we are dealing with here.

μητρανύκτης
Otherwise unattested. Perhaps a speculum, but the διόπτρα already occurs on the eleventh-century list. I lean toward uterine dilator. διαστολεύς, which was one of the terms used for such an instrument in the classical period (see Milne, 81–82) does occur on the list but only, I think, in the sense of "rectal dilator" (see above). So perhaps this new term was evolved to identify the uterine dilator.

ὀξεῖα
Surely a scalpel; cf. Paul 6.86, ὀξεῖα σμίλη.

ὀξυλαβίδιον
The ὀξυλάβη is attested as a kind of tongs, cf. *Suda, s.v.* Ἥφαιστος. The present piece therefore would be a small forceps.

ὀδοντοξύστης / odontoxister
A tooth scaler; cf. Pollux IV, 181; Milne, 138.

ὀστεγχύτης
Otherwise unattested. On the analogy, of μητρεγχύτης and *otemquites* (see App. II below, *s.vv.*). The name should mean "bone irrigator" rather than an "irrigator made of bone."

ὀσταναλαβεύς
Otherwise unattested. Apparently the same as ὀστάγρα ("bone forceps"), which also occurs on the eleventh-century list.

ὀφθαλμοστάτης / ostalmostater
Otherwise unattested. An eye instrument; an eyelid retractor? (see Paul 6.21; M–S, 41–42 and Taf. VIII, 6, 7).

παραστολεύς / parastoleus
Otherwise unattested. I suggest that a blunt hook or retractor (τυφλάγκιστρον) is meant on the basis of Galen (ed. Kühn), 2.523 (παραστέλλων τὴν γαστέρα) and Oribasius 45.6.6 (τυφλαγκίστροις μεγαλοκαμπέσι παραστέλλειν). The term τυφλάγκιστρον seems unattested after Paul, so perhaps παραστολεύς replaced it.

περιξύστης / perixister
Not in Milne, but elsewhere attested as a rugine for scraping bone; cf. e.g., Oribasius 46.11.29.

περιλαβεύς / peribabeos
Otherwise unattested. If not a forceps, perhaps an instrument of reduction.

πλευροπρίστηρ / pliroprister
Otherwise unattested. A rib saw. Ribs were sawed out in several operations (Paul 6.77, 88; Celsus VII, 4); see also ἐντεροφύλαξ above.

πολυ⟨πο⟩σφάκτης
Otherwise unattested. Possibly a knife to deal with polyp (cf. ἐμβρυοσφάκτης, App. II below, s.v.), but then the instrument would probably be the same as the ῥινοσπάθιον below. Another possibility is that the term = πολυποξύστης, a combination rugine/forceps for removal of polyp (see Milne, 93–94). This alternative is preferable because the πολυποξύστης does not occur elsewhere on the eleventh-century list, but does show up on the ninth-century list (olipoxister). So also LSJ.

πρασιά / prasia
Otherwise unattested. One can only guess. Many instruments draw their names from vegetables, fruits, etc., e.g., βάλανος, διπύρηνον, σικύα, φακωτός. If this instrument derives its name from the leek (πράσον), it might be, e.g., some sort of knife or dissector if an analogy is drawn with its leaves. On the other hand we might have here a ladder-like instrument of reduction (Hipp., Art. 42, 78) the shape of which suggested a bed of leeks (πρασιά).

πύαλος
Not found among the étui treated by Milne. A trough or bathing tub in which surgeons bathed patients after surgical treatment of enterocele (Paul 6.65).

ῥαφίδες
One of two items occurring in the plural on the lists (cf. ἄγκιστρα). Perhaps needles for suturing tissues (cf. Paul 6.107, ῥαφαῖς) as opposed to bandages. See Milne's discussion (pp. 74–75).

ῥινοτορίνιον / rinotorine
Milne has ῥινάριον, ῥίνη, and ῥίνιον; the present spellings are otherwise unattested (and may therefore be corruptions (so LSJ). In any case, a surgical file seems intended.

ῥινοσπάθιον / rinuspatium
Otherwise unattested. The σπαθίον is a knife (see App. II below, s.v.); so the present piece would be a scalpel for work on the nose, probably a πολυπικὸν σπαθίον.

σαλπιν̈
"Fraglich" in Schöne's view. I believe that σαλπίγγιον or "bellows" is meant. Galen in his treatise on anatomical operations (ed. Kühn, 2.717) mentions the device which he compares to οἱ τῶν χρυσοχόων φυσητῆρες. Now a smith's bellows was used to treat volvulus (see Milne, 108) so it is not at all out of place on a list of surgical instruments. And indeed the ninth-century list includes the fisiter.

σαρκολάβον / sarcolabon
A tumor forceps (see App. II below, s.v.). The classical name, μύδιον, does not occur on the lists.

σίφων
Drainage tube for hydrocele; see Galen (ed. Kühn), 10.988.

σκυθομήλη
A probe (μήλη) of some sort but what σκυθ- stands for is anyone's guess.

σκηνορράφιον
Cf. κυνορράφιον. A needle of some sort. If σκην = σκύνιον (skin above the eyes, Pollux 2.66), then perhaps a fine needle for suturing in this area.

σταφυλολαβίς
Another name for σταφυλάγρα; see App. II below, s.v.

τετραπίαλος / tetrafixos
"Fraglich," according to Schöne. A four-part trough? Cf. πύαλος.

ὑπερβιβαστήρ
Cf. epibastes. An instrument of reduction?

fenicus
Schöne suggests σφηνίσκος is meant. If so, the term commonly designated a wedge or a pledget in Byzantine times (see App. II below, s.v.). It is once used by Hippocrates in the sense of a wedge-shaped cautery (Milne, 119).

ostanaboleos (ὀστaναβολεύς)
Otherwise unattested. The same as the ἀναβολεύς or bone lever. Perhaps the compound came into use to distinguish the bone lever from (assuming they were different) a lever used to remove sling bullets which was also called ἀναβολεύς (Paul 6.88.9).

malium
"Fraglich," according to Schöne. I guess = μήλιον or "small probe," although this name is not attested in the literature. Note that the eleventh-century list has λεπτομήλη, which would mean the same thing.

cefaloclases (κεφαλοκλάστης)
Otherwise unattested. A cranioclast. The eleventh-century list has ἐμβρυοθλάστης.

epibastes (ἐπιβιβαστήρ)
Cf. ὑπερβιβαστήρ above.

incliridium
If = ἐγχειρίδιον, as Schöne suggests, then a type of instrument case; see Isidore, Etym. IV, XI, 1 and Milne, 168–70 who, however, supplies no name.

nasticium
If = ναρθήκιον, then a splint (see App. II below, s.v.)

deltarium (δελτάριον)
A delta-shaped instrument. A cautery?

APPENDIX II

A PRELIMINARY LIST OF BYZANTINE SURGICAL INSTRUMENTS AND PARASURGICAL ITEMS

As I prepared this study, I took care to note down the names of surgical instruments and related gear which I encountered in Byzantine medical texts. These I present here in alphabetical order with references to illustrations of the Classical Period whenever possible. I do not pre-

tend that I have discovered every name or that I have
listed all textual references to those names which occur
here. Even so, I do not believe that many names or important references have been omitted. For this reason it
seemed to me that such a list might be of use, especially
as I know of no other such list available to students of
Byzantine medicine.

ἀβάπτιστον (*sc.* τρύπανον)
Drill with collar guard. Paul 6.90. See Milne, Pl. XLII.

ἄγκιστρον / angistrum
Sharp retractor/hook. Orib. 44.8.1 *et passim* (50.48.6 =
τυφλάγκιστρον); Paul 6.5 *et passim* (6.18, ἄγκ.
μικροκαμπές); S (9th and 11th). Cf. κιρσουλκός, τυφλάγκιστρον. See Milne, Pl. XXIV.

ἀγκτήρ
A suture if not a clamp (see Milne's discussion, pp. 162–
63). Paul 6.107.

ἀγκυλότομον
Tonsil knife. Paul 6.30, Cf. ἀντιοτόμον. See M–S, Taf.
IV, 12.

αἰγιλωπικὸν καυτήριον
Cautery for treating aegilops. Paul 6.22.

αἱμαρροιδοκαύστης
Caustic forceps for hemorrhoids. Paul 6.79. See Milne,
Pl. XXXII, 2.

ἀκανθοβόλος
Pharyngeal forceps. Paul 6.32. See Milne, Pl. XXXII, 1.

ἀκίς
Needle. S (11th).

ἀκμάδιον
Conical crucible (see App. I above, *s.v.*). S (11th).

ἄμβη
Instrument of reduction. Paul 6.114.

ἀμφισμίλη
Probe with olivary enlargements. Michael Italicus, *Lettres
et discours*, ed. P. Gautier, (Paris 1972), 114. Cf. διπύρηνον. See Milne, Pl. XI, 1.

ἀναβολεύς
Bone lever, Orib. 45.6.6 (ἡ καμπὴ ἀναβολέως). Lever for
extracting weapons, Paul 6.88. Cf. μοχλίσκος, *naboleus*.
See Milne, Pl. XLI, 1.

ἀναρραφικὸν σμιλίον
Knife for operation on the eyelid. Aetius 7.71; Paul 6.8
et passim. See M–S, Taf. V, 5.

ἀντιβολάδιον / antiboladium
Bone lever? (see App. I above, *s.v.*). S (9th and 11th).

ἀντίθετοι
See ἐκκοπεύς.

ἀντιοτόμον / antiothomum
Tonsil knife (App. I above, *s.v.*). S (9th and 11th). Cf.
ἀγκυλοτόμον.

ἀντόπτρα
Probably a speculum (see App. I above, *s.v.*). S (11th).

ἁπλή
See σμίλη.

ἀ⟨πο⟩ξυστήρ
A raspatory (see App. I above, *s.v.*). S (11th).

ἀρίς / aridion
Bow-drill. Orib. 46.11.7; S (9th and 11th). See R. Caton,
JHS, 34 (1914), Pl. IX, 23.

αὐλίσκος
Lead tube to prevent contractions and adhesions, Paul,
6.81. Bronze or horn tube to convey medicaments, Orib.
44.12.2 (αὐλ. εὐθύτρητον); the tube of a clyster, Orib.
8.24.62, 8.37.3; tube of a clyster fitting into a catheter,
Aetius 6.34; curved bronze tube serving as a guard for a
cautery, Orib. 44.20.39. Cf. μοτός, σωλήν, σωληνάριον.

βάραθρον (ἢ ὄργανον) Ἱπποκράτους
Machine for reducing dislocations. Orib. 49.3.27, 49.27;
Paul 6.117.

βελόνη
Surgical needle. Orib. 45.18.15 *et passim*; Paul 6.12 *et passim*; Leon III, xx.

βελουλκός
Forceps for extracting weapons. Paul 6.88. See Milne, Pl.
XLIV.

βλεφαροκάτοχον / blefarocatochon (*sc.*μύδιον)
Eyelid forceps. Paul 6.8; S (9th and 11th).

βλεφαρόξυστον
Raspatory for treatment of opthalmia. Paul 3.23.

βλεφαροτόμον
Probably = ἀναρραφικὸν σμιλίον (see App. I above, *s.v.*).
S (11th).

βούγλωσσον
A cautery? (see App. I above, *s.v.*). S (11th).

βρόχος
Ligature. Paul 6.79 *et passim*, Michael Italicus, *loc. cit.* (note
38 above); cord for reductions, Paul 6.118.

γαμμοειδὲς καυτήριον
Gamma-shaped cautery. Paul 6.62, 6.66 (γαμμοειδὴς
καυτήρ).

γλωσσοκάτοχον / glossocathocon
Tongue depressor. Orib. 44.11.13; Aetius 8.48; S (9th
and 11th). Milne, Pl. XX, 6.

γλωσσοκόμον Νυμφοδώρου
Instrument of reduction. Orib. 49.4.23, 49.21, 46.1.76
(γλωσσοκόμιον).

γλωσσοκόμος
A splint. Orib. 46.1.73.

γομφωτήρ
A chisel. Orib. 44.20.15 (ἐκκοπεὺς τῶν στενῶν καὶ πάχος
ἱκανὸν ἐχόντων).

γραμμιστήρ / grammister
Perhaps a stylus (see App. I above, *s.v.*). S (9th and 11th).

γραφεῖον
Stylus. Aetius 8.36.

deltarium (δελτάριον)
See App. I above, *s.v.*; S (9th).

δέλτος
Medicine box. St. Basil, PG, 31, col. 1444.

δεσμός
Bandage? Michael Italicus, *loc. cit.* (note 38 above).

διαστολεύς
Probably a rectal speculum (see App. I above, *s.v.*). Paul 6.78; S (11th). Cf. ἑδροδιαστολεύς. See Milne, Pl. XLVI, 1.

διέδριον
A type of chair? *Varia Graeca Sacra*, 36, 25.

διόπτριον
See μικρὸν διόπτριον.

διόπτρα / διόπτρον
Vaginal speculum. Paul 6.73; S (11th); Psellus, Ποίημα Ἰατρικόν 1189 (διόπτρον).

διπύρηνον / diripinium.
Probe with olivary enlargements. Orib. 45.18.25; Paul 6.13 *et passim*, 6.77 (διπ. εὔκαμπές of tin or bronze); S (9th and 11th). "Eyed" types; Paul 6.25 (τρῆμα διπ.).

δίφρος
See μαιωτικὸς δίφρος.

διωστήρ / dioster
Impellent. Paul 6.88; S (9th and 11th).

δοῖδυξ
Pestle. Paul 3.59 *et passim*; used like a hammer, Orib. 44.10.4.

δρεπανοειδὲς . . . ὄργανον
Fistula knife. Leon V, xix. Cf. συριγγοτόμον.

ἐγχειρίδιον
Instrument case. Isidore, *Etym.* IV, XI, I; S (9th) has *incliridium*, see App. I above, *s.v.*

ἑδροδιαστολεύς
Rectal speculum. Orib. 44.20.66; Paul 6.78. Cf. διαστολεύς, μικρὸν διόπτριον.

ἐθειρολόγος
Epilation forceps (see App. I above, *s.v.*). S (11th). Cf. τριχολαβίς, -ον.

ἐκκοπεύς / etcopetis.
Chisel. Orib. 44.20.12; Paul 6.43 *et passim*; S (9th and 11th). In some cases chisels were used in pairs, the one to steady the other (ἀντίθετοι); see Paul 6.77, 6.90, 6.108 and Milne's discussion pp. 122–23. Cf. γομφωτήρ, φακωτὸς ἐκκ., σμιλωτὸς ἐκκ. See L. J. Bliquez (note 2 above), 12.

ἔλασμα
The flat part of an instrument; e.g., μήλης. Orib. 44.8.3; μηνιγγοφύλακος, Orib. 44.8.2; καυτηρίου Orib. 44.20.3; κατιάδος, Orib. 44.11.4.

ἐλασμάτιον
Probe (of tin). Orib. 50.10.7.

ἐμβρυοθλάστης
Cranioclast. S (11th). Cf. *cefaloclases*. See M–S, Taf. VI, 1.

ἐμβρυοσφάκτης
Spike for dispatching a fetus. S (11th).

ἐμβρυοτόμον / enbriotomum
Perforator for the fetal cranium. S (9th and 11th). See M–S, Taf. IV. 6.

ἐμβρυουλκός
Embryo hook. Paul 6.74; S (11th); Psellus, Ποίημα Ἰατρικόν 1187. See Milne, Pl. L, 1.

ἐνετήρ
Clyster. S (11th). Cf. κλυστήρ.

ἐντε⟨ρο⟩φύλαξ
Guard (see App. I above, *s.v.*). S (11th). Cf. μηνιγγοφύλαξ.

εὐμενιστήρ
Blunt dissector. Paul 6.5, 6.36. Cf. λαβίδιον. See Milne 24, 84–85.

epibastes (ἐπιβιβαστήρ)
See App. I above, *s.v.*

ἐπίδεσμος
Bandage. Orib. 46.1, *passim*; Paul 6.99; Leon VI, x, etc.

ἐπίκοπον / epicopo / ἐπικόπιον
Block. Orib. 44.20.77; Paul 6.67; S (9th and 11th).

ἐπικρουστικὸν φλεβοτόμον
A type of phlebotome. Aetius 6.8. See Milne, Pl. VIII, 3.

ἐπικρούστιον
Very likely = ἐπικρουστικὸν φλεβ.; see App. I above, *s.v.*

Ἑρμῆς
See κίων Ἑρμῆς.

Etfolocus
S (9th), "fraglich."

ἡλωτὸς καυτήρ
Nail-shaped cautery. Paul 6.66.

ἡμισπάθιον
A type of knife. Orib. 44.20.57 (ἡμίσπαθον), 44.20.66; Paul 6.71, 6.78. Cf. σπαθίον. See M–S, Taf. IV, 7, 8.

θυία
Mortar. Aetius 7.101 *et passim*. Cf. ἰγδίον.

ἰγδίον
Mortar. Paul 3.59 (lead) *et passim*.

ἱμάς
Thong for extension. Paul 6.118.

ἱπωτήριον
Papyrus tent to hold σωληνάριον, Orib. 50.9.8; bougie, Orib. 44.20.61, 44.21.9; a plaster, Orib. *Ecl. med.* 51.10.

ἱπωτρὶς σπάθη
Instrument of reduction. Orib. 49.18.9, 49.33.4–5.

ἴρις
Ear clyster. Paul 6.73. Cf. ὠτικὸς κλυστήρ, *otemquites*.

ἴσκαι
Ignited medullary wood of walnut tree. Paul 6.49.

καθετήρ
Catheter. Paul 6.59; Leon VI, iv; *Typikon*, 1270; Psellus, Ποίημα Ἰατρικόν, 1369. Cf. σωληνάριον. See Milne, Pl. XLV, 1, 2.

καλαμὶς πτεροῦ ὀρνιθείου
Shaft of a bird's feather used in place of a σωληνάριον. Orib. 50.9.8.

καλαμίσκος / calamiscos
Drainage tube, Paul 6.50, S (9th and 11th), cf. σίφων, μοτός; a tube used in weapons extraction, Paul 6.88. See Milne, Pl. XXXIX, 2, 3.

κάλαμος
Insufflator. Orib. 44.21.9, 8.13.1 (of bronze or a natural reed). See also χύτρα. See Milne, Pl. XL, 4.

κατιάς / κασία / cacias
A type of phlebotome. Orib. 44.11.3; Aetius 8.48; Paul 6.74; S (9th and 11th).

καυλοκλυστήρ
A type of clyster (see App. I above, s.v.). S (11th).

καυτήρ / καυτήριον
Cautery. Orib. 50.7.4; Aetius 6.24 (πλατύτερον καυτ.); Paul 6.45 et passim, 6.77 (κ. σιδηροῦν), 6.42 (λεπτὸν καὶ ἐπιμηκὲς κ.), 6.54 (λεπτὸν καυτ.), 6.50 (λεπτὸν σιδηροῦν κ.), 6.48 (μακρὸν καυτ.); St. John Climacus, PG, 88, cols. 1168–1169 (καυστήρ); Leon II, ii et passim; Typikon, 1274 (σίδηρα καυτηριῶν, as though there were a καυτηριά). Cf. the following, special types: αἰγιλωπικόν, γαμμοειδές, ἡλωτός, μαχαιρωτός, μηνοειδές, πλινθωτός, πυρηνοειδές, συριγγιακός, τριαινοειδές, φακωτός, ψυχροκαυτήρ, and a cautery fitting in a tube, s.v. αὐλίσκος. See Milne, Pl. XL, 1.

κέρας
Tube of clyster. Orib. 8.32.7. Cf. κλυστήρ.

κέστωρ / κέστρος / cestros
See App. I above, s.v.; S (9th and 11th).

κεφαλικὸν σφυρίον
Surgical hammer. Orib. 46.11.19. Cf. σφυρά.

cefaloclases (κεφαλοκλάστης)
Cranioclast (see App. I above, s.v.). S (9th). Cf. ἐμβρυοθλάστης.

κιρσουλκός
Retractor for varicose veins. Orib. 45.18.5 (ἄγκιστρα τῶν σφόδρα μικροκαμπῶν, καλουμένων δὲ κιρσουλκῶν, γαμμοειδῆ κατὰ τὴν καμπήν).

κίων ὁ λεγόμενος Ἑρμῆς, κίων τοῦ Ἐφεσίου Ἡρακλείδου
Instrument of reduction. Orib. 49.4.39, 49.4.48.

κλίμαξ
Instrument of reduction. Paul 6.114.

κλυστήρ
Clyster; see Oribasius, book 8, for all sorts of data. Orib. 8.24.62: straight (εὐθύτρητος) and side (παράτρητος) bore; Paul 6.52; Leon V, ix; S (11th). Theophanes Nonnos (Bernard) I, 290. Cf. ὠτικὸς κλυστήρ, αὐλίσκος, κέρας, otemquites. Milne, Pl. XXXVIII, 1–2.

κοπάριον
Probe. Paul 6.62 et passim, 6.85 (λεπτόν), 6.78 (τετρημένον). Cf. ὑδροκηλικὸν κοπάριον.

κουφιστήρ
Ring pad around trephine opening. Orib. 46.19.11.

κόραξ
Curved knife. Orib. 44.7.5. Cf. ὀξυκόρακον.

κυαθίσκος / quiatiscos
Scoop, Paul 6.40 (κυαθίσκος μήλης); S (9th and 11th). Cf. τραυματικὴ μηλωτίς. See L. J. Bliquez, "Roman Surgical Instruments in the Johns Hopkins University Institute of the History of Medicine," 56 (1982), nos. 19–24 (pp. 205–9).

κύαθος
Spoon. Orib. 45.29.26 et passim, Ecl. med. 38.4 (κ. . . . πλῆθος τριωβόλου); Aetius 6.63 et passim. See L. J. Bliquez, "Roman Surgical Instruments" (op. cit.), s.v. κυαθίσκος, no. 5 (p. 200).

κυκλίσκος, (sc. ἐκκοπεύς)
Hollow chisel/gouge. Orib. 46.21.17; Paul 6.90.

κυνορράφιον
See App. I above, s.v.; S (11th).

κυρτίς
Strainer. Paul 7.20. See Milne, 165.

λαβή / λαβίδιον τοῦ σμιλίου
Blunt dissector. Orib. 45.6.6, 45.17.6; Aetius 6.1.

λαβίς / λαβίδιον
Forceps (see App. I above, s.v.). Aetius 6.91, 7.21 (λαβίδιον); S (11th).

λεπτάριον
See App. I above, s.v.; S (11th).

λεπτομήλη
Sound (see App. I above, s.v.). S (11th).

λημνίσκος
Pledget; Orib. 44.11.5, 50.49.1 (λ. στενόν); Aetius 6.1; Paul 6.73. Bandage; Orib., Ecl. med. 97.41.

λιθοτόμον / litothomum
Knife/hook combination for lithotomy. Paul 6.60; S (9th and 11th). Cf. λιθουλκός.

λιθουλκός
Stone extractor. Orib. 45.6.6; Paul, 6.60. See Künzl, Hassel, Künzl, BJb, 182 (1982), 47, nos. 17, 18.

λικώνυμος
Ligature (?). Michael Italicus, loc. cit. (note 38 above).

μαιωτικὸς δίφρος
Chair for birthing and fumigation. Orib. 10.19.

malium
Small probe? (see App. I above, s.v.).

μασχαλολαβεύς / mascalolabeos
Instrument of reduction? (see App. I above, s.v.). S (9th and 11th).

μάχαιρα / μαχαίριον / macherium
Scalpel. St. John Climacus, PG, 88, cols. 1168–1169 (μάχαιρα); S (9th and 11th). Cf. σμίλη, etc. See Milne, Pls. V-VI.

μήλη / mele
Probe. Orib. 44.8.2 et passim (πλάτυ μήλης), 44.13.20 (πύρην μήλης); Aetius 6.91 (μήλης ἔριον ἐχούσης); Paul 6.9 et passim; S (9th and 11th). Cf. λεπτομήλη, μηλωτίς, σπαθομήλη, πυρηνομήλη. See Milne, Pls. X-XIII; M–S Taf. I, 2–8.

μηλωτίς / μηλωτρίς
Ear probe. Orib. 44.7.16 *et passim*, 44.21.12 (μ. ἐπ' ἄκρου τρῆμα ἔχουσα), 44.19.5 (of tin or lead to explore fistula), 44.20.53 (τῆς μ. πυρήν; see Milne's discussion, p. 7.); Aetius 8.25 (μηλωτρίδι ἔριον παρειλήσας); Paul 6.13 *et passim*; S (11th); Michael Italicus, *loc. cit.* (note 38 above). Cf. τραυματικὴ μηλωτίς. See Bliquez, "Roman Surgical Instruments" (*op. cit.*), *s.v.* κυαθίσκος.

μηνιγγοφύλαξ / meningofilax
Guard. Orib. 44.8.2. *et passim*; Paul 6.77 *et passim*; S (9th and 11th). Cf. ἐντεροφύλαξ. See Milne, Pl. XL, 3.

μηνοειδὲς καυτήριον / μηνοειδὴς καυτήρ
Lunated cautery. Orib. 50.7.4; Paul 6.57. Cf. καυτήριον. See L. J. Bliquez, "An Unidentified Roman Surgical Instrument in Bingen," *JHM*, 36 (1981), 219–20, and Fig. 1.

μητρανύκτης
See App. I above, *s.v.*; S (11th).

μητρεγχύτης / metrochites
Uterine irrigator. S (9th and 11th).

μικρὸν διόπτριον
Rectal speculum. Orib. 44.20.66. Cf. διαστολεύς.

μοτοφύλαξ
Bandage to keep a μοτός in place. Orib. 44.7.8 (πτυγμάτιον δίπτυχον ἢ τρίπτυχον), 44.20.74 (μοτοφυλάκιον).

μότος / μοτάριον
Shredded lint tampons. Orib. 44.7.8, 44.20.74; Paul 6.28.

μοτός
Tube to prevent contractions and adhesions, Paul 6.25; a tent, Paul 6.25 (ἐλλυχνιωτὸν μοτόν); a drainage tube, Aetius 6.1. Cf. σωλήν, καλαμίσκος. See Milne, Pl. XXXIX, 1.

μοχλίσκος
Bone lever. Paul 6.106 (iron preferred). Cf. ἀναβολεύς.

μύδιον
Tissue forceps. Orib. 50.9.7 *et passim*; Aetius 8.64; Paul 6.70 *et passim*. Cf. σαρκολάβον. See Milne, Pls. XXVIII, XXIX.

naboleus
Cf. ἀναβολεύς.

νάρθηξ / ναρθήκιον
Splint. Orib. 44.20.74; Paul 6.99 *et passim*, 6.92 (splint for the jaw).

nasticium
Probably = ναρθήκιον; S (9th).

ξυστήρ / xister / ξυστήριον
Raspatory. Orib. 46.9.4; Paul 6.90, 6.12 (ξυστήριον). Cf. ἀποξυστήρ, περιξυστήρ.

ξύστρα
Strigil or scraper for removing hair. Aetius 6.63.

ὀδοντάγρα / odontagra
Tooth forceps. Paul 6.28 *et passim*; S (9th and 11th). Cf. ὀστάγρα, ῥιζάγρα, σταφυλάγρα. See H. Cüppers, *Kranken- und Gesundheitspflege in Trier und dem Trierer Land von der Antike bis zur Neuzeit* (Trier, 1981), 40 (Abb. 22).

ὀδοντοξύστης / ὀδοντοξυστήρ / odontoxister
Tooth scaler (see App. I above, *s.v.*). S (9th and 11th).

olypoxyster
See πολυποξύστης.

ὀξεῖα (*s.c.* σμίλη)
See App. I above, *s.v.*; S (11th).

ὀξυκόρακον (*sc.* σμιλίον)
Curved knife. Paul 6.87, Cf. κόραξ.

ὀξυλαβίδιον
Small forceps; see App. I above, *s.v.*

ὄργανον
Instrument of reduction, of which the following types are attested: τὸ τοῦ τέκτονος (Orib. 49.4.8; 49.24); τὸ τοῦ Ἀνδρέου (Orib. 49.4.8); τὸ Φιλιστίωνος (Orib. 49.4.38).

ὄργανον . . . τρία σμιλία ἴσα
Scarifier. Paul 6.41.

ὀστάγρα / osteagra
Bone forceps. Orib. 44.8.7; Paul 6.74; S (9th and 11th); *Typikon*, 1270. Cf. ὀδοντάγρα, ῥιζάγρα, σταφυλάγρα, ὀσταναλαβεύς. See Milne, Pl. XLIII.

ostanaboleos
Bone lever; see App. I above, *s.v.*; S (9th).

ὀσταναλαβεύς
See App. I above, *s.v.*; S (11th).

ὀστεγχύτης
Bone irrigator; see App. I above, *s.v.*; S (11th).

ὀφθαλμοστάτης / ostalmostater
See App. I above, *s.v.*; S (9th and 11th).

παρακεντήριος / paracenteter
Couching needle. Paul 6.21; S (9th and 11th). See Milne, 69–71 and Pl. XVI, 2–7.

παραστολεύς / parastoleus
See App. I above, *s.v.*; S (9th and 11th).

περιλαβεύς / peribabeos
See App. I above, *s.v.*; S (9th and 11th).

περιξύστης / perixister
Raspatory. Orib. 46.11.29 (περιξυστήρ); Paul 6.25; S (9th and 11th).

πιλάριον
Cap or bandage for hydrocephalus. Aetius 6.1.

πλάτυ
The spatula on a probe. See μήλη.

πλευροπριστήρ / pliroprister
Rib-saw (see App. I above, *s.v.*). S (9th and 11th).

πλινθίον τοῦ Νειλέως
Instrument of reduction. Orib. 49.4.23, 49.8.

πλινθωτὸς καυτήρ
Brick-shaped cautery. Paul 6.66.

πολυπικὸν σπαθίον
Polyp knife. Orib. 45.6.3; Paul 6.23 *et passim*, 6.25 (πολ. σπαθ. τῷ μυρσηνοειδεῖ ἀκμαίῳ). Cf. ῥινοσπάθιον. See Milne, Pl. VIII, 1; M–S, Taf. IV, 13.

πολυποξύστης
Forceps/rugine combination for polyp. Paul 6.25; S (9th), *olypoxister*. See Milne, Pl. VIII, 1.

πολυ⟨πο⟩σφάκτης
Probably a forceps/rugine combination; see App. I above, *s.v.*

πολυποτόμον
Πολυπικὸν σπαθίον. Leon III, ii.

πρασιά / prasia
See App. I above, *s.v.*; S (9th and 11th).

πριαπίσκος
A tent. Orib. 44.20.72, *Ecl. med.* 15.1; Paul 6.72.

πρίων / pionin
Saw. Orib. 44.20.18; Paul 6.77 *et passim*; S (9th and 11th). See Milne, Pl. XLI, 3: M–S, Taf. III, 1.

πτέρον
See καλαμίς, σύριγξ.

πτερυγοτόμον / pteriotimum
Pterygium knife. Aetius 7.62; Paul 6.15 *et passim*. See M–S, Taf. VIII, 11.

πύαλος
Bathing tub (App. I, above, *s.v.*). Paul 6.65; S (11th).

πυουλκός
Pus extractor. Orib. 44.12.2. (with a wide bore); S (11th).

πυρήν
Olivary enlargement on the end of a probe (see *s.vv.* μήλη, μηλωτίς) or a needle (see Paul 6.21).

πυρηνοειδὲς καυτήριον
Olivary cautery. Orib. 45.19.1; Paul 6.2 *et passim*, 6.47 (λεπτόν); Aetius 6.50.

πυρηνομήλη
Probe with olivary enlargement. Paul 6.42. See Milne, Pl. XI, 1,3,5.

ῥαφίς
Needle (see App. I above, *s.v.*). S (11th).

ῥίζαι
Ignited roots. Orib. 10.11.

ῥιζάγρα / rizoagra
Stump forceps. Paul 6.88; S (9th).

ῥινάριον
File. Paul 6.28; Aetius 8.32 (iron, with an olivary enlargement); S (9th and 11th) ῥινοτορίνιον / rinotorine. See Milne, Pl. XVI, 1.

ῥινεγχύτης
Nasal syringe. Aetius 6.96.

ῥινοσπάθιον / rhinuspatium
Polyp knife. S (9th and 11th). Cf. πολυπικὸν σπαθίον.

σαλπίγγιον (?)
See App. I above, *s.v.* σαλπιν̄. S (11th).

σανίδιον
Splint. Orib. 44.20.74 (of limewood).

σαρκολάβον / sarcolabon
Tumor forceps. Orib. 45.10.2; Paul 6.17 *et passim*. Cf. μύδιον. See M–S Taf. X, 3.

σιδήριον
Lancet; see M. Delehaye, *Les Saints stylites* (Brussels, 1923), 219.

σίδηρον
See καυτήρ.

σίδηρος
Scalpel; see Theophanes Nonnus (Bernard), II 66.

σικύα
Bleeding cup. Orib. 7.15–18 (glass, horn, bronze, various shapes); Aetius 6.28 (κουφή); Paul 6.41; Schol. Nicandri *Theriaca* 921 (iron); Leon VII, xvii, xx.

σίφων
Drainage tube. (See App. I above, *s.v.*). S (11th).

σκηνορράφιον
Needle. (See App. I above, *s.v.*). S (11th).

σκολόπιον
A knife. Orib. 50.5.4, 50.9.3 (σκόλοψ στενός); Paul 6.50.

σκολοπομαχαίριον
Another name for σκολόπιον. Paul 6.6 *et passim*. See M–S, Taf. III, 3.

σκυθομήλη
See App. I above, *s.v.*; S (11th).

σκυλισκωτὸς (*sc.* ἐκκοπεύς)
Gouge. Paul 6.90. Cf. κυκλίσκος.

σμίλη, etc.
Scalpel. Orib. 45.21.2; Paul 6.39, 6.86 (ὀξεῖα σμίλη), 6.77 (σ. κατὰ τὸ οἰκεῖον σχῆμα); Orib. 44.20.4 (σμιλίον), Aetius 7.82 (σμιλίον στενόν), Paul 6.12 *et passim*; Aetius 6.1, 8.48 (σμιλάριον); S (9th, *hismilarium*, and 11th, σμήλα). Cf. ἀναρραφικὸν σμιλίον, κόραξ, μαχαίριον, λαβή. See Milne, Pl. V.

σμιλωτόν (*sc.* ὄργανον)
Tooth scaler. Paul 6, 28. Cf. ξυστήριον.

σμιλωτὸς ἐκκοπεύς
Chisels for bone work. Orib. 44.20.74; 46.11.17.

σπάθη
Block. Orib. 44.20.18. See also ἱπωτρίς.

σπαθίον
Knife. Paul 6.6 *et passim*. Cf. πολυπικὸν σπ.; σπ. συριγγοτόμον.

σπαθιοτήρ
See Milne, 141; = ὑποσπαθιστήρ.

σπαθομήλη / spatomele
Spatula probe. Orib. 44.11.13; S (9th and 11th); Michael Italicus, *loc. cit.* (note 38 above). See μήλη, πλάτυ μήλης. See Milne, Pls. XII, XIII.

σπαρτίον
Cord. Leon II, xxii.

σπλήν
Compress. Paul 6.115.

σπόγγος
Sponge. Orib., *passim* books 44 and 45; Paul 6.41 *et passim*; St. John Climacus, PG, 88, 1168–1169; Leon V, ix.

σταφυλάγρα
Uvula forceps. Paul 6.31 *et passim*. Milne, Pls. XXX, XXXI.

σταφυλεπάρτης
Perhaps σταφυλάγρα, but see Milne, 89. Paul 3.26.

σταφυλοκάτοχος
σταφυλάγρα. Aetius, *apud* J. G. Schneider, *Nicandri Alexipharmaka seu De venenis in potu cibove homini datis eorumque remediis carmen* (Halle, 1792), *ad* 511 (p. 243).

σταφυλοκαύστης / stafilocautes
Forceps for application of caustic. Paul 6.31, 6.79; S (9th and 11th).

σταφυλολαβίς
σταφυλάγρα (see App. I above, *s.v.*). S (9th).

σταφυλοτόμον / stafilotomon
Uvula knife. Paul 6.31; S (9th and 11th).

στοματοδιαστολεύς
Device to keep the mouth open. Orib. 44.11.13.

στομαΐ
S (11th) "fraglich."

συριγγιακὸς καυτήρ
Cautery for fistula. Leon II, xxii.

συρίγγιον
Tube for scarification. Paul 6.87 (bronze or iron).

σύριγξ πτέρου σκληροῦ
Same as συρίγγιον. Paul 6.87.

συριγγοτόμον / syringotomum
Fistula knife. Orib. 44.20.57; Paul 6.52 (ὀρθόν), 6.78 (σπαθίον συριγγοτόμον, δρέπανος τοῦ συριγγ.); S (9th and 11th).

σφηνάριον
Wedge to keep the mouth open. Orib. 44.11.13 (of oak).

σφηνίσκος
Pledget. Aetius 7.82, Paul 6.7, 6.81; = σφηνάριον, Orib. 8.6.21.

σφυρά
Hammer. Orib. 46.21.20; Paul 6.90. Cf. κεφαλικὸν σφυρίον. See S. Zervos, *Les Bistouris, les sondes et les curettes chirurgicales d' Hippocrate* (Athens, 1932), 53, Fig. 42.

σωληνάριον
Tube for preventing adhesions and contractions. Orib. 50.9.8 (bronze or tin); Paul 6.91 (lead); catheter, Paul 6.57 (lead); part of fumigation apparatus, see χύτρα. Cf. σωλήν.

σωλήν
Tube for preventing adhesions and contractions. Orib. 44.20.72 (lead or tin), Paul 6.55 (lead); drainage tube, Orib. 44.5.12 (tin); a box or pipe for keeping a broken limb straight, Paul 6.106 (wood or clay). Cf. μοτός, αὐλίσκος.

ταινία
Strap for retracting flesh. Orib. 44.20.18.

τελαμών
Bandage, Orib. 10.18.15; tourniquet, Orib. 7.9.1 (εὔτονος); = ταινία, Orib. 44.20.18.

τετραπίαλος / tetrafixos
See App. I above, *s.v.*; S (9th and 11th).

τετρημένον
See κοπάριον.

τραυματικὴ μηλωτίς
Scoop for removal of impacted weapons, Orib. 46.11.26; Paul 6.88 (κυαθίσκος τ. μ.).

τριαίνα ἢ τριαινοειδὲς καυτήριον
Trident-shaped cautery. Paul 6.48.

τρῆμα
Eye of a probe. See μηλωτίς.

τρίσπαστον 'Απελλίδος ἢ 'Αρχιδήμους
Triple pulley for reductions. Orib. 49.4.23, 49.23.

τριχολαβίς / τριχολάβον / triclolabon
Tweezers. Paul 6.13 *et passim*; S (9th and 11th). Milne, Pl. XXVI.

τρύπανον / tripanin / τρυπάνη
Drill. Orib. 46.11.7 (ἀκμὴ τοῦ τρυπ.) *et passim*, 44.20.12 (τρυπάνη); Paul 6.77 *et passim*. See Milne, Pl. XLII, 3–5.

τυφλάγκιστρον
Blunt retractor. Orib. 45.18.9 *et passim*, 45.6.6 (τυφλ. μεγαλοκαμπές); Aetius 8.66; Paul 6.62 *et passim; Varia Graeca Sacra*, 36, 25. See Milne, Pl. XXIII, 3, 4.

ὑδροκηλικὸν κοπάριον
A dissector; see Milne, 85; M–S 24–25. Paul 6.62, 6.82 (ἐπικαμπές).

ὑπερβιβαστήρ
See App. I above, *s.v.*; S (11th).

ὕπερον
Instrument of reduction. Paul 6.114, 6.118.

ὑποσπαθιστήρ
Periosteal elevator. Paul 6.6; Psellus, Ποίημα 'Ιατρικόν 1334. Cf. σπαθιστήρ. See M–S, Taf. III, 3.

φακωτὸς or φακοειδὴς ἐκκοπεύς
Lenticular. Orib. 46.21.20; Paul 6.90. See Milne, Pl. XL, 2.

φακωτὸς καυτήρ
Lentil-shaped cautery. Paul 6.66.

Fisiter (φυσητήρ)
A bellows. S (9th).

φλεβοτόμον / flebotomum
Phlebotome. Orib. 50.5.4; Paul 6.5 *et passim*; St. John Climacus, PG, 88.1168–1169; Leon I, i; *Typikon*, 1270. Cf. ἐπικρουστικόν, κατιάς. See M–S, Taf. IV, 9.

χαράκτης
Trephine? (see Milne, 131–33). S (11th).

χερνιβόξεστον χαλκοῦν
Bronze washbasin. *Typikon*, 1270.

χοινικίς
Trephine. Paul 6.90; S (11th). See J. Como, *Germania*, 9 (1925), 160 (Abb. 6, 1–5).

χύτρα (+ καλαμὸς + σωληνάριον)
A fumigation apparatus. Orib. 10.19.1–4; Aetius 16.80.

ψαλίς / psallidium
Scissors. Orib. 43.36.42 *et passim*; Paul 6.58 *et passim*; S (9th and 11th). See Milne, Pl. X, 5.

68
69   ψυχροκαυτήρ
70   Caustic applicator? Paul 6.58, 6.87; Leon VII, xiv. (ψυχρὸς
71   καυτήρ). Cf. σταφυλοκαύστης.
72
     otemquites (ὠτεγχύτης)
     Ear syringe. S (9th). Cf. ὠτικός κλυστήρ.

ὠτικὸς ἴρις
Ear syringe. Paul 6.73.

ὠτικὸς κλυστήρ
Ear syringe. Orib. 8.24.65; Paul 6.59.

ASPECTS OF BYZANTINE MATERIA MEDICA*

JERRY STANNARD

Byzantine materia medica, although not coterminous with Byzantine medicine in general, was certainly one of its more prominent subdivisions. Many different kinds of texts, varying greatly in size, date, style and credibility were concerned, wholly or partially, with medicaments as the primary means of promoting health. The heterogeneous nature of those texts is such that some have been ignored by students of Byzantine medicine while others would scarcely be recognized as practical medical texts by physicians and pharmacists today. For that reason, it may be convenient to examine some of the major components of Byzantine materia medica and to determine their relations, one with another, within the wider context of Byzantine medicine.

Prior to our discussion of some of the characteristic features of Byzantine materia medica, a few remarks on sources and their utilization are required. These remarks, however, are not those of the *Quellenforscher*, bent on establishing a textual tradition or the reconstruction of a lost *Urtext*. Rather, they are designed to call attention to one of the most pervasive characteristics of Byzantine materia medica, viz., the reliance of Byzantine writers on earlier written sources and the frequency with which the same authorities and their claims were copied, recopied, paraphrased and excerpted century after century.[1]

In Byzantine texts on materia medica a reference to a written source, especially in the form of a personal name, for example, Hippocrates or Galen, was not the act of historical scholarship that today is associated with a learned footnote. Such a reference, it is true, sometimes furnishes a useful clue to the sources used by late Byzantine writers. But sometimes it appears as if a citation to an earlier writer was a ritualistic performance reflecting, in part, the traditionalism inherent in Byzantine medicine.

Hippocrates and Homer, as one would expect, were almost venerated by medical writers and, in the case of Hippocrates, for good reason. Leaving aside the question concerning the authorship of the texts traditionally ascribed to Hippocrates, there is little doubt that the observations contained in some of those texts provided valuable insights into the nature of disease and hence guidelines for therapy. On the other hand, citing the equally magical name of Homer was of questionable value with respect to therapeutic practice. For similar reasons references to Orpheus, Democritus, Poseidonius, and others were more a show of learning than an indication of how to minister to the sick.

References to the earlier, well-known Greek and Greco-Roman physicians are more readily understood. This applies especially to Dioscorides and Galen, but to others as well. Some of their writings, not merely extracts available in a florilegium, must have been readily available for consultation judging by the frequency of citation and the fidelity with which those passages agree with the original.[2] Even earlier Byzantine medical writers are sometimes cited by their successors, for example, Oribasius, Theophilus, Aitios, John Myrepsus and Jacob Psychrestus are all mentioned, favorably one might add, by later compilers.

In addition to citing sources and authorities by name, there are also references to anonymous oral

[The reader is referred to the list of abbreviations at the end of the volume.]

*I am grateful to Miss Mary Kay, Head, Reference Department, University of Kansas Libraries, and her staff for assistance in obtaining some of the materials necessary for the completion of this study.
[1] As an example, see the parallel passages assembled by A. Sideras, "Aetius und Oribasius," *BZ*, 67 (1974), 110–30.

[2] See J. M. Riddle, "Pseudo-Dioscorides' *Ex herbis femininis* and Early Medieval Medical Botany," *JHB*, 14 (1981), 43–81.

sources,[3] rustics,[4] books whose titles can no longer be ascertained,[5] and the vague references to *hoi Indoi, hoi Persai, hoi palaioi*, and the like. Finally there is a large but elusive class of references, typified by such phrases as *hos tines phasi* and *hos legetai*. Whether the passages introduced by such phrases are genuine references to information current at the time or mere literary formulae requires further research.

Last is a group of pseudonymous texts. The attribution of a text, often rather small, to an identifiable figure was a well known literary device in both the East and the West. Hence there are several texts on materia medica that were attributed to Hippocrates, Galen, Dioscorides, Aitios, Simeon Seth and others.[6] None of these is now accepted as genuine.[7]

It is important, then, to recognize the dependence of Byzantine writers upon their predecessors. This applies particularly to descriptions of plants and plant substances which, in fact, make up the bulk of the composita. As the writings of Aitios and Paul indicate, they often repeated, sometimes with only the slightest verbal modifications, descriptions of simplicia drawn from Galen's abridgments of Dioscorides or from the latter's *De materia medica*.[8] There is little evidence in such descriptions that the Byzantine compilers possessed any additional information, with the result that the contemporary reader of Aitios or Paul was reading an account already over 500 years old. While plant species do not normally change very much in so short a period, their geographical distribution, and hence market availability, may have changed dramatically. Silphium is a good example.[9] According

to Pliny the Elder, it was already rare in the first century A.D.[10] Yet Leon and Alexander include it as an ingredient in composita without any hint that it might be rare or even unprocurable.[11]

With this by way of background, it is time to examine five other prominent aspects of Byzantine materia medica.

A convenient starting point is the recipe literature. For this is, in terms of size, one of the largest single components of the literature on materia medica.[12] By that very fact, it reveals the attitude towards drugs and the reliance placed upon them.[13]

I. RECIPES

Recipes played the same role in Byzantine medicine as they do in modern folk medicine.[14] They were, so to speak, the distillate of traditional wisdom. They were the tangible evidence that diseases and other complaints were capable of being cured, for, after all, what other meaning can be placed on such phrases, usually at the conclusion of a recipe, as: "this has been tried," "he will be cured," or "you will be amazed." Other phrases of similar intent perhaps exaggerated the efficacy of the remedy.

The sheer mass of recipes, whether or not accompanied by magical devices,[15] gave the impres-

---

[3] ἐγώ γοῦν οἶδά τινα, ὅς . . . ἔφασκε Alexander (ed. Puschmann), II, 485.

[4] Alexander identified his sources for useful medical information as παρ' ἀγροίκου (II, 563 Puschm.) and παρὰ Κερκυραίου ἀγεοίκου (II, 565 Puschm.) Dialectal forms of plant names are likewise credited παρὰ τοῖς ἰδιώταις (Delatte, *Anecdota*, II, 283.13; 300.14; cf. also 345.12 . . . οἱ ἰδιῶται καλοῦσι).

[5] The source for the Mousarion collyrium is described by Alexander (II, 15 Puschm.) ἐκ τοῦ ἱερατικοῦ τόμου.

[6] As an example of such pseudonymous texts, see H. Schöne, ed., "Hippokrates Π. φαρμακῶν," *RhM*, 73 (1920), 434–48.

[7] See Delatte, *Anecdota*, II, pp. 339, 385, 456, 466.

[8] *De simplicium medicamentorum temperamentis ac facultatibus*, in Galen (ed. Kühn), XI, 379–892; XII, 1–377.

[9] Asafoetida, the congealed sap of silphium, was also known under other names, for example, λάσαρον καὶ λάσαρ ὁ ὀπὸς τοῦ σιλφίου, Delatte, *Anecdota*, II, 290.7. It was probably obtained from one or both of two closely related species, *Ferula narthex* Boiss. and *Scorodosma foetidum* Bunge. See, Vladimir Vikentiev, "Le Silphium," *BIE*, 37 (1954), 123–50.

[10] *NH* 19.15.39.

[11] Leon Philosophus, *Conspectus medicinae* I, 8 (in Ermerins, p. 97); Alexander, I, 407 Puschm.

[12] E. Jeanselme, "Sels médicamenteux et aromatiques," *BullSocFrançHistMédical*, 16 (1922), 324–34; *id.*, "Sur un aide-mémoire de thérapeutique byzantine," *Mél. Ch. Diehl*, I (Paris, 1930), 147–70; A. P. Kousis, "Quelques considérations sur les traductions en grec des oeuvres médicales . . . par Constantin Melitiniotis," Πρακτ.Ἀκαδ.Ἀθ., 14 (1939), 205–20; *id.*, Ἐκ τῶν Μητροδώρας περὶ τῶν γυναικείων παθῶν τῆς μήτρας, Πρακτ. Ἀκαδ.Ἀθ., 20 (1945), 46–68; Emile Legrand, "Formulaire Médical de Jean Staphidas," in his *Bibliothèque Grecque Vulgaire*, II (Paris, 1881), 1–27. Miscellaneous recipes are noted in Ch. Daremberg, "Notices et extraits des manuscrits médicaux grecs," *AMSL*, 2 (1851), 24–37. Because of a Byzantine substratum in late Coptic *Rezeptliteratur*, cf. Walter Till, "Koptische Rezepte," *BSACopt*, 12 (1949), 43–54 and *id.*, *Die Arzneikunde der Kopten* (Berlin, 1951). For Western medieval analogues, cf. J. Stannard, "Rezeptliteratur als Fachliteratur," *Scripta* (Brussels), 6 (1982), 59–73.

[13] For useful supplementary references to the use of and value placed upon drugs and drug therapy at the popular level, see J. H. Magoulias, "The Lives of the Saints as Sources of Data for the History of Byzantine Medicine in the Sixth and Seventh Centuries," *BZ*, 57 (1964), 127–50.

[14] J. Stannard, "Albertus Magnus and Medieval Herbalism," in James Weisheipl, ed., *Albertus Magnus and the Sciences* (Toronto, 1980) 355–77.

[15] Cf. the series of "Recettes magiques" edited by A. Delatte, *Anecdota*, I, *passim*.

sion that, provided the enumerated ingredients were available, prepared and administered in the manner stipulated, there was, ready at hand, one or more means of combating a disease. The plurality of recipes for the same complaint, often in succession, seemed to demonstrate that there was a variety of procedures, all equally efficacious. The conclusion that *we* would reach, viz. that such a sequence was a virtual admission that none was predictably reliable, was apparently not drawn. The usefulness of these recipes, however, was not confined to curing diseases or healing wounds. They also provided one with the means of averting misfortunes, prognosticating the future, and a wide range of techniques applicable to daily life, either at home or when traveling abroad.[16]

Because of the wide range of processes and events that could be corrected or controlled by following a recipe, it is impossible to even guess at their number. They occur in profusion, as one might expect, in the general medical treatises, from Oribasius to Actuarios. In addition they occur, though with a lesser frequency, in lexica, herbals, and dietetic texts. Finally, of course, there were the recipe collections themselves. But even here, there is considerable variety in the individual recipes. Many were straightforward statements of what to prepare and how to administer it for a specific medical problem, for example, gout, fever, headache, and the like. Others, however, were more akin to what we would call *secreta*, that is, pieces of useful information, not generally known, relating to the solution of mundane problems, for example, how to rid the house of mice,[17] how to disguise gray hair,[18] or the means of exorcising demons[19] or predicting the sex of an unborn child.[20]

II. LEXICAL

A second aspect of Byzantine materia medica, prominent in itself but also related to the authoritarianism noted earlier, is a concern with nomenclature and other lexicographical issues.[21] That concern with words was not restricted, however, to glossaries, many of which have been published in the past half century.[22] The same attention to orthography, etymology, and synonymies is also evident in the recipe literature and in the descriptions of simplicia that are scattered throughout the several medical texts.

A concern with words might appear, at first glance, somewhat sterile from a medical point of view. But, despite the inevitable excesses of some authors, such a concern was meant to serve a practical purpose. To what extent it did so, however, is difficult to judge in the absence of evidence concerning the use of those lexica by physicians and apothecaries in the course of their daily professional work.[23] But the time and effort expended in preparing lexica, especially the multilingual ones, was probably justified.

Classical, that is, Attic Greek, the *koine*, and some vernacular dialects came together in Byzantium. Over the centuries that polyglot was infiltrated by many non-Greek loan words, some of which were later accepted and functioned as if they were truly Greek.[24]

As a result of this linguistic admixture, various problems arose concerning the vocabulary of materia medica. As older words lost currency and were

---

[16] In addition to Delatte, *Anecdota*, II (cf. note 4 above), see H. J. Magoulias, "The Lives of Byzantine Saints as Sources of Data for the History of Magic in the Sixth and Seventh Centuries A.D.," *Byzantion*, 37 (1968), 228–46. Means of averting the potential dangers of traveling are indicated in numerous ways. For example, see G. Dagron et J. Rougé, "Trois horoscopes de voyages en mer," *REB*, 40 (1982), 117–33.

[17] Margaret H. Thomson, ed., *Textes grecs inédits relatifs aux plantes* (Paris, 1955), p. 111.9–19.

[18] Kousis, "Quelques considérations" (note 12 above), 213.1–4. Three recipes for darkening the hair are given by Alexander, I, 453 Puschm.

[19] Sp. Kabasilas, Λαογραφικὰ σύλλεκτα, Λαογραφία, 2 (1911), 645–54; Delatte, *Anecdota*, I, 111.1–18. For a modern parallel, cf. L. Arnaud, "La baskania ou le mauvais oeil chez les grecs modernes. II. Exorcismes quérisseurs," *EO*, 15 (1912), 518.

[20] E. Legrand, *Bibliothèque* (note 12 above), II (1881), 16.452–55; A. Delatte, *Anecdota*, I, 451.19–22.

[21] Cf. J. Stannard, "Byzantine Botanical Lexicography," *Episteme*, 5 (1971), 168–87.

[22] A. Delatte, "Le Lexique de botanique du Parisinus graecus 2419," *BiblFacPhilosLettLiège*, 44 (1930), 59–101; *id.*, *Anecdota*, II, 273–454 [15 lexica]; Margaret H. Thomson, *Textes grecs* (note 17 above), 125–77 [3 lexica]. Much earlier, Vilh. Lundström published two other lexica: "Botaniska lexika från den grekiska medeltiden," *Göteborgs Högskolas Årsskrift*, 15 (1909), 42–52; *id.*, "Ett persiskt-grekiskt medico-botaniskt lexikonfragment," *Eranos*, 12 (1912), 170–74.

[23] It is tempting to think that the ἐπιστήκων or the πημεντάριοι attached to the Pantokrator Hospital had access to a receptarium in order to prepare the many different compounds for patients of both sexes who suffered from a variety of illnesses and wounds. Cf. P. Gautier, ed., "Le typikon du Christ sauveur Pantocrator," *REB*, 32 (1974), 1–145.

[24] For example, ζουλάπιον (Arab. *julab*), used by Planudes, *De morborum materie*, 30 (Ideler, II, p. 321.9). For similar reasons, μαατζοῦν (Arab. *matzun*) i.e., an electuary, "encore usitée aujourd'hui chez le peuple grec," A. Kousis, "Quelques considérations" (note 12 above), p. 217. Cf. also πημεντάριος (Lat. *pigmentarius*, note 23 above). For further examples, see G. Meyer, "Die lateinischen Lehnworte im Neugriechischen," *SBWien*, Phil.-hist. K., 132/3 (1895), 1–84.

supplemented, then supplanted, by newer words, lexica were required in order to stay abreast of medical terminology, and, at the same time, to read with understanding the older authorities, especially Dioscorides and Galen.

The perplexity created by the fluid vocabulary of materia medica can be illustrated in many ways—for example, the profusion of synonyms, Greek and non-Greek alike,[25] for a single substance, scribal errors based on similarities of sound and/or spelling of words denoting medical substances, and the fact that, even today, the denotata of some of those terms is an educated guess.[26]

The ambiguity that resulted was not a mere academic challenge, for it may well have made a difference whether, for example, *ammoniakon* was thought to mean a mineral or a gum resin,[27] or whether *peristereon* meant a bird or a plant,[28] or *chelidonion* a bird, a mineral *or* a plant.[29]

Under these circumstances and in the absence of a standardized nomenclature, many physicians prepared lexica for their private use. These must be distinguished from the lexica prepared by literary scholars and professional glossators such as Photios and Hesychios. For while the former are grossly inferior in terms of style, and all of them much smaller, they have the merit of being restricted, for the most part, to the vocabulary of medicine and allied disciplines. This should not be taken to mean, however, any significant advance in medical lexicography. For, despite the praiseworthy purpose for which these smaller lexica were compiled, they are studded with errors of one kind or another. The most important, for our purpose—and I think I also speak for the nameless patients of those physicians—is the high number of incorrect synonyms for plants, portions of which served as ingredients in literally hundreds of composita. It would be uncharitable to catalogue those incorrect synonyms here, but it is worth emphasizing if only to call attention to the possibility of serious consequences when the names of medicinal substances were misunderstood.

III. Medicinal Substances

It is but a short step from the words used to denote medicinal substances to an examination of the substances themselves. The vast majority described in Byzantine texts on materia medica as having therapeutic properties can be identified with some assurance.[30] Of that number many are also known today, though not always as medicinal substances. Some of them, garlic and parsley for example, are used as seasoning agents. Others, for example thyme and rue, are grown in modern herb gardens, while others, such as the lily or daffodil, are known as ornamentals. Still others, such as frankincense and myrrh, are used for liturgical purposes much as they were in Byzantium. Finally, of course, many of the substances listed as ingredients in Byzantine recipes are still employed as primary foodstuffs: tuna, goose, wheat and barley, cheese, bread, and wine. Moreover, nearly every one of the substances mentioned in our texts is also used in modern folk medicine, and often for similar purposes. Most of the substances found in Byzantine materia medica, however, have long since been abandoned in modern *Schulmedizin*.

For a variety of reasons—uncertainty concerning the precise identification of some substances, the ambiguities of the lexical synonymies and, above all, the absence in antiquity of any chemical means of describing mineral substances—it is idle to speculate on the number of therapeutic substances referred to in our texts. But even if certainty were reached concerning their identification, it is un-

---

[25] Three of the lexica edited by Delatte (*Anecdota*, II, pp. 393–454) contain synonyms in Latin, Italian, Turkish and Arabic.

[26] A selection of neologisms and rare words pertaining to Byzantine materia medica will be found in Jeanselme, "Un aide-memoire" (note 12 above), *passim*.

[27] Ἀμμωνιακόν was a gum resin derived from *Dorema ammoniacum* D. Don. Used medicinally for its pungent odor, the fumes were inhaled; hence the frequent gloss θυμίαμα. Ἅλς ἀμμωνιακός, known to Byzantine glossators as ἅλας ἀμμωνιακόν, was a natural, crystalline, mineral substance whose composition probably varied depending upon the water-soluble impurities. Because the two substances were not always distinguished, a post-classical name, λεοντόγαλα, was coined (Delatte, *Anecdota*, II, 306.12).

[28] Περιστερεών, sometimes περιστερά in the lexica, usually meant a plant, probably *Verbena* sp., hence the synonymy ἱερὰ βοτάνη. The form περιστερεὼν ὄρθιος or ὀρθός was presumably an attempt to distinguish the plant from the common dove. The latter occurs rarely as a medicament and not at all in the medical lexica. Dioscorides' effort to explain the name (IV, 59 Wellmann) was abbreviated by Galen, XII, 98 K. For further details, cf. J. Stannard, "Magiferous Plants and Magic in Medieval Materia Medica," *Maryland Historian*, 8 (1977), 33–46.

[29] Due to the similarity between χελιδών, χελιδόνιον and χελιδονία these terms became confused, as they had in Latin. In fact, the confusion in late Greek reflects the Latin, cf. χελιδόνιον τὸ μικρόν· κελιδώνια μηνόρε and χ. τὸ μέγα· κ. μαϊόρε, Delatte, *Anecdota*, II, 416.16–17.

[30] Cf. B. Langkavel, *Botanik der späteren Griechen vom dritten bis driezehnten Jahrhunterte* (Berlin, 1866). (Langkavel's study must be used with caution). For supplementary data and modern scientific nomenclature, cf. J. Stannard, "Identification of the Plants Described by Albertus Magnus, *De vegetabilibus*, Lib. VI," *Res Publica Litterarum*, 2 (1979), 281–318.

likely that all of them would have been available at any one time in a given place.

It is more compendious, therefore, to divide the medicinal substances into five large groups and provide a few illustrations of each.

(i) Substances of Plant Origin

Since several examples of plant substances that were used therapeutically have been noted above, it will suffice to make but a few general observations. Approximately 450 different species of plants can be identified in the materia medica. This includes all the major taxa, including mosses, ferns, algae and even fungi. The greatest emphasis, however, was on the seed-bearing plants whose seeds, foliage and roots accounted for most of the botanicals whether used as medicaments, as seasoning agents, or as primary foods. In many instances it appears that a pronounced aroma or taste was the most important rationale for its use, unless, of course, the older authorities could be cited as having used that species for a specific purpose. But it was the exotica, transshipped via the Near East, that dominated the recipes—cinnamon, pepper, ginger, cloves and sugar. These, the so-called spices, were usually available only in the dried commercial form. Various passages suggest that their quality varied considerably. This may have been due to political and economic events which periodically disrupted trade. Despite the efforts of the commercial guilds, uniform quality was probably not always achieved.

(ii) Substances of Animal Origin

As in the case of plants, some portion of most of the common animals—sheep, goat, ass, for example—was used for some medicinal purposes. This included not only mammals but birds, fish, reptiles and amphibia. But the use of animal products extended well beyond the vertebrata. A wide range of insects, arachnids, crustacea, molluscs, and other phyla were also employed.[31] By and large, most of the animal substances long ago disappeared from medical practice, and one suspects that part of the reason for this was that while it may have been difficult to authenticate, it was all too easy to falsify crocodile dung, hyena gall, rabbit brain, and the like.

(iii) Substances of Mineral Origin

It is even more difficult to summarize the therapeutic uses of mineral substances for, in many cases, their descriptions permit only a tentative identification. Depending upon the impurities, inorganic as well as organic, plus physical processes such as weathering, what passed for *nitron* or *adarke* in one region may have been quite different with respect to color, odor, texture and weight in another region.[32] It was their physical properties and physiological action that determined the medicinal uses, particularly the water-insoluable minerals and metallic ores. Nonetheless, one can specify a few of the more frequently used mineral substances. Leaving aside coral and amber, whose animal and plant origin respectively were apparently unknown, this includes sulfur, various iron, lead, copper and arsenic compounds, argillaceous clays, and a host of precious and semi-precious gem stones whose virtues were enumerated in lapidaries.[33]

(iv) Praeparata

The fourth class, praeparata, can be dismissed more quickly, but not because those substances were unimportant. It is rather the case that the items falling within this class—wine, vinegar, olive oil, butter, barley meal, cheese, bread and the like—were, and are, household items known to all.[34] Each of the aforementioned was used for therapeutic purposes, either singly or as an ingredient in composita. To some of them specific properties were attributed. Butter, for example, possessed, according to Paul, a digestive and a dispersive or discutient property. For that reason it was useful for buboes and other swellings.[35]

(v) Composita

The last class, composita, can be dealt with even more quickly, for there is no simple way of discussing several hundred compound drugs in one paragraph. Suffice it to say our texts provide accounts

[31] J. Théodoridès, "Intérêt scientifique des miniatures zoologiques d'un manuscrit byzantin," *Acta Biologica Debrecina*, 7/8 (1969–70), 265–72, 8 figs.

[32] Cf. M. Japhet, "Etude sur les principales eaux minérales de l'Asie mineur," *AnnSocHydrolClimatolMéd de Paris*, 23 (1877–78), 316–80.

[33] Cf. M. Psellos, *De lapidibus*, in Ideler, I, 244–47. (The recent edition by P. Galiani, *Michele Psello, De lapidum virtutibus* [Firenze, 1979] was not available to me.) Extracts from the Ps.-Hippocratic Ἑρμηνεία περὶ ἐνεργῶν λιθῶν are printed by Legrand, *Bibliothèque*, II, (1881), p. xxiii.

[34] E. Jeanselme et L. Oeconomos, "Aliments et recettes culinaires des Byzantins," *ProcInternCongrHistMed, London, 1922,* (Anvers, 1923), 155–68.

[35] Paul (ed. Heiberg [*CMG* IX, 1] I, p. 201).

of how to prepare and administer them, possible modifications, admissible substitutions, and the purpose or purposes served by each. Not infrequently this is accompanied by remarks concerning dosage and potential side effects. Many of those composita, incidentally, bore specific names, for example the Collyrium of Constantine or the Salt of St. Gregory the Theologian.[36] This association of a drug with the name of the person who allegedly introduced it or used it with conspicuous success was a convenient tag for physician and patient alike and acted occasionally, no doubt, as a testimonial.

IV. Dietetics

The fourth aspect concerns dietetics. Throughout antiquity and the Middle Ages, there was an intimate relation between materia medica and dietetics. This was due partially to the dangers inherent in one of the most obvious of alternatives to drug therapy, surgery. Emphasis was thus often placed on the adoption of a regimen, of which diet was only one, albeit a conspicuous, part. But the close relations between materia medica and dietetics were further strengthened by the fact that the same substance—depending, of course, on how it was prepared, administered, and the amount— might function sometimes as a foodstuff or as a seasoning agent, at other times as a medicament. Herbs are good examples, but so too are some of the vegetables, for example onion, beet, or cabbage. Even to fruits and nuts there were attributed specific therapeutic properties. But pride of place went to barley. In the form of a thin soup or a thick gruel flavored with various ingredients, a barley tisane was, one is tempted to say, standard bill of fare.[37]

Because of the emphasis placed on dietetic advice as a means of curing specific diseases as well as averting future complaints, it is not surprising that a sizable literature developed.[38] The writings falling within this class vary considerably, from Anthimus' almost illiterate letter to the Emperor Theodoric[39] to Simeon Seth's painfully scholastic

analysis of nearly 200 items, many of which were part of everyday living.[40]

There is little need at this point to summarize the substances discussed by the medico-culinary writers, for there is a high correspondence between substances eaten for nourishment and those eaten to correct an imbalance or cure a disease. In the process of describing these substances and enumerating their virtues, attention was sometimes directed to the proper season to eat nuts, for instance, or certain species of fish or fowl. When reduced to rules, that information could be connected with calendaric and astrological data.[41] By so doing, a mystique *and* a rationale was provided, not only for dietetic advice but for a wide class of magical recipes and rituals designed to alleviate suffering.

V. Paramedical Data

The last aspect, which for want of a better term I shall call "paramedical data," is also the most difficult to keep within bounds. Those paramedical data that I shall concentrate on here include amulets, talismans, incantations, and other techniques, all of which had, in addition to these medicinal uses, a further range of religious and magical uses.[42] Admittedly, only a thin line separates magic and religion, and an even more tenuous line separates folk beliefs from the grosser forms of superstition in which supernatural agents are either involved or implicated. My purpose here is not to settle the long-standing controversy of where to draw the line but to call attention to the medical aspects thereof. A simple example will illustrate the problem. For both epilepsy and gout there was a large assortment of simplicia and composita from which to choose;[43] moreover, various diets and regiminary

---

[36] For τὸ Κωνσταντίνου κολλούριον cf. Ermerins, 135–37. For St. Gregory's salt, cf. E. Jeanselme, "Sels médicamenteux et aromates pris par les Byzantins au cours des repas," *BullSoc-FrançHistMédical*, 16 (1922), 327. Gregory's role as a healer even extended to praying to him for health and prosperity, cf. Legrand, *Bibliothèque*, II (1881), p. xx.

[37] Cf. E. Darmstädter, "Ptisana," *Archeion*, 15 (1933), 181–201.

[38] Cf. Delatte, *Anecdota*, II, pp. 455–99.

[39] *Anthimi De observatione ciborum ad Theodoricum regem francorum epistula*, ed. E. Liechtenhan (Berlin, 1963) [*CMG* VIII, 1].

[40] *Simeonis Sethii Syntagma de alimentorum facultatibus*, ed. B. Langkavel (Leipzig, 1868).

[41] Cf. Hierophilus, πῶς ὀφείλει διαιτᾶσθαι ἄνθρωπος ἐφ' ἑκάστῳ μηνί, in Delatte, *Anecdota*, II, 456–66. (A different version is printed by Ideler, I, 409–17.) The same calendaric orientation underlies Theodore Prodromus, *Mensium adornatio* (Ideler, I, 418–20).

[42] Cf. G. Schlumberger, "Amulettes byzantins anciens destinés à combattre les malefices et maladies," *REG*, 5 (1892), 73–93; V. Laurent, "Amulettes byzantines et formulaires magiques," *BZ*, 36 (1936), 300–15; and F. Pradel, "Griechische und süditalienische Gebete, Beschwörungen und Rezepte des Mittelalters," *RVV*, III:3 (1907), 253–403.

[43] For epilepsy, the peony (*Paeonia officinalis* Retz.) was the most popular simplex, partly due to Galen's endorsement (XI, 859 K.), partly because of its prominent role in late Greco-Roman astrology. (cf. A. Olivieri, "La peonia nell'astrologia greca," *RIGI*, 21 [1937], 139–56.) Among the many recipes for composita, cf. Alexander (ed. Puschmann), I, 545–49; Kousis, "Quelques con-

procedures such as baths were also advised.[44] But in addition, amulets, periapts, and semi-precious stones carried on one's person were also thought to be of avail.[45] Generalizing from this example, it is clear that some people regarded the employment of amulets and the like as not essentially different from the use of poultices, decoctions, and clysters.[46] This was especially the case when the amulet was fashioned of a natural product that, in other instances, was regarded as a common medicament or foodstuff. This explains in part, I believe, the frequency with which laurel and olive leaves were

employed in medico-magical rituals, some of which had a healing function.

To conclude, it has been my intention to emphasize the most notable aspects of Byzantine materia medica and to provide a few illustrations of each. If space permitted, several other less obvious features would have been included, for example the several different, but ultimately interrelated philosophic theories that provided the rationale of drug action and hence explained why a particular substance was thought to be efficacious for a specific purpose. But since a discussion of such theoretical issues is restricted, on the whole, to a limited range of texts, it has been excluded here. It would also have been desirable to enlarge upon the physical operations and technological processes by means of which the raw or crude substances were prepared for administration and/or capable of being stored away for an indefinite period of time. Finally, I have not thought it necessary to enumerate the diseases and complaints for which drug therapy was recommended, the wide range of therapeutic forms available at the time, or the many alternatives to drug therapy. It is sufficient to say that the Byzantine physician had at his disposal one or more means of treating nearly every complaint with which he was faced. For that purpose texts were required, and it is presumably to such texts that Alexander of Tralles was referring when he stated that by following his recipes it was unnecessary to search further.[47]

The University of Kansas

sidérations," 212.20; 213.2; 214.23 etc. For gout, many simplicia were employed, including *Colchicum autumnale* L., the source of colchicine, clinically recognized as specifically effective for gout. There are also many recipes for the preparation of composita, e.g., Alexander (ed. Puschmann), II, 517–47; Kousis, 214.7; M. H. Thomson (note 17 above), p. 73, etc.

[44] Alexander (ed. Puschmann), I, 541–45 recommended a wide range of regiminary measures for epilepsy. A few dietary counsels are recorded by S. Seth (ed. Langkavel) pp. 29.20; 47.15; 109.3; 123.13. For gout, Alexander recommended baths (II, 511–13 Puschm.) and some dietary restrictions (II, 508–10 Puschm.). Alexander, II, 531 Puschm. and Seth, 38.14–19 favor the use of chickpeas (*Cicer arietinum* L.) in the diet. For further details, cf. G. Schmalzbauer, "Medizinisch-Diätetisches über die Podagra aus spätbyzantinischer Zeit," *JÖBG*, 23 (1974), 229–43.

[45] Because the neuro-physiological cause of epilepsy was unknown, a supernatural origin was accepted, on the basis of which epileptics were shunned (cf. F. J. Dölger, "Der Ausschluss der Besessenen von Oblation und Kommunion," *Antike und Christentum*, 4 (1974), 110–29). As a consequence, magical devices were commonly recommended (cf. Alexander I, 557, 561, 567 [Puschm.]; Delatte, *Anecdota*, I, 486.11; 618.17), though rational therapy was still attempted (A. Philipsborn, "ΙΕΡΑ ΝΟΣΟΣ und die Spezial-Anstalt des Pantokrator-Krankenhauses," *Byzantion*, 33 (1963), 223–30). In general, see E. Jeanselme, "L'epilepsie sur le trône de Byzance," *BullSocFrançHistMédical*, 18 (1924), 225–74.

[46] Anna Chatzenikolaou, Μετάλλινα μαγικὰ εἰκονίδια Κωνσταντίνου καὶ Ἑλένης, Ἐπ.Ἑτ.Βυζ.Σπ., 23 (1953), 508–18.

[47] Alexander, II, 109 Puschm.

EARLY BYZANTINE PHARMACOLOGY

John Scarborough

Introduction

The study of Byzantine drug lore presents the modern scholar with several problems. At first glance, it would appear that Oribasius, Aetius of Amida, Alexander of Tralles, and Paul of Aegina have simply replicated data and nomenclature found in the works of Dioscorides, Galen, and other earlier Greek and Roman accounts of herbs and herbals, medicinal minerals, and animal products employed in the manufacture of drugs. Yet when one investigates carefully the Greek texts of all four of these major so-called compilers in the history of early Byzantine medicine, one soon discovers that there are indeed duplications from Greco-Roman authorities in consideration of drugs and drug lore, but that the theory of drug-action has shifted in an important manner, and also that substances used in pharmacy have been augmented, both in number and in kind. This new theory of pharmacology, based firmly upon scattered statements from a wide range of Galenic writings, can be nicely illustrated with the lengthy prologue by Aetius of Amida to his *Medical Books* (the *Tetrabiblon*).[1] Moreover, when one compares "borrowing" by Oribasius, Aetius, Alexander, and Paul, from Galen and earlier authorities, one discerns significant variations in syntax and, most importantly, a clear consideration of medicinal substances in their own right, rather far removed from the copyist epithet often given to these early Byzantine medical writers. Oribasius and Alexander, in particular, submit drug recipes that show a command of the ancient texts and personal experience with pharmaceuticals.

We are also fortunate in being able to link the allegedly formal aspects of early Byzantine drug lore with data that the non-physician might know—

at least in late Roman and Byzantine Egypt. Many papyri, especially those contained in the collection called the *Papyri Graeci Magicae*,[2] show how drugs and pharmaceuticals were used in numerous nonmedical contexts, but of great importance among these papyrological citations is the assumption of common knowledge of the *kyphi* and *krisma* recipes, also significant in the formal works by Byzantine physicians on pharmacology. Early Byzantine pharmacy drew upon classical heritages—from the Hippocratics through Galen—but it also shows a clear development of its own, seen best in a reworked drug theory and in the augmentation of particular substances employed as pharmaceuticals. This sophisticated pharmacy is also paralleled in the papyri,[3] but these documents are, of course, shorn of theory, which may or may not have penetrated into the ranks of Egyptian priests, soothsayers, and purported experts in magic.[4]

The Historical Background of Greek and Roman Pharmacy to Galen

Drug lore is the first aspect of Greek medicine that can be documented, since spices and presumed pharmaceuticals turn up in the Linear B tablets of Mycenaean Greece and Crete.[5] After the

[The reader is referred to the list of abbreviations at the end of the volume.]

[1] Aetius I *prooemium* (ed. Olivieri [*CMG* VIII 1], pp. 17–30).

[2] See esp. *PGM*, IV, 2307–9; XII, 401–45; XXXVI, 322–32.

[3] Marie-Hélène Marganne, *Inventaire analytique des papyrus grecs de médecine* (Geneva, 1981). Magical papyri are excluded.

[4] E.g., *PGM*, XII, 401–45. Cf. H. Harrauer and P. J. Sijpestein, *Medizinische Rezepte und Verwandtes* (Vienna, 1981); K. Sudhoff, *Ärztliches aus griechischen Papyrus-Urkunden* (Leipzig, 1909); H. I. Bell, A. D. Nock, and H. Thompson, *Magical Texts from a Bilingual Papyrus in the British Museum* (London, 1931 [Proceedings of the British Academy, Vol. XVII]). Unfortunately, the rich lore and medical equivalencies in E. A. E. Reymond, *From the Contents of the Libraries of the Suchos Temples in the Fayyum*, Part I: *A Medical Book from Crocodilopolis P. Vindob. D. 6257* (Vienna, 1976), cannot be trusted. A new edition with translation and commentary of P. Vindobonensis D. 6257 is in preparation at the Oriental Institute of the University of Chicago.

[5] See esp. L. R. Palmer, *Interpretation of Mycenaean Greek Texts* (Oxford, 1963), Nos. 163–168 [pp. 269–73], and J. Chadwick, *Documents in Mycenaean Greek*, 2nd ed. (Cambridge, 1973), Nos.

passing of the Mycenaeans, there is good indication of a common knowledge of *pharmaka* (at least
those that were involved in application of simples
for minor wounds, and those that were deemed
potent in spells and incantations) in Homer's ep-
ics,[6] so that drug lore probably flourished among
the Greeks of the Homeric Age, much as it would
later.[7] Lyric poetry has left us with some isolated
mentions of drugs and salves,[8] and there is firm
evidence that certain drugs were well known among
the Greeks in the fifth century B.C., suggested by
puns in Aristophanes and other non-medical writers.[9] It is not until the fifth and fourth centuries
B.C. that a separate study of medical plants was made
a part of formal medical practice, and the Pseudo-
Aristotelian *Problems* probably mirror the same
sources for drugs and drug theory that appear also
in several books of the Hippocratic *corpus*.[10] Diocles of Carystos (a contemporary of Aristotle)[11]
studied plants for their pharmaceutical properties,
and the study of botany received a canonical form
in Theophrastus' *Historia plantarum* and *De causis
plantarum* (both c. 300 B.C.);[12] Book IX of *Historia
plantarum* is our first extant herbal in Greek.[13]

Theophrastus carefully classifies plants by their
leaves, roots, seeds, stems, and growing season, and
the methodologies of his master, Aristotle, show
brilliantly in the taxonomy and morphology.[14]

Although there is good evidence for the study of
pharmacy in the Hellenistic era, our available texts
for the period consist of fragmentary remains of
the drug lore of Apollodorus (*fl.* c. 250 B.C.),[15] and
such notables as Herophilus and Erasistratus (both
fl. 270–260 B.C.),[16] as well as the two poems on toxicology by Nicander of Colophon (*fl.* c. 130 B.C.)
called *Theriaca* and *Alexipharmaca*.[17] Nicander stole
his data from the lost works of Apollodorus, who
had made a detailed study of toxic substances, poisonous snakes, scorpions, spiders, and insects,[18]
apparently in the manner of Peripatetic natural
history,[19] but it would be Nicander's obtuse poems
that became standard "textbooks" in toxicology,
employed by almost all medical authorities from
his own time through the European Renaissance.[20]

Theophrastus struggled with the problem of how
drugs were to be classified, and he provides an extremely muddled system in *Historia plantarum* IX.[21]
Much of his data is derived from a professional class
of *rhizotomoi*, whose firsthand experience Theophrastus records in several instances.[22] Yet the definition of *poa* ("herb") remains hopelessly vague,
since Theophrastus' overriding methodology demanded first attention to morphology and taxonomy, not to the medical properties of any particular plant or drug made from a plant. A foggy notion

103, 105, and 107 [pp. 224, 228, and 231]. A few, scattered studies
have begun to appear on these texts and similar ones, e.g., Anna
Sacconi, "La mirra nella preparazione degli unguenti profumati
a Cnosso," *Athenaeum*, n.s. 47 (1969), 281–89; C. P. W. Warren,
"Some Aspects of Medicine in the Greek Bronze Age," *Medical
History*, 14 (1970), 364–77; and R. Janko, "Un 1314: Herbal
Remedies at Pylos," *Minos*, 17 (1981), 30–34.

[6] E.g., Homer, *Odyssey* X, 304–6, 316–17, and 391–94, among
many references.

[7] Cf. Homer, *Iliad* VIII, 306–8, with Dioscorides IV, 64.1 (ed.
Wellmann, II, p. 218).

[8] When Sappho, Frg. 96 (var. eds., trans. D. A. Campbell, *Greek
Lyric*, I [Cambridge, Mass., 1982], p. 120 [Loeb]), writes "the
dew is shed in beauty, and roses bloom and tender chervil and
flowery melilot," one immediately perceives a long-lived close
acquaintance with herbs and flowers. Sappho, Frgs. 105, 143,
189, and 210 (Campbell, pp. 132, 156, 180 and 192) mention
hyacinth, chick peas, nitrum, and fustic. Cf. Theognis 537 and
1193 (squill and spiny broom); Simonides 10 (myrtle); Hesiod,
Works 41 (asphodel), etc., among many references.

[9] E.g., Aristophanes, *Lysistrata* 89, and *Peace* 712 (puns on the
uses of the pennyroyal [*Mentha pulegium* L.]). Discussion in Scarborough, "Nicander II," 74–75 with nn. 239–54.

[10] J. Scarborough, "Theoretical Assumptions in Hippocratic
Pharmacology," in F. Lasserre and P. Mudry, eds., *Formes de pen-
sée dans la collection hippocratique: Actes du IVᵉ Colloque international
hippocratique (Lausanne . . . 1981)* (Geneva, 1983), 307–25.

[11] W. Jaeger, *Diokles von Karystos*, 2nd ed. (Berlin, 1963), 186–
236. The fairly extensive fragments of Diocles' writings are collected in M. Wellmann, ed., *Die Fragmente der sikelischen Ärzte
Akron, Philistion und des Diokles von Karystos* (Berlin, 1901), 117–
207.

[12] F. Egerton, ed., *Edward Lee Greene: Landmarks of Botanical
History* (Stanford, California, 1983; 2 vols.), I, 128–211.

[13] J. Scarborough, "Theophrastus on Herbals and Herbal
Remedies," *JHB*, 11 (1978), 353–85.

[14] Egerton, ed., *Greene* (n. 12 above), I, 169–89. O. Regenbogen, "Theophrastos," *RE*, Supplementband VII (Stuttgart, 1940),
cols. 1354–1562, esp. 1435–79 (botany).

[15] M. Wellmann, "Apollodorus (69)," *RE*, Vol. I, part 2 (Stuttgart, 1894), col. 2895, and (same author), "Das älteste Kräuter-
buch der Griechen," in *Festgabe für Franz Susemihl* (Leipzig, 1898),
1–31. J. Scarborough, "Nicander's Toxicology, I: Snakes," *PH*,
19 (1977), 3–23 (3–4, with nn. 8–19).

[16] P. M. Fraser, *Ptolemaic Alexandria* (Oxford, 1972; 3 vols.), I,
353, and II, 519 n. 116, and 627 n. 472 [Herophilus]. R. Fuchs,
"Eine neue Receptformel des Erasistratos," *Hermes*, 33 (1898),
342–44.

[17] Nicander (ed. and trans. Gow and Scholfield) is the best
edition available, with a translation quite often based on shrewd
guesswork—openly admitted by the editors.

[18] Scarborough, "Nicander's Snakes" (n. 15 above), 3–4, and
(same author), "Nicander II" *passim*.

[19] Scarborough, "Nicander II," 5–6. Wellmann, "Kräuter-
buch" (n. 15 above), 28.

[20] E.g., a late Greek manuscript (Bologna, Bibl. Univ. Codex
3632, esp. fol. 417) of the late fifteenth or early sixteenth century. Scarborough, "Nicander II," 4, with nn. 4–8.

[21] Egerton, ed., *Greene* (n. 12 above), I, 180–81. Scarborough,
"Theophrastus" (n. 13 above), 356–57.

[22] Theophrastus, *HP* IX, 8 *passim*; 11.7 and 9; 15.2; 16.3; 18.3
and 10; and 20.4.

of toxicology does appear in Book IX of *Historia plantarum*,[23] but Theophrastus and his sources seem unaware of a basic theory that would explain the differences among drugs. Some hints of an embryonic theory of toxicology do, indeed, appear in the Pseudo-Aristotelian *Problems*, as well as certain tracts of the Hippocratic *corpus*, but there is more of an attempt to collect data than to propose a logical and careful hypothesis about how and why drugs "work" as they do. Nicander's poems also reflect this attention to the collection of details, and the lack of a cohesive theory to link them together, and the fragments of other Hellenistic pharmacologists likewise suggest a haphazard and often erroneous set of prescriptions, or—in the cases of Herophilus and Erasistratus—an attempt to set down specific treatments for particular ailments, in the classic manner of the Hippocratic writers.

Dioscorides of Anazarbus (*fl. c.* A.D. 65) attempted to change the chaos of pharmacology into an ordered system.[24] He seems to have invented a "drug affinity" methodology for the study of pharmaceuticals, quite similar to the modern concepts underlying pharmacognosy, but this non-alphabetical, non-humoral theory demanded precise observation of plants in their varying growing seasons as well as extreme accuracy in the physician's observations concerning which drugs were useful against which specific ailments and diseases. Dioscorides' *Materia medica* certainly became a classic handbook, quoted by almost all later writers on pharmacy (both Greek and Latin, as well as Arabic) for nearly 1800 years.[25] He includes nearly 600 species of plants in the *Materia medica*,[26] compared with approximately 450 species in the Hippocratic *corpus*,[27] the 550 species recorded by Theophrastus,[28] and the 300 plant names given by Nicander.[29] Dioscorides' listings encompass many drugs introduced into Greco-Roman pharmacy from the

Far East,[30] showing the expansion of trade and geographic knowledge in the Hellenistic era and in the first decades of Roman imperial rule in the eastern Mediterranean.[31] His rejection, however, of both the poetic form of relating knowledge of drugs (illustrated by the difficult hexameters of Nicander) and also the apparently standard manner of listing simples in alphabetical order,[32] led in turn to the discarding of Dioscorides' classification system by later pharmacologists, including the chalcenteric Galen.[33] Dioscorides' drug lore tapped not only the formal sources of pharmacology, as they might be found in earlier written records, but also folk medicine, acknowledged from time to time in the *Materia medica*.[34] Moreover, he insists that the would-be pharmacologist has to know his plants, not from book-learning, but by patient and lengthy observation of herb growth as they changed form, shape, and color through differing seasons in various geographic locations as he knew them generally in the eastern Mediterranean litoral.[35] Added to the demand of painstaking observation of reaction to drugs by actual patients, these two requirements by Dioscorides soon led to modifications, including a return to alphabetical listings and pharmaceutical poetry.[36] While respecting Dioscorides for his obvious learning and meticulous attention to botanical details, Galen rejected the "drug affinity" system, while retaining (at least he says he does) Dioscorides' admonition to know the plants from personal experience. And it would be Galen, not Dioscorides, who would provide the beginning models for Byzantine drug lore.

GALEN'S PHARMACY

Galen of Pergamon (A.D. 129-prob. 210) looms as one of the most influential writers in the entire history of medicine.[37] His summary of all aspects

---

[23] Theophrastus, *HP* IX, 16.4–7. Scarborough, "Theophrastus" (n. 13 above), 376–77 with nn. 131–35.

[24] Scarborough and Nutton, "Preface," 189–90. J. M. Riddle, "Dioscorides," *DSB*, Vol. IV (New York, 1971), 119–23. Riddle's *Dioscorides* (Austin, Texas [in press]) explicates in brilliant detail Dioscorides' "drug affinity" system.

[25] J. M. Riddle, "Dioscorides" in *Catalogus* IV, 1–143. Scarborough and Nutton, "Preface," 187–88.

[26] J. Stannard, "Byzantine Botanical Lexicography," *Episteme*, 5 (1971), 168–87 [171].

[27] My "count" differs sharply with that of Stannard (*ibid.*), who suggests about 225 spp. [p. 170].

[28] Regenbogen, "Theophrastos" (n. 14 above), col. 1467. Egerton, ed., *Greene* (n. 12 above), I, 96 gives 500 as his "count."

[29] Based on Nicander, ed. and trans. Gow and Scholfield.

[30] E.g., ginger (*Zingiber officinale* Roscoe) among several. J. I. Miller, *The Spice Trade of the Roman Empire* (Oxford, 1969), 53–57.

[31] J. Scarborough, "Roman Pharmacy and the Eastern Drug Trade," *PH*, 24 (1982), 135–43.

[32] Scarborough and Nutton, "Preface," 212–13.

[33] *Ibid.*, 190–91.

[34] *Ibid.*, 189 with nn. 10 and 13.

[35] Dioscorides, *Preface* 7 (ed. Wellmann, I, p. 4; trans. Scarborough and Nutton, "Preface," 196–97).

[36] E.g. the medical poetry of Damocrates (quoted by Galen) and most of the drug lists by Galen.

[37] The literature on Galen is enormous, but only a few works are based securely on the Greek texts. Recommended are: V. Nutton, "The Chronology of Galen's Early Career," *CQ*, n.s. 23 (1973), 158–71, and [same author], "Galen and Medical Auto-

of medicine and related matters, including philosophy and pharmacology, exerted a heavy sway over physicians and medical commentators well into the nineteenth century,[38] and one may gauge his prolixity and learning by the simple task of counting the volumes (20) represented by the Kühn edition of Galen.[39] Since his drug lore influenced later writers, especially in the Byzantine East, so heavily, one necessarily must consider Galen's pharmacology in some detail in order to perceive how early Byzantine drug theory might be similar to and different from the presumed blueprints laid down in several of his treatises which consider pharmaceuticals in particular.

Galen's drug lore is scattered throughout the massive number of works left under his name, but much of his approach to pharmacology, herbs, and treatments through pharmaceuticals is concentrated in *Mixtures and Properties of Simples,*[40] *Compound Drugs Arranged by Location of Ailment,*[41] *Compound Drugs Arranged by Kind,*[42] *Antidotes,*[43] and similar tracts, some of which may be spurious.[44] Galen quotes from dozens of earlier Greek and Roman pharmacologists—including Dioscorides—and although Galen insists one had to know plants and drugs personally,[45] many of the recipes, prescriptions, and treatments are filched from earlier authorities,[46] most often through previous collections of recipes compiled by Andromachus (physician to Nero [A.D. 54–68]), Asclepiades the Pharmacist (prob. *fl.* c. A.D. 50), and Criton (physician to Trajan [A.D. 98–117]). He includes all of the famous simples, known from the time of Theophrastus, but adds no new herbs to the varieties already known to Dioscorides.

In *Mixtures and Properties of Simples* I–V,[47] Galen sets out in an incredibly verbose fashion his composite theory of drug action, based upon degree of cold and hot, moist and dry, with subtle sub-classifications generally measured according to the senses of taste, touch, and smell. Not surprisingly, these 329 Kühn pages will not form the foundation of Byzantine adaptation of Galen's drug theories, as will be suggested below with the consideration of the Preface to Aetius' *Medical Books*. Galen proposes his arguments upon what he says are the "best authorities," and *Simples* I–V is replete with name-dropping of the worthies of the pharmaceutical past, from Diocles, Hippocrates, and Theophrastus, through Dioscorides and Asclepiades. What emerges in this involuted summary is the famous "drugs by degrees" system,[48] which would retain its hold on western pharmacy until the nineteenth century. Only in the beginning of Book VI of *Simples* does Galen speak in specific about drugs, and then only after a Preface to Book VI in which he warns against misleading authorities (for example, Pamphilus)[49] who were not experts in plants, and in which he re-lists the reliable sources (a long list that includes Dioscorides)[50]— but Galen lets us know that none of his predecessors understood drugs as well as he does. Then follows the listing of drugs, beginning with "On Shrubby Wormwood and Absinthe and their Particular Kinds."[51] Unlike the extreme clarity of Dioscorides, we read a muddled catalogue of properties generally based on locale. *Simples* VI, 2[52] is "On Agnus Castus," *Simples* VI, 3 is "On Dog's Tooth Grass" [*agrōstis*],[53] VI, 4 is "The Four Kinds of Alkanet" [*anchousa*],[54] VI, 5 is "The Agaric 'Root'"

biography," *Proceedings of the Cambridge Philological Society,* 18 (1972), 50–62; J. Scarborough, "The Galenic Question," *SA,* 65 (1981), 1–31, and (same author), "Galen and the Gladiators," *Episteme,* 5 (1971), 98–111; J. Ilberg, "Aus Galens Praxis," *Neue Jahrbücher für das klassische Altertum,* 15 (1905), 276–312 (rptd. in H. Flashar, ed., *Antike Medizin* [Darmstadt, 1971], 361–416); J. Mewaldt, "Galenos (2)," *RE,* Vol. VII, part 1 (Stuttgart, 1910), cols. 578–91; F. Kudlien and L. G. Wilson, "Galen," *DSB,* Vol. V (New York, 1972), 227–37; W. D. Smith, *The Hippocratic Tradition* (Ithaca, New York, 1979), 61–176; J. Kollesch, "Galen und die Zweite Sophistik," in Nutton, ed., *Galen: Problems,* 1–12; and— above all—Temkin, *Galenism,* 10–50 ("The Portrait of an Ideal").

[38] Temkin, *Galenism,* 134–92 ("Fall and Afterlife").

[39] The texts of Galen in *CMG* are a small proportion of the works contained in the Kühn ed., which is badly marred by corruptions. To the listing in H. Leitner, *Bibliography to the Ancient Medical Authors* (Bern, 1973), 38–39, can now be added: Nutton, ed., *Galen On Prognosis;* and De Lacy, ed., *Galen On the Doctrines of Hippocrates and Plato.*

[40] Ed. Kühn, XI, 379–892, and XII, 1–377 (in 11 books).

[41] Ed. Kühn, XII, 378–1007, and XIII, 1–361 (in 10 books).

[42] Ed. Kühn, XIII, 362–1058 (in 7 books).

[43] Ed. Kühn, XIV, 1–209 (in 2 books).

[44] *Theriac to Piso* (ed. Kühn, XIV, 210–94 [possible]), *Theriac to Pamphilus* (ed. Kühn, XIV, 295–310 [certainly spurious]), *Easily-Obtained Drugs* (ed. Kühn, XIV, 311–581 in 3 books [certainly spurious]).

[45] Galen, *Mixtures and Properties of Simples* VI, preface (ed. Kühn, XI, 797). Scarborough, *Medicine,* 128–30.

[46] Fabricius, 62–100.

[47] Ed. Kühn, XI, 459–788.

[48] See discussion of Aetius with nn. 149–68 below.

[49] Ed. Kühn, XI, 793–94.

[50] *Ibid.,* 794 and 797.

[51] *Simples* VI, 1 (ed. Kühn, XI, 798–807). Scarborough and Nutton, "Preface," 225–27 (wormwoods).

[52] Cf. Dioscorides I, 103. This is *Vitex agnus-castus* L. (ed. Kühn, XI, 807–10).

[53] Scarborough and Nutton, "Preface," 219 (dog's tooth grass: *Cynodon dactylon* [L.] Pers.). ed. Kühn, XI, 810–11.

[54] Ed. Kühn, XI, 811–13. Cf. Dioscorides IV, 23. This is *Anchousa tinctoria* L.

[*agarikos*],[55] and so on, so that by the end of Book VI of *Simples*, Galen has reached *iota* in what has become an alphabetical listing of simples (all plants) with some properties given according to "heating" and "cooling." Books VII and VIII[56] complete the alphabetical listing of herbs and their properties by their classes of heating and cooling qualities. *Simples* IX, 1.1–4 is "Earths,"[57] IX, 2.1–21 "Stones,"[58] and "Things Mined as Drugs" [*metallika pharmaka*] is *Simples* IX, 3.1–40.[59] Most of these substances are in alphabetical order, with some exceptions suggesting possible corruptions in the Greek texts. *Simples* X is what we would call "animal products," and much as had Dioscorides often prescribed blood for various ailments, so too does Galen extrapolate on this "humor" as a drug along with a number of other materials presumably classed with blood because they emerge from animals; the listing in and of itself is instructive, not so much for what Galen recommended, but for the substances he found listed in his sources (Xenocrates seems to be a major authority).[60] After listing various animal bloods (dove, bat, rabbit, deer, rooster, male goat, lamb, bear, bull, green frog, crocodile and lizard),[61] one reaches a "dairy product" listing (milk, cheese, butter, rennet, seal rennet),[62] followed by biles, perspiration, urine, saliva, and various kinds of animal and bird dungs and manure.[63]

In Book XI of *Simples*, Galen lists other "animal products,"[64] ranging from the flesh of poisonous snakes, marrow, and the liver of a mad dog,[65] to spider webs, blister beetles, cicadas, castor, brains of various animals, eggs, and charred crabs.[66] *Simples*

XI, 2 is a collection of oddments that could be labeled "products of the sea useful in medicinals,"[67] and here are sponges, garum, coral, various sorts of salts and salt products including *asphaltos*.[68] Unlike the herbs and plants of *Simples* VI–VIII, which are given alphabetically, Galen's animal products and sea-medicines seem entered according to another pattern, perhaps ultimately derived from Dioscorides or earlier data found in some of the Hippocratic texts. In sum, Galen lists about 440 different plants in his accounting of herbs in *Simples* I–VIII, and about 250 other substances in the remaining books as useful in making drugs. Indeed, there are caustic remarks concerning the drugs of Xenocrates, especially the varieties of dung, but Galen *does* list them, and one can presume that such materials had long standing in ancient pharmacology, verified by a comparison with medicinals suggested by writers in the Hippocratic *corpus*, Dioscorides, as well as the magical papyri.[69]

Once the alphabetical and non-alphabetical listings of drugs are completed in *Simples*, Galen apparently decides to approach pharmaceutical lore in another way in the ten books we have as *Compound Drugs Arranged by Location of Ailment*.[70] These ten books were written after Galen had put down the *Method of Healing*,[71] whereas the *Simples* predates it.[72] Galen's struggle with drugs—and how to classify them—can be discerned through the successive attempts he made to provide lucid catalogues: first is his *Properties of Cleansing Drugs*, writ-

---

[55] Ed. Kühn, XI, 813–14. As this is a shelf-fungus, the passage shows Galen's ignorance. G. Maggiulli, *Nomenclatura micologica latina* (Genoa, 1977), 85–87. Cf. Dioscorides III, 1.

[56] Ed. Kühn, XII, 1–158.

[57] *Ibid.*, 165–92.

[58] *Ibid.*, 192–208.

[59] *Ibid.*, 208–44.

[60] *Simples* X, preface (ed. Kühn, XII, 245–53).

[61] *Simples* X, 2–6 (ed. Kühn, XII, 256–63).

[62] *Simples* X, 2.7–12 (ed. Kühn, XII, 263–75).

[63] *Simples* X, 2.13–29 (ed. Kühn, XII, 275–308). *Simples* X, 2.15 (ed. Kühn, XII, 284–88) ends with Galen noting that "drinking the urine of a prepubescent boy is not recommended," and *Simples* X, 2.16 (ed. Kühn, XII, 288–90: on salivas) has a rare direct quotation from Nicander (*Theriaca* 86). *Simples* X, 2.17 (ed. Kühn, XII, 290) summarizes why one uses such materials. Cf. Paul of Aegina VII, 3, *s.v.* κόπρος (ed. Heiberg, II, 228).

[64] Ed. Kühn, XII, 310–77.

[65] *Simples* XI, 1.1 (snakes, esp. the *echidnē*: Scarborough, "Nicander's Snakes" [n. 15 above], 7–8); XI, 1.3 (marrow); and XI, 1.10 (rabid dog's liver). ed. Kühn, XII, 311–23, 311–33, and 335.

[66] *Simples* XI, 1.23 (spider webs); XI, 1.44–45 (blister beetles); XI, 1.36 (cicadas); XI, 1.15 (castor); and XI, 1.31 (brains, kid-

neys, and eggs). Ed. Kühn, XII, 343, 363–64, 360, 337–41, and 349–55. Charred or burned crabs, or more accurately the ashes of crabs, are prescribed in *Simples* XI, 1.24 (ed. Kühn, XII, 356–59). See J. Scarborough, "Some Beetles in Pliny's Natural History," *Coleopterists Bulletin*, 31 (1977), 293–96 ("Spanish Fly" and beetles of Lyttinae) and (same author), "Nicander II," 13–14, 20–21, 73–80 with nn. 134–45, 215–30, and 237–325 (blister beetles, descriptions, and purported remedies for the ingestion of "Spanish Fly" in classical antiquity); and (same author), "The Drug Lore of Asclepiades of Bithynia," *PH*, 17 (1975), 43–57 (51: castor).

[67] Ed. Kühn, XII, 369–77.

[68] *Simples* XI, 2.11 (sponges); XI, 2.12 (garum); XI, 2.3 (coral); and XI, 2.5–10 (salts and salt products). Ed. Kühn, XII, 376, 377, 370–71, and 372–75. For garum, see R. I. Curtis, "In Defense of *Garum*," *CJ*, 78 (1983), 232–40, and [same author] "The Garum Shop of Pompeii," *Cronache Pompeiane*, 5 (1979), 5–23. For sponges, see J. Théodoridès, "Considerations on the Medical Use of Marine Invertebrates," in M. Sears and D. Merriman, eds., *Oceanography: The Past* (New York, 1980), 734–49 (esp. 734–36).

[69] Cf. *PGM*, I, 224–25; IV, 1439–40, 2574–75, 2585, 2651; VII, 486; XII, 410, 414.

[70] Ed. Kühn, XII, 378–1007, and XIII, 1–361.

[71] *Drugs by Location* I, 1 (ed. Kühn, XII, 378).

[72] Ilberg, *Schriftstellerei*, 89.

ten before A.D. 169;[73] then Galen wrote the second of his "drug books," *Simples*, probably in the 170s, number six on the list of the works as suggested by Ilberg, after Galen's return to Rome in 169;[74] *Location* was written sometime in the period between A.D. 180 and 193, preceded by *Compound Drugs Arranged by Kind*.[75] Even though Ilberg shows that *Drugs by Kind* was composed before *Drugs by Location*, the Kühn edition places *Location* previous to *By Kind*, so that the following synopsis proceeds according to the unfortunately erroneous order (which has become traditional) set down in the Kühn volumes. Both *Drugs by Location* and *Drugs by Kind* indicate Galen's continual efforts to obtain clarity in description of medicinals, and Ilberg rightly notes that these two collections of drug lore came from Galen's pen very close to one another in time, perhaps in the two or three years preceding the fire in the Temple of Peace in A.D. 192.[76]

The arrangement of drugs in *Location*, so Galen writes,[77] is inspired by the example of Hippocrates, and would seem to show an order of the simplest sort: a beginning with affections of the head would lead, naturally enough, to ailments to be treated as one proceeds down from the head through other parts of the body (each with its own malfunctions: *tou kamnontos krasis hē te tou paschontos moriou physis*[78]), a manner called in the later Latin tradition, *a capite ad calcem*. What follows in *Drugs by Location* is a series of suggestions for various problems, indicative more of an "upper class" practice and a culling of beauty-care manuals than of Galen's original intent to organize drug lore in a logical head-to-toe pattern. Titles of the sections delineate the subject matter of *Drugs by Location*, almost in contradistinction to what Galen has said he wants to do in the short preface: "Alopecia," "On Hair Loss," "On the Coloring of Hair," "Drugs for Broken Hair," "Thin Hair," "On Hair that is Dying," and "Dandruff."[79] Much of this material comes from quoted extracts of Criton's books on drugs,[80] in turn extracting earlier sources on pharmaceuticals under the names of Archigenes, Cleopatra, and Apollo-

nius.[81] Book II of *Drugs by Location* has recipes from a number of sources on "illnesses of the head,"[82] but most of the prescriptions for ear and nose problems are in Book III,[83] and the list of "authorities" has expanded to include Damocrates (recipes in poetry), Heras, Apollonius, Archigenes, Andromachus, Xenocrates, Harpalus, Harpocrates, Solon the Dietician, Zoilus the Ophthalmologist, Asclepiades, Charixenus, Antonius Musa, Heraclides of Tarentum, etc.[84] Eye diseases and numerous *kollyria* recipes comprise *Location* IV,[85] and more "beauty aids" for eye-bruises and black eyes begin *Location* V,[86] followed by lachrymal fistulas,[87] and salves, ointments, and plasters for the forehead, along with a great number of mouthwashes, dentifrices (Damocrates' poems) and treatments for various tooth problems.[88] Stomach soothers and gargles form Book VI,[89] congestion relievers and arteriaces are Book VII,[90] but *Drugs by Location* IX contains a melange of remedies, including internal treatments for jaundices and affections of the spleen, followed by hemorrhoids, priapism, anal suppositories, and finally a recipe for the treatment of "uterine suffocation."[91] Book X provides recipes for the treatment of kidney problems, gout, sciatica (*ischias*), and arthritis,[92] and at one point where a poem of Damocrates is being quoted for a cure of sciatica, there is clear indication that an illustrated text has been consulted.[93] *Compound Drugs Arranged by Location of Ailment* does not emerge as a complete and coherent tract on drug lore, but seems to be a potpourri of recipes collected and loosely grouped by external parts, emphasizing the head, with sections on gout, sciatica, and the like that might formally qualify the work as a "head-to-toe" treatise.

The third of Galen's massive pharmaceutical

[81] Fabricius, 198–99 (Archigenes), 180–83 (Apollonius).

[82] Ed. Kühn, XII, 498–598.

[83] *Ibid.*, 599–695.

[84] Fabricius, 189–90 (Damocrates), 183–85 (Heras), 180–83 (Apollonius), 198–99 (Archigenes), 185–89 (Andromachus the Younger), etc. M. Wellmann, "Beiträge zur Quellenanalyse des Älteren Plinius," *Hermes*, 59 (1924), 129–56 (140–42; Xenocrates; 142–43: Solon).

[85] Ed. Kühn, XII, 696–803.

[86] *Ibid.*, 804–93.

[87] *Ibid.*, 820–22.

[88] *Ibid.*, 889–93 (Damocrates' poems).

[89] Ed. Kühn, XII, 894–1007.

[90] Ed. Kühn, XIII, 1–115.

[91] *Ibid.*, 228–320. "Uterine Suffocation": *Location* IX, 10 (ed. Kühn, XIII, 319–20). Cf. *PGM*, VII, 260–71, and Soranus, *Gynecology* III, 50 (ed. Ilberg, pp. 127–28).

[92] Ed. Kühn, XIII, 321–61.

[93] *Ibid.*, 351.

[73] Ed. Kühn, XI, 323–42. Ilberg, *Schriftstellerei*, 77.

[74] Ilberg, *Schriftstellerei*, 89.

[75] *Ibid.*, 20–23 and 84.

[76] *Ibid.*, 84.

[77] *Drugs by Location* I, 1 (ed. Kühn, XII, 381).

[78] *Ibid.* (ed. Kühn, XII, 378).

[79] *Drugs by Location* I, 2–9 (ed. Kühn, XII, 381–497).

[80] On Criton, physician to Trajan (A.D. 98–117), see E. Kind, "Kriton (7)," *RE*, Vol. XI, part 2 (Stuttgart, 1922), cols. 1935–38, and J. Benedum, "Kriton," *RE*, Supplementband XIV (Stuttgart, 1974), cols. 216–20.

works is titled *Compound Drugs Arranged by Kind*.[94] It seems that Galen had been attacked by other physicians for his earlier writings on drugs,[95] which had omissions and faulty principles of organization; it also seems apparent that he wrote *Drugs by Kind* late in life, after the fire at the Temple of Peace in A.D. 192.[96] He will stick by his "system of degrees" as developed in the *Simples*, but he has shifted somewhat as he begins to write this "third approach" to drugs, taking up the venerated "treatment by contraries."[97] What follows in the seven books of *Drugs by Kind* is compilation accompanied by commentary, interspersed by recipes, and the remedies "work" according to the theory of treatment by contraries. An odd sort of fuzziness characterizes the initial chapters of *Drugs by Kind* I, but there is a greater care with sources than one finds in Galen's earlier treatises on pharmacy, illustrated by the subtitles: "A White [Plaster] from [White] Pepper, as Compounded by Attalus and Heras," followed by "Attalus, as Quoted by Andromachus, on the Compounding of a White [Plaster] for a Small Wound by a Rabid [Dog] and for Wounded *Neura*."[98] Heras was an authority on rabies,[99] but Galen is concentrating his attention in Book I of *By Kind* on the white color of the plasters under discussion, and he ends the book with a quotation from Damocrates' medical poem, "On the White Plaster."[100] Green plasters occupy Galen in *By Kind* II, 2–4 (Kuhn, XIII, 470–99), but *By Kind* II, 3 (Kuhn, XIII, 496) shows that Galen is *not* arguing that the similarities of color give certain "related" plasters their effectiveness, but that their similarity of properties (*dynameis*) provide their usefulness—even though he condemns Andromachus for taking color as a guide. *By Kind* II, 5 (Kuhn, XIII, 499–503) is "Drugs That Can be Wiped Away Quickly," and here are salves and oily ointments as cited (without specific recipes) from Criton, Heras, Archigenes, Philip, Menecrates, and other authorities. *By Kind* II–IV contain a large number of suggestions on plasters, drugs for wounds of the *neura*, and drugs for promoting the healing of wounds and ulcerations, as well as plasters and ointments that helped form scar tissue (cicatrization), culled

from a number of sources.[101] Book V of *By Kind* (Kuhn, XIII, 763–858) might be titled "Multi-Purpose Drugs," and Galen gives a dazzling display of his purported knowledge of pharmaceuticals—or at least his command of the written sources that have recorded such multiple-use drugs. In *By Kind* V, 1 (Kuhn, XIII, 763–65), Galen restates his basic, underlying theory of drugs by describing them all, in the first place, as characterized by the hot, the cold, the dry, and the wet, and then, consequently, considering the compounding from simples of these drugs according to their dominant quality; this, in turn, would indicate how these compound medicinals would perform according to their "thinning" properties, "thickening" properties, "promotion of scarring" properties, induction of flesh-growth properties, and so on. Only in this way, Galen insists, can one comprehend why drugs work as they do. Formulas abound. Authorities appear in a rapid blur, and the list of names cited in Book V of *By Kind* indicates which sources Galen had at his disposal, and will provide part of the pattern through which Byzantine medical writers would use *their* sources—whether through Galen or independently.[102]

Book VI of Galen's *Compound Drugs Arranged by Kind* (Kuhn, XIII, 859–945) takes up the subject of multi-use plasters. First comes a "Preface" (*By Kind* VI, 1 [Kuhn, XIII, 859–62]) in which Galen notes that the previous book of *By Kind* has considered the plasters called *poluchrēstoi*, designated as

---

[94] Ed. Kuhn, XIII, 362–1058 (in 7 books).
[95] *By Kind* I, 1 (ed. Kuhn, XIII, 363).
[96] *By Kind* I, 1 (ed. Kuhn, XIII, 362).
[97] *By Kind* I, 1 (ed. Kuhn, XIII, 367).
[98] *By Kind* I, 13–14 (ed. Kuhn, XIII, 414–27).
[99] *By Kind* I, 16 (ed. Kuhn, XIII, 431–42: Heras on hydrophobia, accompanied by Xenocrates).
[100] *By Kind* I, 19 (ed. Kuhn, XIII, 455–57).

[101] Ed. Kuhn, XIII, 503–762.
[102] Heras of Cappadocia, Epigonus, "from the Temple of Hephaestus at Memphis" (a plaster made from dittany [Kuhn, XIII, 778–80]), Hicesius, Criton quoting Heras, Criton quoting Hicesius, Andromachus, Criton quoting the recipe of the "Medicine of Machairon" for the healing of all kinds of wound (Kuhn, XIII, 796–97), Criton quoting Damocrates, Asclepiades (*By Kind* V, 4 [Kuhn, XIII, 801–2] along with a recipe compounded by Galen), Phylacus quoting Diophantus the surgeon, Andromachus on green plasters (quoting Evagrius, Epicurus, Alcimonius or Nicomachus), Heraclides of Tarentum quoting Hicesius, Philoxenus, Damocrates' poem on making a plaster from dittany (*By Kind* V, 10 [Kuhn, XIII, 820–23]), Asclepiades quoting Aristarchus of Tarsus (V, 11 [Kuhn, XIII, 824–25]), Andronius, Terentius, Areius, [Scribonius] Largus (Kuhn, XIII, 828), Threptus, Hierax of Thebes, Lucius, Magnus of Philadelphia, Gaius of Naples, Agathinus, Mnesitheus, Apollophanes. Nicolaus, Petronius, Agathocles, Achilla (Kuhn, XIII, 834), Isidorus, Alcimion quoting Apollonius Archistator on the "pill that acts like a scalpel" (Kuhn, XIII, 835), Glaucius, Tiberius Caesar, Phanius, Antipatrus, Publius, Philinus, Melitonus, Apollonius of Tarsus, Asclepiades quoting Marcellus, Xenocrates from his work *Drugs from Vetch* (Kuhn, XIII, 846), a recipe of Serapis "set up on metal plates: a fleshmaker" (Kuhn, XIII, 847), Tryphon, Heliodorus, Ptolemy, Eunomus, Theotropus quoting Areius, Apelles, and Cleobulus. Galen has gained most of these names and recipes through the collections of Andromachus, Asclepiades, and Criton.

those preparations to be "laid on" for treatment of open sores, ulcers, and the like, either to cause them to heal rapidly, or to cause them to remain open, according to the course of therapy prescribed by the physician. Galen says he has observed the compounding of such drugs during his frequent travels, and how he will, now, record some further "wide-use" plasters, but only after he has verified their efficacy in his own experience with patients. These plasters are those which are employed for flesh that is rotting or semi-putrified, and he will begin with plasters made from herbs. But instead of a formula designated by some geographic location, Galen starts his account by quoting Criton's "Plaster from Herbs" (*By Kind* 2 [Kühn, XIII, 863–64]), with measurements. One wonders what happened to Galen's gathered drug lore, presumably recorded from his travels, when he proceeds to explain why *Criton's* formula would contain poppies (*mēkōn*: *Papaver* spp.), black henbane (*hyoskyamos*: *Hyoscyamus niger* L.)—these would give the "cold"— and the scarlet pimpernel (*anagallis*: *Anagallis arvensis* L.), which would provide the "drying property." Following in *By Kind* VI, 1 (Kühn, XIII, 869–73) is a "Squill Plaster" (*skilla*: *Urginea maritima* [L.] Baker), again probably from Criton's collection, and Galen commends this formula provided one tempers it with wax (Kühn, XIII, 871). After discussing further recipes from Criton and Andromachus,[103] Galen proceeds to the vexed question of weights and measures: after his valuable discussion of how weights and measures are calculated in Italy, Greece, Alexandria, and Ephesus, it seems clear enough that Galen is rather frustrated by the inexactitude of the formulas he has received in the pharmacological sources, and especially by the inexact equivalences that seem to thwart his reproducing the formulas to his satisfaction.[104] Adromachus continues to supply Galen with the listed

plaster recipes, until one reaches "A Tyrian Plaster" (*By Kind* VI, 12; [Kühn, XIII, 915–23]), which turns out to be another medical poem by Damocrates, not an original formula from Phoenician Tyre as might have been recorded by Galen.[105] The confused nature of Galen's drug formulas in *By Kind* may be illustrated by an example from the listings of *malagmata*, "emollient" or "soft" plasters. *By Kind* VII summarizes *malagmata* with an apparent strained classification system, as Galen tries to distinguish them from other plasters,[106] and Galen's quotation from Heras on a compound called the *kērelaion* shows how Galen's written sources had confused the specific names of these drugs—and by implication why the best of the Byzantine writers on pharmacy did *not* use Galen as an exact blueprint:

> *Kērelaion*: Praised by Heras above all among Drugs. "Take freshly defibered clear fat, 44 [Roman] ounces, 24 ounces of beeswax, 6 ounces of cerussite,[107] 6 ounces of massicot,[108] and dissolve together the dry ingredients, and shortly they will become congealed." Heras said "the beeswax and the clear fat are the softening properties." Thus if some beeswax would be mixed with a little oil, you will make what is called by the doctors a *kērelaion*, a wax-oil.[109] But clearly the oil ought not to be called either the squeezings of unripe grape [*to omphakinon*] or oil of unripe olives,[110] nor should one assume the addition of the oil of palm leaves.[111]

The remainder of *By Kind* VII[112] continues in this confusion, with numerous quotations from Damocrates, Andromachus, Asclepiades (probably the "Younger," or Pharmacion), and other names now familiar from other Galenic drug books. One may suspect textual corruptions in the Kühn Greek, but interpolations do not explain away the rampant disorder in drug classifications, except for the broad categories of plasters, emollients, earths, herbal simples, and the like. Even though Galen has a reasonably clear theory of drug action, it is smothered by the numerous and often contradic-

---

[103] Of interest in terms of preparation technique is "A Plaster from a Whetstone," i.e., a powdered compound rubbed on a whetstone (ed. Kühn, XIII, 874–82; cf. Dioscorides I, 98). Criton also provides Galen with a formula from Heras (*By Kind* VI, 3 [Kühn, XIII, 882–83]), another by Serapion (*By Kind* VI, 4 [Kühn, XIII, 883–84]), and another by Andromachus (*By Kind* VI, 5 [Kühn, XIII, 884–85]). Galen seems to take some data directly from Andromachus (quoting Isidore of Antioch) on a plaster for gangrene (*By Kind* VI, 6 [Kühn, XIII, 885–86]). Then Galen tells us he will take up other sorts of plasters, arguing at some length that one ought not to be ignorant of the good data at one's fingertips—unlike so many in his day (*By Kind* VI, 7 [Kühn, XIII, 889]), and then we receive a formula (again from Andromachus) for the Egyptian *Phaia*[?] Black[?] Plaster (*By Kind* VI, 8 [Kühn, XIII, 890–91]), a good example of an excellent compound ignored by physicians (Kühn, XIII, 891).

[104] Ed. Kühn, XIII, 895–97.

[105] *By Kind* VI, 12 (Kühn, XIII, 915–23).

[106] *By Kind* VII, 1 (Kühn, XIII, 946–51).

[107] $PbCO_3$, lead carbonate, or "white lead" (*Psimythion*). Preparation of white lead: Theophrastus *On Stones* 56. Preparation of white lead salves: *Geoponica* XVII, 7.2; XVIII, 15.3; and VII, 15.18 (ed. Beckh, pp. 473, 494 [from Didymus], and 203 [from Sotion]). Cf. Dioscorides V, 82 and 88.

[108] PbO, lead monoxide (*lithargyros*). Cf. *PGM*, XII, 194; Nicander *Alexipharmaca*, 594; Galen, *Drugs by Kind* I, 5: "Plasters Made from Lead Monoxide" (Kühn, XIII, 394–98).

[109] This is Galen's "cooling wax salve" in *Hygiene* VI, 14.8 (ed. K. Koch, *Galeni De sanitate tuenda* [Leipzig, 1923; in *CMG* V 4, 2], p. 195).

[110] Theophrastus, *On Odors* 15. Dioscorides I, 30.

[111] *By Kind* VII, 2 (Kühn, XIII, 952–53).

[112] *By Kind* VII, 4–16 (Kühn, XIII, 958–1058).

tory quotations from earlier sources, and Galen's attempts to "explain" why various drugs might be included in the works of Criton, Andromachus, Damocrates, and others, are often surprisingly feeble. Galen generally has not actually sought out the drugs he prescribes—as he likes to boast—but has availed himself of a rich doxographical tradition in Greco-Roman pharmacy, a tradition that was exploited earlier by Criton in the reign of Trajan,[113] and by Dioscorides in the middle of the first century. Unlike Dioscorides, however, Galen did not simply survey his predecessors' work,[114] but excerpted those tracts in large swatches. Once the early Byzantine pharmacologists had analyzed Galen's "Drug Books," they were forced to rearrange, streamline, and "edit them" rather heavily, even though Galen remained a venerated fountainhead of drug lore. It is very significant that Byzantine medical writers, from Oribasius through Paul of Aegina, quite frequently sought out the "original" writings on drugs from earlier Greco-Roman antiquity, and did not continue the pharmaceutical doxography illustrated by Galen's summaries in the late second century.

ORIBASIUS AND PHARMACOLOGY

Oribasius functioned as court physician to the Emperor Julian (A.D. 361–363), but he had been friend and confidant of Julian before the eventful months of 360 and 361 that led to his elevation to the undisputed possession of the imperial purple. Oribasius had prepared a synopsis of Galen's works at Julian's request, while the future emperor served Constantius as Caesar in Gaul.[115] In 360—again at the request of Julian—he compiled a second work that summarized not only Galen but also many other medical authorities, and we have forty books plus a number of fragments of the original seventy in this *Medical Collection*. From the *Medical Collection*, one may gauge how Galen's pharmacology was employed by Oribasius, and one may also discern some skillful rearrangements, reclassifications, and fresh juxtapositions as Galen is quoted directly. In many respects, Oribasius' use of Galen's works provides a reasonable measure of what tracts by Galen were known in the mid fourth century, and the numerous quotations from all three of Galen's massive

pharmacological books show that they all should probably be included within the "genuine" Galenic corpus. *Antidotes* is also excerpted,[116] but not to the extent that Oribasius uses Galen's *Mixtures and Properties of Simples* (593 citations), *Drugs by Location* (206 citations), and *Drugs by Kind* (62 citations). *Theriac to Piso* does not appear among the quoted extracts.

These raw numbers (almost 600 extracts from Galen's *Simples*, just over 200 from *Location*, and 62 from *By Kind*) may suggest a basic pattern for Oribasius' adaptation of Galenic pharmacology. In the first place, Galen's *Simples* had laid down a fairly precise theory of drug "properties," and this tract also included almost all of the listed medicinals known to Greco-Roman pharmacy; secondly, since Oribasius does not quote Damocrates' medical poems (nor any medical poetry at all), this would suggest that Oribasius valued *Location* and *By Kind* (in which Damocrates' poems bulk large) less than *Simples*, or, that medical poetry had fallen out of fashion by Oribasius' day; third, since Galen had given a fairly complete listing of pharmaceuticals in *Simples*, first listed alphabetically (the plants) and then "classed" by source (animals, minerals), Oribasius apparently assumed Galen's *Simples*, combined with the rearranged alphabetical listing of drugs taken from Dioscorides' *Materia medica*,[117] would provide the important substances used in pharmaceutical therapy; Galen's two other books on drugs (*Drugs by Location* and *By Kind*) did not offer a significant improvement in perceptions of drug lore. Moreover, Galen's *Location* and *By Kind* merely repeated the substances (using other authorities) previously listed in his simples, so that there was no quantitative improvement in Galen's nearly 450 drugs contained in his *Simples* that could not be gained by the more streamlined listing of pharmaceuticals from Dioscorides. Oribasius can thus assume his pharmacology would include all of the over 600 "standard" drugs by a judicious combination of Galen and Dioscorides, as well as careful quotations from other authorities directly from their works. Oribasius' arrangement of drugs most likely resulted from the requirements of an active and personal practice of medicine—particularly seen in the quotations of Galen's *Simples* in *Medical Collection* XV—and his adaptation of drug lore became a standard method in medical botany and

---

[113] See n. 80 above, and J. Scarborough, "Criton, Physician to Trajan: Historian and Pharmacist," in J. Eadie and J. Ober, eds., *Festschrift Chester Starr* (Washington, D.C., 1984) in press.

[114] Scarborough and Nutton, "Preface," 190.

[115] Oribasius, *Medical Collection* prooemium 1–2 (ed. Raeder, I, 4).

[116] Raeder, IV, 327 (nine citations).

[117] Oribasius, *Medical Collection* XI–XIII (ed. Raeder, II, 80–180).

pharmacology still followed in modern times.[118]

Galen's *Simples* had developed a tight theory of pharmaceutical action, based upon primary "qualities" (viz. properties) of particular classes of drugs, followed by a second set of secondary "qualities," and then a third classification of tertiary properties.[119] Galen had argued that the Hot, Cold, Wet, and Dry were common to all substances, and that changes came to matter through either active or passive influences.[120] This, in turn, explained the effects of all drugs.[121] Following from this premise, Galen can then argue for "secondary" properties and "tertiary" properties from the pharmaceutical effects derived from combinations and mixtures of the "primary" properties, as such would be perceived by the senses.[122] There is, however, a vagueness to Galen's "tertiary" qualities/properties, and Harig has shown that Galen meant merely "local effects" in his "tertiary level," that is, local effects of the "secondary qualities."[123] Thus in the beginning of Book V of *Simples*, Galen can make the statement that it is better to classify pharmaceutical compounds by their *eidē* ("species" or "kinds"),[124] apparently meaning their "useful effects" in pharmacy as they are perceived by the senses. By way of illustration, Galen writes that it is more accurate to say that wheat-meal plaster is a balance between the Wet and Hot,[125] rather than to list the plaster's qualities/properties as pus-producing, soothing, cathartic, and relaxing.[126]

Oribasius does some very significant things with Galen's drug theory, and the following can only be suggestive. In quoting from Galen's *Simples* V, 2,[127] Oribasius merely excerpts what Galen has to say about the "utility of drugs" (*peri chreias tōn pharmakōn*), the basic statement of how one understands drug action. Oribasius has, in effect, extracted exactly those passages from Galen's verbose

description of drug properties which are precise and clear: "The utility of drugs among men is often from this alone: the heating, cooling, drying, and the moistening, or from the combination of effects as produced [by these properties]." Oribasius includes Galen's assumptions that such physical properties as condensation of drugs, rarification, and so on, would also be explained by the underlying theory of *stoicheia/dynameis*, but the repetitive passages following line 5 (Kühn, XI, 707) are not quoted. *Medical Collection* XIV, 4 (Raeder, II, 184–85), is not a continuation of Galen's *Simples* V, but begins with an excerpt from *Simples* III, 11 (Kühn, XI, 564–65), titled by Oribasius "How One Determines the Elementary Property of the Full Compound by Comparison with an Exactly Balanced Substance." *Simples* III, 11 is employed here because Galen has defined a "moderate *krasis*" (a "balancing," or in archaic English, a "temperament"), and such is determined by the sense of touch. *Medical Collection* XIV, 4.1–3, is extracted from Galen's *Simples* III, 11, but *Medical Collection* XIV, 4.4 is from *Simples* III, 13 (Kühn, XI, 571). Oribasius again has skipped an incredibly verbose and repetitive section of Galen's *Simples*, and extracts exactly those passages which summarize precisely what Galen means in terms of his mid-way *krasis*, after Galen has provided an excellent illustration of the cooling properties of rose oil in *Simples* III, 11. Oribasius has shown his shrewd adaptation and rearrangement of Galen, and the *Medical Collection* becomes an attempt to give Galen a clarity—using his own words—lacking in the original texts. Oribasius also has digested an enormous quantity of Galen's writing, no mean feat in itself, and has simplified Galen's tripartite "intensity theory" of drugs so that the original notion is preserved for the employment of future physicians and pharmacologists. In fact, as Harig has argued, Oribasius' quotations of Galen's *Simples* ensured the preservation of the most essential parts of Galen's theory, shorn of the vague and generally unsatisfactory extension of the theory into a "tertiary" level of effects.[128]

Oribasius exhibits great care in citing his sources. One would expect him to cite materials as he had found them quoted in earlier compendia of recipes, such as are found in Galen's *Drugs Arranged by Location of Ailment* and *Drugs Arranged by Kind*. A few examples of sources cited by name, compared to the sloppy manner of Galen's use of recipe col-

---

[118] G. Harig, "Die Galenschrift "De simplicium medicamentorum temperamentis ac facultatibus" und die "Collectiones medicae" des Oribasios," *NTM*, 7 (1966), 1–26 [4].

[119] See G. Harig, *Bestimmung der Intensität im medizinischen System Galens* (Berlin, 1974), *passim*.

[120] Galen, *Elements According to Hippocrates* I, 9 (ed. Kühn, I, 485), and *Commentary on Hippocrates' On the Nature of Man* I, 7 (ed. J. Mewaldt, *Galeni In Hippocratis de natura hominis* [Leipzig, 1914; in *CMG* V 9, 1], p. 22).

[121] Galen, *Simples* I, 8 (ed. Kühn, XI, 397).

[122] Galen, *Simples* III, 13, and V, 2 (ed. Kühn, XI, 573 and 709–10).

[123] Harig, *Intensität* (n. 119 above), 110–15.

[124] Galen, *Simples* V, 1 (ed. Kühn, XI, 704–6).

[125] Galen, *Simples* V, 2 (ed. Kühn, XI, 712).

[126] Galen, *Simples* V, 2 (ed. Kühn, XI, 711–12).

[127] Oribasius, *Medical Collection* XIV, 3 (ed. Raeder, II, 184) = ed. Kühn, XI, 706–7.

[128] Harig, "Oribasius" (n. 118 above), *passim*.

lections by Criton, Andromachus, and Asclepiades the Pharmacist, will suggest Oribasius' meticulous care and insistence on quoting *directly* from the original work. It will be recalled that Galen cites Xenocrates for a number of animal-derived drugs,[129] and one would, presumably, expect Oribasius to pick up these citations and record them somewhere in the *Medical Collection*. Except, however, for some scholia recording parallel passages from Xenocrates, Galen, and Dioscorides,[130] and one fragmentary quotation (twenty-one lines) from Xenocrates' "Plasters Made from Whelk [*kēryx*] and murex [shellfish],"[131] Xenocrates appears only in a lengthy, direct quotation from *Foods from Water Animals*,[132] which fits neatly into Oribasius' "elementary" books on preparation and recommendation of healthy foods. Here are how one classifies fish and shellfish,[133] and a catalogue of agreeable and disagreeable fish in the diet. No bloods, rennets, or dungs appear in Oribasius' quotations from Xenocrates, and one is again struck by the display of good judgment in the employment of an earlier source, quoted directly and not through an intermediary. Other quoted authors receive similar treatment (for example, the obscure Heraclas),[134] so that Oribasius has "gone to the sources," unlike his verbose model, Galen.

There is ample evidence throughout Oribasius' writing—*Medical Collection*, [*Medical*] *Synopsis for Eustathius*, and [*Medical*] *Books for Eunapius*—not only that he had read and assimilated the writings of many authorities of medicine in the Greco-Roman tradition, but also that his medical practice included much personal knowledge of pharmaceuticals, which he was pleased to share with his son, and with his friend Eunapius. A few examples will illustrate. *Medical Collection* IX, 27 (= *Synopsis for Eustathius* III, 79 [Raeder, II, 30, and Raeder, ed., *Synopsis*, 89]) is "Plasters from the Husks of Wheat." He tells us that one can use the "leftovers" of the wheat by pounding the husks, and the plaster (made from combining the pounded husks with a honey-

vinegar mixture and a gum ammoniac [here probably *Ferula communis* L. or *F. marmarica* Asch. & Taub.; less likely *Dorema ammoniacum* D. Don.]) would be useful as a warming plaster for various skin ailments as well as liver and spleen problems. No source is discernable here, and there is only a slight resemblance to the mention of gum ammoniac by Dioscorides;[135] the suggestions by Dioscorides for *ammōniakon* in *Materia medica* III, 84 (Wellmann, II, 100–102) overlap with those by Oribasius only in terms of being useful for ailments of the liver and spleen (*Materia medica* III, 84.3 [Wellmann, II, 102]), but there is no combination with pounded husks of wheat. It is signifcant that Aetius borrows this account of the plaster of pounded wheat husks directly from Oribasius.[136] Thus, it is apparent that Oribasius was a skilled drug compounder in his own right, also shown by other adapted and "original" medicines.[137] Characteristic of Oribasius' command of drug compounding is his direct simplicity and general avoidance of complicated mixtures that might require exotic ingredients.

Oribasius was also well acquainted with Dioscorides' *Materia medica*, but he—like Galen before him—decided that Dioscorides' precise and difficult system of drug affinities was either too cumbersome for practical use,[138] or too diffuse as it stood. *Medical Collection* XI–XII (Raeder, II, 81–159) is an alphabetized listing of the simples in Dioscorides' *Materia medica* (456 substances, including some of Dioscorides' "animal products," for instance, *stear* ["fat"]), and *Medical Collection* XIII (Raeder, II, 160–80) is "From Dioscorides on the Properties [*Dynameis*] of 'Mined' Drugs [*Metallika*] and their Preparation" (88 medicinals, including various stones and earths). Oribasius has carefully alphabetized 544 pharmaceuticals as contained in Dioscorides' *Materia medica*, and there is, indeed, a succinct clarity that would be absent in Dioscorides' original tract. One can suppose that Oribasius drew up this listing, or one may assume that he took a previously-compiled alphabetical listing and simply reproduced it. Given Oribasius' normal habit of citing almost all of his sources by name, it seems unlikely that he had borrowed the alphabetical register of

---

[129] Galen, *Simples* X preface (ed. Kühn, XII, 245–53).

[130] Oribasius, *Medical Collection* XI A 54, and XV (ed. Raeder, II, 89, 293, and 296).

[131] Oribasius, *Medical Collection* XV, 3 (ed. Raeder, II, 296–97.).

[132] Oribasius, *Medical Collection* II, 58 (ed. Raeder, II, 47–57).

[133] Oribasius, *Medical Collection* II, 58. 11–13 (ed. Raeder, II, 48).

[134] Oribasius, *Medical Collection* XLVIII, 1–18 (ed. Raeder, III, 262–68). See also C. L. Day, *Quipus and Witches' Knots: The Role of the Knot in Primitive and Ancient Cultures, with a Translation and Analysis of "Oribasius De Laqueis"* (Lawrence, Kansas, 1967), 107–31.

[135] Dioscorides III, 48.3 (ed. Wellmann, II, 62). Cf. Pseudo-Dioscorides, III, 84 (ed. Wellmann, II, 101).

[136] Aetius III, 178 (ed. Olivieri [*CMG* VIII 1], p. 350).

[137] E.g., Oribasius, *Synopsis for Eustathius* III, 77 (Raeder, p. 88) = *Medical Collection* IX, 25 (Raeder, II, 28–29): "A Plaster Made from Beer-Yeast."

[138] Scarborough and Nutton, "Preface," 190.

Dioscorides from an unknown source, and the accuracy of the quotations would indicate that Oribasius had performed this onerous task himself. If so, it may be quite probable that Oribasius' alphabetical text of Dioscorides is the archetype of many later manuscripts of the Greek "alphabetical" Dioscorides, including the justly famous Vienna text of A.D. 512.[139]

FROM ORIBASIUS TO AETIUS

Although it can be argued that Theodorus Priscianus' *Euporiston* could be included in the scope of early Byzantine medicine (Priscianus was court physician in the reign of Gratian [A.D. 375–383]), the text was written in Latin, as befitted the court of a western Roman emperor.[140] Moreover, the fascinating farrago of drugs and folklore that make up the *De medicamentis* by Marcellus Empiricus (*fl.* as *magister officiorum* under Theodosius I [A.D. 379–395]),[141] will not be considered here, since the work is in Latin, and belongs more to the history of pharmacy in early medieval western Europe. Caelius Aurelianus (*?fl.* c. A.D. 450) has left us a masterpiece of compression—also in Latin—of the best of the Methodist physicians, and the drug lore of Soranus of Ephesus assumes a major importance.[142] And the compendium of Cassius Felix, called *De medicina*, was published in A.D. 447, with the *a capite ad calcem* therapeutics of Galen summarized in Latin guise.[143] One would like to know more about Hesychius of Damascus (*fl.* A.D. 430 in Byzantium), the father of Psychestrus, Asclepiodotus, and Palladius,[144] but as important as were these medical practitioners in the fifth century, we learn about them through isolated quotations in later authors and from summaries as contained in the *Suda* and Photius' *Library*.[145] Alexander of Tralles (V, 4 [Puschmann, II, 163]) gives us a tantalizing bit about Psychestrus' therapy using a "liquifying diet,"[146] and all of these names, excepting Alexander of Tralles, were associated with some residence or study at Alexandria, which continued to be a famous center for medical education of many varieties.[147] It is only with Aetius of Amida, who had indeed spent time in Alexandria,[148] in the early sixth century that one again can assess the next stages of development in early Byzantine pharmacology.

AETIUS OF AMIDA

Drug theory begins Aetius' account of medical practice. In fact, the lengthy *Preface* to Book I of Aetius' *Medical Books* (Olivieri, I, 17–30) is entirely devoted to theoretical pharmacology. The complete *Preface* emerges from Galen, but in a deftly arranged manner from several different Galenic passages, generally from *Mixtures and Properties of Simples*, with the first eighteen lines quoted from *Simples*, prooemium VII (Kühn, XII, 2–4). Even in English translation, one is able to detect Aetius' subtle yet crucial modulations of Galen's original, as well as the important reorganization of vital passages from Galen's pharmacological theory, so that clarity could replace imprecision:

> The variations of the individual effects of drugs are due to each of them being to a certain sufficiency [*tō epi tosonde*: "to a certain degree" is the modern expression] hot or cold or dry or wet, or each having fine [or "small"] or coarse [or "large"] particles [or "parts"]. The extent/measure of the degree, however, of the attachments [lit. "fastenings-together"] in each of the drugs cannot be expressed with truthful accuracy. But we have attempted to encompass and characterize them with adequately clear terms and definitions for use in medical practice [*eis tēn cheian tēs technēs*]. We are demonstrating that there is one kind [*hen genos*] of drugs which is [*aphiknoumenon*: lit. "arriving at" or "coming into"] a same *krasis* as our bodies, when it has received some *archē* of both change and alteration [*alliōsis*] from the hot in this kind of drugs, and, that there is another kind of drugs which is hotter. From this, it seems to me that four orders [*taxeis*] can be made: the first is indistinct [*asaphē*] to the senses, [and] detecting it necessarily comes through pure reason [*logos*]; the second is distinct and perceivable to the senses; the third is rather hot, but not to the point of burning; the fourth and last is the corrosive or caustic kind of drugs.[149] Likewise also for the cooling kind of drugs, the first order must come from pure reason in demonstrating its coldness, the second is cooling detectable by the senses, the third is rather cold, and the fourth causes

[139] Vienna, Österreichische Nationalbibliothek MS Gr. 1.

[140] V. Rose, ed., *Theodori Prisciani Euporiston* (Leipzig, 1894).

[141] Marcellus (ed. Liechtenhan).

[142] Caelius Aurelianus (ed. and trans. Drabkin).

[143] V. Rose, ed., *Cassii Felicis De medicina* (Leipzig, 1879).

[144] Hunger, "Medizin," 292. Temkin, "Byzantine Medicine," *DOP*, 16 (1962), 100 = *Double Face of Janus*, 205–6.

[145] On Jacob Psychestrus: R. Asmus, *Das Leben des Philosophen Isodorus von Damaskios aus Damaskos* (Leipzig, 1911), esp. 72–75.

[146] Cf. Alexander of Tralles, ed. Puschmann, I, 74, and reffs. Puschmann, II, 162 n. 1.

[147] Hunger, "Medizin," 292. Temkin, "Byzantine Medicine," 101–2 = *Double Face of Janus*, 206–7.

[148] Aetius I, 131, and II, 3 (ed. Olivieri [*CMG* VIII 1], pp. 65 and 154).

[149] *Pharmaka kaustika*. Galen, *Simples* V, 15 (ed. Kühn, XI, 754). Zopyrus in Oribasius, *Medical Collection* XIV, 57.1 (ed. Raeder, II, 226).

necrosis.[150] Analogous in these definitions are also the wetting and drying drugs.[151]

Galen (*Simples* VII, 10.1) then proceeds to speak of catnip (*kalaminthos*: *Nepeta cataria* L.),[152] writing "catnip is basically of small particles and has a hot and dry *krasis*, and is from the third order with both qualities."[153] Aetius, however, does not continue with *Simples* VII: the next twelve lines in the *Preface* to Book I of the *Medical Books* come from Galen, *Simples* III, 13 (Kühn, XI, 571–72):

> Thus let there be set down a clear instruction of these very degrees [or sufficiencies]: in the first order [*taxis*] of cooling drugs would be placed rose oil or the rose (*Rosa gallica* L., and related spp.) itself; in the second would be placed rose-juice [*ho to rhodou chylos*]; and in the third and fourth orders we would include—for good reason—the very cold drugs: hemlock (*kōneion*: *Conium maculatum* L.), the juice of the opium poppy (*mēkōneion*, viz. opium from *Papaver somniferum* L.), mandrake (*mandragoras*: either *Mandragora officinarum* L. [mandrake], or *Atropa belladonna* L. [deadly nightshade]), and black henbane (*hyoskyamos*: *Hyoscyamus niger* L.). Concerning the hot drugs, dill (*anēthon*: *Anethum graveolens* L.) and fenugreek (*tēlis*: *Trigonella foenum-graecum* L.) are in the first order; the drugs which appear next to them are in the second order; and in the third and fourth orders we would include the caustic and corrosive drugs. And in the same manner in regard to the wetting and drying drugs, one begins with a drug of moderate and proportionate [*krasis*], [and] we will make orders [*taxeis*] one after the other until the farthest extremes [*akroi*]. For some use of such knowledge is not unimportant in the medical practice [*methodos*].

Aetius now drops Galen's *Simples* III, 13 (which goes on to grumble about the general ignorance of doctors in such matters), and switches to an adaptation of *three lines* from Galen's *Simples* IV, 4 (Kühn, XI, 632), in which Aetius writes: "One should also use the sense of taste, and retain in the memory the peculiarity of each quality of the juices" (Olivieri, I, p. 18, lines 15–17); and then Aetius shifts again to four, slightly modified lines from Galen, *Simples* I, 39 (Kühn, XI, 453), ". . . as, for example, when such a substance [*sōma*: lit. "body"] is laid on the tongue, it greatly dessicates, contracts, and deeply roughens it, such as unripe wild pears (*achrades aōroi*: probably *Pyrus pyraster* Burgsd., or *P. amygdaliformis* Vill.), Cornelian cherries (*krana*: *Cornus mas* L.), and

the like; every such substance is called sour [or "astringent": *stryphnon*] since it is intensely bitter [*austēron*]" (Olivieri, I, p. 18, lines 17–20). With some slight syntactical adaptations, Aetius has provided a lucid account of Galen's basic pharmacological theory, using Galen's own words and phrases, but judiciously selected and rearranged so that the reader understands (as best as he would be able) this system of drug classification "by intensity" or "by degree." What has been muddled, scattered, and often repeated in Galen's original texts, has now been compacted, edited, and streamlined. The remainder of Aetius' *Preface* to Book I of his *Medical Books* shows a similar ability, and Galen's enormously influential classification of drugs "by degrees" has emerged in the form in which it would be used by countless physicians and pharmacists until well into the eighteenth and nineteenth centuries.

Once Aetius has completed his redaction of Galen's drug theory, he then proceeds to list alphabetically 418 medicinals of plant origin, almost all quoted from Galen, but with an occasional passage from Rufus, Dioscorides, and Oribasius.[154] Book II lists, in part alphabetically, 195 medicinals,[155] an occasional clipped, simplified recipe of drugs derived from metals (lit. "things mined"), stones, earths, and a wide spectrum of "animal products" (from milk to insects); most entries are quoted from Galen, Oribasius, and Dioscorides, but there are a few citations from Rufus, Antyllus, and Theophrastus. Book II, 196–271 returns to the "drugs by degrees" system[156] and now "fits" the 613 substances into the various grades of heating, cooling, drying, and moistening medicinals, followed by a discussion of the properties (*dynameis*) of foods.[157] Then Aetius turns his attention again to the definition of Galen's puzzling "large" and "small" particles as they relate to the properties of foods,[158] but the source is Oribasius, not Galen. With Book III,[159] Aetius begins to list formulas and recipes for cathartics and similar drugs, and his arrangement of simples in the first two books is explained: one has to be acquainted with the basic components—and the theory of how such ingredients would "work"—before the pharmacologist-physician could

---

[150] Galen, *Bloodletting* 4 (ed. Kühn, XI, 265).

[151] Aetius I *prooemium* (first eighteen lines) (ed. Olivieri [*CMG* VIII 1], pp. 17–18).

[152] A rare form. Cf. Nicander, *Theriaca* 60.

[153] Ed. Kühn, XII, 4.

[154] Aetius I, 1–418 (ed. Olivieri [*CMG* VIII 1], pp. 30–146.

[155] Aetius II (ed. Olivieri [*CMG* VIII 1], pp. 147–255).

[156] Ed. Olivieri (*CMG* VIII 1), pp. 223–55.

[157] Aetius II, 239 (ed. Olivieri [*CMG* VIII 1], pp. 237–38).

[158] Aetius II, 240–241 (ed. Olivieri [*CMG*, VIII 1]), 237–40.

[159] Ed. Olivieri (*CMG* VIII 1) pp. 256–355.

proceed into prescription of pharmaceuticals by a combined class of action. In Book IV,[160] Aetius takes up formal dietetics, quoting heavily from Galen's *Hygiene*,[161] and one also reads the expected admonitions about exercise and a generally healthy regimen to maintain a healthy body. His earlier discussion of the properties of foods now "fits," as he can suggest which foods would do the best service in the diet, according to the theoretical constructs laid down in Book II, 239–241.[162]

Books V and VI take up diagnostics and the venerated theory of the humors,[163] and some common diseases that can be elucidated through these theories. Only occasional pharmaceuticals appear as they are appropriate to the discussions, but Aetius' major sources have shifted to lengthy quotations from Aretaeus of Cappadocia as well as Galen and Oribasius. Book VII is one of the finest accounts of ophthalmology written in ancient and medieval times,[164] and the discussion is replete with collyria recipes drawn mostly from Galen and Oribasius. Although Aetius does not mention cataract couching, there are clear descriptions of sixty-one eye diseases, showing close acquaintance with the essential anatomical structures.[165] Book VIII is a mixture of materials on inflammations, various plasters, and the like, with many details drawn from Galen's *Compound Drugs Arranged by Place of Ailment*. And although Aetius' complete *Medical Books* are in sixteen books (hence the traditional title of *Tetrabiblon* of the *Biblia iatrika hekkaideka* from the customary division in manuscripts into four *tetrabibloi* to every four *logoi*), one lacks competent modern, well-edited Greek texts,[166] and therefore the pharmacy that teems in the last eight books cannot be accurately assessed. Famous, of course, is Book XVI with its splendid summary of gynecology and obstetrics, but the most often cited Ricci

translation is based on the Cornarius *Latin* translation of 1542,[167] and the most recently edited Greek text suffers from a number of inadequacies.[168]

ALEXANDER OF TRALLES

As Aetius of Amida had carefully redacted earlier pharmacology, so also Alexander of Tralles reworked much of the earlier data into a lengthy compendium of suggested treatment of diseases by their symptomatology, explained through a general pathlogy that assumed a causation of illness from morbid humors. Alexander was born in A.D. 525, and was the son of a physician named Stephen. Our main data for Alexander's family comes from Agathias' *Histories* V, 6.3–6,[169] and Stephen had fathered five sons, all of whom became prominent in their professions: Anthemius, the architect-engineer who designed the magnificent St. Sophia; Olympius, a gifted lawyer; Metrodorus, a pre-eminent grammarian; Dioscurus, a doctor, ". . . who lived out his life in his native city in which he carried on the practice of medicine with great success;"[170] and Alexander, who "lived in Rome, summoned to hold high position."[171] Agathias implies that Alexander's fame had not reached the ears of Justinian, whereas both Anthemius and Metrodorus were well known to the emperor. After much travel and experience, Alexander settled in Rome and died in A.D. 605.

Of all the Byzantine physicians, Alexander of Tralles has exercised the greatest attraction for modern medical historians, due to his direct experience with the practice of medicine, vividly and frequently recorded in his extant books on various aspects of medical treatment. Two relatively modern translations (in French and German) of Alexander's works have been produced, and both Puschmann and Brunet are impressed by what they perceive as the "strikingly modern" approach by Alexander to medicine and pharmacy.[172] Alexander does represent a sharp contrast to the arid scholasticism of Aetius, but both Oribasius and Paul of Aegina were clearly practicing physicians, and

---

[160] Ed. Olivieri (*CMG* VIII 1) pp. 356–408.

[161] E.g., Aetius IV, 1 (ed. Olivieri [*CMG* VIII 1], pp. 358–59), and Galen, *Hygiene* I, 1 (ed. Koch [n. 109 above], p. 3); and Aetius, IV, 36 (ed. Olivieri, pp. 378–79) and Galen, *Hygiene* III, 3 (ed. Koch, pp. 85–86).

[162] Ed. Olivieri (*CMG* VIII 1), pp. 237–40.

[163] Ed. Olivieri (*CMG* VIII 2), pp. 1–249.

[164] Ed. Olivieri (*CMG* VIII 2), pp. 250–399.

[165] See Emilie Savage-Smith, "Byzantine Ophthalmology" (above in this volume), esp. nn. 61–69.

[166] Barely serviceable "modern" texts of various books of Aetius' *Tetrabibloi* include: G. A. Kostomiris, ed., *Aetiou Logos dōdekatos* (Bk. XII) (Paris, 1892); S. Zervos, ed., *Aetio Amidēnou Logos dekatos kai tritos ē Aetiou Amidēnou Peri daknontōn zōōn kai iobolon* (Bk. XIII) in *Athēna*, 18 (1905), 241–302; and S. Zervos, ed., *Aetiou Amidinou* [sic] *Logos dekatos pemptos* (Bk. XV) in *Athēna*, 21 (1909), 3–144. Bk. XI is in the Daremberg and Ruelle edition of Rufus, pp. 85–126.

[167] J. V. Ricci, trans., *Aetios of Amida: The Gynaecology and Obstetrics of the VIth Century A.D.* (Philadelphia, 1950).

[168] S. Zervos, ed., *Aetii Sermo sextidecimus et ultimus* (Leipzig, 1901).

[169] R. Keydell, ed., *Agathiae Myrinaei Historiarum* (Berlin, 1967; *CFHB*, II), p. 171.

[170] *Ibid.*

[171] *Ibid.*

[172] Alexander (trans. Brunet), Vol. I. Puschmann, ed., Alexander, I, 75–87, 287–88.

their writings show a sense of the clinic as do those by Alexander. It will not, however, be accurate to describe Alexander of Tralles as a "modern" any more than to designate Galen as such; but Alexander is, indeed, humane and conscientious in his practice, meticulous in his prescriptions, and careful with his command of earlier authorities in medicine. Drugs are scattered throughout Alexander's books, given as recipes for the treatment of specific diseases, usually through the long-lived "treatment by contraries." The occasional complexity of Alexander's drug prescriptions (using 495 different pharmaceuticals) are justified by conflicting symptoms, and many medicinals are recorded as efficacious as verified by personal observation and experience. A critical attitude toward his numerous written sources is characteristic throughout Alexander's works, illustrated by the following, which appears in Book V, 4, "On Viscous Humors and Thick Masses Found in the Lung:"

> This is a true statement by Galen on Archigenes:[173] "He was but a man and it would be difficult for him not to make mistakes in many things, being completely ignorant, making bad judgments, and who provided carelessly written accounts." And I would not have said this about such a learned man, unless Truth itself had not inspired me and urged me on, and did I not believe that keeping silent was sinful. For a doctor who does not speak his opinion commits a great sin and through his silence is greatly to be condemned. But one ought to follow that which Aristotle says he has stated: "Plato is my friend, but the Truth is also my friend; between the two, one must choose the Truth."[174]

Alexander does not devote any of his tracts specifically to drugs, but pharmaceutical therapy is very prominent throughout the various subdivisions, for example, fevers, headaches, what we would call "nervous diseases," melancholia, ophthalmology, the rightly famous "Letter on Intestinal Worms," lung diseases, cholera, gout,[175] and so on. Many of the drug recipes seem original, although the particular ingredients have all been used and defined in Greek, Roman, and earlier Byzantine pharmacy. There are occasionally "new names" applied to certain substances, and this can be illustrated by

Alexander's "Armenian Stone," which is part of a recipe in *On Fevers* VII [Quartans] (Puschmann, I, 429). Earlier Greek sources—including the *Papyri Graecae Magicae* XII, 201—had noted the use of *ios chalkou* ("verdigris," or copper oxyacetate, approximately $[C_2H_3O_2]_2Cu \cdot Cu[OH]_2 \cdot 5H_2O$), but Alexander's *Armeniakos lithos* has taken the place of *ios chalkou*. This "new" substance had been foreshadowed in Dioscorides, *Materia medica* V, 90, and if we understand the geological chemistry the "Armenian Stone" is a combination of copper oxyacetate, azurite $(2CuCO_3 \cdot Cu[OH]_2)$, and malachite $(CuCO_3 \cdot Cu[OH]_2)$.[176] Roman and Byzantine pharmacy could substitute one "kind" of copper oxyacetate for another, and it is probable that Alexander knew the "Armenian Stone" in the same role as had been played by verdigris in earlier prescriptions. The remainder of the recipe "On the Armenian Stone" suggests that Alexander's "new" pharmacy consisted of rearrangement of ingredients according to his experience:

> The stone, which is called "The Armenian," given washed or unwashed in a dosage of 4 *keratia* [c. 800 mg./12 grains] works well for all forms of quartan fever, since it [performs] as no other for the evacuation of black bile. Washed in water, it completely purges the lower bowels, but unwashed it is an emetic which does not cause too much heating, unlike the others. But if some [of your patients] regard the solution of "the stone" with disgust, make little pills using the following ingredients:
> - 4 *grammata* [c. 4.6 grams/4 scruples/80 grains] of *pikras* [an aloe-honey mixture][177]
> - 3 *grammata* [c. 3.5 grams/3 scruples/60 grains] of *epithymon* [lesser dodder, *Cuscuta epithymum* (L.) Murr.][178]
> - 1 *gramma* [c. 1.2 grams/1 scruple/20 grains] of *agarikon* [prob. a tree mushroom of *Boletus* spp.][179]
> - 1 *gramma* of *Armeniakos lithos*
> - 5 "berries" of *karyophylla* [cloves, *Eugenia caryophyllata* Thunb.; here the sun-dried, unopened flowerbuds][180]
> - 5 *grammata* [c. 5.9 grams/5 scruples] of *skammōnia* [scammony, *Convolvulus scammonia* L.][181]

---

[173] More-or-less Galen, *Drugs by Location* II, 1 (ed. Kühn, XII, 535).

[174] Alexander (ed. Puschmann), II, p. 155; French trans. by Brunet, III, 124–25.

[175] Alexander (ed. Puschmann), I, 290–439 (fevers; in 7 books); I, 465–507 (headaches); phrenitis, lethargy, epilepsy, etc. (I, 508–91); melancholia (I, 591–612); ophthalmology (II, 2–70); intestinal worms (II, 586–600); lung diseases (II, 146–244); cholera (II, 320–34); gout (II, 500–86).

[176] Cf. D. Goltz, *Studien zur Geschichte der Mineralnamen in Pharmazie, Chemie und Medizin von den Anfängen bis Paracelsus* (Wiesbaden, 1972; *SA* Beiheft 14), 146–47.

[177] Juvenal VI, 180, and Galen, *Hygiene* VI, 10.19 (ed. Koch [n. 109 above], p. 188).

[178] Dioscorides IV, 177 (ed. Wellmann, II, pp. 326–27). Galen, *Hygiene* VI, 7.18 (ed. Koch [n. 109 above], p. 182).

[179] Maggiulli, *Nomenclatura* (n. 55 above), 85–88.

[180] Paul of Aegina VII, 3 (ed. Heiberg, II, 211). A. F. Hill, *Economic Botany*, 2nd ed. (New York, 1952), 445–46. J. W. Purseglove, E. G. Brown, C. L. Green, and S. R. J. Robbins, *Spices* (London, 1981; 2 vols.), I, 237 ("fruits").

[181] Theophrastus, *HP* IV, 5.1, and IX, 1.3. Nicander, *Alexipharmaca* 565. Dioscorides IV, 170 (ed. Wellmann, II, 318–19).

Mix with juice of *kitrion* (citron, *Citrus medica* L.),[182] or with *krokomēlon* (a jam made from quince [*Cydonia oblonga* Mill.] and saffron [*Crocus sativus* L.]), or with *rhodomēlon* (a jam made from roses [*Rosa gallica* L.] and quince),[183] or with *rhodomeli* (rose-honey mixture). The dose is 2 *grammata* [c. 2.4 grams/2 scruples/40 grains].[184]

It is significant that an alchemical papyrus from late Roman or Byzantine Egypt also has the combination of water and verdigris,[185] so that Alexander has recorded a common association of "washing" the "green rust" that is copper oxyacetate. The remaining substances in the recipe are known from earlier Greco-Roman sources, and even though the cloves appear exotic, they were known in Roman pharmacy in the first century,[186] but with the close links in the traditions between Cosmas Indicopleustes and Alexander,[187] it seems that this peculiar *hapax legomenon* may reflect a special connection with the spice trade from the Far East. The text of Alexander, *On Fevers* VII [Quartans] (Puschmann, I, 429 and 431) shows a careful assessment of drugs in the context of the ancient humoral pathology, and it appears that this recipe—and many others by Alexander—was compounded after a lengthy experience with patients who exhibited quartan fever. Alexander's pharmacy indicates that Byzantine drug lore was anything but repetitive and static: it shows a continual attempt by the best of the early Byzantine physicians to utilize the traditional pharmacopoeia in new patterns, while retaining the theoretical context of Hippocratic and Galenic medical theory.

Theophilus Protospatharius and Paul of Aegina

Before considering the lucid summary of pharmacology by Paul of Aegina (*fl.* in the 640s in Alexandria),[188] the works of Theophilus Protospatharius should be mentioned. Although there has been debate concerning the century in which Theophilus practiced medicine,[189] the dating by

Krumbacher seems to have stood up to scrutiny; we may thus continue to assume that Theophilus lived during the reign of Heraclius (A.D. 610–641). Whenever one dates Theophilus, there can be little doubt about his masterful conglomeration of the ancient medical classics with the Byzantine Christian outlook, nicely exemplified by his *On the Structure of the Human Body*,[190] which fuses Galen's demiurge and teleology in *Use of Parts* with a continually emphasized *ho demiourgos theos hēmōn*.[191] Of interest for Byzantine pharmacy is the short fragment of Theophilus' *On Excrements*,[192] indicating a continued use of dungs in medicinals. And of fundamental interest in the fresh approaches of Byzantine medical practice and diagnosis is Theophilus' *On Urines*,[193] which became the probable ancestor of so many Byzantine works on the topic.

The seventh of Paul's *Seven Books* is devoted solely to drugs and pharmaceuticals and represents a culmination of the Greek, Roman, and early Byzantine search for clarity in drug lore. In the first six books, Paul does indeed give a great number of prescriptions as treatments for diseases, but in the seventh, he gathers all of the 600 plants and 80 non-botanical ingredients into a crisply clear alphabetical catalogue. First, he pens a precisely worded introduction to drug theory, adapted from Oribasius and Aetius:

On the Mixtures [*kraseis*] of Substances as Indicated by Their Tastes. It is not adequate to judge from the smell concerning the *krasis* of things perceived by the senses. Substances without odors are made up of large particles, but it is not clear whether they are hot or cold. And things which do have an odor, to a certain extent, are made up of small particles and are hot. But the degree of the smallness of their parts, or of their heat, is not apparent, because of the inequality of their substance. And still more uncertain it is to judge them according to their colors, since with every color are found hot, cold, drying, and wetting substances. In tasting, however, all parts of the substances undergoing tasting come into contact with the tongue and stimulate the sense of taste, and thus one can judge clearly their properties in their *kraseis*. Astringents, therefore, contract, obstruct, condense, dispel, and thicken; and added to all of these properties, they are cold and drying. That which is acidic cuts, divides, thins, removes obstructions, and cleans without making heat; but that which is acrid is like the acidic in being thinning and purging, but it differs from it: the acidic is cold, and the acrid is hot; moreover, the acidic repels, but the acrid attracts, consumes, dissolves, and promotes scab [or scar] formation. Similarly, that which is

[182] Dioscorides I, 115.5 (ed. Wellmann, I, 109). Galen, *Simples* VII, 12.19 (ed. Kühn, XII, 77).

[183] Cf. Alexander (ed. Puschmann), I, 479, 503, 523, 613, and II, 371, 495, 567 [further reffs. to the rose-quince jam]; and cf. Alexander, I, 327, 383, 415, 613, and II, 61, 275, 371, 591, 593 [further reffs. to rose-honey].

[184] Alexander (ed. Puschmann), I, 429 and 431 (Greek text).

[185] *PGM*, XII, 193–201.

[186] Pliny, *Natural History* XII, 30.

[187] The "Cosmas," to whom the *Fevers* is dedicated (Puschmann, I, 289) is probably Cosmas Indicopleustes, whose father was an early medical teacher of Alexander (Puschmann, I, 83, following Meyer, *Botanik*, II, 384).

[188] Hunger, "Medizin," 302.

[189] *Ibid.*, 299.

[190] Ed. Greenhill.

[191] Hunger, "Medizin," 299.

[192] Ideler, I, 397–408.

[193] Ideler, I, 261–83.

bitter cleans the pores, is cleansing and thinning, and cuts the thick humors without any heat perceived by the senses. What is wet is cold, thick, and promotes condensation, contraction, blockage, necrosis, and torpidity. By contrast a salty substance contracts, strengthens, preserves as in pickling, and dries without detectable heat or coldness. What is sweet relaxes, "cooks" [viz. promotes "coction"], softens, and lessens density; and what is oily moistens, softens, and relaxes.[194]

On the Orders and Degrees of the *Kraseis* [adapted from Oribasius and Aetius]. A moderate drug is of the same *krasis* as that to which it is applied, so that it does not dry, moisten, cool, or heat, and it should not be called dry, wet, cold, or hot. But that which is drier, moister, hotter, or colder, is thereby known from its dominant property [*dynamis*]. It will be satisfactory to make—for practical use—four orders [*taxeis*] according to the dominant property, naming the substance hot as appropriate to the first order, when it would heat indistinctly and it would require reason to demonstrate its property; likewise this would be true for the cold, dry, and wet, when the dominant property requires reason to demonstrate its existence, and it has no strong or apparent property as perceived by the senses. And such substances as are clearly those having drying, wetting, heating, and cooling properties may be said to be in the second order. Such substances which have these properties, but not to an extreme degree even though they are strong, may be said to be in the third order, but such substances as those which are hot enough to cause scarring or burning are in the fourth order. Similarly, such substances as those which are so cold as to cause necrosis are also in the fourth order. Nothing, however, is found drying in the fourth order that does not burn: for that which dries to an extreme degree [*akrōs*] also always burns, for example, chalcopyrite [prob. $CuFeS_2$],[195] rock alum [a ferrous sulfate],[196] and quicklime [CaO].[197] But a substance may be in the third order of dessicants without being caustic, such as those substances which are sharply astringent, *e.g.* the juice of unripe grapes, sumac [*Rhus coriaria* L.],[198] and alum [prob. a potash alum: $KAl(SO_4)_2 \cdot 12H_2O$].[199]

Comparing this concise summary with the attempts by Galen to bring some sort of order and clarity into the chaos of drug lore delineates the Byzantine ability in choosing essentials and explicating them with great precision. Galen had posed

questions and—having rejected the brilliant "drugs-by-affinity" system of Dioscorides—attempted an ordering for pharmaceuticals; but Galen had failed to provide a satisfactory method, even though he perceived three separate approaches evinced in his *Simples*, *Drugs by Location*, and *Drugs by Kind*. Oribasius had excerpted much of Galen, and had shown a method of extraction of drug theory.[200] Aetius of Amida had further refined the attempts by Galen to comprehend medicinals by a "system of degrees," but even though there is a judicious care in the lengthy preface on drugs and drug lore in Aetius, *Medical Books* I, there remains a muddled character and a somewhat jagged result from the painstaking juxtaposition of the carefully chosen extracts of Galen's drug theory. Alexander knows his Galen, but chooses to concentrate on the practical aspects of drug lore, so that one does not find a specific "book" on pharmaceuticals either in Alexander's separate tracts on fevers, or in his extant Twelve Books on Medicine: the theory of drugs is embedded in the recipes recorded. Paul's distillation of classical drug theory has finally captured the essence, and it has the characteristics of filtration and the reworked theory seen earlier in Oribasius and Aetius. Paul is also deeply learned in the medical classics, but his compilation bears the marks of an age skilled in ensuring that adaptation accompanied a creative synthesis borne of direct clinical experience combined with venerated assumptions applied to the "modern" age of Heraclius and the Arab invasions of Egypt, Palestine, Syria, and beyond. In the broader historical and cultural context, the early Byzantine physicians should be viewed as part of the same tendencies which produced the brilliant compactions of Roman law from the *Codex* of Theodosius through the *Institutes*, *Digest*, and *Novella* of Justinian.

APPENDIX: THE PAPYRI AND BYZANTINE MEDICINE ON MULTI-INGREDIENT INCENSE. *KYPHI* AND *KRISMA*

Among several hundred medicinals mentioned in the collection of Greek and Coptic papyri known as the *Papyri Graecae Magicae*,[201] occur the names

---

[194] Paul of Aegina VII, 1 (ed. Heiberg, II, p. 185).

[195] Dioscorides V, 74 and 100. *PGM*, XII, 195 and 399. Goltz (n. 176 above), 156–57 (μίσυ).

[196] Χαλκῖτις most often $Fe_4(OH)_2(SO_4)_5 \cdot 18H_2O$, as in the χαλκῖτις στυπτηρίη of the Hippocratic *Wounds* 14 (ed. Littré, VI, p. 416); ἄνθος αἰγυπτίη χαλκοῦ ὀπτὸν, στυπτηρίη αἰγυπτίη ὀπτη. Dioscorides V, 99. Goltz (n. 174 above), 154–55.

[197] Here τίτανος, as contrasted to the usual ἄσβεστος. Goltz (n. 176 above), 171.

[198] Theophrastus, *HP* III, 18.3. Dioscorides I, 108 (ed. Wellmann, I, pp. 101–2).

[199] Here the common στυπτηρία, as in Aristotle, *Historia Animalium* 547a20.

[200] E.g., Oribasius, *Medical Collection* XIV, 5 and 11 (ed. Raeder, II, 185–86 and 193), extracted from Galen, *Simples* I, 38, and V, 26–27 (ed. Kühn, XI, 450–51, and 785–87). Behind Oribasius, *Medical Collection* XIV, 5.1–2 (ed. Raeder, II, 185)—as quoted by Galen—are Plato, *Timaeus* 65B-66C, and Theophrastus, *De causis plantarum* VI, 4.1.

[201] My "count" is 425 different herbs, minerals, insects, dungs, etc. An English translation of the entire *PGM*, with commentar-

of two kinds of multi-ingredient incense, *kyphi* and *krisma*.[202] The anonymous writers apparently presume that their readers would know the ingredients for these two incenses, much as they have assumed a knowledge of the numerous medicinal plants, insects, minerals, and other animals employed in a curious mixture of rational and irrational medical-cum-magical prescriptions.[203] These papyri generally emerge from late Roman and Byzantine Egypt, and one may be sceptical of claims that Greek medicine had made its way into the everyday traditions of the native Egyptians, but it also must be recalled that a common knowledge of plants and animals among ancient peoples would be "taken for granted,"[204] a factor often ignored by modern scholars, who presume a constant specialized expertise, analogous to modern medicine and pharmacy. The magical papyri, however, afford a rare glimpse into the actual "medicine of the masses" (at least in Roman and Byzantine Egypt), and this medicine has great affinity to the religious/magical medicine explicated by Gary Vikan in this collection of essays.[205] If, however, the "upper class" pharmaceutical sources had not recorded the exact names of plants and herbs,[206] one would be reduced to learned speculation concerning ingredients, particularly in the cases of drugs compounded from a number of substances. *Kyphi* and *krisma* show a sophistication of both compounding drugs among the so-called common folk, and they also indicate a developing history of their own, destroying the accepted mythology of modern medical historians that ancient medicine developed to a certain point, and then remained utterly static for countless centuries. By contrast to this assumption, the Greek texts show that Egyptian priest-physicians—and their non-Egyptian Greek, Roman, and Byzantine medical counterparts—were in a continual process of "improving the product." One is able to trace *kyphi* from the first century through the mid seventh century, and the mentionings in the magical papyri indicate that such compounds were available far beyond the urban centers of the Roman and Byzantine Empires.

Dioscorides is well acquainted with Egypt, and his *Materia medica* has the first Greek record of *kyphi*, a multi-ingredient incense that not only was to be burned for its heavy and pungently aromatic odor, but which also was an effective medicinal salve—one could even eat it for presumed benefits. Dioscorides writes that in the Egypt of his day (the mid first century) there were many formulas for *kyphi*, and that he is setting down only one of them (*Materia medica* I, 25 [Wellmann, I, pp. 28–29]), and he lists ten ingredients with measures: ½ *xestēs* [c. ½ pint] of nut grass [*kyperos*: *Cyperus rotundus* L.]; ½ *xestēs* of ripe juniper berries [*Juniperus communis* L.]; 12 *minae* [c. 11 lbs.] of raisins, "the seeds having been removed"; 5 *minae* [c. 4.5 lbs.] of purified pine resin [*rhētinē apokekatharmenēs*]; 1 *mina* [c. 15 oz.] of sweet flag [*kalamos arōmatikos*: *Acorus calamus* L.]; 1 *mina* of camel's thorn (oil) [*aspalathos*: *Alhagi camelorum* Fisch.]; 1 *mina* of camel grass (oil) [*schoinos*: *Cymbopogon schoenanthus* Spreng.]; 12 *drachmai* [c. ¾ lb.] of myrrh [*smyrna*: *Commiphora* spp.]; 9 *xestai* [c. 9 pints] of old wine; and honey as part of the preparation instructions, viz.:

> Having removed the seeds from the raisins, pound and triturate them with the wine and the myrrh, and having pounded and sifted the rest of the ingredients, combine them all to soak for one day; then, having boiled the honey until it has a glutinous consistency, mix it carefully with the melted pine resin, and then having carefully pounded together the rest of the ingredients, put up for storage [this incense] in an earthenware vessel.[207]

Dioscorides does not say if other *kyphi* recipes in his time were more complicated, or if they had more ingredients, but Plutarch, *Isis and Osiris* 383E(80)–384C lists a *kyphi* formula with sixteen ingredients. Ten are the same as in Dioscorides' recipe (honey, wine, raisins, nut grass, pine resin, myrrh, camel's thorn oil, two sizes [large and small] of juniper berries, and sweet flag), but Plutarch's list adds six more ingredients: hartwort (*seselis*: *Tordylium officinale* L.), mastic (*schinos*: *Pistacia lentiscus* L.), Dead Sea bitumen (*asphaltos*: $C_nH_{2n}O_n$ + V, Ni, Mo [traces]), rush (*thryon*: *Juncus glaucus* Sibth.), spinach dock (*lapathon*: *Rumex patientia* L.), and cardamon (*kardamōmon*: *Elettaria cardamomum* [L.] Maton.). Unlike a similar recipe, reduced to a medical poem by Damocrates,[208] Plutarch provides no measures, nor does he give any instructions for the preparation of the *kyphi*. He simply writes that "the ingredients

---

ies, will shortly appear (ed. H. D. Betz, and a team of a dozen scholars), to be published by the University of Chicago Press.

[202] *PGM*, IV, 1313–14, 2971; V, 221; VII, 538, 873.

[203] Paralleled in the Greek texts known as the *Cyranides*. Dimitris Kaimakis, ed., *Die Kyraniden* (Meisenheim am Glan, 1976).

[204] G. E. R. Lloyd, *Science, Folklore and Ideology* (Cambridge, 1983), 119–35.

[205] See G. Vikan, "Art, Medicine and Magic in Early Byzantium" above in this collection of essays.

[206] Esp. Theophrastus in *HP* and *De causis plantarum*, and Dioscorides in his *Materia medica*.

[207] Dioscorides I, 25 (ed. Wellmann, I, pp. 28–29).

[208] Damocrates in Galen, *Antidotes* II, 2 (ed. Kühn, XIV, 117–19).

are not compounded haphazardly, but whenever the drug-preparers [*myrepsoi*] are mixing these substances, sacred writings are read to them."[209] Since the *Suda* mentions a work by Manetho called *Preparation of Kyphi-Recipes*,[210] Plutarch probably gained his listing of the sixteen ingredients from this lost book,[211] which suggests that Dioscorides' first-century *kyphi* recipe represented a pared-down version of earlier Ptolemaic Egyptian listings for *kyphi*, in turn derived from very ancient Egyptian origins.[212] "They use *kyphi* in both drinks and ointments,"[213] so Plutarch says, and even though he gives some farfetched speculation on why this incense should have been so valued as a drug, Plutarch has recorded an important detail: *kyphi* was commonly consumed in a drink.

Paul of Aegina III, 28.2 (ed. Heiberg, I, p. 206) mentions a *kyphi*, called "the lunar" (*kyphi selēniakon*), which is termed *chrisma selaniakon* in the papyri.[214] Paul writes that, in addition to being used to give a pleasant (if heavy) odor, it is to be rubbed into the forehead as a salve. Oribasius had recorded a formula for a "lunar kyphi" with twenty-five ingredients,[215] while Paul's detailed recipe for the "lunar incense-salve" has twenty-eight ingredients.[216] Some of the ingredients overlap with those given by Dioscorides and Plutarch quoting Manetho, and the anonymous authors of the magical papyri indicate that by the fourth century, some *kyphi* recipes had become known by the more specific *chrismata*, perhaps to suggest their medical use as oily unguents and incenses, but not as drinks or an "edible" drug.[217] Yet the compiler of the papyrus can assume his reader would "know" the ingredients of this complicated incense-salve, and Oribasius and Paul seem to presume an equivalence of *kyphi* with *krisma*, which may indicate that the *kyphi* label had, indeed, become the more "Hellenic" *krisma* outside Egypt. The function, however, of the late Roman and early Byzantine *kyphi-chrismata* generally followed the hallowed Egyptian pattern, while adding an ever more impressive array of ingredients, exotic and local. Paul III, 28.2, is illustrative:

> Another incense-salve of 28 ingredients, called "the lunar"
> 7 *ounkiai* [c. 191 grams] of *bdellion*: bdellium, either the aromatic gum of the Haddi tree, or, the bdellium of the Mukul "myrrh" tree (*Commiphora erythraea* Engl. var. *glabrescens* Engl., or, *C. mukul* Engl.)
> 7 *ounkiai* of *helenion*: either calamint [= basil thyme], or elecampane [= horseheal] (either *Satureja calamintha* [L.] Scheele, or *Inula helenium* L.)
> 2 *ounkiai* [c. 55 grams] of *schoinos*: camel grass (*Cymbopogon schoenanthus* Spreng.)
> 5 *ounkiai* [c. 136 grams] of *sphagnos*: horehound [= false dittany] (*Ballota acetabulosa* [L.] Bentham)
> 50 small juniper berries (*arkeuthides mikrai*): *Juniperus communis* L.
> 5 *ounkiai* of *kardamōmon*: cardamon (*Elettaria cardamomum* [L.] Maton.)
> 7 *ounkiai* of *aspalathos*: camel's thorn oil (*Alhagi maurorum* Medik.)
> 5 *ounkiai* of *kassia syrinx*: cassia "quill" (*Cinnamomum cassia* Blume.)
> 2 *ounkiai* of *nardostachys*: spikenard oil (*Nardostachys jatamansi* DC)
> 5 *ounkiai* of *kyperos*: nut grass (*Cyperus rotundus* L.)
> 4 *ounkiai* [c. 109 grams] of *asphodelos rhiza*: asphodel root (*Asphodelus ramosus* L.)
> 4 *ounkiai* of *brathu*: savin (*Juniperus sabina* L.)
> 3 *ounkiai* of *kyparissos* (*sperma*): cypress seeds (*Cupressus sempervirens* L.)
> 3 *ounkiai*. [c. 82 grams] of *nardos Keltikē*: valerian (*Valeriana celtica* L.)
> 3 *ounkiai* of *malabathron* (*meta tōn phyllōn*): Indian cassia + leaves (*Cinnamomum tamala* [Buch.-Ham] Nees. & Eberm.)
> 3 *ounkiai* of *rhoda xēra*: dried roses (prob. *Rosa gallica* L.)
> 2 *ounkiai* of *kostos*: costus (*Saussurea lappa* C. B. Clarke)
> 2 *ounkiai* of *krokos*: saffron crocus (*Crocus sativus* L.)
> 7 *ounkiai* of *ladanon*: gum labdanum (*Cistus ladaniferus* L.)
> 7 *ounkiai* of *symrna*: myrrh (*Commiphora myrrha* [Nees.] Engl.)
> 2 *litrai* [c. 655 grams] of *staphis* (*enkigartistheisos*): pitted, dried grapes = raisins (prob. *Vitis vinifera* L.)
> 2 *litrai* of *ischas liparos*: dried, fat figs (*Ficus carica* L.)
> 8 *ounkiai* of *strobilos*: kernels of the stone pine (prob. *Pineus pinea* L.)
> 1 *litra* [c. 327 grams] of *terebinthinē*: Chian turpentine from terebinth (*Pistacia terebinthus* L.)
> 7 *ounkiai* of *styrax*: storax gum (*Styrax officinalis* L.)
> 1 *litra* of *phoinikoi liparoi*: dates of the date palm (*Phoenix dactylifera* L.)
> 5 *litrai* of *meli*: honey [c. one and two-thirds kilograms] *oinos euōdes to akroun*: fragrant wine as is sufficient

[209] Plutarch, *Moralia: Isis and Osiris* 383E(80).

[210] *Suda*, M no. 142 (ed. Adler, Vol. III, p. 318).

[211] Thus this is Frg. no. 87 in W. G. Waddell, ed. and trans., *Manetho* (Cambridge, Mass., 1940 [Loeb: in vol. *Manetho. Ptolemy: Tetrabiblos*], pp. 202–5).

[212] G. Ebers, "Ein Kyphirecept aus dem Papyros Ebers," *Zeitschrift für ägyptische Sprache und Altertumskunde*, 12 (1874), 106–11. Further reffs. in J. G. Griffiths, ed., with trans. and comm., *Plutarch's De Iside et Osiride* (Cambridge [for Univ. Wales Press], 1970), 569 n. 4.

[213] Plutarch, *Moralia: Isis and Osiris* 384B(80): τῷ δὲ κῦφι χρῶνται καὶ πώματι καὶ χρίματι.

[214] *PGM*, VII, 873.

[215] Oribasius, *Synopsis for Eustathius* III, 220 (ed. Raeder, p. 121).

[216] Paul of Aegina VII, 22.5 (ed. Heiberg, II, p. 394).

[217] Cf. Galen, *Hygiene* VI, 4.6 (ed. Koch [n. 109 above], p. 177).

Oribasius' "lunar salve" has almost all of the same ingredients and measures as seen here in Paul's recipe: Paul has added only the gum labdanum, saffron crocus, and the Indian cassia. One can presume that once mixed, this salve-incense would be doled out carefully and would have lasted for several months.

Paul VII, 22.1 (ed. Heiberg, II, p. 393) makes it clear that early Byzantine pharmacy placed the *kyphi* among perfumes, but he also tells us that the aromatic function is a minor one for especially the *kyphi*: one uses them as drugs, to be taken internally for the production of accumulation of mucus, and as preventative measures during times of epidemics, as well as for freeing up the lungs and for liver ailments caused by cold. Following are four recipes: perfume of roses, perfume of lilies, the "Great *Kyphi*, called 'The Solar'" (36 ingredients), and the 28-ingredient "lunar *kyphi*" given above in detail. Dioscorides had been one of the first Greco-Roman physicians to recognize the usefulness of the traditional Egyptian multi-ingredient incense recipes, and the *kyphi/krismata* soon occupied an important place in Roman pharmacy, as evinced by Damocrates' poem as quoted by Galen. And Paul, in the seventh century, probably indicates why these curious, quasi-folkloric incenses should have been regarded as very useful by formal pharmaceutics: *kyphi* occupied a place between drugs prepared as lozenges to be dissolved in the mouth, and those drugs thought to be true antidotes.[218]

University of Kentucky

---

[218] Paul of Aegina VII, 22.1 (ed. Heiberg, II, p. 393).

ASAF'S *BOOK OF MEDICINES*: A HEBREW ENCYCLOPEDIA OF GREEK AND JEWISH MEDICINE, POSSIBLY COMPILED IN BYZANTIUM ON AN INDIAN MODEL*

Elinor Lieber

Like all medieval Jewish medical works, the Hebrew *Book of Medicines*, attributed to Asaf the Sage, is predominantly based on Greek concepts. However, as far as I know, it is the only work in any language in which aspects of medicine are also systematically presented in the light of Jewish ideas. Such treatment is not even found in the Bible or Talmud, the bases of Jewish thought: these works contain no *systematic* consideration of medical matters, and those discussed are regarded primarily from the legal point of view.[1]

In ancient Israel the Biblical declaration: "*I am the Lord that healeth thee*" (Exodus 15:26), was generally interpreted in the most literal terms. This attitude was reinforced by the sad story of King Asa, who called in the doctors when he was sick (II Chronicles 16:12–13), as contrasted with the healing of King Hezekiah, who trusted to God alone (II Kings 20:1–11). Yet the Bible provides an alternative view, since it is also maintained that if two men fight and one is injured, the other must "cause him to be thoroughly healed" (Exodus 21:18–19). Thus there was always a place for professional medicine, and the Talmud shows that while one school of rabbis maintained that "men have no power to heal," this was opposed by others who claimed that "a man should not speak thus," since, from the above verses of Exodus, "we learn that permission has been given to the physician to heal."[2]

Yet, while the practice of medicine came to be tolerated, medical writings in Hebrew were far longer proscribed. A story from Mishnaic times, often subsequently repeated, refers to a possibly legendary work, a *Book of Medicines* (*Sefer Refuot*) said to have been suppressed by King Hezekiah—a move with which later rabbis concurred.[3] In any case, apart from the book of the same name attributed to Asaf, the dating of which is by no means certain, no Hebrew medical work is known prior to the tenth century.

Moreover, few medical writings by Jews in languages other than Hebrew are known from before that date. The earliest extant treatises of this kind are by Isaac Israeli (c. 855–955), who wrote in Arabic. However, Galen (129–after 210) refers a number of times to Rufus of Samaria, a contemporary Jewish physician who produced commen-

[The reader is referred to the list of abbreviations at the end of the volume.]

*This paper was prepared with the help of an award from the Wellcome Trust, London, which is gratefully acknowledged. I also thank Professor C. Carmichael of Cornell University for his most constructive criticism.

[1] According to Jewish tradition the Pentateuch constitutes the Written Law while the Talmud, including the Mishnah, represents the main body of the Oral Law. The Mishnah, a collection of oral laws based on the Bible, was completed around the end of the second century of this era. Two versions of the exegesis of the Mishnah by numerous scholars, the "Babylonian" and the "Jerusalem" Talmuds, were written down in the fifth and seventh centuries, respectively. English trans.: *The Mishnah*, ed. and trans. H. Danby (Oxford, 1950); *The Babylonian Talmud*, ed. I. Epstein (London) (hereafter, *BT*).

[2] See *BT* Berakhot 60a. This also cites a prayer to be said by the patient before submitting to bloodletting, which includes the words, "Thou art a faithful healing God, and thy healing is sure." On the subject in general see G. Vermes, *Jesus the Jew* (Philadelphia, 1981), 59–60; and I. Jakobovits, *Jewish Medical Ethics* (New York, 1959), chap. I.

[3] Baraita to Pesaḥim 4, 8. Danby, *Mishnah*, note 7 to 141. Also *BT* Pesaḥim 56a = Berakhot 10b.

taries on Hippocratic works in Greek[4] while, according to Arab sources, a Syrian Jewish physician
named Māsarjawaih not only translated a medical
encyclopedia, the *Pandects* of Ahrūn, from Syriac
to Arabic around A.D. 684, but he also added two
treatises of his own.[5] Thus he is one of the first
translators of medical works into Arabic, and also
the earliest known medical writer in that language.
However, like almost all Jewish medical authors,
Isaac Israeli based himself almost exclusively on
Greek medical concepts, and provided no Jewish
content whatsoever; and the same was almost certainly true of Rufus and Māsarjawaih. This trend
was later epitomized by the medical works (all written in Arabic) of Maimonides (1135–1204), the
greatest Jewish philosopher and theologian.[6]

In this, Jewish medical writers resembled their
Christian and Muslim colleagues in Byzantium and
the medieval Islamic world. Byzantine Christians
continued the ancient Greek pagan tradition of
medicine, largely in the form of commentaries on
Hippocratic works or, like Paul of Aegina in the
seventh century, produced medical encyclopedias,
in conformity with the general Byzantine trend of
compiling encyclopedias of classical learning.[7] The
Arabs, on the other hand, lacked ancient written
traditions of any kind. Thus, in the eighth century,
in the lands newly conquered by Islam, they
mounted a fresh, though now bloodless, campaign. With the revelation of the Koran they had
become a "People of the Book," like the Jews and
the Christians. Now they made a conscious attempt
to acquire, like them, an ancient tradition of book-
learning. Through their Syrian Christian subjects
and allies they were able to procure that large part
of the ancient Greek heritage of philosophy, medicine, and science which the Syrians already pos-

sessed,[8] and were now prepared to translate into
Arabic for their new masters. By the tenth century
the Muslims had achieved their aim. Selected works
on all these subjects, including almost the whole
Galenic corpus, were available in Arabic.[9]

Yet, as far as medicine was concerned, the Christians and Muslims, like the Jews, had always faced
a quandary. While recognizing the need for medical practice, the key for one lay in the New Testament, for the other in the Koran.[10] A compromise
solution, which was eventually to be adopted by all
three religions, had already evolved by the sixth
century—through the early Syrian translators, many
of them monks, who had studied medicine in Alexandria and elsewhere. Medical literature would
be based on ancient Greek writings (a principle
which continued to form the theoretical basis of
Western medicine up to very recent times), but it
was to be entirely free of theology. Whereas medical parallels continued to be invoked in theological
debates, religion was not to be used either to support or to oppose the views expressed in medical
works.[11] This was only made possible by the fact
that Greek medicine—like much of Aristotelian
philosophy—makes practically no allusion to pagan beliefs, nor, on the whole, do its basic tenets
conflict with monotheistic ideas.[12]

---

[4] *Galeni in Hippocratis Epidemiarum Libr. VI, Comm. I–VIII*, ed.
E. Wenkebach and F. Pfaff, *CMG* V 10, 2, 2 (Berlin, 1956), esp.
213, 289, 293, 413.

[5] See Sezgin, *Geschichte, III*, 166–67, 206–7, 224–25.

[6] On these works see E. Lieber, "Galen: Physician as Philosopher, Maimonides Philosopher as Physician," *BHM*, 53 (1979),
268–85. However, in one medical work Maimonides did introduce a purely theological polemic, which was originally found
in one of his philosophical works. See J. Schacht and M. Meyerhof, "Maimonides against Galen on Philosophy and Cosmo-
gony," *Bull. Faculty of Arts, Cairo University*, 5 (1939), 53–88.

[7] See O. Temkin, "Byzantine Medicine: Tradition and Empir-
icism," *DOP*, 16 (1962), 95–115 (= *Double Face*, 202–22). On
Byzantine encyclopedias in general, see P. Lemerle, *Le Premier
Humanisme byzantin* (Paris, 1971), 267–307, and on their medical
encyclopedias, L. Thorndike, *A History of Magic and Experimental
Science*, 8 vols. (New York, 1923–58), I, 566–93.

[8] According to J. Tkatsch, *Die arabische Uebersetzung der Poetik
des Aristoteles*, I (Vienna, 1928), 54 and 56, the Syrian Christians
were already using Aristotelian logic in the third century for
their schismatic disputes, and they began to translate philosophical works into Syriac in the fifth century at the latest. However, the earliest known Syriac translations of Greek medical
works are those of Sergios of Reš'ainā (d. 536). It is probably
not by chance that Sergios, though a Jacobite, had Nestorian
leanings (*ibid.*, 66), that the later translators of Greek medical
works into Arabic were mainly Nestorians, and that Nestorian
missionary activity was so strongly associated with all aspects of
medicine. Medicine conformed with their particular religious
beliefs, even though it was pagan Greek medicine which they
did so much to propagate.

[9] See *ibid.*, 55 and T. J. de Boer, *The History of Philosophy in
Islam*, trans. E. R. Jones (London, 1903), 10–30. On the translations of Galen, see, "Hunain ibn Isḥaq ueber die syrischen
und arabischen Galen-Uebersetzungen," ed. and trans. G.
Bergstraesser, AbhKM, 17 (1925).

[10] Among Muslims this was expressed in a small number of
works from highly orthodox circles, expounding the so-called
Medicine of the Prophet. See Ullmann, *Medizin*, 185–89; F. Klein-
Franke, *Vorlesungen ueber die Medizin im Islam* (Wiesbaden, 1982),
SA, Beiheft 23, 109–32.

[11] Such "separation of Church and State" in medical literature was of course an entirely unwritten rule. I know of no actual reference to it in the writings of the time.

[12] While Byzantine medicine on the whole, "in spite of its
Hellenistic origins and traditions saw its duty of healing the sick
in strictly Christian terms" (A. Sharf, *The Universe of Shabbetai
Donnolo* [Warminster, 1976], 104), this attitude is not reflected

This trend in medical writing was reinforced by the fact that during the ninth and tenth centuries Byzantium too experienced a general revival of Greek learning, although here, unlike the Muslim endeavor, it also comprised historical and literary works.[13] As with the Muslims, however, the intention seems primarily to have been an attempt to unearth and absorb an ancient tradition; for by this period the Byzantines had almost lost contact with their own ancient culture, in its original form. Despite their Christian beliefs, they now felt the need to revert to their pagan Greek roots.

Hence, throughout the medieval world the goal was adherence to tradition rather than originality of thought. Yet the Muslims soon started to build on this alien foundation, and to make use of their newly-found knowledge for their general advancement. In the medical field they produced encyclopedic and other works in which ancient Greek experience was adapted to their own time and place.

In Byzantium, however, the ancient tradition was mainly copied and conserved. Yet the general search for roots undoubtedly influenced the small Jewish communities living in Apulia, deep in the south of Italy, which in the ninth to eleventh centuries re-mained under Byzantine rule.[14] Here Greek was still a living language,[15] in addition to Latin. However, the Jews also knew Hebrew, although only now did it become the vehicle for secular writings. Details of the everyday life of the Jews in Oria, one of these Apulian communities, are provided by the Hebrew *Book of Genealogies* (*Sefer Yuḥasin*), written by Ahimaʿats in 1054. It also shows that their spiritual center lay with the Jewish communities in Muslim lands, with which they had close personal ties. In this way, as well as through the numerous Muslim invasions of southern Italy, they were influenced by developments in both Byzantium and the Islamic world.[16]

The *Book of Genealogies* was but one of a number of Hebrew works which appeared in Byzantine Italy over this period. One might almost speak of a Hebrew mini-Renaissance, which resembled its Greek counterpart insofar as it included historical writings, as well as works on philosophy and medicine. While the *Book of Genealogies* seeks only to establish a local historical tradition, the other works we possess in this group go further in seeking out cultural roots. As far as non-medical works were concerned, an attempt was made to adapt the ancient Jewish written tradition to secular purposes. But even here the tradition followed was not Jewish alone, for ever since Hellenistic times it had been closely interwoven with strands of Greek culture.

These trends are plainly evident in another Hebrew historical work from Italy,[17] probably from the Byzantine south,[18] this time by an anonymous author. It appeared in 953,[19] and came to be known as the *Book of Yosippon* (*Sefer Yosippon*). Though dealing with the general history of the Jews up to the author's own time, it is largely based on Latin versions of the works of Josephus (37/8–after 100).

---

in the medical literature. Yet, as an example of such Christian influence, the sixth-century Alexander of Tralles is said by Sharf (104–5) to "prescribe prayers together with his potions," in his medical encyclopedia. This claim is based on the inclusion of a monotheistic incantation in one of the many magical prescriptions in the work. The recipe is quoted in full by Thorndike [n. 7 above], I, 583–84), who merely comments that it shows "Jewish or Christian influences." Such prescriptions may, however, have been handed down for centuries or even millenia, and were often accompanied by pagan incantations which, in this case, included an adjuration to the plant to heal the patient. Like any ancient adjuration or oath, it contains an invocation to supernatural forces and a curse, to ensure that the oath be kept. In this work by a respected Christian physician an invocation to pagan gods would clearly not be appropriate. It has therefore assumed a more acceptable monotheistic form, through the replacement of their names by Hebrew synonyms for the name of the Deity, although "mother earth" still remains. Similarly, the example of Lot's wife is now invoked as a curse. (For corresponding changes in Arabic and Persian literature, see G. Strohmaier, "Ḥunayn ibn Isḥāq et le Serment Hippocratique," *Arabica*, 21 [1974], 318–23). This Judaic mutation may indicate that the prescription once passed through Jewish hands, or may merely be due to the fact that Jews were supposed to be adept at magic. In any case, the absence of any purely Christian reference clearly denotes that such an incantation cannot be taken as a sign of Christian religious influence on Byzantine medical writings. Temkin, "Byzantine Medicine," p. 110 = *Double Face of Janus*, 215–16, presents an exceptional example of the converse tendency in a medical work, whereby a certain Theophilus (? seventh century) opposes the Biblical, as well as the Homeric concept of the primary seat of the soul, in favor of the medical (Galenic) point of view.

[13] See Lemerle, *Le Premier Humanisme* (n. 7 above), 29 f.

[14] On Byzantine Jewry in general, see J. Starr, *The Jews in the Byzantine Empire 641–1204* (Athens, 1939); A. Sharf, *Byzantine Jewry from Justinian to the Fourth Crusade* (London, 1971).

[15] The vexed question of the knowledge of Greek in Byzantine southern Italy in general is summarized in G. Rohlf's review of St. C. Caratzas, "L'origine des dialectes néo-grecs de l'Italie méridionale," *BZ*, 52 (1959), 99–104. As regards the Jews see Sharf, *Donnolo* (n. 12 above), 97–8.

[16] *The Chronicle of Ahimaaz*, trans. M. Salzman (New York, 1924), *passim*.

[17] The work has never been translated. Critical edition of the text with commentary: *The Josippon (Josephus Gorionides)*, ed. D. Flusser, 2 vols. (Jerusalem, 1978 and 1980).

[18] *Ibid.*, II, 84–98.

[19] *Ibid.*, II, 79–84. The Byzantine origin and this dating have both been contested by Golb, in N. Golb and O. Pritsak, *Khazarian Hebrew Documents of the Tenth Century* (Ithaca, New York, 1982), 89, note 47.

Josephus, who had been a leader of the Jewish revolt against the Romans in Palestine, was captured by Vespasian, the Roman commander. However, he predicted that Vespasian would soon become Emperor, and after this indeed came to pass, he was released and honored by Vespasian,[20] subsequently spending the rest of his life in Rome, where he wrote his historical works.

Hence Josephus, as he himself notes, was considered as a traitor by the Jews,[21] who ignored his writings for centuries, even though these favored the Jewish point of view. The Church, on the other hand, "embraced the outcast."[22] In their Greek and Latin versions his writings were always of interest to Christians, including the Byzantine chroniclers, since they constituted an excellent source of the history of Israel and Rome in and around the time of Jesus. In the ninth century his main works were summarized in the *Bibliotheca* of Photius.[23] With the *Yosippon*, however, some kind of Hebrew version finally appeared, obviously intended for Jews.

In Byzantium, as in the medieval Islamic world, there were many Jewish physicians,[24] yet so far they lacked any tradition of medical writing. By the beginning of the tenth century medical and philosophical works by the celebrated Isaac Israeli had appeared in Arabic, and now books of this kind in Hebrew were to be written in Byzantine southern Italy by a physician named Shabtai bar Abraham, usually known as Donnolo. Donnolo himself tells us most of what we know about his life.[25] He was born at Oria and in 925, at the age of twelve, was taken captive by Arab raiders, together with others, Jews and Christians, from the town. He was eventually ransomed, and then set himself to study astronomy, astrology and medicine, for which purpose he traveled widely within the Byzantine Empire. He could probably read Greek and Latin, as

well as Hebrew, and he possibly also knew Arabic. Apart from his books, he became a well-known practitioner, and his name was even linked with the legendary founding of a "medical school" in Salerno, although there is no evidence that he ever had any connection with that city.[26]

Donnolo produced a treatise on pharmacy known as *The Book of Mixtures* (*Sefer ha-Mirqaḥot*) around the year 970.[27] This is not only the oldest extant medical treatise in Hebrew to which some kind of date can be given, it is also the oldest medical work of any kind from medieval Italy. In his Introduction Donnolo states that the book was designed to instruct the physicians of Israel in the art of dispensing medicines "according to the wisdom of Israel and Byzantium."[28] Yet nothing specifically Jewish is found in the work, which appears to be simply a Hebrew version of a typical Greek pharmaceutical text. Thus, although "the wisdom of Israel" may be an allusion to those apocryphal medical works mentioned in the Bible and Talmud, it is far more likely that it refers to the *Book of Medicines* attributed to Asaf, in which much of the same Hebrew botanical terminology is found.

Donnolo also wrote on astronomy and astrology, which in those days were inextricably linked, and on their connection with medicine.[29] However, even from the purely medical point of view, his most interesting work is that usually known as the *Ḥakhmoni*, a philosophical commentary on the mystical *Book of Creation* (*Sefer Yetsira*). Donnolo's was only one of the many commentaries on this anonymous Hebrew philosophical work, which was probably composed between the third and sixth centuries of the present era. However, it differs from the others in that it develops a theological argument along purely medical lines. In discussing Genesis 1:26–27, the creation of man in God's image, Donnolo uses analogies with the anatomy, physiology, and

[20] Josephus, *Jewish War* III, 392–408; IV 622–29 (Loeb, II, 686–91; III, 184–87 [Cambridge, Mass., 1926–65]). Suetonius, *Vespasian* V, 6. See also note 106 below. On the life of Josephus in general, see T. Rajak, *Josephus* (London, 1983).

[21] Josephus, *Jewish War* III, 434–39. See S. Dubnov, *History of the Jews*, trans. M. Spiegel, 6 vols. in 3 (New York and London, 1967–69), Vol. I, 782–83; E. Schuerer, *The History of the Jewish People in the Age of Jesus Christ*, new English version, ed. and revised G. Vermes and F. Millar, Vol. I (Edinburgh, 1973), 490–91, 494.

[22] *The Latin Josephus*, I, ed. F. Blatt (Copenhagen, 1958), 9–16.

[23] Photius (ed. Henry), I, pp. 32–35 and 155–58 [Cod. 47, 48, and 76], and V, 141–55 [Cod. 238].

[24] See Sharf, *Donnolo* (n. 12 above), 108–10.

[25] *Il commento di Sabbatai Donnolo sul Libro della Creazione*, ed. D. Castelli (Florence, 1880), 1–4; Sharf, *Donnolo* (n. 12 above), 7–10.

[26] M. Steinschneider, *Donnolo. Pharmakologische Fragmente aus dem zehnten Jahrhundert* (Berlin, 1868), 9.

[27] Text: *ibid.*, Suppl. G. Brecher, I–VI; translation: 124–53. Text only: S. Muntner, *R. Shabtai Donnolo*, 2 sections (Jerusalem, 1949), I, 7–23. *Ibid.*, 8 note 12, followed by Sharf, *Donnolo* (n. 12 above), 109, suggests a date between 970 and 980, since Donnolo claims to have written the work after "forty years" of experience. However, this experience might well have started while he was still in his teens. Moreover, the Jewish use of the number "forty" is often allegorical, referring to the years of wandering in the Wilderness, and thus merely denoting a long and weary period. Hence the true date of composition might be up to ten years earlier.

[28] Steinschneider, *Donnolo* (n. 26 above), Suppl., p. I. Muntner, *R. Shabtai*, I, 8.

[29] Sharf, *Donnolo* (n. 12 above), 4, 14–32.

even with the pathology of the body,[30] which seem largely to be based on the *Book of Medicines*, and contain a number of medical terms found only in that work. Interspersed with these are numerous Biblical quotations. A brief extract from this part of Donnolo's work, (without any reference to it) seems to be included in the *Yosippon*.[31]

A long fragment of a "Practica," a treatise on the diagnosis and treatment of diseases, is often attributed to Donnolo,[32] since it is found in the same manuscript as his *Book of Mixtures*. However, this manuscript also contains part of the *Book of Medicines*, and the fragment may well belong to the latter. Like the *Book of Mixtures* it is purely Greek in content, with no specifically Jewish features.

The *Book of Medicines* attributed to Asaf the Sage is a far more important and substantial medical work than anything so far described. This too may well be a product of Byzantine Italy in the ninth or tenth centuries, but as nothing definite is known about its authorship, provenance or dating, I have left its consideration to the last. It is an extraordinary work in many respects, not least because, as has already been noted, it breaks the "rules," and not only incorporates Jewish theological—and essentially Biblical—concepts, but even uses them to reinforce ancient Greek medicine.

This very long work has never been published in full,[33] and I am at present preparing the first critical edition of the text from all the known manuscripts, together with a translation and commentary. The present description is thus solely a progress report, and in view of the many difficulties involved in this task, only a few of which can be touched upon here, any conclusions presented are tentative indeed.

The longest version of the work opens with the statement that it is a "Book of Medicines." From this it derives its name, which is somewhat misleading since it seems to imply that the work is merely a collection of prescriptions. In fact it is a rambling encyclopedia, covering almost every aspect of ancient medicine, other than surgery. As such it fits in with the general Byzantine encyclopedic tradition of this period, and it certainly follows the great ancient and medieval tradition of medical encyclopedias in Greek, Latin, Sanskrit, Chinese, Syriac and Arabic, which were always based on much earlier material.

The Introduction consists of a legendary account of the beginnings of medicine, taken in part from the *Book of Jubilees*,[34] one of the group of Biblical pseudepigrapha which contains the story of Noah. It claims that the work which it introduces represents a version of a "Book of Medicines" which was written down by Noah after the Flood from the words of Raphael, God's healing angel, and was then given by Noah to his son Shem. Thus medicine acquired Semitic ancestry, but it was then copied by "ancient sages" throughout the world, who carried on the tradition. Among these the "sages" of India, Greece, Egypt and Mesopotamia are specifically mentioned, but only four of them are named: Hippocrates, "Asaf the Jew," Dioscorides, and Galen. Apart from Asaf, of whom we know nothing, these were probably the three names in Greek medicine most familiar to medieval readers. If they have intentionally been placed in chronological order, it may denote that Asaf was supposed to have lived between the time of "Hippocrates" and that of Dioscorides, that is, at some period between the fifth century B.C. and the first century A.D. Yet no historical physician, Jewish or other, is known by this name.

Although most of the work claims to represent the medical teachings of Asaf as based, like those of the other sages, on the *Book of Medicines*, some of the sections are presented in the name of an equally unknown Yoḥanan. In both cases the teachings are reported as though they had been set down by a hearer, possibly a pupil. No clue as to its date of composition has yet been found in the contents, nor even in scribal additions. Moreover, despite assertions that the work was mentioned by others at much earlier dates,[35] I have so far been

[30] Castelli, *Il commento* (n. 25 above), 10–19; Muntner, *R. Shabtai* (n. 27 above), I, 24–38, esp. 25–35. This part of the work is discussed and partly quoted by Sharf, *Donnolo* (n. 12 above), chaps. 4 and 5.

[31] Flusser, *Josippon* (n. 17 above), II, 81.

[32] See Sharf, *Donnolo* (n. 12 above), 96–97. Text: Muntner, *R. Shabtai* (n. 27 above), I, 109–44.

[33] The only extract published which has been critically edited is L. Lieber, "The Covenant Which Asaf . . . and Yoḥanan . . . Made with Their Pupils," *Muntner Memorial Volume*, ed. J. O. Liebowitz (Jerusalem, 1983) 83–87 (Hebrew and English). Other extracts: Hebrew: S. Muntner, "Asaph Harofe, Sefer Harefuoth," *Koroth*, 3 (1965), 396–422, and most subsequent issues till 6 (1972), 28–51; A. Melzer, *Asaph the Physician—The Man and His Book* (Ann Arbor, 1980), 93–251; English: A. Bar-Sela and H. E. Hoff, "Asaf on Anatomy and Physiology," *JHM*, 20 (1965), 358–89; Hebrew and English: S. Pines, "The Oath of Asaph the Physician," *Proceedings of the Israel Academy of Sciences and Humanities*, 5 (1975), 224–26 and 258–59.

[34] *The Apocrypha and Pseudepigrapha of the Old Testament*, ed. R. H. Charles, II, *Pseudepigrapha* (Oxford, 1964), 27–28, "The Book of Jubilees," X, 1–16.

[35] L. Venetianer, *Asaf Judaeus, der aelteste medizinische Schriftsteller in hebraeischer Sprache*, 3 pts. (Budapest, 1915–17), Part I, 26–39.

unable to corroborate any indubitable reference before about 1200.[36]

Greater or lesser parts of the book have now been found in eighteen manuscripts, mainly from European libraries,[37] the longest extending to some 350 folios. None are dated and few possess the name of the copyist. However, a number of them have recently undergone expert paleographical examination, and of these the earliest seems to date from the twelfth or the early thirteenth century.[38] Most appear to be of European origin, from the Mediterranean area. They vary greatly in the extent and order of their subject matter, and none possesses any table of contents. Moreover, unlike most other encyclopedic works, they lack any formal bibliographical division into books, chapters and so on, so that it is practically impossible to determine the true extent of the work, even in its most complete form. It no doubt appeared in many versions, some of which may have grown by accretion, while others were abridged.

The book as we have it contains at least three types of material. Items which appear to be original, or whose source has yet to be discovered, are found within the main body of the text. They seem largely to have been composed at the time of the main compilation, although they are undoubtedly based on much older material. Interspersed with them, however, are paraphrased abridgments of easily-identifiable Greek works, such as the Hippocratic *Aphorisms* and the *Materia medica* of Dioscorides. Finally, there are the clinical sections, on diagnosis and treatment, including various collections of prescriptions, much of which may have been added later.

The medical concepts expressed throughout the work are basically Greek and Hippocratic in origin. However, the more original parts of this work, unlike the purely medical writings of Donnolo, contain a large amount of Biblical analogy, some of which, as we shall see, never rises to the surface. As far as I know, the *Book of Medicines* is unique

among Jewish, Christian or Muslim[39] medical works in thus incorporating theological ideas.

As hinted in its Introduction, the book also shows traces of ancient Egyptian, Indian and Syriac elements, while Persian and occasional Arabic influences vary greatly with the different manuscripts. On the whole, however, Arabic medicine plays little or no part in the work, and is mainly expressed in a few technical terms, which may have been added later. Perhaps this accounts for the relative lack of Galenic concepts, while the preponderance of Hippocratic material is a sign that European influence predominates. In any case, a remarkable feature is the virtual absence of astrological material or references to magical practices.[40]

The work differs from most Greek encyclopedias of medicine, and resembles the Arabic works, in its attention to anatomy and to the ancient equivalent of physiology, including embryology. Yet Arabic anatomy is almost entirely Galenic. In the Hebrew work the section on anatomy proper limits itself to the constituent parts of the "members" (*evarim*) which, by ancient Hebrew definition[41] are those parts of the body which contain bones and "vessels" (*gidim*)[42] and are covered by flesh. The internal organs are described in a separate section, and mainly from the point of view of their func-

---

[36] *The Commentary of Rabbi David Kimhi on Hosea*, ed. H. Cohen (New York, 1929), chap. 14, 8; pp. 113–114.

[37] The main manuscripts are (Hebrew) Bodleian Cat. Neubauer 2138; Munich Staatsbibliothek 231; Florence Laurenziana Plut. 88.37; British Museum Or. 12252.

[38] Bodl. 2138. For this I am most grateful to Professor I. O. Lehman of the Hebrew Union College, Cincinnati, Dr. Colette Sirat of Paris, and Professor M. Beit-Arié of Jerusalem. See also J. Shatzmiller, "Doctors and Medical Practices in Germany," *Proc. American Acad. for Jewish Research*, 50 (1983), 149–64. Munich 231, which was hitherto generally thought to be the oldest, is probably a sixteenth-century copy.

[39] Excluding, of course, the works on "Prophetic medicine" mentioned above.

[40] In one section the signs of the zodiac are named for each month; a handful of prescriptions utilize magic, but these are almost certainly later additions to the original collections of recipes.

[41] *BT* Ḥullin 128b and *Tosefta*, ed. M. S. Zuckermandel (Pasewalk, 1877–82), Ohalot 1, 7 (Hebrew), cf. Ezekiel 37:6; as is Job 10:11.

[42] An example of the pseudo-archaic language found in the *Book of Medicines* is the unqualified use of the entirely non-specific anatomical term *gid* (plural: *gidim*) throughout the work. As in the Bible (Ezekiel 37:6; Job 10:11) it may indicate any elongated, but not necessarily hollow, structure in the body, including vessels of all kinds, nerves, sinews, tendons and, when qualified, even the penis. As such it seems to correspond with the ancient Egyptian term *mt* (see H. Grapow, *Grundriss der Medizin der alten Aegypter, I. Anatomie und Physiologie* [Berlin, 1954], 20 and 72), and perhaps with the Akkadian *šer'ānu* (see A. L. Oppenheim, "On the Observation of the Pulse in Mesopotamian Medicine," *Orientalia*, 31 [1962], 27–33). However, in the context discussed here, which is certainly derived from Ezek. 37:6, the term probably refers only to the most essential of these elements, the blood vessels and nerves. In the Mishnah and Talmud a more specific term, *vrid*, corresponding with the Greek *phleps* (see I. M. Lonie, *The Hippocratic Treatises "On generation,"* . . . [Berlin and New York, 1981], 105), is used without qualification to denote the blood vessels in general. In Job 30:17 the term *oreq* in its context seems to indicate a "vessel" which "does not rest," and hence perhaps an artery. The same term, when qualified as "pulsating," is the commonest way of differentiating an artery from a vein in medieval Hebrew (and Arabic) medical works, but the terms *vrid* and *gid* are also used in this fashion.

tion. This is probably the oldest arrangement of a specifically anatomical text, and traces of it are even found in the Galenic scheme regarding the subject matter and order of anatomical teaching.[43] In all other respects, however, Galenic anatomy reflects an approach differing entirely from that of the *Book of Medicines*. Though ostensibly human, it was based on observations obtained from the dissection of animals for anatomical purposes, whereby the tissues and organs were systematically exposed, layer by layer, in order to reveal their relationships. The anatomical and "physiological" sections of the Hebrew work, on the other hand, reflect a view of animal anatomy familiar to the ordinary man in former times, when nearly everyone took some part in the slaughter of animals for food. Immediately the animal was killed, the organs were removed from the body in order to preserve the flesh from decay. Hence the anatomy of the "members"—of the bony parts covered by vessels and flesh—was that of the limbs and of the empty cadaver. Since the organs were rapidly removed, their relationship to one another, and to the cadaver itself, remained vague, and this was even mirrored, as has been seen, in works based essentially on anatomical dissection.

Hence this was the aspect of the body observed after slaughter according to the Jewish dietary laws,[44] methods which had been practiced and perfected for centuries before they were first written down in the Mishnah in the second century A.D. In the Talmud we also find instructions for examining the cadaver and organs—to ensure that the meat is fit for consumption—and these were continually supplemented and revised. Such procedures must clearly have resulted in a profound knowledge of animal anatomy, even if it were never recorded as such.

At first sight the sections of the *Book of Medicines* dealing with anatomy, "physiology" and "pathology" seem to be a confused mass of Greek and Jewish concepts. Yet, as we shall see, there is not only method in this apparent madness, there are also

amazing flashes of insight. My first example of Greek-Jewish interaction in this work is probably the most interesting of all, because it has produced such a remarkable offspring. It is the account of the blood vessels, which forms part of the anatomical section.[45] Its highly unusual nature was first recognised in 1933 by Dr. I. Simon of Paris;[46] but his finding has been almost totally ignored. Since it is stated in the description that the blood "goes around" the body and then "returns to the heart," he considered this to be an account of the actual circulation of the blood. The author, according to Simon, was Asaf, an unknown Jewish physician from around the seventh century, who had thus forestalled William Harvey (1578–1657)[47] by some nine hundred years—although Simon felt that Asaf could not have appreciated the true significance of his discovery.

However, Simon's interpretation of this section of the work is based on one manuscript alone. Still more important, he does not identify the individual vessels in the description, and so cannot justify his conclusions on an anatomical basis. It seems to me, therefore, that the whole matter warrants entirely fresh consideration.[48]

The account opens by stating that it concerns "those vessels (*gidim*)[49] which convey the soul in the blood to all the body." It then describes how "the abundance of the blood" flows from vessels in the neck down to the heart. From there the blood "goes around" the body to the different parts, then "returns to the heart," and leaves it once again. It is not said, however, to proceed to the lungs, which receive no mention at all. Nor is it clear whether the blood actually returns from the limbs, or is partly or wholly absorbed there.

Since the archaic and non-specific Biblical term

---

[43] See E. Lieber, "Galen in Hebrew: the Transmission of Galen's Works in the Mediaeval Islamic World," in Nutton, ed., *Galen: Problems*, 167–86, esp. 172–73.

[44] See Mishnah Tractate Ḥullin. This tradition of slaughter is said to be based on the commandment at Sinai (Deuteronomy 12:21), "Thou shalt kill . . . as I have commanded thee," and on the prohibition of eating blood found in Genesis 9:4 and Leviticus 17:10–14. . For summaries of these laws and procedures see *Julius Preuss' Biblical and Talmudic Medicine*, trans. F. Rosner (New York, 1978), 501–6 and 103; *Encyclopaedia Judaica*, vol. 14 (Jerusalem, 1971), *s.v. Shehitah*, cols. 1337–44.

[45] For trans. see Bar-Sela and Hoff, "Asaf on Anatomy" (note 33 above).

[46] I. Simon, *Asaph Ha-Iehoudi* (Paris, 1933), 41 and 45.

[47] Harvey's account of the circulation was first published in 1628, as *De motu cordis et sanguinis*. See W. Harvey, *An Anatomical Disputation concerning the Movement of the Heart and Blood in Living Creatures*, trans. G. Whitteridge (Oxford, 1976), (hereafter: Harvey, *De motu cordis*, Whitteridge). On his discovery see: W. Pagel, *William Harvey's Biological Ideas* (Basel, New York, 1967), hereafter: Pagel, *WHBI*; G. Whitteridge, *William Harvey and the Circulation of the Blood* (London, New York, 1971); *William Harvey and His Age*, ed. J. J. Bylebyl (Baltimore, 1979).

[48] I shall be publishing a special study of this Hebrew account of the vessels, which will include the text, a translation, a full anatomical interpretation, and a comparison with Harvey's findings.

[49] See note 42 above. In this account the term is translated as "vessels" since here, when unqualified, it clearly denotes the blood vessels alone.

gid is used to denote all the vessels, and as none of them are actually named, it would at first seem impossible to identify the vessels concerned. As an anatomical description it thus seems primitive indeed, an impression which probably accounts for its totally unjustified neglect. Yet the difficulty in recognizing what is actually described seems mainly to lie in the fact that it is presented in a very different form from other known works of this kind, ancient or medieval. These are generally based on systematic dissection of the vessels, in animals or man, for anatomical purposes, or else describe the vessels as a guide to bloodletting procedures. However, this purely medical Hebrew account appears to be founded on a knowledge of the cadaver of animals slaughtered for food, and hence includes only those vessels which remain in the body after the organs have been removed. Once this unusual presentation is recognized, each of the vessels described can be identified in modern anatomical terms. This is possible, despite the lack of any guiding nomenclature, since, surprisingly enough, the direction of flow in each vessel is, with one exception, correctly described. On account of this hemodynamic approach, the arteries and veins can be distinguished from one another, and both types of vessel are obviously thought to contain blood.[50] The blood is thus said to be repeatedly carried to the heart by vessels essentially corresponding with the veins and it flows from the heart to the periphery in vessels identifiable as the aorta and its branches.

Yet this is by no means a layman's account, for it is certainly influenced in part by some of the most ancient Greek descriptions of the vessels. In its phraseology and in purely anatomical details it shows affinities with that of Diogenes of Apollonia, which dates from the fifth century B.C. and is probably the oldest known systematic account of the vessels.[51] In many respects it also resembles certain descriptions found in the Hippocratic work *Bones*,[52] particularly those which themselves resemble the work of Diogenes.

It has of course long been claimed that certain Hippocratic writings already showed an awareness

of the circular motion of the blood, although this view has also been hotly disputed.[53] However, the Greek anatomical accounts are more or less static descriptions of the vessels, and those few Hippocratic treatises which actually allude to the motion of the blood do not so much as hint at a circulatory system beginning and ending in the heart.

The central function of the heart in relation to the vascular system seems to have been recognized by the ancient Egyptians,[54] and it was firmly established by Plato and Aristotle,[55] as part of the belief in the general primacy of the heart in the body. The two latter, however, likened the vessels to a centrifugal system of irrigation canals.[56] These carried the blood from a central source, the heart, to the periphery of the body. Since the blood, with all its contents, was thought to be wholly absorbed by the tissues—like the water in an irrigation canal—there could be no question of a circulation. This basic idea of the function of the vessels was to be adopted by Galen,[57] and by almost all physicians up to the time of Harvey and even beyond. However, like Galen they generally rejected the idea of the centrality of the heart, claiming that this organ played only a minor role in the cardiovascular system. The liver was the main point of distribution of the blood (with its "nutriment") to the body, via the veins, and hence the greater part of the blood was thought to bypass the heart.[58] The heart "gave rise" to the arteries alone, whose task it was to bring "spirit" (*pneuma*) to the body.[59]

Yet, from very early times Platonic and, above all, Aristotelian ideas greatly influenced both medical and non-medical concepts of the cardiovascular system. In the sixteenth century in particular, the widespread adoption of these theories in philosophical and theological works resulted in a general diffusion of the belief in the central position

[50] As suggested by Aristotle (*Parts of Animals* III, 5; 667b–668a), and demonstrated by Galen (*An in arteriis natura sanguis contineatur*, chap. 2 [ed. Kühn, IV, 707]), who was, however, so inconsistent about this, that most of his followers adopted the view that the veins contained much blood and a little spirit, while the converse held for the arteries. That both types of vessel are full of blood is fundamental for any concept of the circulation.

[51] Aristotle, *Historia animalium* III, 2; 511b, 31–512b, 11.

[52] Hippocrates (ed. Littré), IX, 168–97.

[53] The polemic has been superbly presented in Harris, *Heart* 29–96. See also Lonie, "*On Generation*" (n. 42 above), 87–97.

[54] *The Papyrus Ebers*, trans. B. Ebbell (Copenhagen, 1937), XCIX and C, 114–15, 117.

[55] Plato, *Timaios* 70 A-B; Harris, *Heart*, 118–21. Aristotle, *Parts of Animals* III, 4; 665b–666a. Harris, *Heart*, 122.

[56] Plato, *Timaios* 79A; Aristotle, *Parts of Animals* III, 5; 668a.

[57] Galen, *Natural Faculties* III, xv (trans. Brock, 324–27).

[58] According to Galen most of the blood in the vena cava in the chest went straight up to the throat. See Galen, *Parts* VI, 4 (trans. May, I, 286), and Galen, *Hippocrates–Plato* VI, 5, 2 (ed. De Lacy, II, 389). The heart proper was thought to consist only of the ventricles.

[59] On Galen's ideas on the cardiovascular system, which are scattered throughout his works, see A. R. Hall, "Studies on the History of the Cardiovascular System," *BHM*, 34 (1960), 391–413; Harris, *Heart*, 267–396; and the excellent diagram in Scarborough, *Medicine*, fig. 13, p. 118.

of the heart, which led in its turn to various theoretical concepts of circular movement within the
cardiovascular system. It is possible that these ancient Greek theories and their later developments
affected our Hebrew account directly or indirectly,
just as much later they influenced Harvey.[60] There
is certainly no doubt that Harvey based his arguments directly on Aristotelian logic, and he freely
acknowledges his debt to Aristotle for many of his
philosophical and medical ideas.[61] These included
a macrocosmic parallel to the circulation of the
blood, based on Aristotle's descriptions of cosmo-
logical cycles,[62] and it is interesting to note that the
Bible, which so obviously influenced the *Book of
Medicines* in general, also describes such a cycle in
Ecclesiastes 1:4–7.

Yet, despite its ancient Greek echoes, the *Book of
Medicines* seems to present a very different view of
the cardiovascular system, remote even from neo-
Galenic ideas. Crude as it appears, we have here
an account of the continuous flow of the blood
around the body for, since the blood leaves the heart
by one route and returns to it by another, there can
be no question of an ebb-and-flow movement. Although here there is no actual allusion to movement in a circle, none of these elements of a true
circulation is found, as far as I know, in any Greek
text, nor in any other work before the mid-sixteenth
century.

According to the modern, physiological definition of the circulation of the blood, all the blood is
continuously pumped around the body through all
the vessels, passing through the heart on the way
to and from the lungs. In our Hebrew account there
are two possible gaps in the circuit. As has been
seen, it is possible that the blood was thought to be
absorbed in the limbs and hence did not return
from there to the heart. Secondly, the lungs are not
mentioned at all.[63] Yet if the blood constantly returns to the heart, how does it flow from the veins

and the right side of the heart to the left side of
the heart and the arteries, without traversing the
lungs? The Hebrew account provides no clue at all
but, provided that the question were ever considered, it is possible that Galenic views were adopted,
so that this route was not anatomically required.
According to Galen the blood could pass from the
veins to the arteries directly through anastomoses
between them. It also flowed from the right side of
the heart to the left through channels in the interventricular septum.[64] However, in view of the non-
Galenic spirit of this account, it is more likely that
the shunt was thought to be effected in a manner
which Aristotle seems to describe.[65]

The first known description of the course of the
blood from the right side of the heart to the left
via the lungs was written in the thirteenth century
by Ibn an-Nafīs, a Muslim physician.[66] It was redis-
covered in Europe three hundred years later, perhaps with the aid of a translation of this Arabic
account.[67] Yet to these pioneers this was no more
than a pulmonary transit, with no hint whatsoever
of circular movement. However, the concept of this
vascular pathway through the lungs, linking the
veins with the arteries, clearly cast doubt on Gal-
en's hypothesis that the blood could pass through
the interventricular septum of the heart. Hence,
although fully accepted by Harvey, it was rejected
by others during and after his time. The function
of the lungs in oxygenating the blood was of course
known no more to Harvey than to the author of
our Hebrew account. Yet some of Galen's varied
notions of the *pneuma* or "spirit," derived from the
air via the lungs, came remarkably close to the
mark,[68] and these were the theories adopted by most
of Galen's successors, and by Harvey among them.

---

[60] See W. Pagel, *WHBI*, and *New Light on William Harvey* (Basel, c. 1976), both *passim*; C. Webster, "William Harvey and the Crisis of Medicine in Jacobean England," in Bylebyl, *Harvey and His Age* (n. 47 above), 1–27, esp. 15 ff.

[61] See H. Ratner, "William Harvey, M.D.: Modern or Ancient Scientist?," *The Thomist*, 24 (1961), 175–208; J. S. Wilkie, "Harvey's Immediate Debt to Aristotle and Galen," *History of Science*, 4 (1965), 103–24.

[62] Harvey, *De motu cordis*, chap. 8 (Whitteridge [n. 47 above], 75–76); cf. Aristotle, *Meteorologica* I, 9, 346b–347a.

[63] Interestingly enough, the identical concept of a partly closed circuit, confined to the trunk—although physiologically impos-
sible—was suggested by Harvey's contemporary, Jean Riolan, the Professor of Anatomy in Paris, to counter Harvey's idea of the circulation. He claimed, moreover, that the blood passed through the interventricular septum of the heart, and only flowed

through the lungs under exceptional circumstances. J. Riolan, *A Sure Guide to Physick and Chyrurgery*, Englished N. Culpeper and W. R. (London, 1657) (= *Encheiridium anatomicum*), 57 and 108.

[64] Galen, *Natural Faculties* III, xv (Brock, 321).

[65] This is based on my personal interpretation of Aristotle, *Historia animalium* III, 3, 513b, 1–33, which will be presented in the paper referred to in n. 48 above.

[66] See M. Meyerhof, "Ibn An-Nafis (XIIIth cent.) and His Theory of the Lesser Circulation," *Isis*, 23 (1935), 100–120; J. Schacht, "Ibn al-Nafīs, Servetus and Colombo," *Al-Andalus*, 22 (1957), 317–36.

[67] See Meyerhof, *ibid.*, and Schacht, *ibid*. The Arabic account is said to have been translated into Latin in the sixteenth cen-
tury, but this version has never been found, see C. D. O'Malley, "A Latin Translation of Ibn Nafis (1547) Related to the Problem of the Circulation of the Blood," *JHM* 12 (1957), 248–53. Plagiarism on the part of Servetus is refuted by O. Temkin, "Was Servetus Influenced by Ibn an-Nafīs?," *BHM*, 8 (1940), 731–34.

[68] As rightly suggested by Harris, *Heart*, 338.

However, not until Harvey was the pulmonary transit conceived of as part of the general movement of the blood around the body.[69] Yet to Galen, and to those who for centuries followed his lead in this matter, a circulation would have been "unnecessary" on purely physiological grounds, and hence could not be discovered.

In the Hebrew description, however, the blood as a whole serves to convey the soul, rather than the spirit, around the body. Since the soul, unlike the spirit, does not depend directly on the lungs, the latter are of no special importance in the context of the vascular system. Perhaps that is why, like some other organs, such as the alimentary tract, they receive no mention at all, even though they may well have been thought to take part in the circular motion of the blood. Nor is their absence surprising in such a description, based on animal slaughter, in which, as we have seen, the vascular connections of the organs in any case tend to be vague.

This Hebrew work thus essentially provides an account of the progress of the soul in the blood around the body, from the hemodynamic point of view, as it proclaims in its opening phrases, in which an "abundance" (*šefa*) of the blood is said to enter the heart via the veins. This is an extraordinary declaration: it is diametrically opposed to Galenic physiology, which on principle claims that the mass of the blood never enters the heart. It is even more remarkable that the identical observation regarding the "abundance" (*copia*) of the blood entering the heart, and its subsequent development along purely hemodynamic lines, constituted, as Harvey tells us himself, the discovery of the circulation of the blood.[70]

It is not generally realized, however, that to arrive at this triumphant conclusion Harvey had first to close the anatomical gap left by Galen and almost all his successors. In a work published earlier, the *Lectures on Anatomy*, Harvey had already reverted to the Aristotelian idea that the vena cava "begins" in the heart rather than in the liver. Hence,

according to Harveian hemodynamics, all the blood in the vena cava would have to enter the heart—in total opposition to the Galenic point of view.[71]

In *De motu cordis*, having announced his discovery, Harvey then justifies it on teleological grounds: blood cooled in the extremities is forced back to the heart, there to "seek again both heat and spirit."[72] Yet in a work published later, *On the Generation of Animals*, Harvey plays down the importance of the spirit and even downgrades the heart, in favor of the predominance of the blood, containing the soul. "Spirit" is now merely the "instrument" of the soul and, as he rightly maintains, the only purpose of the heart is to "receive this blood . . . and drive it forth again into every part throughout the whole body."[73] The concept of the preeminence of the soul in the blood, and of its distribution throughout the body, was no product of Galenic physiology. For Harvey, as for the Hebrew account, it sprang from "the Scriptures": from the idea expressed in Leviticus 17:11, that "the soul of the flesh is in the blood."[74]

And this same Biblical verse serves to explain the hemodynamic approach of our Hebrew account, some seven hundred years before Harvey. For Leviticus 17:11 forms part of the Biblical laws (Genesis 9:3–4 and Leviticus 17:10–14) which prohibit the eating of blood in general, including the blood in the flesh. However, Leviticus 17:13 allows flesh to be eaten if the blood has been poured out, and this proviso constitutes the basis of Jewish methods of slaughtering animals for food. These were devised and perfected over the millennia, with the aim of rapidly killing the animal, exsanguinating it as fast and completely as possible and yet, as already stated

---

[69] M. Neuburger, "Zur Entdeckungsgeschichte des Lungen-kreislaufes," *Arch. f. Gesch. Med.* 23 (1930), 7–9, followed by Meyerhof, "Ibn An-Nafis," and by Pagel, *WHBI* (n. 47 above), 51 and 136, have stressed the essential fact that the so-called pulmonary circulation is in fact no circulation on its own, since it does not begin and end in the same place. It only forms part of the general circulation of the body as a whole.

[70] See Harvey, *De motu cordis*, chaps. 8 and 10 (Whitteridge [n. 47 above], 75 and 85). But see Pagel's comments, *WHBI* (n. 47 above), 224 on the similar observation by Vesalius in 1543, and its possible influence on Harvey.

[71] *The Anatomical Lectures of William Harvey*, ed. G. Whitteridge (Edinburgh, London, 1964), 75r, 258–59. For Galen's views see n. 58 above.

[72] Harvey, *De motu cordis*, chap. 15 (Whitteridge [n. 47 above], 109).

[73] *William Harvey's Disputations Touching the Generation of Animals*, trans. G. Whitteridge (Oxford, 1981), chap. 51, pp. 245–46 and chap. 71, p. 382, and see C. Webster, "Harvey. De generatione," *British Journal for the History of Science*, 3 (1967), 262–74.

[74] Harvey, *Generation of Animals* (ed. Whitteridge), chap. 51, p. 243; chap. 52, p. 257. Here Harvey, however, uses the term "life" (*vita*), which does not strictly correspond with the Hebrew *nefeš* (soul), used in the Bible (and in the Hebrew description of the blood vessels), nor with the Vulgate (*anima*) and Septuagint (*psyche*). "Life" is found, however, in the King James English version, which first appeared in 1611, when Harvey was a young man. The same applies to Genesis 9:4, which is usually translated as Leviticus 17:4, although the latter text here is exceedingly corrupt. On this mis-translation in another context, see J. O. Liebowitz, "Annotation on Fulton's *Servetus*," *JHM*, 10 (1955), 232–38.

by Maimonides in the twelfth century,[75] inflicting on it the minimum suffering and pain. This was basically achieved by very rapidly severing the common carotid arteries in the neck. The animal lost consciousness almost immediately, and the blood from the whole of the body then drained off through these vessels.

Exact details regarding these slaughtering procedures, the subsequent obligatory examination of the carcass and the actual excision of certain vessels from the flesh,[76] were handed down over the generations, and were known to the public at large. They were written down and openly discussed by the rabbis, who were ultimately responsible for adherence to the rules, and who often knew something of medicine. The ritualization of slaughter led to its systematization, but it did not prevent the development of its techniques. Thus, by the Middle Ages the experience accumulated over the ages had produced such a grasp not only of vascular anatomy but, above all, of hemodynamics, that when appended, as here, to medical knowledge, it was possible to presage the circulation of the blood.

In this respect Harvey's views are still closer to our Hebrew account, since he supports his case for the Biblical concept of the soul in the blood with evidence along very similar lines: "I have proved by the frequent dissection of living animals . . . that when the animal was already dying and no longer breathing, the heart continued to pulsate for a while and kept some life in itself."[77] This constitutes the hemodynamic basis of the Jewish method of slaughter, whereby maximum exsanguination occurs in the minimum time. Moreover, already in *De motu cordis*, together with experimental findings confirming his theory of the circulation of the blood, Harvey had presented empirical observations regarding the evacuation of the blood in animals slaughtered under different conditions, which, as he noted, were well known to butchers.[78] Yet, apart from the author of the Hebrew account, their significance does not seem to have been appreciated by the medical world, other than Harvey. And Harvey alone verified this empirical knowledge by scientific experiment.

Thus, while these remarkable resemblances be-

tween the two concepts of the vascular system are not coincidental, there is no reason whatsoever to believe that Harvey knew, directly or indirectly, of this Hebrew account. Both are based on a similar approach and on similar sources, which were neglected by most other physicians. Apart from the customary Greek background, both authors applied their medical knowledge to the Bible, on the one hand, and to empirical findings on the other.

Yet, though this Hebrew account presages Harvey's discovery, it does not forestall it. It presents only a very crude scheme of the cardiovascular system, omitting the lungs and lacking any description of the actual workings of the heart. Many centuries before Harvey, however, it already offers some astonishing insights. Like so much of the *Book of Medicines*, it appears to be the fruit of a blend of Jewish and Greek concepts, tempered by the genius of the anonymous author.

In the "physiological" sections of the *Book of Medicines* the body is said to be formed from the four humors and four qualities—hot, cold, wet, and dry—and the state of health or disease depends on their balance, or on the condition of the "spirit." These are common medieval concepts, generally taken from the writings of Galen, but ultimately based on Hippocratic works, such as the *Nature of Man*. In the *Book of Medicines*, however, such Greek "physiological" theories form a pastiche with Jewish ideas, taken mainly from the Bible. Yet, in addition to this open relationship, there is sometimes also a hidden dimension. This is an esoteric device for "those in the know"; but it must be stressed that it holds no mystical significance whatsoever. To be "in the know" one must merely recognize certain key words or phrases in the text as coming from the Bible, and then be able to identify the source. The verse thus referred to, and often its context as well, serves as a kind of scholarly note, deepening one's understanding of the text. This is an aspect of a very ancient literary practice, used in many languages, and known as *cento*, or as the "rhetorical style," and in Hebrew as *melitsah*.[79] But while in the normal way *melitsah* is employed in a text which is of Jewish significance alone, here it is

---

[75] Moses Maimonides, *The Guide of the Perplexed* III, 48, trans. S. Pines (Chicago, 1963), 599.

[76] See note 44 above.

[77] Harvey, *De generatione*, chap. 51 (Whitteridge [n. 73 above], 243).

[78] Harvey, *De motu cordis*, chap. 9 (Whitteridge [n. 47 above], 81–83).

[79] This is also known as the "mosaic style," "in which minute fragments of the ancient texts are combined into new wholes," but often, as here and in the Bible, it also contains another very important element—play upon words in every conceivable form. See C. Rabin (to whom I am indebted for the reference), "The Ancient in the Modern," in *Language and Texts*, ed. H. H. Paper (Ann Arbor, 1975), 149–79. For Greek and Latin see *OCD, s.v. cento* ([Oxford, 1970], pp. 220–21).

intended to supplement the Biblical parallels to pagan Greek concepts.

The possible presence of this complex literary form must be taken into account throughout the first part of the work, but here I shall provide only a single example. This concerns the interaction of Greek and Jewish concepts of "spirit," in its role as a kind of physiological entity. In such a context the Greek term *pneuma* which, since about the fourth century B.C., was considered as essential to life,[80] would be translated as "spirit" or "breath." It can also mean "wind," like the Hebrew term *ruah*, which similarly denotes "spirit" but does not mean "breath," for which there is a separate term. According to the *Book of Medicines*, the *ruah* (spirit) in the body originates in the four winds (*ruhot*, plural of *ruah*). There is no doubt about this latter translation, since in this particular case the *ruhot* are specifically said to be natural forces. Yet we cannot understand why the spirit should arise from "the four winds," unless we realize that the phrase simply serves as a clue for the reader, a pointer to a specific Biblical verse concerning the winds and the spirit. The allusion can only be to the four winds mentioned in Ezekiel's vision of the resurrection of the slain in the valley of dry bones (Ezekiel 37:1–14). Here the prophet proclaims: "From the four winds come, O spirit, and blow upon these slain that they may live" (Ezekiel 37:9).[81]

The recall of this verse and its context thus demonstrates the existence of a Biblical concept of the spirit as essential to life ("And I shall put my spirit into you and you shall live"), which resembles the Greek view mentioned above, but is not identical with it. It is taken from the account of the resurrection of man, since the concept appears here, but not in the far better-known story of the creation of man found in Genesis 2:7. For in Genesis God created the first man by blowing into him breath (*nešamah*), so that he "became a living soul." Ezekiel, on the other hand, speaks of those who have lived but were slain. God first lays on their dry bones the "vessels" (*gidim*) and flesh, and covers them with skin (verse 6).[82] Yet the bodies still need spirit (*ruah*)

for their actual revival. Since God initiated the first creation with the breath, but not spirit, he fittingly allots the task of blowing in the spirit to the winds (*ruhot*).

This interpretation—that breath was required to create a "living soul," whereas spirit is needed for the body's resurrection—may underlie Paul's distinction between the "natural body" and the "spiritual body," the former being that of the first man, a "living soul," while the last man is "a quickening spirit" (I Corinthians 15:35–45). However, Paul was no physician, whereas in the *Book of Medicines* "spirit" is used in a physiological sense, as an actual component of the body, essential to life. One may therefore postulate that the reference to Ezekiel has still wider medical connotations. Since the first man did not pass through the fetal stage, his breathing had to be initiated by God's own breath. From this the vital spirit was obtained, for it was thought to be normally acquired from the breath. In the act of dying, however, the slain lost their spirit (cf. Eccles. 12:17). The winds thus "blew in" the spirit of life which stimulated both breathing and the heart, and the bodies were revived. And such a spirit moving the heart is actually mentioned in the section of the *Book of Medicines* describing the anatomy of the heart.

These verses from Ezekiel seem also to have influenced Donnolo's theological commentary, and it is just this part of the commentary which, as has been noted above, was incorporated in the *Book of Yosippon*. However, other parts of this same section of Donnolo's work are clearly based on the *Book of Medicines*, although that work is never mentioned by name. It is quite possible that Donnolo was aware of the hidden reference it contains to the book of Ezekiel, in which case the extract from his commentary found in the *Yosippon* would ultimately be derived from the *Book of Medicines*.

An entirely different aspect of Greek-Jewish interaction is found in the long medical oath, said to have been sworn to Asaf and to Yohanan by their pupils.[83] While this shows many affinities with the Hippocratic Oath, it is not taken from it directly. It also resembles, for example, God's covenant with the people of Israel in Deuteronomy and, like the Hippocratic Oath itself, it contains parallels with many other non-medical documents of this type. From the literary point of view it constitutes a remarkable mosaic of Biblical phrases.

The paraphrased version of the Hippocratic *Aphorisms* is almost complete, and may have been

---

[80] See Harris, *Heart*, 106 ff.

[81] Unfortunately in the English Bible the term "breath" rather than "spirit" is used for the Hebrew *ruah* in this verse and throughout the passage, wherever it is associated with the human body. Thus the Hebrew distinction between "spirit" (*ruah*) and "breath" (*nešamah*) is lacking there, as in the Septuagint, where the Greek term *pneuma* is used. The term *nešamah* does not occur in this passage, but in Genesis 2:7, for example, the English Bible correctly translates it as "breath."

[82] See note 41 above on the "members" of the body which, as has been seen, are the only parts to be described in the purely anatomical sections of the *Book of Medicines*.

[83] See note 33 above.

composed directly from the Greek. It appears to be based on a Greek version which can be traced back to a group of manuscripts of the work which was known to Galen,[84] but was not used as the basis for his own commentary on this Hippocratic work. Being essentially a paraphrase, the Hebrew text obviously diverges somewhat from the original, but in many cases its arrangement and meaning are so much clearer that it may well be of value for purposes of textual criticism.

The Hebrew version of the *Materia medica* of Dioscorides is a paraphrase of a substantial part of the work, comprising about one-third of all the botanical items in the first four books. The order of these items corresponds roughly with that of the Greek non-alphabetical texts, but I have not yet been able to compare this version with those in Greek or other languages. Many of the plant names are given not only in Hebrew, but also (in Hebrew transcription) in Greek, Latin, and Syriac, and occasionally in Arabic or Persian. Some of these may well have been added later, but the Syriac names are so numerous that it has been suggested that the Hebrew version was taken from the Syriac translation of the work, which was made in the ninth century[85] but has since been lost.

The remainder of the *Book of Medicines* deals mainly with clinical medicine, and contains little original material, but endless prescriptions in various collections. Otherwise, treatment is mainly dietetic and Hippocratic in nature, and surgery is hardly mentioned at all. Byzantine and, in some manuscripts, perhaps Salernitan material may well be included, but a specifically Jewish element is practically absent from this part of the work.

Superficially, this Hebrew work bears some resemblance to an anonymous, undated Syriac medical encyclopedia, also known as the *Book of Medicines*. Yet it lacks the essentially Galenic content of the Syriac work[86] and, moreover, differs from it, and from the general Greco-Arabic encyclopedic tradition, in the form of its presentation. In this respect it resembles only some of the oldest Indian medical encyclopedias. It must, however, be stressed that as far as its concepts are concerned, the Hebrew work shows few similarities with specifically Indian thought.

The ancient Indian medical encyclopedias constitute different recensions of the same basic material, which goes back to the first century A.D. or even before. In their present form, however, they date from many centuries later.[87] The two earliest, attributed to Caraka and named after Suśruta, respectively,[88] are those which structurally resemble the *Book of Medicines*. However, as far as can be judged from the few descriptions and extracts which have appeared in European languages, the greatest similarity is shown by a Tibetan medical encyclopedia, the *rGyud bzhi*. Though showing Chinese and other influences, it is probably based on a much older Indian medical work, from which it was adapted and translated around the eighth century.[89]

Like these Indian works, the *Book of Medicines* is presented as the teachings of an ancient sage—and one who is historically unknown. Like them, too, it harks back to the supernatural origins of medicine—in the one case emanating from God via Noah, and in the other case from the Indian gods. Each also provides a subsequent "history" of medicine, as well as a medical oath.[90] None of these features is present in any other known medical encyclopedia, of western or eastern origin.

I have tried to make out that the *Book of Medicines* aims to demonstrate the existence of a true Jewish medicine, that is, to convince the Jewish reader that the Jews, like the Greeks, possess medical roots. If this indeed be the case, didactic encyclopedias of this kind, covering almost all aspects of their own, indigenous medicine, would provide a highly suitable pattern for the work, even though the concepts expressed are entirely different in na-

[84] This Hebrew version contains a fragment, taken mainly from the Hippocratic work *Sevens*, which has been added on to the end of Book VI of the *Aphorisms*. It is found in only two of the extant Greek manuscripts of the work. See *Hippocrates* (ed. Littré) I, 401 ff. and *Hippocrates* (ed. and trans. Jones), IV, 217.

[85] I. Loew, *Die Flora der Juden*, 5 vols. in 4 (Vienna, 1824–34), IV, 167–69.

[86] E. A. Wallis Budge, ed., *Syrian Anatomy, Pathology and Therapeutics*, 2 vols. (London, 1913). According to C. Brockelmann's review of Wallis Budge, *ZDMG*, 68 (1914), 185–203, it is mainly a "Plagiat" of Galen's *De locis affectis*. For further Galenic citations see J. Schliefer, "Zum Syrischen Medizinbuch," *Zeitschrift für Semitistik*, 4 (1926), 70–122, 161–95; *ibid.*, 5 (1927), 195–237; *ibid.*, 6 (1928), 154–77, 275–99.

[87] J. Filliozat, *The Classical Doctrine of Indian Medicine*, trans. D. R. Chanana (Delhi, 1964), 26 and 14; R. E. Emmerick, "Ravigupta's Place in Indian Medical Tradition," *Indologica Taurinensia*, 3–4 (1975–76), 209–21.

[88] A number of English translations exist of these works and their commentaries, but none is satisfactory.

[89] See J. Filliozat, *Fragments de textes koutchéens de médecine et de magie* (Paris, 1948), 33–34. The work and its commentaries are described in Jampal Kunzang, *Tibetan Medicine in Original Texts* (London, 1973; Berkeley, 1976); E. Finckh, *Foundations of Tibetan Medicine*, Vol. I, trans. F. M. Houser (London, 1978).

[90] For the Indian "history of medicine," see *The Suśruta-Saṃhitā*, Fasc. I, trans. A. F. R. Hoernle (Calcutta, 1897), 1–13. For the Indian medical oath, *ibid.*, 13–17, and in the version of the Caraka Saṃhitā, see I. A. Menon and H. F. Haberman, "The Medical Students' Oath of Ancient India," *Medical History*, 14 (1970), 295–99.

ture. The Indian encyclopedias were themselves perhaps based on far earlier, Persian models, of which nothing is known; and if so the *Book of Medicines* may take after a common, ancient Persian source. It is more likely, however, that the Hebrew work followed a Persian or Arabic version of one of these Indian works. The *Suśruta Saṃhitā* had already been translated into Arabic by about the eighth century, while well before the tenth century the Caraka recension had passed into Arabic from Persian.[91] As regards the Tibetan encyclopedia, the Hebrew work might have been modelled on some Persian or Arabic translation of a common Indian source. However, in the eighth century Nestorian monks from Persia, versed in the literature of ancient Greek medicine, were present in Tibet,[92] and it is possible that they also translated into Syriac Tibetan medical works.

Since the *Book of Medicines* differs in so many respects from other encyclopedias based on Greek medicine, it is not surprising that there has been much speculation regarding its authorship, provenance and dating. In the last century it was generally held to be a pseudepigraphical compilation from around the tenth century.[93] However, since the appearance of the first substantial study of the work, by Venetianer in 1916, the prevailing view has been that it indeed represents the teachings of Asaf, a hitherto unknown Jewish physician. He is thought to have lived in Persia, Palestine, or Mesopotamia, at some time between the third and seventh centuries, although the work was later re-edited and much material added.[94]

Little objective testimony, internal or external, has so far been presented in support of any of these theories but, on hardly weightier evidence, I personally favor the older view—that this is a pseudepigraphical work, which in some versions was abridged and in others continued to grow by accretion. In this and other ways, such as the fact that the authors' names, though reported, are false, it seems to imitate not only the Indian medical works, but also Israelite non-medical writings from before A.D. 70, and the Biblical pseudepigrapha in particular. These last have been described as "a sort of literary onion which must be peeled, layer by layer, not without tears,"[95] an apt designation indeed for the *Book of Medicines* or, in fact, for the two earliest Indian medical encyclopedias, which also appear to be pseudepigraphical works of this kind.

It is of course possible that the *Book of Medicines* incorporates medical writings from the great Jewish centers of learning in Palestine and Mesopotamia during or before the early Byzantine period, although no evidence exists that they produced any medical works. In the seventh century most of these areas came under Muslim rule but, as has been seen, they remained accessible to the Jews of Byzantine Europe. Yet, just as the language of the work would appear to be a pseudo-Biblical Hebrew from a much later period,[96] so the overwhelming impression is obtained that, while many of the items are taken from ancient Greek writings, others were skillfully composed in medieval times, as a synthesis of Greek and Jewish—predominantly Biblical—concepts. The aim was to simulate ancient Hebrew medical writings, although works of this nature may never have existed at all. "Asaf" represented the Jewish Hippocrates, and Greek, mainly Hippocratic, concepts were carefully chosen to coincide with Jewish ideas. These items were then interspersed with Hebrew versions of genuine ancient Greek works. The latter may even have included translations of the writings of Greek Jewish physicians, such as Rufus of Samaria.[97] It is likely, moreover, that the same author or editor was responsible for determining the Indian encyclopedic form of the work.

[91] They seem to be mentioned in the tenth-century Arabic work, *The Fihrist of al-Nadīm*, ed. and trans. B. Dodge, 2 vols. (New York, London, 1970), II, 710. See also Ullmann, *Medizin*, 103–7.

[92] See C. I. Beckwith, "The Introduction of Greek Medicine into Tibet in the Seventh and Eighth Centuries," *Journal of the American Oriental Society*, 99 (1979), 297–313. On the Nestorians in Tibet, see *Mélanges offerts au R. P. Ferdinand Cavallera* (Toulouse, 1948), J. Dauvillier, "Les Provinces chaldéennes 'de l'extérieur' au Moyen Age," 260–316.

[93] See M. Steinschneider, *Die hebraeische Uebersetzungen des Mittelalters* (Berlin, 1893), 650.

[94] Venetianer, *Asaf Judaeus* (n. 35 above), I, 26 and 39, suggests Mesopotamia in the seventh century at the latest; S. Muntner, *Introduction to the Book of Assaph the Physician* (Hebrew) (Jerusalem, 1957), 39, 50, prefers Palestine or Mesopotamia before 650. The most recent and extreme views—with which I can in no way concur—are those of Melzer, *Asaph* (n. 33 above): "Asaph wrote his book in the middle of the 3rd century, somewhere in Persia" (p. 72), probably in Jundišapur (p. 63). "His chosen student-aide was one Jochanan ben Zavda" (p. 72). "The Munich manuscript [231] is a faithful copy of the original book of Asaph" (p. 72). Some 200 years later a Jewish "Jundishapurian learned professor . . . corrected and completed the manuscript. It is his edition which was extensively copied and publicized" (p. 78), in particular as the Oxford manuscript 2138 (p. 79).

[95] See M. Smith, "Pseudepigraphy in the Israelite Literary Tradition," in *Pseudepigrapha*, I, ed. K. von Fritz (Geneva, 1972), 191–227, esp. 195.

[96] On this form of Hebrew as used in the Middle Ages see, Rabin, "The Ancient in the Modern" (n. 79 above), esp. 153. For Melzer's very different views, see *Asaph* (n. 33 above), 73–80 (English) and 352–379 (Hebrew). My thanks are due to Dr. Hadassah Shy, of Beersheba University, for her linguistic assistance.

[97] As suggested by Muntner, *Introduction* (n. 94 above), 171–74.

To this basic structure, however, other material, with a more contemporary flavor, was then added over the years.

As with the writings of Donnolo and the *Book of Yosippon*, certain Greek and Latin terms seem to have been transcribed into Hebrew in an Italianized form[98] and on this and other counts the work may well be a product of Italy, and probably of Byzantine Italy. It has even been suggested that Donnolo had a hand in the work,[99] but this seems unlikely in view of Donnolo's particular astrological interest, and of his adherence to the traditional view that medical works were to be divorced from religion—in both cases in marked contrast with the *Book of Medicines*. Thus, since he almost certainly alludes to material found in the latter work, it would seem to have been in existence before his time, that is, by the beginning of the tenth century at the latest.

Not only is the true author entirely unknown, but the attributions of the work to sages named Asaf and Yoḥanan are equally obscure. No less puzzling is the fact that each is occasionally called an "astrologer" in the text, despite the virtual absence of astrology in the work.

It is impossible to discuss here all the suggestions which have been offered regarding the name Asaf, whereas the choice of "Yoḥanan," as representing the author of certain parts of the work, has been practically ignored. As far as Asaf is concerned, the name occurs several times in the Bible, as one of the Levite singers who ministered to the service in the time of King David and then in the Temple. Moreover, a number of Psalms are attributed to him. However, II Chronicles 29:30 refers to the Levites singing "the words of David and of Asaf the Seer (predicter)." This may have some connection with the fact that the term *āšipu* denotes a particular type of ancient Mesopotamian healer, one who practiced divination.[100] Moreover, Asaf, son of Berakhyahu, as he is called in several places in the *Book of Medicines*, was in Muslim legend indeed a sage, the vizier of King Solomon.[101] The Hebrew verb *asaf* itself denotes "gathered," or "collected," and hence could refer to a compiler. In the spirit of *melitsah* the possibility of such a play on the name

may also have helped to determine its choice. Yet, all these associations, on their own, would scarcely justify the use of a name of no great Jewish significance to designate an expounder of Jewish-Greek medicine, on a par with Hippocrates and Galen.

I shall therefore throw into the ring an entirely new theory, which provides an additional basis for the names of both "sages." Not only has it some "medical" connotation, but it lies within the Jewish historical tradition. It will be suggested that, like the *Yosippon*, the *Book of Medicines* is ultimately attributed to Josephus, but now in the role of sage, diviner and healer. Certainly Josephus lived in the period apparently ascribed to Asaf in the "historical" introduction to the work, yet today he is known from his works as a soldier and historian alone. It will be recalled, however, that his writings were preserved for posterity mainly through Christian interest, and two medieval Christian texts refer to him in the guise of an astrologer. The first is a Syriac fragment in which Asaf, "the writer and historian of the Hebrews," is said to have written a history of the zodiac, and to have named the signs in Aramaic.[102] Nothing of this is found in the *Book of Medicines*. The reference must be to a Greek work, and Asaf has surely been confused with Josephus, who wrote mainly in Greek, although his native tongue was probably Aramaic.[103] The other, a Latin manuscript composed by a Christian monk, is essentially a cosmographical text, with a section on the planets but no medical content.[104] Although much of it is said to be taken from a work by "Asaf the Jew," the historical aspects seem to be based largely on the Latin Christian versions of the writings of Josephus, and perhaps also on the *Yosippon*.

Parallel with these works, Christian legends representing Josephus as sage, astrologer, diviner, and even healer, were current in Europe before the tenth century and for hundreds of years thereafter.[105] His fame in these roles ultimately springs from his various successful predictions, about which he tells us

[98] E.g., the transcription of the Italian *flemma* for "phlegm," as already noted by M. Steinschneider, *Hebraeische Bibliographie*, 19 (1879), 38; and see M. Treves, "I termini Italiani di Donnolo e di Asaf (sec. X)," *Lingua Nostra*, 22 (1961), 64–66.

[99] The suggestion was long ago refuted by M. Steinschneider, *Zur pseudepigraphischen Literatur des Mittelalters* (Berlin, 1862), 81.

[100] A. L. Oppenheim, "Man and Nature in Mesopotamian Civilization," *DSB*, XV, Suppl. I, 634–66, esp. 643.

[101] *Encyclopaedia of Islam*, new ed., I (Leiden, London, 1960), *s.v.* Āṣāf b. Barakhyā, 686.

[102] A. Mingana, "Some Early Judaeo-Christian Documents in the John Rylands Library. Syriac Texts," *Bulletin John Rylands Library*, 4 (1917), 59–118; J. H. Charlesworth, ed., *The Old Testament Pseudepigrapha*, I (London, 1983), "Treatise of Shem," trans. J. H. Charlesworth, 473–86.

[103] Josephus, *Jewish War* I, 3. Similarly, some of Aesop's fables found in Syriac texts are attributed to Josephus, due to confusion of their names in Syriac: A. Baumstark, *Geschichte der syrischen Literatur* (Bonn, 1922), 26.

[104] Partly transcribed by A. Neubauer, "Assaph hebraeus," *Orient und Occident*, 2 (1864), 657–76 and 767–68. On the basis of this text Neubauer claimed that the Hebrew *Book of Medicines* was the translation of a Latin work by a Christian called Asaf.

[105] See H. Lewy, "Josephus the physician," *JWarb*, 1 (1937), 221–42.

in his writings, and above all, from that made to Vespasian,[106] which has been mentioned above. As authoritative a work as the Talmud then retails a very similar story,[107] although here it is attributed to a figure far more respected among Jews than Josephus—to his contemporary, the Jewish "sage" Yoḥanan ben Zakai.[108] This version, however, goes on to say that Yoḥanan also managed to reduce a sudden swelling of Vespasian's foot, by means of a spell. This purely legendary, "medical" addition was then, in its turn, attributed to Josephus by Christian sources. It is already reported around the year 1000 by Landolfus Sagax, a Christian chronicler from southern Italy; but the leg now belongs to Vespasian's son Titus, and it is said to be actually cured of a disease. Landolfus probably took the story from a cycle of Christian legends,[109] and it must have been adapted from Jewish sources still earlier. As relating to Josephus it should therefore have been available to the author of the *Book of Medicines* by the tenth century or even before.

The attribution of healing powers to a wise rabbi like Yoḥanan is wholly appropriate, but it is not in character with Josephus who, indeed, mentions no incident of such a kind in his works. Thus, although the story led to his widespread reputation as a healing sage throughout the Middle Ages,[110] it may be significant that in the *Book of Medicines* neither Asaf nor Yoḥanan are actually called physicians. When given a title, Asaf is most often known as a sage, while Yoḥanan is an astrologer. This would of course conform with the Biblical tradition,

whereby God alone was the healer. However, by about 1200 the book is already attributed to "Asaf the Physician."[111]

This complex association of Josephus and Yoḥanan, and their connection with the work, may be taken still further. In Hebrew script "Yosef" the Hebrew name of Josephus, is almost identical with "Asaf," and in fact in several manuscripts of the work the name "Asaf" is occasionally copied as "Yosef." Moreover, the name Yoḥanan ben Zakai can easily be confused with that of an even more celebrated Yoḥanan: the apostle John son of Zebedee or, in Hebrew, Yoḥanan ben Zabda; and in the oath found in the *Book of Medicines*, Yoḥanan, the supposed part-author, is even called by this name.

The attribution of the work to Asaf the sage and to an astrologer called Yoḥanan, may thus in both cases be derived from this tangled skein of Judeo-Christian legend, all ultimately referring back to Josephus. Similarly, in this same period, after centuries of Jewish neglect, the bare bones of the latter's own writings were fleshed out in Hebrew and resurrected as the *Book of Yosippon*.

The author of the *Yosippon* clearly appreciated the pro-Jewish nature of the works of Josephus, and thought it time to lift the ban. However, the name of Josephus is never mentioned.[112] It is still felt prudent to attribute his works not to Yosef ben Mattitiahu—the full Hebrew name of Josephus—but to another Yosef, Yosef ben Gorion, to whom Josephus briefly refers as one of his important military colleagues.[113] Though as far as we know he did not write books, it is much more important in this case that he did not defect to the Romans, and hence did not shame his people. Thus the title, the *Book of Yosippon*, which was later ascribed to the work, though generally considered to be derived from the Greek name of the historian Josephus,[114] probably refers in fact to another "Josephus," the Greek name of Yosef ben Gorion.

For the very same reason, the *Book of Medicines* was not attributed directly to Josephus, not even in his role as sage, astrologer, or healer. His name was transformed into "Asaf," with its venerable connotations, in the Bible and elsewhere, as sage, astrologer and healer through divinatory powers.

This is an exoteric hypothesis but, in the Jewish

---

[106] His earlier predictions included one made in a dream. (*Josephus*, I, [Loeb, trans. Thackeray], *The Life* 208 [42]). Josephus himself claims that once Vespasian had acknowledged his general gift for predicting the future, (*Jewish War* III, 403–7), he called Josephus "a minister of the voice of God" (IV, 626); and "Thus Josephus won his enfranchisement as the reward of his divination, and his power of insight into the future was no longer discredited" (IV, 629).

[107] *BT* (n. 1 above), Gittin 56a. See Lewy, "Josephus the Physician" (n. 105 above).

[108] See Dubnov, *History* (n. 21 above), I, 803–4, which provides a somewhat apologetic and yet adulatory picture of Yoḥanan's part in the war, and thus in itself illustrates the general Jewish attitude towards him over the generations. He was admired not only for his piety and learning, but because, even before the fall of Jerusalem to the Romans (which he is said to have predicted), "he was preparing for the social and spiritual rehabilitation of the nation that would be politically shattered." This attitude must be contrasted with that of the worldly, "Hellenistic" Josephus, who after the war lived in luxury in Rome. See also note 20 above.

[109] See Lewy (n. 105 above), on the origins of this story, cited by Landolfus Sagax, *Historia miscella*, ed. Fr. Eyssenhardt (1869) IX, 2, p. 194.

[110] Lewy (n. 105 above), not only speaks of "Josephus the physician," but he goes as far as to claim that he appeared to the medieval reader as a kind of "court physician."

[111] See note 36 above.

[112] See Flusser, *Josippon* (n. 17 above), I, 299 note 2, and II, 69.

[113] Joseph ben Gorion was put in control of Jerusalem during the war, together with the high priest. *Jewish War* II, 563.

[114] Flusser, *Josippon* (n. 17 above), II, 69.

tradition of *melitsah*, so prevalent in the *Book of Medicines*, it may well find support in a Biblical play upon words. For Genesis 30 seems to furnish still another association between the names Yosef and Asaf—perhaps even in a "medical" context.[115] According to verses 1–8, Rachel was barren, and her first two sons were in fact borne by her maid. Finally, however, God granted her a son of her own, upon which she said (verse 23), in the words of the Authorized Version: "God has taken away my reproach," and in a less picturesque, literal translation: "God has gathered up (*asaf*) my shame." The next verse continues: "And she called his name Joseph (*Yosef*) saying: God adds (*yosef*) to me another son." And when associated with the *Yosippon*, it seems to indicate to the reader "in the know" that the past "shame" of Josephus should now also be forgiven, even though his works are still ascribed to "another son," that is, to another Yosef. Whether or not this be the case, the author of the *Book of Medicines* must have been well aware that Josephus was no medical man; hence the work was similarly ascribed to "another son," another Yosef, this time entitled "Asaf."

Among Jewish medical works in Hebrew and Arabic the *Book of Medicines* is unique in trying to establish Jewish roots in its particular field. Yet, as

has been seen, it in no way denies the validity of pagan Greek concepts. On the contrary, it produces Jewish and even Biblical credentials for their use. Perhaps this apologetic aspect of the work was partly a reaction to a general backlash to non-priestly medicine, which seems to have been prevalent in the Byzantine world at this time. Donnolo himself had his offer of medical aid rebuffed by Nilus the monk, with the words that Jesus alone was his healer.[116] Even the *Book of Medicines* surrenders at times to this trend. Before the students of medicine swear their medical oath to Asaf and Yoḥanan, their teachers, they receive a solemn warning from them, composed in true *melitsah*, as a mosaic of phrases from the Bible:

And now put your trust in the Lord your God:
a true God, a living God.
For it is he who kills and makes live;
who wounds and who heals.[117]

Even Asaf and Yoḥanan, with all their enthusiasm for ancient Greek thought, must remind their pupils that the ultimate healer is God and not man.

Green College, Oxford

[115] I am most grateful for this suggestion to Professor D. Berger of Brooklyn College, New York, who is obviously one of "those in the know."

[116] *Nili junioris vita* VII, 50. PG, vol. 120, col. 92C–93A.
[117] These phrases bring to mind Ps. 115:2–11; Isaiah 36:7 = II Kings 18:22; and Deuteronomy 32:39.

EARLY MEDIEVAL LATIN ADAPTATIONS
OF BYZANTINE MEDICINE IN WESTERN EUROPE

Gerhard Baader

If one surveys the state of medical knowledge in late antiquity and in the early Middle Ages in western Europe, it is deplorable. Greek scholarship had vanished in most of Italy.[1] By the fifth century, the attempt to establish a medical literature in Latin, on a level comparable to that of the second century (in Greek), had failed. Technical medical texts, as contrasted to those written in Vulgar Latin,[2] had little influence. The so-called African medical writers are not representative: the standards are not, for example, Caelius Aurelianus, but anonymous Vulgar Latin texts, full of superstition and folk medicine, suggestive of this time of crisis for the Roman Empire in the West, growing in intensity since the third century. Generally, one can say that after the loss of knowledge of Greek in medicine during the fifth and especially the sixth century, doctors who knew a little Greek translated—into Vulgar Latin—medical tracts for their colleagues who knew no Greek nor any medical works. The so-called Lombard medical literature was created by these northern Italian translators, at the court of Theodoric and in nearby locations.[3] This is the overwhelmingly popular medical literature of the time and of the early Middle Ages.

Most of the important medical works of antiquity, from the Hippocratic corpus to Galen, had not been translated. An exception was Dioscorides, but this resulted in no widespread tradition.[4] This can also be said about two treatises of the Hippocratic corpus, found in the Codex Ambrosianus G 108 inferior, originally written in Ravenna, or in the Codex Parisinus Latinus 7027, also of Italian origin, or in a Fulda manuscript, today in the Library of Bodmer.[5] From the Hippocratic corpus, one finds a single tract with a truly widespread tradition, that is, the Hippocratic *Aphorisms* and Galen's commentary on them,[6] and sometimes Byzantine commentaries on the *Aphorisms* appear to have taken the place of Galen. Regarding Galen's works, the same state existed for them as for the Hippocratic corpus:[7] their tradition is also limited to the Milan manuscript.

This Milanese manuscript is of great importance, since it not only contains early translations of Galen, but it also has Byzantine commentaries on those works, compiled by the iatrosophist Agnellus, and translated by Simplicius in Ravenna during the sixth century. Although these Byzantine commentaries are found only in the Milan manuscript, they provide hints of the important Byzantine influence one must consider for northern Italy and occasionally France in the sixth century. This links with other evidence. One finds the Byzantine physician Anthimus as an immigrant at

[The reader is referred to the list of abbreviations at the end of the volume.]

[1] For the decline of Greek scholarship in Italy generally from the fifth century, see P. Courcelle, "Les Lettres grecques en occident de Macrobe à Cassiodore," BEFAR, 159 (1948), 129–36; see also G. Baader, "Zu den Aufgaben der medizinhistorischen Forschung auf dem Gebiet der Geschichte der mittelalterlichen Medizin in der Gegenwart," *Actes du XXVIe Congrès International d'Histoire de la Médecine (Plovdiv, 20–25 aout 1978)*, I (Sofia, 1980), 85–88.

[2] G. Baader, "Lo sviluppo del linguaggio medico nell'antichità e nel primo medioevo," *AR*, n.s. 15 (1970), 1–19 (esp. 6 f.).

[3] *Ibid.*, 10 f. See also I. Mazzini, "Il latino medico in Italia nei secoli V e VI," *La cultura in Italia fra Tardo Antico et Alto Medioevo: Atti del Convegno tenuto a Roma . . . del 12 al 16 Novembre 1979* (Rome, 1981), 433–41.

[4] G. Baader, "Die Anfänge der medizinischen Ausbildung im Abendland bis 1000," *Settimane di studio del Centro Italiano di studi sull'altro medioevo*, 19 (1971), 669–742 (esp. 691).

[5] *Ibid.*, 685–87, and I. Mazzini, "De observantia ciborum: Un'antica traduzione latina del pesudo-ippocratico (I.II) (editio princeps)," *Romanobarbarica*, 2 (1977), 287–93.

[6] Baader, "Anfänge" (n. 4 above), 687–89.

[7] Cf. A. Beccaria, "Sulle tracce di un antico canone latino di Ippocrate e di Galeno I.II," *Italia medioevale e umanistica*, 2 (1959), 1–56, and 4 (1961), 1–75.

the court of Theodoric.[8] He had to flee from the court of Zeno to Ravenna due to his traitorous dealings with the Franks. In France, a physician named Reovalis, who had been trained in Constantinople, is mentioned as being at Poitiers in 590, the episcopal seat,[9] but he appears to have been an exception in this region. Anthimus wrote a short tract to Theodoric, *De observatione ciborum*, in the Vulgar Latin of the day, which was full of Hellenisms but also replete with German words.[10] One may presume Galen and Dioscorides as sources for Anthimus, but Byzantine medical writers do not seem to have been employed by him.

More important than Anthimus were the translations of ancient medical compendia, especially those compiled by Oribasius in the fourth century in Constantinople, and by Alexander of Tralles, who practiced medicine in Rome during the second half of the sixth century. The influence of Byzantine medicine in early medieval Europe[11] is illustrated by the two sixth-century translations of Oribasius produced in northern Italy, at Ravenna or at a location nearby. Although the older translation is included in two manuscripts, dating from the end of the sixth century or the beginning of the seventh (originating in Italy), and in one Fleury manuscript dating from the end of the eighth or the beginning of the ninth century (which was later in Chartres), traces of this older translation are rare: besides excerpts in a St. Gall manuscript of the ninth century, one can only suppose that the *editio princeps* of Schott goes back to an earlier manuscript that is no longer extant. The second translation, conjectured by Mørland as also of the sixth century,[12] was apparently more influential: eight manuscripts (dating from the ninth through the twelfth centuries, as well as a few of later date), from Italy, France, and Germany, show that it had been copied several times. Nevertheless, its influence was minimal: one finds only traces of its use in medical glossaries of the early Middle Ages,[13] but no traces of the second translation of Oribasius are found in the Latin compendia of this era. The

influence of Alexander of Tralles seems to be stronger, but only in certain respects. The translation of his compendium is contained *in toto* in a French manuscript from Angers, in one of Cassinese origin, and in the Fleury manuscript (which also has the older translation of Oribasius), and the impact of Alexander was more significant than that of Oribasius: Alexander's dietetics had become integrated into the main corpus of tradition by which ancient dietetics were transmitted to the early Middle Ages.[14] Even so, the influence of Alexander of Tralles was indirect, and dietetics was but a small portion of the transmitted material.

Regarding Paul of Aegina, the third book of his medical encyclopedia was translated into Vulgar Latin during the sixth century in northern Italy.[15] The influence, however, either of Paul's third book or of his sixth, the famous *Surgery*, was almost negligible. It was not translated into Latin in late antiquity or early medieval times, and Paul had no direct influence comparable to Oribasius or Alexander of Tralles. Thus it is not surprising that in the actual surgery of early medieval Europe none of the instruments and difficult procedures in surgery described by Paul was known. In the West, operations are limited to cauterization, bloodletting, the excision of polyps and removal of hemorrhoids, and perhaps sometimes depressing cataracts, as known through literary and iconographic sources.[16]

In summarizing these traces of Byzantine medicine in sixth-century northern Italy, one fact needs emphasis: no Byzantine medical writings of significant originality were translated into Vulgar Latin, and these are the treatises which Temkin has characterized as having a new combination of empiricism and tradition.[17] What was translated were two kinds of Byzantine medical treatises. First were commentaries on important works of ancient medicine, usually written by the so-called iatrosophists, and these tracts frequently are scholastic and stiff. Latin translations of such commentaries were limited (if one omits the single instance of the Hip-

[8] Anthimus (ed. Liechtenhan), preface, ix f.

[9] G. Baader. "Gesellschaft, Wirtschaft und ärztlicher Stand im frühen und hohen Mittelalter," *Medizinhistorisches Journal*, 14 (1979), 176–85 (esp. 179).

[10] Baader, "Sviluppo" (n. 2 above), 11 f.

[11] Baader, "Anfänge" (n. 4 above), 689–91; and G. Baader and G. Keil, *Medizin im mittelalterlichen Abendland* (Darmstadt, 1982), 12 (Einleitung).

[12] Cf. H. Mørland, "Die lateinischen Oribasiusübersetzungen," *SOsl*, suppl. 5 (Oslo, 1932), 43–51.

[13] *Glossae medicinales* (ed. Heiberg), e.g., 5, 3–6; 10, 4–5, etc.

[14] A. Beccaria, *I codici di medicina del periodo presalernitano (secoli IX, X e XI)*, Storia e letteratura 53 (Rome, 1956), 468. An edition of this text is in preparation by M. Machleb (Med. diss., Berlin). The dietetic corpus generally will be analyzed by F.-D. Groenke in his Med. diss. (Berlin) on the dietetic calendars of the early Middle Ages.

[15] Baader, "Sviluppo" (n. 2 above), 13.

[16] Baader, "Anfänge" (n. 4 above), 700 f.

[17] O. Temkin, "Byzantine Medicine: Tradition and Empiricism," *DOP*, 16 (1962), 97–115 (esp. 97) = *Double Face of Janus*, 202.

pocratic *Aphorisms*) to the Milanese manuscript. Secondly, there were compendia of ancient medical writings, never quite independent from their sources, but which show their differences each through their author's own style. Although the traditions of these translated compendia are more widespread than those of the commentaries, their influence is limited, and their only importance lies in parts incorporated into the corpus of tradition (for example, medical dietetics) for the process of transmission of medical knowledge in the early Middle Ages.

The popular medical literature of early medieval Europe includes two other kinds of Byzantine medical tracts—translated or rewritten into Latin—the newly enlarged versions of important ancient medical works, which had close connections with the commentaries, and short manuals from Byzantine sources which, in their original form, had been abridged into epitomes and condensations, shorn of theory.

One may illustrate the first of these two other kinds of Byzantine medical tracts with the only translation of a Galenic work that had any real impact in the early Middle Ages, Galen's *Therapeutics for Glaucon*. Mentioned by Cassiodorus, this treatise is part of a corpus of tradition of six books, and became one of the most popular guides to therapy in early western medieval Europe.[18] Yet only the first chapter of the first book shows that it is a loose translation of Galen's writing, and the remaining chapters have no relation at all to the purported Galenic original. These chapters are nothing more than part of an enlarged version of the Latin translation—but not of Galen. Their origins, however, may be discerned; for example, chapter 52, "On the Four Stages of the Origin of the Fevers," is an enlarged version of the preface *ante rem* of a Byzantine manual on pulse and urine by an otherwise unknown Alexander.[19] Having mentioned the kinds and stages of the fevers, Alexander lists the signs that must be known for a correct prediction of the course of the diseases followed by fever, for instance the pulse or urine, as well as the influence of the climate and region, as known from Hippocrates. At the end of the preface, without any connection with the preceding text, Alexander says that to give drugs at the right moment will ensure suc-

cess in therapy. This is the major point of Galen's Byzantine compiler: he employs the parts of the preface of the unknown Alexander to stress that the knowledge of the four stages of fevers is the basis of every efficient therapy. Such examples show not the Galenic original, but an enlarged Byzantine version translated into Vulgar Latin in sixth- and seventh-century northern Italy. This is nothing more than a Byzantine adaptation of Galen's doctrines, which have been transmitted in this form by such tracts into western Europe. The widespread tradition of this treatise, incorporated into a cohesive corpus of writings on therapeutics, indicates that this expanded Latin version of a presumably Galenic tract was an important textbook of therapy in the early Middle Ages.

The second kind of Byzantine medical tract appropriated for an unsophisticated medical practice in the early medieval West was the Byzantine medical manual, which had been previously reduced to an epitome and shorn of theory. This form is typical of many diagnostic—or, more accurately, prognostic—texts in numerous Latin manuscripts which, in turn, have separate parts with their own textual traditions,[20] or which became incorporated into the body of didactic letters and short didactic treatises, also possessing textual traditions of their own.[21] One may refer again to the Byzantine tract *On Pulses and Urines* by the unknown Alexander, which had been translated twice into Vulgar Latin in the early Middle Ages.[22] Sphygmology had been a prominent and sophisticated method of prognosis and diagnosis in the medical works up to the end of the second century,[23] as suggested by the important works by Galen on the subject.[24] None of these tracts was translated into Latin, as contrasted to the short manual on urine by Alexander, which is arranged according to the fevers and the

[18] Baader, "Anfänge" (n. 4 above), 694–97.
[19] M. Stoffregen, *Eine frühmittelalterliche Übersetzung des byzantinischen Puls- und Urintraktats des Alexandros: Text-Übersetzung-Kommentar* (Diss. med., Berlin, 1977), 137–46.

[20] G. Baader and G. Keil, "Mittelalterliche Diagnostik: Ein Bericht," in C. Habrich, F. Marguth, and J. H. Wolf, eds., *Medizinische Diagnostik in Geschichte und Gegenwart. Festschrift für Heinz Goerke zum 60. Geburtstag* (Munich, 1978 [*Neue Münchner Beiträge zur Geschichte der Medizin und Naturwissenschaften: Medizinhistorische Reihe*, 7/8]), 124–29.
[21] W. Wiedemann, *Untersuchungen zu dem frühmittelalterlichen medizinischen Briefbuch des Codex Bruxellensis 3701–15* (Med. diss., Berlin, 1976), 46–81; and V. Scherer, *Die "Epistula de ratione ventris vel viscerum": Ein Beitrag zur Geschichte des Galenismus im frühen Mittelalter* (Med. diss., Berlin, 1976), 13–30a.
[22] Stoffregen, *Alexandros* (n. 19 above), 24–59.
[23] Baader and Keil, "Diagnostik" (n. 20 above), 122; and J. A. Pithis, *Die Schriften Περὶ σφυγμῶν des Philaretos: Text-Übersetzung-Kommentar* (Husum, 1983 [Abh. zur Geschichte der Medizin und Naturwissenschaften, 46]), 11–30.
[24] Stoffregen, *Alexandros* (n. 19 above), 147–50; and Pithis, *Philaretos* (n. 23 above), 27–31.

individual diseases. Although it seems to follow the pattern of almost every ancient medical manual (for example, the pseudo-Galenic *Medical Definitions*) in its ordering from "head to toe" and the distinctions between acute and chronic diseases, *On Pulses and Urines* does not reproduce the pattern generally employed in the earlier Greco-Roman manuals.[25] One can understand why Alexander did not use Galen's books on the pulse: they were heavily theoretical.

Alexander based his manual on Galen's isagogic treatises, such as *On Pulses for Beginners* and mainly on *Therapeutics for Glaucon*. Alexander's methodology can be seen in the first chapter of his tract, almost nothing more than an excerpt taken from the second chapter of the first book of Galen's *Therapeutics for Glaucon*. Galen's textbook was mainly oriented towards the clinic, but Alexander made extracts from it only as it referred to the semiotics of the pulse. Every theoretical concept is missing—for example, the lore of the different mixtures of the humors. Yet Alexander is following the different descriptions of illness and the pulses which are typical for them, so that in descriptions of the pulses, Alexander quite often alters Galen, particularly when Alexander adds short definitions of the pulses, found nowhere in Galen, not even in the isagogic textbook *On Pulses for Beginners*.[26] In *Therapeutics for Glaucon*, Galen says that the daily fevers show an equality in the extent, in the density, and in the velocity of their pulses, calling this kind of pulse σύμμετρος, that is, balanced in its three dimensions, length, breadth, and depth. These pulses, therefore, are the simplest ones. In Alexander, this pulse is called "simple," and he gives a definition of this simple pulse wrenched from its context, not found anywhere in the works of Galen. This simple pulse is introduced again in the expanded version of Galen's *Therapeutics for Glaucon*, as we see it in the Latin translation.[27] Similarly, Alexander speaks about an unequal pulse. In Galen one reads that a pulse has an inequality according to certain features of its extent, its velocity, its dimness, and its density in comparison to its beat.[28] At the end of the chapter, however, Alexander shows he has not understood Galen at all: Galen had written (as adapted also by Alexander) that red

urine is typical of the daily fevers, but at the end of the first chapter Alexander says that nearly white urine is typical of the daily fevers. In Galen one reads that this nearly white urine is only typical of the daily fever that follows bubo, and in every daily fever it is the equality of the pulse that is typical for each of them. By omitting the last word, ὁμαλότης, Alexander has misunderstood the whole sentence.[29] In the second chapter of his *On Acute Fevers*, Alexander uses Galen's terminology, if he takes steady (συνεχής), and acute as synonyms. In a similar way, Galen uses ὁμότονος, "having the same force," and ἀκμαστικός, "vigorous at its climax," as synonyms for the unremitting fever. Alexander distinguishes between ἀκμαστικός, ὁμότονος, and παρακμαστικός, "after the climax," with definitions that cannot be found in Galen. Such definitions and distinctions are not only in Alexander, but also in other Byzantine texts, for example, the treatise on fevers by Pseudo-Philoponus in the Codex Mosquensis 466 (fol. 161ᵛ), where the acmastic, the homotonous, and the paracmastic fevers are distinguished.[30] The detailed and sophisticated differentiations with no intention of application to practice and bereft of any new observations, coupled with the loss of the theoretical basis found in Galen, are typical elements in such Byzantine manuals. In their condensed form, these manuals were designed for reception by the unsophisticated medicine of western Europe in this era.

These characteristics are even more prominent in the second part of the tract, which considers urine. Among Galen's writings, there is none on urine: all tracts on urine included by Chartier and Kühn in their editions of Galen are spurious.[31] The hints one finds in the Hippocratic writings on the prognostic importance of urine refer only to single and specific descriptions of diseases,[32] and they are not part of a sophisticated system, as had been the case with Galen's pulse lore. After Galen's time, however, pulse was replaced by urine as employed in the practice of prognosis. It is only then that one finds for the first time in Byzantine medical writers separate treatises dealing with urine. Magnus, Theophilus Protospatharius, and Stephen of Athens show a systematic urine lore. Urine physiology was based upon humoral pathology, especially the

[25] Stoffregen, *Alexandros* (n. 19 above), 151.
[26] *Ibid.*, 153–61.
[27] *Ibid.*, 156.
[28] *Ibid.*, 155 f.

[29] *Ibid.*, 163 f.
[30] *Ibid.*, 164 f.
[31] Baader and Keil, "Diagnostik" (n. 20 above), 123.
[32] *Ibid.*, 122.

notion of concoctions, which underpinned the theory of its ἀποστάσεις, which are distinguished according to the colors of the urine, its consistency and its insoluable precipitates, characterized as *hypostaseis*, *enaioremata*, and *nephelai*, to which the sense of smell was added as a tool in medical diagnostics.[33]

In addition to this sophisticated urine lore, one soon finds in Byzantine medical writing short epitomes of urology, probably used for an unsophisticated diagnostics. These are either anonymous or ascribed to Galen, and include little more than clipped information on the color of the urine, its *hypostaseis*, clouds found in it, criteria of similarity to other urines, and whether such signs are constant or not. With such criteria as are associated with diseases accompanied by fevers (or not), one could make diagnoses for headache, phthisis, elephantiasis, pneumonia, liver complaints, and podagra; or one could predict if an illness would be lengthy or might end in death.[34]

Standing between these simple epitomes of urine lore and the scientific and theoretical tracts on urine, are the Byzantine manuals on urine which omit a detailed uroscopy; typical of these is Theophilus. Although the colors of the urine, its compactness and its insoluble parts are treated in more detail than in the epitomes on urine, these manuals are closer than the scientific compendia to the lower levels of medical prognosis. For if one compares the manuals with the sophisticated compendia, they show a loss of pathophysiology; if, on the other hand, one compares them with the clipped epitomes on urine, one does not find any hint of the process and consequence of the disease, characteristic in the urine epitomes.[35]

It is significant that in early medieval Europe, none of the elaborate compendia on urine were translated or adapted. Only manuals and epitomes on urine are found as parts of the prognostic corpora of the tradition. Worse, in contrast to Byzantium, no compendium with theoretical pathophysiology was available. In the East, if a physician used urine epitomes in his practice, compendia were available for further information. In western Europe, only manuals with reduced theory were at hand. Such a manual is the second part of the

translation by the unknown Alexander of the tract on pulses and urines. Although one finds an arrangement according to the fevers in the first chapter, as well as prognostic method using uroscopy, urine lore occupies a secondary role. Beyond the second chapter, especially in the second part of the tract arranged according to diseases, uroscopy receives the primary function. Although Alexander attempts to compose a manual on pathological diagnostics by arranging the single chapters according to individual diseases, he cannot substantiate his claim to a more theoretical view of uroscopy: these chapters are more similar to the urine epitomes than to the scientific tracts on the subject. One example will illustrate the manner of abridgment. One reads in Galen that black and livid urine is a bad sign because of its coldness, based upon humoral pathology; in Alexander, one reads only that livid urine indicates a worsening[36] of the headache, in the same manner as he has said in the chapter on acute fevers that black or livid urine is a bad sign.[37]

One finds the same state in another medical treatise of early western medieval Europe: the so-called pseudo-Galenic urine lore. As we have it in Alexander, one must assume a Byzantine original, since in his prologue *praeter rem* the translator not only delivers a panegyric on Galen, but also says explicitly that he has translated this manual from the Greek into Latin.[38] At least the prologue *ante rem* appears to stem from a Byzantine Greek original, and the author of this pseudo-Galenic urine lore attempts to provide a theory of the urine's origin and its coction before giving practical instructions for uroscopy: one must observe the colors of the urine, its precipitates, whether the patient urinates with pain, and whether the patient has control of his urine. Here the author gives a superficial and shallow view of pathophysiology which has no connection whatever with the actual contents of the tract. The work is nothing more than a collection of urine epitomes. The author focuses his attention only on an elaborate ordering of these summaries: twelve paragraphs of the preface are followed by twelve paragraphs which outline the colors of the urine. In the next twelve paragraphs, the author discusses exceptions that include apostema, syntexis or diseases of the brain or of the

[33] *Ibid.*, 122–24.
[34] Ideler, II, 304. Cf. Baader and Keil, "Diagnostik" (n. 20 above), 123 f.
[35] G. Keil, *Die urognostische Praxis in vor- und frühsalernitanischer Zeit* (Med. Hab. schr., Freiburg Br., 1970), 22 f.

[36] Stoffregen, *Alexandros* (n. 19 above), 199.
[37] *Ibid*, 175.
[38] Keil, *Praxis* (n. 35 above), 23.

nerves, and the next twelve paragraphs abstract how one evaluates the colors of the urine, in turn followed by six paragraphs that deal with the precipitates of urine.[39] Generally, one can say that the main portion of this pseudo-Galenic urine lore is linked to an unlearned medical practice that lacks theoretical concepts. The tradition of this text is limited to two manuscripts of Italian origin dated in the end of the eighth or the ninth century.[40] Only in the more recent manuscript have four sections been added to the pseudo-Galenic urine lore, and these are generally identical with parts of Alexander's treatise.[41] With the ninth-century additions, the semiotics of fever have been introduced into the treatise, but in a very unrefined form. It appears that for this ninth-century material no Greek original can be assumed, as suggested by the confusing separation of a number of items from Alexander's ordering. For example, this is the case in the summary of acute fevers. Alexander says that in treating acute fevers, signs of impending death are white, spumous, or red urines, but that greater urine flow than usual, or watery urine, or nosebleed are signs of shivers. In the addition of the pseudo-Galenic urine lore, these two aspects are divided into two epitomes, whereby nosebleed is incorporated wrongly into the first abstract instead of the second.[42]

These rules of urine found here are not only part of Alexander's treatise, but also form the nucleus of the very widespread texts on uroscopy in early medieval western Europe, the so-called pseudo-Galenic rules of urine. Although there are parallels to Alexander, the later authors assume no theoretical foundations. The ordering of these rules is, therefore, very simple and schematic: after mentioning the leading symptom (for instance, for a fever), the author gives data on the urine, but before giving the prognosis, the author considers the accompanying symptoms.[43] As shown above, such rules of urine have their exact models in Byzantine medicine, and their Byzantine origin is without doubt. One can find these kinds of precepts on urine not only in Alexander, but also in other Byzantine Greek texts, as suggested previously. It is impossible, however, to delineate most of the urine rule tracts of this type which are found

in Latin manuscripts from the eighth to the fifteenth centuries—those that do not show any trace of Salernitan or post-Salernitan uroscopy, exactly parallel to that of Byzantium. Most of the later Byzantine texts remain unknown or have not been investigated. Yet one must assume that these urine rules, which were part of the usual manuals of uroscopy in early medieval western Europe, had been altered numerous times or that new rules had been added. These manuals bear witness to an unsophisticated and primitive practice of uroscopy in western Europe, unlike the level of uroscopy in Byzantine medicine. Among the Byzantines, there were always excellent tracts on uroscopy available, as well as the simplified manuals which were in common use.

Although uroscopy was the most important diagnostic method in the early Middle Ages, one can cite other diagnostic tools and texts of this era which were also Byzantine in their origin. Part of the tradition of the corpus of diagnostics is the *Capsula eburnea*, found also in the Corpus of tradition II, which likewise includes didactic letters and other short didactic tracts on medicine.[44] The Byzantine Greek original of the *Capsula eburnea* is known from several manuscripts, and Sudhoff published the text from the Codex Vindobonensis med. Graecus 8 of the fifteenth century.[45] In the preface, it is stated that this text was found in the tomb of Hippocrates, hidden in a casket made of ivory. This Byzantine legend precedes a prognostic text in which, for the first time, pathologic apostaseis (that is, nipples or cutaneous eruptions) are used to predict the course of the disease, or to predict death. In their patterns of simplicity, these maxims resemble the rules on urine. Having mentioned the leading symptom of the disease, the author adds the outer shape of the small blisters or blebs and other cutaneous eruptions, which can be identified without omitting the accompanying symptoms. At the end, the prognosis—death—is given. One finds a therapy only in a few cases. The *Capsula eburnea* was translated into Vulgar Latin, and it must have been greatly popular:[46] it shows a very widespread tradition which can be compared with the pseudo-Galenic rules on urine. In sixteen manuscripts, dating from the ninth to the eleventh century, it is

---

[39] *Ibid.*, 23–25.

[40] *Ibid.*, 32.

[41] Stoffregen, *Alexandros* (n. 19 above), 167–218 *passim*, and 223–25.

[42] *Ibid.*, 170 f.

[43] Keil, *Praxis* (n. 35 above), 32–40.

[44] Scherer, *Epistula* (n. 21 above), 14 f.

[45] K. Sudhoff, "Die pseudohippokratische Krankheitsprognostik nach dem Auftreten von Hautausschlägen, 'Secreta Hippocratis' oder 'Capsula eburnea' benannt," *SA*, 9 (1916), 79–116 (esp. 85 f., and 106–8).

[46] Baader and Keil, "Diagnostik" (n. 20 above), 124–26.

included or mentioned generally under the names of Hippocrates or Democritus.[47]

In a Corpus I of the manuscript tradition, containing mostly didactic letters and other similar short tracts, one finds a Latin pseudo-Hippocratic letter on hematoscopy,[48] also present in the Corpus II of the tradition of prognostic texts. This method of employing the visible state of the blood, gained through phlebotomy, to prognosticate the exit of a disease, also hearkens back to Byzantine origins.[49] The extant text, however, does not represent a translation of a Greek original: it is an adaptation of this topic into the form of a didactic letter, written—as the language and Germanic words indicate—in the western Frankish kingdom during the seventh or eighth century.[50] The textual tradition of this pesudo-Hippocratic letter on hematoscopy is limited to two manuscripts of the ninth century.

The influence of Byzantine medicine in the West did not only have importance for commentaries on Hippocrates and Galen, or expanded revisions of their works or prognostic tracts, but that influence also was in the manner by which the Latin compendia had not adapted Byzantine medical works: in the short treatises that had made their way into the West, such as the rules for urine and urine lore, one may detect a role in the training of physicians in the monasteries and the primitive medical practice in those institutions.

One may notice dietetic tracts, arranged according to the order of the month, a pattern not found in the Greek medical literature earlier than Byzantine times.[51] Together with the dietetic excerpts of Alexander of Tralles, they had become part of the dietetic corpus of medical tradition, the most important dietetic texts of the early Middle Ages.[52] In this same tradition, which also includes the letter on hematoscopy, are found surgical texts which have their origins in Byzantine medicine. One of them is a list of surgical tools, and Bliquez has emphasized its Byzantine background.[53] The other is

a questionary under the title *Surgery of Heliodorus*,[54] having nothing to do with Heliodorus, but a textbook employed in the teaching of medicine. Such textbooks are known on the papyri from the second century and later, and in the Geneva Papyrus 111, one finds fragments of a textbook of surgery.[55] In addition to the Vulgar Latin, both Latin texts are so poor that very few could have used them. Thus one can address only the bookish tradition of these late Greek manuals: only a very few of the instruments used in Byzantine surgery have survived, and almost none of the surgical procedures described earlier seem to have been employed in early medieval western Europe. Within the listings and instruments described, one finds the lancet for bloodletting and the technique for bloodletting.[56] This important surgical technique is contained in a didactic letter on phlebotomy which shows a widespread textual tradition. Fifteen Latin manuscripts transmit this text anonymously under the names of Hippocrates, Galen, or Heliodorus,[57] and they date from the eighth through the eleventh century. In the textual traditions, the bloodletting letter is inserted into both Corpora I[58] and II[59] of the known didactic letters and short didactic tracts. The bloodletting letter is partially arranged by means of questions, in the manner of the *Surgery of Heliodorus*. One cannot, however, ascertain the direct Greek original from which this text had been rendered, although there are many Greek didactic letters on phlebotomy of Byzantine origin which can be compared to it.[60] The Byzantine letter on bloodletting was, however its origins are traced in future research, an introduction to this important surgical technique for early medieval western Europe.

Another didactic letter, which includes a primitive anatomy and a mutilated pathophysiological theory of concoction, belongs more in the class of

---

[47] Beccaria, *Codici* (n. 14 above), 447.

[48] Wiedemann, *Untersuchungen* (n. 21 above), 67, and D. Blanke, *Die pseudohippokratische "Epistula de sanguine cognoscendo"* (Med. diss., Bonn, 1974), *passim*.

[49] Cf., for example, Oribasius, *Medical Collection* VII, 4.11 (ed. Raeder, I, p. 202) and *Synopsis* I, 9.6 (ed. Raeder, p. 10), based on Galen, *Bloodletting Therapy* 14 (ed. Kühn, XI, 291, 15 through 292, 5); but see also the one-page epitome on phlebotomy in Ideler, I, 293.

[50] Blanke, *Epistula* (n. 48 above), 21 f.

[51] E.g., Ideler, I, 409–29.

[52] See note 14 above.

[53] H. Schöne, "Zwei Listen chirurgischer Instrumente," *Hermes*, 38 (1903), 280–84. For the Latin text, see also R. Laux, "Ars

medicinae: Ein frühmittelalterliches Kompendium der Medizin," *Kyklos*, 3 (1930), 424 ff., and H. E. Sigerist, "Die 'Lecciones Heliodori'," *SA*, 13 (1921), 146 ff.

[54] H. E. Sigerist, "Die 'Cirurgia Eliodori'," *SA*, 12 (1920), 1–9.

[55] *Ibid.*, 8f. See also J. Kollesch, *Untersuchungen zu den pseudo-galenischen Definitiones medicae* (Berlin, 1973 [Akademie der Wissenschaften der DDR. Zentralinstitut für Alte Geschichte und Archäologie: Schriften zur Geschichte und Kultur der Antike, 7]), 39.

[56] See notes 52 and 53 above.

[57] Beccaria, *Codici* (n. 14 above), 451.

[58] Wiedemann, *Untersuchungen* (n. 21 above), 53–56.

[59] Scherer, *Epistula* (n. 21 above), 16 f.

[60] Diels, *Handschriften*, III, 49. See also R. Czarnezki, *Ein Aderlasstraktat angeblich des Roger von Salerno samt einem lateinischen und einem griechischen Texte zur "Phlebotomia Hippocratis"* (Med. diss., Leipzig, 1919), 31 f.

theoretical writings than many others previously discussed. This anatomical-coction letter is transmitted to the early medieval western tradition similarly to the manner of adaptation of the letter on bloodletting: the anatomy and coction letter is integrated into both Corpora I and II of the western tradition. Ten manucripts dating from the ninth through the eleventh century, and four of later dates, suggest a widespread textual tradition.[61] The text itself is an adaptation of various sources. The poor anatomy of the digestive and respiratory organs appears to have been lifted from Latin sources of late antiquity—for example, Vindicianus.[62] Yet some indirect knowledge of Galen must be presumed, since the author shows a dim command of Galen in the passages where he treats humoral pathology and the theory of digestion.[63] This abridgment and deformed exposition of the theory is the basis of the author's theory of fevers, known since the time of Hippocrates.[64] Yet in his consideration of fevers, humoral pathology, and digestion, as well as in the following section on the four humors,[65] the author diverges more and more from Galen, and the anonymous writer discusses fevers in relation to the humors and the elements, employing the fevers to diagnose different diseases. Needless to say, the author's prognostic analyses do not occur in Galen. It seems that other sources were more important for this writer, perhaps sources which summarized and analyzed Galenic works. Such other sources can only be Byzantine, as shown for example by the author's connection of burning fever with a superabundance of yellow bile.[66] Thus one can presume other Byzantine sources for pathophysiological notions found only in this treatise.

It should be emphasized that these adapted texts do not represent the best works of Byzantine medicine. The short, little texts with truncated theory already present in their Greek originals (as compared with the Greek medical texts composed before the end of the second century) were the basic foundations in the medicine of early medieval Europe for pathophysiology, humoral pathology, surgery, therapy, and prognosis—for example, urognostics or hematoscopy. The summarization and epitomizing of medical knowledge found in this aspect of Byzantine medicine, as well as the loss of the best tracts of Greek medicine from classical antiquity, are certainly major reasons for the low standards of medicine in western Europe in this era.

A basic question can now be posed: Were these adaptations of Byzantine medicine, mostly in the sixth century in northern Italy (belonging more, therefore, to late antiquity than to early medieval Europe) the only traces of Byzantine medicine in early medieval western Europe?

To answer this question it will be helpful to look at the adaptation of other aspects of Greek than medical writings, especially Byzantine literature in the West. One fact needs emphasis: almost nowhere in western Europe did there exist a tradition of Greek learning during these centuries.[67] Generally, there was knowledge of Greek by single individuals, or there were regions—southern Italy or Sicily—where Greek remained the mother tongue of part of the population, and which thereby were bilingual. A lack of a tradition of Greek learning applies also to the Irish savants of the eighth and ninth centuries, particularly those present at the court of Charlemagne: they had little interest in Greek or Byzantine medicine.[68] The sources which were integrated into the sevenfold Physica, following the Quadrivium in the Irish model of learning, were the encyclopedias of late antiquity, including Isidorus, and were Latin in origin.[69]

A major problem, however, for each intellectual development in western Europe had been whether it was possible to formulate a technical language in Latin which was as capable as Greek of abstraction. The creation of such a language always occurred when translations were made from Greek into Latin, and for the *Artes* and generally for philosophy, this had resulted with the translation of Greek philosophic texts, from Cicero to Boethius.[70] In this context, it is noteworthy that in early medieval times, the first Byzantine commentaries on Aristotle were transmitted to the West, and similarly there occurred transmission in theology to southern Italy

[61] Scherer, *Epistula* (n. 21 above), 31–56.
[62] *Ibid.*, 88–91, and 100 f.
[63] *Ibid.*, 91–95, and 101 f.
[64] *Ibid.*, 95 f. and 102 f.
[65] *Ibid.*, 96–99 and 103.
[66] Rufus (ed. Daremberg and Ruelle), 605, 26.
[67] B. Bischoff, "Das griechische Element in der abendländischen Bildung des Mittelalters," *Mittelalterliche Studien: Ausgewählte Aufsätze zur Schriftkunde und Literaturgeschichte*, II (Stuttgart, 1967), 246–75.
[68] G. Baader, "Die Entwicklung der medizinischen Fachsprache im hohen und späten Mittelalter," in G. Keil and P. Assion, eds., *Fachprosaforschung. Acht Vorträge zur mittelalterlichen Artesliteratur* (Berlin, 1974), 93 f.
[69] B. Bischoff, "Eine verschollene Einleitung der Wissenschaften," *Mittelalterliche Studien. Ausgewählte Aufsätze zur Schriftkunde und Literaturgeschichte*, I (Stuttgart, 1966), 273–88.
[70] Baader, "Entwicklung" (n. 68 above), 90–93.

with Cassiodorus and the Vivarium, and to France with the translation of Pseudo-Dionysius Areopagita.[71] The state, however, for medicine in the early Middle Ages, was quite different.

For the further development of medicine another translation from the Greek became crucially important. At Salerno in southern Italy, a medicine of a higher level than elsewhere in western Europe existed through the entire early Middle Ages. In the eleventh century, archbishop Alphanus of Salerno—himself a medical practitioner—translated Nemesius' anthropological tract *On the Nature of Man* into Latin, and its language was not that of Vulgar Latin. This translation became crucial in the development of medicine in western Europe because Alphanus created a technical language through his translation of Nemesius' book, which was a combination of Byzantine theology and Galenic physiology, and now the Galenic medical Latin became capable of abstraction. This is one of the preconditions for the reception of Greek medicine in Arabic guise beginning at the end of the eleventh century in southern Europe[72] and elsewhere. This medical language is that which Constantine the African could use to translate Arabic medical writers into Latin for the school at Salerno. The most important of these translations for medical education at Salerno and later are included in the first textbook of medicine, the so-called *Articella*.[73] In addition to the translation from Arabic into Latin, one finds in the *Articella* two translations of Byzantine medical treatises, rendered at Salerno in the eleventh century.[74] They are two diagnostic texts: the excellent urognostic compendium by Theophilus Protospatharius, and the unsophisticated manual of sphygmology by a certain Philaretus.[75] Theophilus and Philaretus were also rendered into the new technical Latin created by Alphanus from Byzantine Greek, and these translations mark a new age in Latin medieval medicine.

Freie Universität Berlin

---

[71] *Ibid.*, 94–96.

[72] *Ibid.*, 96–100. See also G. Baader, "Die Schule von Salerno," *Medizinhistorisches Journal*, 13 (1978), 124–45 (esp. 130 f.).

[73] G. Baader, "Handschrift und Inkunabel in der Überlieferung der medizinischen Literatur," in E. Schmauderer, ed., *Buch und Wissenschaft: Beispiele aus der Geschichte der Medizin, Naturwissenschaft und Technik* (Düsseldorf, 1969 [Technikgeschichte in Einzeldarstellungen, 17]), 23–27.

[74] Baader, "Salerno" (72 above), 134.

[75] Pithis, *Philaretos* (n. 23 above), 187–94.

LIST OF ABBREVIATIONS

Used in this Volume of the

Dumbarton Oaks Papers

AA Archäologischer Anzeiger, Supplement to *Jahrbuch des Deutschen Archäologischen Instituts*

Abh Abhandlungen (followed by name of Academy, abbreviated, and by class: e.g., AbhBerl, Phil.-hist.Kl.)

AbhKM Abhandlungen für die Kunde des Morgenlandes

ActaIRNorv Acta ad Archaeologiam et Artium Historiam pertinentia, Institutum Romanum Norvegiae

ActaSS Acta Sanctorum Bollandiana (1643, in progress)

AEpigr L'Année Épigraphique, Supplement to the *Revue Archéologique*

Aetius (ed. Olivieri) Alexander Olivieri, ed., *Aetii Amideni Libri medicinales I-IV* (Leipzig, 1935 [*CMG* VIII 1]); Alexander Olivieri, ed., *Aetii Amideni Libri medicinales V-VIII* (Berlin, 1950 [*CMG* VIII 2])

Aetius XIII (ed. Zervos) S. Zervos, ed., Ἀετίου Ἀμιδηνοῦ περὶ δακνόντων ζῴων καὶ ἰοβόλων ὄφεων, ἤτοι λόγος δέκατος τρίτος, Ἀθηνᾶ,18 (1906), 241–302

AHR American Historical Review

Alexander (trans. Brunet) F. Brunet, *Médecine et thérapeutique byzantines. Oeuvres médicales d'Alexandre de Tralles*, 4 vols. Vols. 2–4 translation (Paris, 1933–37)

Alexander (ed. Puschmann) Theodor Puschmann, ed. and trans., *Alexander von Tralles*, 2 vols. (Vienna, 1878–79; rptd. Amsterdam, 1963)

AMSL Archives des Missions Scientifiques et Littéraires

AnalBoll Analecta Bollandiana

ANRW Aufstieg und Niedergang der römischen Welt (Berlin and New York, 1972–)

AntCl L'Antiquité Classique

Anthimus (ed. Liechtenhan) Eduard Liechtenhan, ed. and trans. (German), *Anthimi De observatione ciborum ad Theodoricum regem Francorum epistula* (Berlin, 1963 [CML VIII 1])

AOC Archives de l'Orient Chrétien

AR Atene e Roma

AStCal Archivio Storico per la Calabria e la Lucania

BCH Bulletin de Correspondance Hellénique

BEFAR Bibliothèque des Ecoles Françaises d'Athènes et de Rome

BGrottaf Bollettino della Badia greca di Gottaferrata

*BHG*³ *Bibliotheca Hagiographica Graeca*, 3rd ed., ed. F. Halkin, 3 vols. (Brussels, 1957)

BHM Bulletin of the History of Medicine

BIE Bulletin de l'Institut d'Egypte (before 1919: *Egyptien*)

BJb Bonner Jahrbücher

BMGS Byzantine and Modern Greek Studies

BNJbb Byzantinisch-Neugriechische Jahrbücher

BO Bibliotheca Orientalis

Bonn ed. Corpus Scriptorum Historiae Byzantinae, ed. B. G. Niebuhr et al. (Bonn, 1828–97)

ByzF Byzantinische Forschungen

BZ Byzantinische Zeitschrift

Caelius Aurelianus (ed. and trans. Drabkin) I. E. Drabkin, ed. and trans., *Caelius Aurelianus On Acute Diseases and On Chronic Diseases* (Chicago, 1950)

CAH Cambridge Ancient History

CahArch Cahiers Archéologiques

Carnoy A. Carnoy, *Dictionnaire étymologique des noms grecs de plantes* (Louvain, 1959)

Catalogus IV F. Edward Cranz and Paul Oskar Kristeller, eds., *Catalogus Translationum et Commentariorum: Medieval and Renaissance Latin Translations and Commentaries*, Vol. IV (Washington, D.C., 1980)

CBHByz Corpus Bruxellense Historiae Byzantinae

Celsus (ed. Marx) F. Marx, ed., *A. Cornelii Celsi quae supersunt* (Leipzig, 1915 [*CML* I])

Celsus (ed. and trans. Spencer) W. G. Spencer, ed. and trans., *Celsus De medicina*, 3 vols. Loeb Classical Library (Cambridge, Mass., 1935–38)

CFHB Corpus Fontium Historiae Byzantinae

CHG   E. Oder and C. Hoppe, eds., *Corpus hippia-tricorum Graecorum*, 2 vols. (Leipzig, 1924–27; rptd. Stuttgart, 1971)

CIC   *Corpus Iuris Civilis*, 3 vols. (Berlin, 1928–29)
  Subdivisions:
  CI   *Codex Iustinianus*, ed. P. Krüger (Berlin, 1929)
  Dig   *Digesta*, ed. Th. Mommsen and P. Krüger (Berlin, 1928)
  Inst   *Institutiones*, ed. P. Krüger (Berlin, 1928)
  Nov   *Novellae*, ed. F. Schoell and G. Kroll (Berlin, 1928)

CIG   *Corpus Inscriptionum Graecarum*
CIL   *Corpus Inscriptionum Latinarum*
CJ   *Classical Journal*
CMG   *Corpus Medicorum Graecorum*
CMH   *Cambridge Medieval History*
CML   *Corpus Medicorum Latinorum*
CQ   *Classical Quarterly*
CR   *Classical Review*

Cramer (or C.)   J. A. Cramer, ed., *Anecdota Graeca e codd. manuscriptis Bibliothecarum Oxoniensium*, 4 vols. (Oxford, 1835–37; rptd. in 2 vols., Amsterdam, 1963)

CSCO   Corpus Scriptorum Christianorum Orientalium

CTh   *Theodosiani libri XVI cum constitutionibus Sirmondianis et leges novellae ad Theodosianum pertinentes*, ed. Th. Mommsen and P. M. Meyer, 2 vols. in 3 parts (Berlin, 1905)

DACL   F. Cabrol and H. Leclerq, *Dictionnaire d'Archéologie Chrétienne et de Liturgie*

Delatte, *Anecdota*, I and II   Armand Delatte, ed., *Anecdota Atheniensia et alia*, I (Paris, 1927); II: *Textes grecs relatifs à l'histoire des sciences* (Paris, 1939)

Diels, *Handschriften*   Hermann Alexander Diels, *Die Handschriften der antiken Ärzte* (Leipzig and Amsterdam, 1970). Rpts. of three articles (I: "Hippokrates und Galenos"; II: "Die übrigen griechischen Ärzte"; III: "Nachtrag") which appeared in *Abhandlungen der Preussischen Akademie der Wissenschaften*, Phil.-hist. Kl., 1905–1907

Dietz   F. R. Dietz, ed., *Scholia in Hippocratem et Galenum*, 2 vols. (Königsberg, 1834; rptd. as one vol., Amsterdam, 1966)

Dioscorides (trans. Berendes)   J. Berendes, *Des Pedanios Dioskurides aus Anazarbos Arzneimittel-lehre* (Stuttgart, 1902)

Dioscorides (ed. Wellmann)   Max Wellmann, ed., *Pedanii Dioscuridis Anazarbei De materia medica*,

3 vols. (Berlin, 1906–14; rptd. Berlin, 1958)

DSB   *Dictionary of Scientific Biography*

EI   *Encyklopädie des Islams*
EO   *Echos d'Orient. Revue d'histoire, de géographie et de liturgie orientales*

'Επ.'Ετ.Βυζ.Σπ.   'Επετηρὶς 'Εταιρείας Βυζαντινῶν Σπουδῶν
'Επ.'Ετ.Κρητ.Σπ.   'Επετηρὶς 'Εταιρείας Κρητικῶν Σπουδῶν

Ermerins   F. Z. Ermerins, ed., *Anecdota medica graeca* (Leiden, 1840; rptd. Amsterdam, 1963)

Fabricius   Cajus Fabricius, *Galens Exzerpte aus älteren Pharmakologen* (Berlin, 1972)

FGrHist   *Die Fragmente der griechischen Historiker*, ed. F. Jacoby, 3 vols. in 16 parts (1923–58)

Flashar, *Melancholie*   Hellmut Flashar, *Melancholie und Melancholiker in den medizinischen Theorien der Antike* (Berlin, 1966)

Galen (trans. Daremberg)   Ch. Daremberg, *Oeuvres anatomiques, physiologiques et médicales de Galien*, 2 vols. (Paris, 1854–56)

Galen (ed. Kühn, or simply K.)   C. G. Kühn, ed., *Claudii Galeni Opera omnia*, 20 vols. in 22 (Leipzig, 1821–33; rptd. Hildesheim, 1964–65. Cited usually by vol. no. and page

Galen, *De usu partium* (ed. Helmreich)   G. Helmreich, ed., *Galeni De usu partium libri XVII*, 2 vols. (Leipzig, 1907–1909; rptd. Amsterdam, 1968)

Galen, *Doctrines* (ed. and trans. De Lacy)   Phillip De Lacy, ed. and trans., *Galen On the Doctrines of Hippocrates and Plato*, 2 vols. (Berlin, 1978–80 [*CMG* V 4, 1, 2])

Galen, *Natural Faculties* (ed. and trans. Brock)   Arthur John Brock, ed. and trans., *Galen On the Natural Faculties*, Loeb Classical Library (London, 1916)

Galen, *Parts* (trans. May)   Margaret Tallmadge May, trans., *Galen On the Usefulness of the Parts of the Body*, 2 vols. (Ithaca, New York, 1968)

Galen, *Procedures* (trans. Duckworth, Lyons, and Towers)   W. L. H. Duckworth, trans., *Galen On Anatomical Procedures: The Later Books*, ed. M. C. Lyons and B. Towers (Cambridge, 1962)

Galen, *Procedures* (ed. Simon)   Max Simon, ed. (Arabic), *Sieben Bücher Anatomie des Galen*, Vol. I (Leipzig, 1906)

Galen, *Procedures* (trans. Singer)   Charles Singer, trans., *Galen On Anatomical Procedures* (London, 1956)

Galen, *Prognosis* (ed. and trans. Nutton)   Vivian

Nutton, ed. and trans., *Galen On Prognosis* (Berlin, 1979 [*CMG* V 8, 1])

Galen, *Scripta Minora*   J. Marquardt, I. Mueller, and G. Helmreich, eds., *Claudii Galeni Scripta Minora*, 3 vols. (Leipzig, 1884–93; rptd. Amsterdam, 1967)

GCS   Die griechischen christlichen Schriftsteller der ersten [drei] Jahrhunderte (1897–   )

Geoponica (ed. Beckh)   H. Beckh, ed., *Geoponica sive Cassiani Bassi scholastici De re rustica eclogae* (Leipzig, 1895)

Glossae medicinales (ed. Heiberg)   J. L. Heiberg, ed., *Glossae medicinales*, Det Kgl. Danske Videnskabernes Selskab. Historisk-filogiske Meddelelser IX, 1 (Copenhagen, 1924)

GRBS   Greek, Roman, and Byzantine Studies

Harig, *Intensität*   Georg Harig, *Bestimmung der Intensität im medizinischen System Galens* (Berlin, 1974)

Harris, *Heart*   C. R. S. Harris, *The Heart and the Vascular System in Ancient Greek Medicine* (Oxford, 1973)

Hesychius, *Lexicon*   M. Schmidt, ed., *Hesychii Alexandrini Lexicon*, 5 vols. (Halle, 1858–68; rptd. Amsterdam, 1965)

Hippocrates XIII (ed. Joly)   Robert Joly, ed. and trans., *Hippocrate*, Tome XIII: *Des lieux dans l'homme. Du système des glandes. Des fistules. Des hémorroïdes. De la vision. Des chairs. De la dentition* (Paris, 1978)

Hippocrates (ed. and trans. Jones)   W. H. S. Jones and E. T. Withington, eds. and trans., *Hippocrates*, 4 vols. Loeb Classical Library (Cambridge, Mass., 1923–31)

Hippocrates (ed. Littré)   E. Littré, ed. and trans., *Oeuvres complètes d'Hippocrate*, 10 vols. (Paris, 1839–61; rptd. Amsterdam, 1973–82)

Hirschberg, *Geschichte*   Julius Hirschberg, *Geschichte der Augenheilkunde*, I: *Geschichte der Augenheilkunde im Altertum* (Graefe-Saemisch, *Handbuch der gesamten Augenheilkunde*, XII) (Leipzig, 1899)

HO   Handbuch der Orientalistik

HSCPh   Harvard Studies in Classical Philology

Hunger, "Medizin"   Herbert Hunger, "Medizin," in *Die hochsprachliche profane Literatur der Byzantiner*, 2 vols. (Munich, 1978), Vol. II, pp. 287–320

Ideler   J. L. Ideler, ed., *Physici et medici graeci minores*, 2 vols. (Berlin, 1841–42; rptd. as one vol., Amsterdam, 1963)

IEJ   Israel Exploration Journal

IG   Inscriptiones Graecae (Berlin, 1873–   )

IGLSyr   Inscriptions Grecques et Latines de la Syrie, ed. L. Jalabert, R. Mouterde, and Cl. Mondésert, 7 vols. (Paris, 1929–70)

Ilberg, *Schriftstellerei*   Johannes Ilberg, *Über die Schriftstellerei des Klaudios Galenos* (Darmstadt, 1974). Rpts. of four articles which appeared in *Rheinisches Museum* in 1889, 1892, 1896, and 1897

ILChV   Inscriptiones Latinae Christianae Veteres, 3 vols., ed. E. Diehl (Berlin, 1924–31)

ILS   Inscriptiones Latinae Selectae, ed. H. Dessau, 3 vols. (Berlin, 1892–1916)

IRAIK   Izvestija Russkogo Arheologičeskogo Instituta v Konstantinopole

JbAChr   Jahrbuch für Antike und Christentum

JHAS   Journal for the History of Arabic Science

JHB   Journal of the History of Biology

JHBS   Journal of the History of Behavioral Sciences

JHM   Journal of the History of Medicine and Allied Sciences

JHS   Journal of Hellenic Studies

JÖB   Jahrbuch der Österreichischen Byzantinistik

JÖBG   Jahrbuch der Österreichischen Byzantinischen Gesellschaft

John of Alexandria, *Epidemics VI* (ed. Pritchet)   C. D. Pritchet, ed., *Iohannis Alexandrini Commentaria In sextum librum Hippocratis epidemiarum* (Leiden, 1975)

JQR   Jewish Quarterly Review

JRAS   Journal of the Royal Asiatic Society

JRS   Journal of Roman Studies

JThS   Journal of Theological Studies

JWarb   Journal of the Warburg and Courtauld Institutes

Krumbacher   K. Krumbacher, *Geschichte der byzantinischen Litteratur* (Munich, 1890; 2nd ed. Munich, 1897)

Lampe: G. W. H. Lampe, ed., *A Patristic Greek Lexicon* (Oxford, 1961)

Leo (ed. Renehan)   Robert Renehan, ed. and trans., *Leo the Physician: Epitome On the Nature of Man* (Berlin, 1969 [*CMG* X 4])

Lewis and Elvin-Lewis   Walter H. Lewis and Memory P. F. Elvin-Lewis, *Medical Botany* (New York, 1977)

Loeb   The Loeb Classical Library (followed by place and date of publication in parentheses)

LSJ   Henry George Liddell, Robert Scott, and

Henry Stuart Jones, *A Greek-English Lexicon*, 9th ed. (1940) with a supplement (Oxford, 1968)

MAMA   Monumenta Asiae Minoris Antiqua

Marcellus (ed. Liechtenhan)   Max Niedermann, ed., revised by Eduard Liechtenhan as a 2nd ed., *Marcellus: De medicamentis*, trans. (German) by Jutta Kollesch and Diethard Nickel, 2 vols. (Berlin, 1968 [*CML* V])

MélUSJ   Mélanges de l'Université Saint-Joseph, Beyrouth

MémInstCaire   Mémoires publiés par les membres de l'Institut Français d'Archéologie Orientale du Caire

Meyer, *Botanik*   Ernst H. F. Meyer, *Geschichte der Botanik*, 4 vols. (Königsberg, 1854–57; rptd. Amsterdam, 1965)

MonPiot   Monuments et Mémoires, publiés par l'Académie des Inscriptions et Belles-Lettres, Fondation E. Piot

Mulomedicina Chironis (ed. Oder)   Eugen Oder, ed., *Claudii Hermeri Mulomedicina Chironis* (Leipzig, 1901)

Nemesius (ed. Matthaei)   C. F. Matthaei, ed., *Nemesius Emesenus De natura hominis* (Halle, 1802; rptd. Hildesheim, 1967)

Νέος Ἑλλ.   Νέος Ἑλληνομνήμων

Nicander (ed. and trans. Gow and Scholfield)   A. S. F. Gow and A. F. Scholfield, eds. and trans., *Nicander: The Poems and Poetical Fragments* (Cambridge, 1953)

NTM   Schriftenreihe für Geschichte der Naturwissenschaften, Technik und Medizin

Nutton, ed., *Galen: Problems*   Vivian Nutton, ed., *Galen: Problems and Prospects. A Collection of Papers submitted at the 1979 Cambridge Conference* (London, 1981)

OCA   Orientalia Christiana Analecta

OCD   Oxford Classical Dictionary, edited by N. G. L. Hammond and H. H. Scullard, 2nd ed. (Oxford, 1970)

OCP   Orientalia Christiana Periodica

ÖJh   Jahreshefte des Österreichischen Archäologischen Institutes in Wien

ÖJhBeibl   Jahreshefte des Österreichischen Archäologischen Institutes in Wien, Beiblatt

OrChr   Oriens Christianus

Oribasius (ed. and trans. Bussemaker and Daremberg)   U. Cats Bussemaker and Ch. Daremberg, eds. and trans., *Oeuvres d'Oribase*, 6 vols. (Paris, 1851–76)

Oribasius (ed. Raeder)   J. Raeder, ed., *Oribasii*

Collectionum medicarum reliquiae, 4 vols. (Leipzig, 1928–33; rptd. Amsterdam, 1964 [*CMG* VI 1, 1–VI 2, 2]). J. Raeder, ed., *Oribasii Synopsis ad Eustathium. Libri ad Eunapium* (Leipzig, 1926; rptd. Amsterdam, 1964 [*CMG* VI 3])

Palladius (ed. Rodgers)   R. H. Rodgers, ed., *Palladius Opus agriculturae. De veterinaria medicina. De insitione* (Leipzig, 1975)

PAPS   Proceedings of the American Philosophical Society

Paul (trans. Adams)   Francis Adams, trans., *The Seven Books of Paulus Aegineta . . . with a Commentary Embracing a Complete View of the Knowledge Possessed by the Greeks, Romans, and Arabians on All Subjects Connected with Medicine and Surgery*, 3 vols. (London, 1844–47)

Paul (ed. Heiberg)   I. L. Heiberg, ed., *Paulus Aegineta*, 2 vols. (Leipzig, 1921–24 [*CMG* IX 1 and 2])

PBSR   Papers of the British School at Rome

Pelagonius (ed. Fischer)   K.-D. Fischer, ed., *Pelagonius Ars veterinaria* (Leipzig, 1980)

PG   Patrologiae cursus completus, Series Graeca, ed. J.-P. Migne

PGL   See Lampe

*PGM   Karl Preisendanz, ed., *Papyri Graecae Magicae: Die griechischen Zauberpapyri*, 2nd ed. Albert Henrichs, 2 vols. (Stuttgart, 1973–74). Papyri usually cited by 'collection' and line no.

PH   Pharmacy in History

Photius (ed. Henry)   René Henry, ed. and trans., *Photius: Bibliothèque*, 8 vols. (Paris, 1959–77)

PIR   Prosopographia Imperii Romani, 5 vols. (Berlin and Leipzig, 1933–70)

PLRE   Prosopography of the Late Roman Empire, edited by A. H. M. Jones, J. R. Martindale, and J. Morris, 2 vols. (Cambridge, 1980)

PO   Patrologia Orientalis (Paris, 1903–   )

Pollux (ed. Bethe)   Eric Bethe, ed., *Pollucis Onomasticon*, 3 vols. (Leipzig, 1900–37; rptd. Stuttgart, 1967)

Polunin, *Flowers of Europe*   Oleg Polunin, *Flowers of Europe* (London, 1969)

Polunin, *Flowers of Greece*   Oleg Polunin, *Flowers of Greece and the Balkans* (Oxford, 1980)

Πρακτ.'Ακαδ.'Αθην.   Πρακτικὰ τῆς 'Ακαδημίας 'Αθηνῶν

Pseudo-Apuleius (ed. Sigerist)   E. Howald and H. E. Sigerist, eds., *Pseudoapulei herbarius*, in *Antonii Musae De herba vettonica liber. Pseudoapulei herbarius. Anonymi De taxone liber. Sexti Placiti liber medicinae ex animalibus etc.* (Leipzig, 1927 [*CML* IV], pp. 13–225)

QDAP *Quarterly of the Department of Antiquities in Palestine*

RAC *Reallexikon für Antike und Christentum*
RACr *Rivista di Archeologia Cristiana*
RBibl *Revue Biblique*
RE *Paulys Realencyclopädie der classischen Altertumswissenschaft*, new rev. ed. by G. Wissowa and W. Kroll (Stuttgart, 1893–)
REArm *Revue des Etudes Arméniennes*
REB *Revue des Etudes Byzantines*
REG *Revue des Etudes Grecques*
RhM *Rheinisches Museum für Philologie*
RHR *Revue de l'Histoire des Religions*. Annales du Musée Guimet
RIGI *Rivista Indo-Greco-Italica di Filologia, Lingua, Antichità*
ROChr *Revue de l'Orient Chrétien*
RPh *Revue de Philologie, de Littérature et d'Histoire anciennes*
RSBN *Rivista di Studi Bizantini e Neoellenici*
Rufus (ed. Daremberg and Ruelle) Ch. Daremberg and Ch. Émile Ruelle, eds. and trans., *Oeuvres de Rufus d'Éphèse* (Paris, 1879; rptd. Amsterdam, 1963)
RVV Religionsgeschichtliche Versuche und Vorarbeiten

SA *Sudhoffs Archiv* [formerly Sudhoffs *Archiv für Geschichte der Medizin*]
SAMN *Society for Ancient Medicine Newsletter*
Sarton, *Introduction* George Sarton, *Introduction to the History of Science*, Vol. I: *From Homer to Omar Khayyam* (Washington, D.C., 1927); Vol. II in 2 parts: part 1: *From Rabbi ben Ezra to Gerard of Cremona*, and part 2: *From Robert Grosseteste to Roger Bacon* (Washington, D.C., 1931); Vol. III in 2 parts: *First Half of the Fourteenth Century* and *Second Half of the Fourteenth Century* (Washington, D.C., 1947)
SB Sitzungsberichte (followed by name of Academy, abbreviated, e.g., SBBerl)
SC Sources Chrétiennes. Collection dirigée par H. de Lubac et J. Daniélou
Scarborough, *Medicine* John Scarborough, *Roman Medicine* (London and Ithaca, New York, 1969; rptd. 1976)
Scarborough, "Nicander II" John Scarborough, "Nicander's Toxicology, II: Spiders, Scorpions, Insects and Myriapods," *PH*, 21 (1979), 3–34 and 73–92
Scarborough and Nutton, "Preface" John Scarborough and Vivian Nutton, "The Preface of

Dioscorides' *Materia Medica*: Introduction, Translation, Commentary," *TS*, n.s. 4 (1982), 187–227
Scribonius Largus (ed. Helmreich) G. Helmreich, ed., *Scribonii Largi Conpositiones* (Leipzig, 1887)
Scribonius Largus (ed. Sconocchia) Sergio Sconocchia, ed., *Scribonii Largi Compositiones* (Leipzig, 1983)
Sezgin, *Geschichte*, III Fuat Sezgin, *Geschichte des arabischen Schrifttums*, Vol. III: *Medizin-Pharmazie-Zoologie-Tierheilkunde* (Leiden, 1970)
Soranus (ed. Ilberg) J. Ilberg, ed. *Sorani Gynaeciorum libri IV. De signis fracturarum. De fasciis. Vita Hippocratis secundum Soranum* (Leipzig, 1927 [*CMG* IV])
SOsl *Symbolae Osloenses*
StM *Studi Medievali*
StMSR Studi e Materiali di Storia delle Religioni
SubsHag Subsidia Hagiographica, Société des Bollandistes
Suda (ed. Adler) Ada Adler, ed., *Suidae Lexicon*, 5 vols. (Leipzig, 1928–38; rptd. Stuttgart, 1971)

Temkin, *Double Face of Janus* Owsei Temkin, *The Double Face of Janus and Other Essays on the History of Medicine* (Baltimore, 1977)
Temkin, *Galenism* Owsei Temkin, *Galenism* (Ithaca, New York, 1973)
Theophilus (ed. Greenhill) Alexander Greenhill, ed., *Theophili Protospatharii De corporis humani fabrica* (Oxford, 1842)
Theophrastus, *HP* Theophrastus, *Historia Plantarum*
TS *Transactions and Studies of the College of Physicians of Philadelphia*
TU *Texte und Untersuchungen zur Geschichte der altchristlichen Literatur* (Leipzig-Berlin, 1882–)

Ullmann, *Medizin* Manfred Ullmann, *Die Medizin im Islam* (Leiden, 1970)

Vegetius (ed. Lommatzsch) Ernst Lommatzsch, ed., *P. Vegeti Renati Digestorum artis mulomedicinae libri* (Leipzig, 1903)

WByzSt Wiener Byzantinistische Studien
WSt *Wiener Studien, Zeitschrift für klassische Philologie und Patristik*
WZKM *Wiener Zeitschrift für die Kunde des Morgenlandes*

ZDMG *Zeitschrift der Deutschen Morgenländischen Gesellschaft*

INDEX